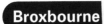 **Broxbourne**

D0785132

Turnford, Broxbourne, Herts, EN10 6AE.
Telephone: 01992 411565

Please remember to return this item by the last
date shown below. You can extend the loan by
telephoning the library.

A fine is charged for each item which is
returned late.

~~NOT TO BE~~
~~TAKEN AWAY~~

 hrc

Churchill Livingstone
Pocket Medical Dictionary

For Churchill Livingstone:

Senior Commissioning Editor: Sarena Wolfaard
Project Development Manager: Gail Wright/Dinah Thom
Project Manager: Samantha Ross
Designer: Judith Wright

Churchill Livingstone
Pocket Medical Dictionary

Edited by

Chris Brooker BSc MSc RGN SCM RNT

Author and Lecturer, Norfolk, UK

FIFTEENTH EDITION

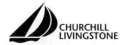

CHURCHILL
LIVINGSTONE

Edinburgh   London   New York   Oxford   Philadelphia   St Louis   Sydney   Toronto   2003

CHURCHILL LIVINGSTONE
An imprint of Elsevier Limited

First edition 1933
Second edition 1935
Third edition 1938
Fourth edition 1940
Fifth edition 1941
Sixth edition 1943

Seventh edition 1946
Eighth edition 1949
Ninth edition 1961
Tenth edition 1966
Eleventh edition 1969
Twelfth edition 1974

Thirteenth edition 1976
Fourteenth edition 1987
Fifteenth edition 2003
Reprinted 2005

Standard Edition ISBN 0 443 07245 0

International Edition ISBN 0 443 07244 2
International Edition of Fourteenth edition 1987
International Edition of Fifteenth Edition 2003

British Library Cataloguing in Publication Data
A catalogue record for this book is available from the British Library

Library of Congress Cataloguing in Publication Data
A catalogue record for this book is available from the Library of Congress

Note
Medical knowledge is constantly changing. Standard safety precautions must be followed, but as new
research and clinical experience broaden our knowledge, changes in treatment and drug therapy may
become necessary or appropriate. Readers are advised to check the most current product information
provided by the manufacturer of each drug to be administered to verify the recommended dose, the
method and duration of administration, and contraindications. It is the responsibility of the practitioner,
relying on experience and knowledge of the patient, to determine dosages and the best treatment for
each individual patient. Neither the Publisher nor the editor assumes any liability for any injury and/or
damage to persons or property arising from this publication.

The Publisher

ELSEVIER your source for books,
journals and multimedia
in the health sciences

Working together to grow
libraries in developing countries

www.elsevier.com | www.bookaid.org | www.sabre.org

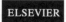 ELSEVIER BOOK AID International Sabre Foundation

The
publisher's
policy is to use
paper manufactured
from sustainable forests

Printed in China

Contents

Preface

Medicine and health care continue to change at a rapid pace and all those concerned need easy access to information from many medical specialties and other healthcare disciplines. The fifteenth edition of the *Churchill Livingstone Pocket Medical Dictionary* aims to meet the needs of a broad group that includes medical students, practising doctors, students of the allied health professions, others working in the medical/health fields, such as medical secretaries and receptionists, and members of the public.

This well-established dictionary has been extensively revised and updated. A team of advisers from academic institutions and many areas of clinical practice have revised existing entries, removed those no longer relevant and written many new entries.

Many subject areas have been expanded or incorporated for the first time including: critical care, complementary medicine, epidemiology, ethics, management, nutrition, occupational medicine, oncology, podiatry, public health and health promotion, quality issues, research and sports medicine. The entries relating to nutrition, occupational therapy, physiotherapy, radiography, and speech and language therapy have been expanded to reflect the increasingly multiprofessional and interprofessional approaches to health care. The pharmacological entries are now more general and most drug entries now relate to drug groups rather than specific drug names. However, further drug information is provided in an appendix. The appendices have been completely revised and new areas have been added.

Appendix 1 contains full page, two colour line illustrations of the major body systems. At the appropriate anatomical term in the dictionary, the reader is directed to the relevant illustration.

Appendix 2 explains about SI units and the metric system and provides useful conversion scales for certain chemical pathology tests and common units of measurement.

Appendix 3 details normal values for blood, cerebrospinal fluid, faeces and urine.

Appendix 4 is a new appendix, providing an overview of the nutrients required for health and well-being.

Appendix 5 introduces the wide-ranging topic of drugs. An overview of drugs and the law is provided with a brief discussion of the main Acts governing the use of medicines in the UK: the Medicines Act 1968, the Misuse of Drugs Act 1971 and the Medicinal Products: Prescription by Nurses Act 1992. Essential information about the measurement of drugs follows. A new feature is information about the drug groups in common use with subgroups, drug examples and clinical indications provided in a table for easy reference.

Appendix 6 lists abbreviations, covering commonly used medical terms, and degrees, diplomas and organizations.

Appendix 7 is a new appendix, providing useful addresses, including web sites. The web sites will help you access the very latest information.

Appendix 8 is a new appendix, providing some common chemical symbols and formulae.

The advisers and I hope that the dictionary will continue to be a valuable resource for students, registered practitioners and all those with an interest in health and health care.

Norfolk, 2003 Chris Brooker

Acknowledgements

The editor would like to thank the following advisers as well as David Llewellyn, Samantha Ross, Dinah Thom, Sarena Wolfaard and Gail Wright.

Panel of advisers

David Assheton MB ChB MRC
Specialist Registrar, Merseyside Hospital, Royal Liverpool University Hospital, Prescott St, Liverpool, UK

Anne Ballinger MD FRCP
Senior Lecturer and Honorary Consultant Physician, Department of Adult and Paediatric Gastroenterology, Barts and the London Queen Mary's School of Medicine and Dentistry, London, UK

Helen Barker BSc SRD MPH PGCE
Senior Lecturer in Dietetics, School of Health and Social Sciences, Coventry University, Coventry, UK

Roger Barker BA MBBS MRCP PhD
University Lecturer and Honorary Consultant in Neurology, Cambridge Centre for Brain Repair and Addenbrooke's Hospital, Cambridge, UK

Mark Batterbury BSc MBBS DO FRCS FRCOphth
Consultant Ophthalmologist and Director of Clinical Studies, St Paul's Eye Unit, Royal Liverpool University Hospital, Liverpool, UK

Philip Benington BDS MSc MOrthRCS FDS(Orth)RCS FDSRCPS
Consultant Orthodontist, Glasgow Dental Hospital and School, Glasgow, UK

Ewen Cameron MA MB BChir MRCP
Specialist Registrar, Department of Gastroenterology, Ipswich Hospital, Ipswich, UK

Andrew Currie BM DCH MRCP(UK) FRCPCH
Consultant Neonatologist, Leicester Royal Infirmary, Leicester, UK

David Gawkrodger MD FRCP FRCPE
Consultant Dermatologist and Honorary Senior Clinical Lecturer
Department of Dermatology, Royal Hallamshire Hospital, Sheffield, UK

Paddy Gibson BSc MB ChB MRCP
Consultant Nephrologist, Department of Renal Medicine, Royal Infirmary of Edinburgh, Edinburgh, UK

Peter Hammond BM BCh MA MD FRCP
Consultant Physician, Department of Medicine, Harrogate District Hospital, Harrogate, UK

Paul Hateley MPH BSc(Hons) DMS RGN RMN OND
Head of Nursing, Pathology and Patient Services, Barts and the London NHS Trust, London, UK

Ariane Herrick MD FRCP
Senior Lecturer in Rheumatology, University of Manchester Rheumatic Diseases Centre, Hope Hospital, Salford, UK

Philip Hopley MB BS(Dist) MRCPsych
Consultant Forensic Psychiatrist, West London Mental Health NHS Trust, London, UK

Diana Hulbert BSc(Hons) MBBS FRCS FFAEM
Consultant, Emergency Department,

Southampton General Hospital, Southampton, UK

Susan Ingamells BSc(Hons) PhD BM MRCOG
Subspeciality Registrar in Reproductive Medicine, Department of Obstetrics and Gynaecology, The Princess Anne Hospital, Southampton, UK

Greg Kelly DipCOT BSc(Hons)Psychology
Lecturer in Occupational Therapy, School of Rehabilitation Sciences, University of Ulster at Jordanstown, Newtownabbey, Co Antrim, UK

Donald L Lorimer BEd(Hons) MChS DPodM SRCh
Former Head of Durham School of Podiatric Medicine, Past Chairman of Council, Society of Chiropodists and Podiatrists, Baldock, UK

Islay M McEwan MSc BSc(Hons) GradDipPhys SRP MCSP
Senior Lecturer in Sports Physiotherapy and Programme Leader MSc Science of Sports Injury, Manchester Metropolitan University, Manchester, UK

Gerald W McGarry MB ChB MD FRCS(Ed. Glas) FRCS ORLHNS
Consultant Otorhinolaryngologist, Department of ENT, Glasgow Royal Infirmary, Glasgow, UK

Alexander McMillan MD FRCP FRCP(Ed)
Consultant Physician, Department of Genitourinary Medicine, Royal Infirmary of Edinburgh, Edinburgh, UK

J Kilian Mellon MD FRCS(Urol)
Professor of Urology, Leicester Warwick Medical School, Leicester General Hospital, Leicester, UK

Cathy Meredith MPH BA DCRt TQFF Cert CT
Senior Lecturer, Division of Radiography, School of Health and Social Care, Glasgow Caledonian University, Glasgow, UK

Jeannette Naish MBBS MSc FRCGP
Senior Lecturer, Department of General Practice and Primary Care, Barts and The London Queen Mary's School of Medicine and Dentistry, University of London, UK

Andrew Nicol BSc MBBS FRCA
Consultant Anaesthetist, Department of Anaesthesia, Barnet Hospital, Barnet, Herts, UK

Marianne Nicolson BSc MD FRCP(Ed)
Consultant Medical Oncologist, Aberdeen Royal Infirmary, Aberdeen, UK

Rowan Parks MD FRCSI FRCS(Ed)
Senior Lecturer in Surgery, Department of Clinical and Surgical Sciences, Royal Infirmary of Edinburgh, Edinburgh, UK

Anne Parry PhD MCSP DipTP
Professor of Physiotherapy and Senior Research Fellow, Professions Allied to Medicine, School of Health and Social Care, Sheffield Hallam University, Sheffield, UK

Helen Richmond MA PGDipE MSc DPSM RM SRN
Senior Lecturer in Midwifery, Anglia Polytechnic University, Chelmsford, Essex, UK

Jillian Riley MSc BA(Hons) RGN RM
Senior Lecturer, Cardio-respiratory Nursing, Thames Valley University, Royal Brompton Hospital, London, UK

Carrock Sewell MB PhD MRCP MRCPath
Consultant Immunologist, Path Links Immunology, Lincolnshire, UK

Anne Shields BA(Hons) RGN OHND
Occupational Health Nurse, Occupational Health Unit, University of Hull, Hull, UK

Christina H Smith BSc MSc PhD
Lecturer, Department of Human Communication Science, University College London, London, UK

Mike Smith MSc PGDipEd RN
Postgraduate Orthopaedic Nursing Course, Nursing Professional Development Unit, Royal Perth Hospital, and Lecturer (adjunct), Faculty of Nursing, Edith Cowan University, Perth, Australia

David Soutar MB ChB ChM FRCS(Ed) FRCS(Glas)
Consultant Plastic Surgeon, Plastic Surgery Unit, Canniesburn Hospital, Glasgow, UK

Andrew Stewart BA MB ChB MRCP MRCPath
Consultant Haematologist, Monklands and Hairmyres Hospitals, Lanarkshire, UK

Quintin van Wyk MB ChB
Specialist Registrar in Histopathology, Department of Histopathology, Royal Hallamshire Hospital, Sheffield, UK

Roger Watson BSc PhD RGN CBiol FIBiol ILTM FRSA
Professor of Nursing, School of Nursing, Social Work and Applied Health Studies, University of Hull, Hull, UK

Jessica White MB BChir MRCP(UK)
Clinical Research Fellow, Department of Medicine, Addenbrooke's Hospital, Cambridge, UK

Simon M Whiteley MBBS FRCA
Consultant in Anaesthesia and Intensive Care, Anaesthetic Department, St James's University Hospital, Leeds, UK

How to use this dictionary

Main entries

These are listed in alphabetical order and appear in **bold** type. Derivative forms of the main entry also appear in **bold** type and along with their parts of speech are to be found at the end of the definition. For example:

amoebicide *n* an agent which kills amoebae—**amoebicidal** *adj.*

Separate meanings of main entry

Different meanings of the same word are separated by means of an Arabic numeral before each meaning. For example:

anastomosis *n* **1** the anatomical intercommunication of the branches of two or more tubular structures, e.g. arteries or veins. **2** in surgery, the establishment of an intercommunication between two hollow organs, vessels or nerves.

Subentries

Subentries relating to the defined main entry are listed in alphabetical order and appear in *italic* type, following the main definition. For example:

alkalosis *n* process leading to low levels of acid (excess of alkali) in the body. *metabolic alkalosis* due to loss of body acids (e.g. vomiting of gastric acid) or excess administration of alkali. *respiratory alkalosis* due to hyperventilation and lowering of carbon dioxide level.

Parts of speech and other abbreviations

The parts of speech follows single word main entries and derivative forms of the main entry, and appears in *italic* type. The parts of speech and other abbreviations used in the dictionary are:

abbr	abbreviation	*npl*	noun, plural
acron	acronym	*opp*	opposite
adj	adjective	*pl*	plural
adv	adverb	*sing*	singular
Am	American	*syn*	synonym
e.g.	for example	*v*	verb
i.e.	that is	*vi*	intransitive verb
n	noun	*vt*	transitive verb

Cross-references

Cross-references alert you to related words and additional information elsewhere in the dictionary. A single symbol has been used for this purpose—an arrow => . Either within or at the end of the definition, the arrow indicates the word(s) you can then look up for related subject matter. For example:

achalasia *n* loss of oesophageal peristalsis and failure of lower oesophageal sphincter relaxation. => cardiomyotomy.

Most drug entries relate to drug groups rather than specific drug names and the cross-reference will be to Appendix 5 for more information. For example:

aminoglycosides *npl* a group of bactericidal antibiotic drugs. => Appendix 5.

Many anatomical terms are cross-referenced to the appropriate figure(s) in Appendix 1 to show the term's position in the body. For example:

aorta *n* the main artery arising out of the left ventricle of the heart. => Figure 8.

Prefixes which can be used as combining forms in compounded words

Prefix	Meaning	Prefix	Meaning
a-	without, not	cata-	down
ab-	away from	cav-	hollow
abdo- ⎱ abdomino- ⎰	abdominal	centi-	a hundredth
		cephal-	head
acro-	extremity	cerebro-	brain
ad-	towards	cervic-	neck
adeno-	glandular	cheil-	lip
aer-	air	cheir-	hand
amb- ⎱ ambi- ⎰	both, on both sides	chemo-	chemical
		chlor-	green
amido-	NH₂ group united to an acid radical	chol-	bile
		cholecysto-	gallbladder
amino-	NH₂ group united to a radical other than an acid radical	choledocho-	common bile duct
		chondro-	cartilage
		chrom-	colour
amphi-	on both sides, around	cine-	film, motion
amyl-	starch	circum-	around
an-	not, without	co- ⎫	
ana-	up	col- ⎬ together	
andro-	male	com-	
angi-	vessel (blood)	con- ⎭	
aniso-	unequal	coli-	bowel
ant- ⎱ anti- ⎰	against, counteracting	colpo-	vagina
		contra-	against
ante- ⎱ antero- ⎰	before	costo-	rib
		cox-	hip
antro-	antrum	crani- ⎱ cranio- ⎰ skull	
aorto-	aorta		
app-	away, from	cryo-	cold
arachn-	spider	crypt-	hidden, concealed
arthro-	joint	cyan-	blue
auto-	self	cysto-	bladder
		cyto-	cell
bi-	twice, two	dacryo-	tear
bili-	bile	dactyl-	finger
bio-	life	de-	away, from, reversing
blenno-	mucus	deca-	ten
bleph-	eyelid	deci-	tenth
brachio-	arm	demi-	half
brachy-	short	dent-	tooth
brady-	slow	derma- ⎱ dermat- ⎰ skin	
broncho-	bronchi		
		dextro-	to the right
		di-/dip-	twos, double
calc-	chalk	dia-	through
carcin-	cancer	dis-	separation, against
cardio-	heart	dorso-	dorsal
carpo-	wrist	dys-	difficult, painful, abnormal

Prefix	Meaning	Prefix	Meaning
ecto-	outside, without, external	intra-	within
electro-	electricity	intro-	inward
em-	in	ischio-	ischium
en-		iso-	equal
end-	in, into, within		
endo-			
ent-	within	karyo-	nucleus
entero-	intestine	kerato-	horn, skin, cornea
epi-	on, above, upon	kypho-	rounded, humped
ery-	red		
eu-	well, normal		
ex-	away from, out, out of	lact-	milk
exo-		laparo-	flank
extra-	outside	laryngo-	larynx
		lepto-	thin, soft
		leuco-	white
faci-	face	leuko-	
ferri-	iron	lympho-	lymphatic
ferro-			
fibro-	fibre, fibrous tissue		
flav-	yellow	macro-	large
feto-	fetus	mal-	abnormal, poor
fore-	before, in front of	mamm-	breast
		mast-	
		medi-	middle
gala-	milk	mega-	large
gastro-	stomach	melano-	pigment, dark
genito-	genitals, reproductive	meso-	middle
ger-	old age	meta-	between
glosso-	tongue	metro-	uterus
glyco-	sugar	micro-	small
gnatho-	jaw	milli-	a thousandth
gynae-	female	mio-	smaller
		mono-	one, single
		muco-	mucus
haema-	blood	multi-	many
haemo-		myc-	fungus
hemi-	half	myelo-	spinal cord, bone marrow
hepa-	liver	myo-	muscle
hepatico-			
hepato-			
hetero-	unlikeness, dissimilarity	narco-	stupor
hexa-	six	naso-	nose
histo-	tissue	necro-	corpse, dead
homeo-	like	neo-	new
homo-	same	nephro-	kidney
hydro-	water	neuro-	nerve
hygro-	moisture	noct-	night
hyper-	above	normo-	normal
hypo-	below	nucleo-	nucleus
hypno-	sleep	nyc-	night
hystero-	uterus		
		oculo-	eye
iatro-	physician	odonto-	tooth
idio-	peculiar to the individual	oligo-	deficiency, diminution
ileo-	ileum	onc-	mass
ilio-	ilium	onycho-	nail
immuno-	immunity	oo-	egg, ovum
in-	not, in, into, within	oophor-	ovary
infra-	below	ophthalmo-	eye
inter-	between	opisth-	backward

xiii

Prefix	Meaning	Prefix	Meaning
orchido-	testis	salpingo-	uterine (fallopian) tube
oro-	mouth	sapro-	dead, decaying
ortho-	straight	sarco-	flesh
os-	bone, mouth	sclero-	hard
osteo-	bone	scota-	darkness
oto-	ear	semi-	half
ova-	egg	sept-	seven
ovari-	ovary	sero-	serum
		socio-	sociology
		sphygm-	pulse
pachy-	thick	spleno-	spleen
paed-	child	spondy-	vertebra
pan-	all	steato-	fat
para-	beside	sterno-	sternum
patho-	disease	sub-	below
ped-	child, foot	supra-	above
penta- } pento- }	five	syn-	together, union, with
per-	by, through		
peri-	around	tabo-	tabes
perineo-	perineum	tachy-	fast
pharma-	drug	tarso-	foot, edge of eyelid
pharyngo-	pharynx	teno-	tendon
phlebo-	vein	tetra-	four
phono-	voice	thermo-	heat
photo-	light	thoraco-	thorax
phren-	diaphragm, mind	thrombo-	blood clot
physio-	form, nature	thyro-	thyroid gland
pleuro-	pleura	tibio-	tibia
pluri-	many	tox-	poison
pneumo-	lung	tracheo-	trachea
podo-	foot	trans-	across, through
polio-	grey	tri-	three
poly-	many, much	trich-	hair
post-	after	tropho-	nourishment
pre- } pro- }	before		
proct-	anus		
proto-	first	ultra-	beyond
pseudo-	false	uni-	one
psycho-	mind	uretero-	ureter
pyelo-	pelvis of the kidney	urethro-	urethra
pyo-	pus	uri-	urine
pyr-	fever	uro-	urine, urinary organs
		utero-	uterus
quadri-	four		
quint-	five	vaso-	vessel
		veno-	vein
radi-	ray	vesico-	bladder
radio-	radiation		
re-	again, back		
ren-	kidney	xanth-	yellow
retro-	backward	xero-	dry
rhin-	nose	xiphi- } xipho- }	ensiform cartilage of sternum
rub-	red		
sacchar-	sugar		
sacro-	sacrum	zoo-	animal

Suffixes which can be used as combining forms in compounded words

Suffix	Meaning	Suffix	Meaning
-able	able to, capable of	-kinesis	motion
-aemia	blood	-kinetic	
-aesthesia	sensibility, sense-perception		
-agra	attack, severe pain		
-al	characterized by, pertaining to	-lith	calculus, stone
-algia	pain	-lithiasis	presence of stones
-an	belonging to, pertaining to	-logy	science of, study of
-ase	catalyst, enzyme	-lysis	breaking down,
-asis	state of	-lytic	disintegration
-blast	cell	-malacia	softening
		-megaly	enlargement
		-meter	measure
-caval	pertaining to venae cavae	-morph	form
-cele	tumour, swelling		
-centesis	to puncture		
-cide	destructive, killing	-ogen	precursor
-clysis	infusion, injection	-odynia	pain
-coccus	spherical cell	-oid	likeness, resemblance
-cule	little	-ol	alcohol
-cyte	cell	-ology	the study of
		-oma	tumour
		-opia	eye
-derm	skin	-opsy	looking
-desis	to bind together	-ose	sugar
-dynia	pain	-osis	condition, disease, excess
		-ostomy	to form an opening or outlet
		-otomy	incision of
-ectasis	dilation, extension	-ous	like, having the nature of
-ectomy	removal of		
		-pathy	disease
-facient	making	-penia	lack of
-form	having the form of	-pexy	fixation
-fuge	expelling	-phage	ingesting
		-phagia	swallowing
		-phasia	speech
-genesis	formation, origin	-philia	affinity for, loving
-genetic		-phobia	fear
-genic	capable of causing	-phylaxis	protection
-gogue	increasing flow	-plasty	reconstructive surgery
-gram	a tracing	-plegia	paralysis
-graph	instrument for writing	-pnoea	breathing
	or recording	-poiesis	making
		-ptosis	falling
-iasis	condition of, state		
-iatric	practice of healing	-rhage	to burst forth
-itis	inflammation of	-rhaphy	suturing

Suffix	Meaning	Suffix	Meaning
-rhoea	excessive discharge	-sthenia	strength
-rhythmia	rhythm	-stomy	to form an opening or outlet
-saccharide	basic carbohydrate molecule	-taxia	arrangement, coordination, order
-scope	instrument for visual examination	-taxis	
		-taxy	
-scopy	to examine visually	-tome	cutting instrument
-somatic	pertaining to the body	-tomy	incision of
-somy	pertaining to chromosomes	-trophy	nourishment
-sonic	sound	-trophy	turning
-stasis	stagnation, cessation of movement	-uria	urine

A

AA *abbr* Alcoholics Anonymous.

AAMI *abbr* age-associated memory impairment.

abacterial *adj* without bacteria. A condition such as inflammation that is not caused by bacteria.

ABCs of proprioception agility, balance and coordination. ⇒ proprioception.

abdomen *n* the largest body cavity.

abdominal *adj* pertaining to the abdomen. *abdominal aorta* that part of the aorta within the abdomen. Smaller arteries branch from it to supply oxygenated blood to abdominal structures, e.g. kidneys ⇒ Figures 9, 19. *abdominal aortic aneurysm (AAA)* a swelling in the abdominal aorta. ⇒ aneurysm. *abdominal breathing* more than usual use of the diaphragm and abdominal muscles to increase the input of air to and output from the lungs. It can be done voluntarily. When it occurs in disease it is a compensatory mechanism for inadequate oxygenation. *abdominal excision of the rectum* an operation sometimes performed for rectal cancer. The rectum is mobilized via an abdominal approach. The bowel is divided well proximal to the cancer. The proximal end is brought out as a permanent colostomy. Excision of the distal bowel, containing the cancer and the anal canal, is completed through a perineal incision. *abdominal reflex* a superficial reflex where the abdominal muscles contract when the skin is lightly stroked. *abdominal regions* where the surface anatomy is divided into nine regions used to describe the location of organs or symptoms, such as pain. ⇒ Figure 18a. *abdominal thrust* ⇒ Heimlich's manoeuvre.

abdominocentesis *n* paracentesis (aspiration) of the peritoneal cavity. ⇒ amniocentesis, colpocentesis, thoracentesis.

abdominopelvic *adj* pertaining to the abdomen and pelvis or pelvic cavity.

abdominoperineal *adj* pertaining to the abdomen and perineum.

abdominoplasty *n* plastic surgical procedure used to tighten the abdominal muscles. Known colloquially as a 'tummy tuck'.

abducens nerve the sixth pair of cranial nerves. They control the lateral rectus muscle of the eyeball, which turns the eyeball outwards.

abduct *vt* to draw away from the median line of the body ⇒ adduct *opp*.

abduction *n* the act of moving, (or abducting) away from the midline ⇒ adduction *opp*.

abductor *n* a muscle which, on contraction, draws a part away from the median line of the body. ⇒ adductor *opp*.

aberrant *adj* abnormal; usually applied to a blood vessel or nerve which does not follow the normal course.

aberration *n* a deviation from normal—**aberrant** *adj*. *chromosomal aberration* loss, gain or exchange of genetic material in the chromosomes of a cell resulting in deletion, duplication, inversion or translocation of genes. *mental aberration* ⇒ mental. *optical aberration* imperfect focus of light rays by a lens.

ability *n* the physical and cognitive capacity to perform a task.

ablation *n* removal. In surgery, the word means excision or eradication (destruction)—**ablative** *adj*.

abort *vt, vi* to terminate before full development.

abortifacient *adj* causing abortion such as the drug mifepristone.

abortion *n* **1** abrupt termination of a process. **2** the induced expulsion from the uterus of the product of conception before viability by medical or surgical means. NB. The preferred term for unintentional loss of the product of conception prior to 24 weeks gestation is miscarriage. *criminal abortion* intentional evacuation of the uterus by other than trained licensed personnel, or where abortion is prohibited by law.

abrasion *n* **1** superficial injury to skin or mucous membrane from scraping or rubbing; excoriation. **2** can be used therapeutically for removal of scar tissue (dermabrasion).

abscess *n* localized collection of pus produced by pyogenic organisms. May be acute or chronic. ⇒ quinsy. *alveolar abscess* ⇒ dento-alveolar abscess. *Brodie's abscess* chronic osteomyelitis occurring without previous acute phase. *cold abscess* one occurring in the course of such chronic inflammation as may be due to *Mycobacterium tuberculosis*. *psoas abscess* ⇒ psoas.

absorption rate constant a value describing the amount of a drug absorbed in a unit of time.

absorptive state the metabolic state immediately after a meal and continuing for about four hours. Absorbed nutrients are used as energy or to build up other substances through anabolic processes such as glycogenesis. ⇒ postabsorptive state.

abuse *n* **1** deliberate injury to another person. It may be either physical, sexual, psychological or through neglect, such as failure to feed or keep clean. The term can apply to any group of individuals, especially those most vulnerable such as children, older people, and those with mental health problems or learning disabilities. ⇒ child abuse, elder abuse. **2** misuse of equipment, drugs and other substances, power and position.

acalculia *n* inability to do simple arithmetic.

accessory motion sliding, gliding or rolling motion that occurs within and between joint surfaces during active or passive joint movement.

Access to Health Records Act (1990) allows access to both paper and computerized health records made after 1991, with certain exceptions, such as where they may cause serious physical or mental harm to a person.

acclimatization *n* the body's ability to adapt physiologically to a variation in environment such as climate or altitude.

accommodating resistance muscle activity during which the resistance provided changes as the muscle moves through its range of motion. Also known as isokinetic activity.

accommodation *n* **1** ability of the lens of the eye to increase its refractive power in order to focus on near objects. **2** decreased sensitivity to stimuli demonstrated by neurons that have been exposed to subthreshold stimuli for long periods of time.

accouchement *n* delivery in childbirth. Confinement.

accountability *n* health professionals have a duty to care according to law. In some countries the statutory body, and/or the professional organization, develop a code of conduct via which each practitioner can accept responsibility and accountability for the professional service delivered to each patient/client. ⇒ duty of care, malpractice, negligence.

accretion *n* an increase of substance or deposit round a central object—**accrete** *adj, vt, vi*, **accretive** *adj*.

acephalous *adj* without a head.

acetabuloplasty *n* an operation to improve the depth and shape of the hip socket (acetabulum); necessary in such conditions as developmental dysplasia of the hip and osteoarthritis of the hip.

acetabulum *n* a cup-like socket on the external lateral surface of the pelvis into which the head of the femur fits to form the hip joint—**acetabula** *pl*.

acetate *n* a salt of acetic acid.

acetic acid an organic acid present in vinegar.

acetoacetate *n* an acidic ketone produced during an interim stage of fat oxidation in the body. Some can be utilized as a fuel by tissues, such as the kidney. In situations where carbohydrate molecules are not available for metabolism, such as in diabetes mellitus or starvation, excess is produced and the high levels in the blood result in ketoacidosis with severe disturbances of pH, fluid and electrolytes.

acetonaemia *n* ⇒ ketonaemia.

acetone *n* inflammable liquid with odour of 'pear drops'; used as a solvent. *acetone bodies* ⇒ ketones.

acetonuria *n* acetone and other ketones in the urine. ⇒ ketonuria—**acetonuric** *adj*.

acetylcholine (ACh) *n* a chemical neurotransmitter released from nerve endings to allow the transmission of a nerve impulse at the neuromuscular junction in voluntary (skeletal) muscle and across synapses in parasympathetic nerves. The nerve fibres releasing this chemical are described as 'cholinergic'. Acetylcholine is broken down into choline and acetate by the enzyme acetylcholinesterase. ⇒ myasthenia gravis.

acetylcholinesterase *n* enzyme that inactivates acetylcholine following the transmission of a nerve impulse across the synapse.

acetyl coenzyme A (*syn* acetyl CoA) an important metabolic molecule involved in many biochemical reactions such as glycolysis.

achalasia *n* loss of oesophageal peristalsis and failure of lower oesophageal sphincter relaxation. ⇒ cardiomyotomy.

Achilles tendinitis inflammation of the Achilles tendon.

Achilles tendon the tendinous termination of the soleus and gastrocnemius muscles inserted into the heel bone (os calcis or calcaneus).

achlorhydria *n* the absence of gastric acid (hydrochloric). Found in pernicious anaemia and gastric cancer—**achlorhydric** *adj*.

acholia *n* the absence of bile—**acholic** *adj*.

acholuria *n* the absence of bile pigments from the urine. ⇒ jaundice—**acholuric** *adj*.

achondroplasia *n* an inherited condition characterized by arrested growth of the long bones resulting in short-limbed dwarfism with a big head. The intellect is not impaired. Inheritance is dominant—**achondroplastic** *adj*.

achromatopsia *n* inability to see colours.

acid *n* any substance that has an excess of hydrogen ions over hydroxyl ions, e.g. hydrochloric acid. They have a pH below 7 and turn blue litmus red. They react with alkalis to form salts plus water.

acidaemia *n* a high level of acid (hydrogen ions) in the blood resulting in a below normal blood pH <7.35 (hydrogen ion concentration >44 mmol/L). ⇒ acidosis—**acidaemic** *adj*.

acid-alcohol-fast *adj* in bacteriology, describes a micro-organism which, when stained, is resistant to decolorization by alcohol as well as acid, e.g. *Mycobacterium tuberculosis*. ⇒ Ziehl–Neelsen technique.

acid–base balance equilibrium between the acid and base elements of the blood and body fluids.

acid-fast *adj* in bacteriology, describes a micro-organism which, when stained, does not become decolorized when washed with dilute acids. *acid-fast bacilli (AFB)* a type of bacteria identified using acid-fast techniques.

acidity *n* the state of being acid or sour. The degree of acidity can be measured on the pH scale where a pH below 7 is acid and pH 6 denotes a weak acid and pH 1 a strong acid.

acidosis *n* process leading to the accumulation of excess acid in the body. *respiratory acidosis* due to hypoventilation and the accumulation of carbon dioxide. *metabolic acidosis* due to the generation of excess acid (lactic acidosis) or depletion of alkali (e.g. diarrhoea). ⇒ acidaemia, ketoacidosis, ketosis—**acidotic** *adj*.

acid phosphatase an enzyme which synthesizes phosphate esters of carbohydrates in an acid medium. An increase of this enzyme in the blood is indicative of cancer of the prostate gland.

aciduria *n* excretion of an acid urine.

Acinetobacter *n* a genus of Gram-negative aerobic bacteria causing infections that include wound infection, pneumonia and meningitis. The micro-organism has developed antibiotic resistance and is a particular danger to critically ill patients having intensive or high dependency care.

acini *npl* minute saccules or alveoli, lined or filled with secreting cells. Several acini combine to form a lobule—**acinus** *sing*, **acinous, acinar** *adj*.

acme *n* **1** the highest point. **2** crisis or critical point of a disease.

acne, acne vulgaris *n* a condition in which the pilosebaceous glands are overstimulated by circulating androgens and the excessive sebum is trapped by a plug of keratin, one of the protein constituents of human skin. Skin bacteria then colonize the glands and convert the trapped sebum into irritant fatty acids responsible for the swelling and inflammation (pustules) which follow. A tetracycline is the drug of choice.

acneiform *adj* resembling acne.

acoustic neuroma a benign tumour (schwannoma) affecting the eighth cranial nerve (vestibulocochlear nerve) as it passes through the skull into the brainstem, causing problems in hearing and balance.

acquired immune deficiency syndrome (AIDS) a term used to denote a particular stage of infection with human immunodeficiency virus (HIV). The Centers for Disease Control and Prevention (CDC) define AIDS as the development of an AIDS-defining illness in a patient with HIV infection. A low CD4+ T cell count of less than 200 per µL (or less than 14% of lymphocytes) in an HIV-positive person is also regarded as AIDS-defining, regardless of symptoms or opportunistic infections.

acrocephalia; acrocephaly *n* a congenital malformation whereby the top of the head is pointed and the eyes protrude, due to premature closure of sagittal and coronal skull sutures—**acrocephalic, acrocephalous** *adj*.

acrocephalosyndactyly *n* a congenital malformation consisting of a pointed top of head, with fusion of fingers and/or toes. ⇒ Apert's syndrome.

acrocyanosis *n* coldness and blueness of the extremities due to circulatory disorder—**acrocyanotic** *adj*.

acrodynia *n* acute, painful reddening of the extremities such as occurs in erythroedema polyneuropathy.

acromegaly *n* enlargement of the hands, face and feet, occurring due to excess growth hormone in an adult, almost always from a pituitary adenoma—**acromegalic** *adj*.

acromicria *n* smallness of the hands, face and feet.

acromioclavicular *adj* pertaining to the acromion process (of scapula) and the clavicle.

acromion *n* the point or summit of the shoulder: the triangular process at the extreme outer end of the spine of the scapula—**acromial** *adj*.

acrophobia *n* morbid fear of being at a height.

acrosome *n* structure surrounding the nucleus of a spermatozoon. It contains lytic enzymes, which when released by many spermatozoa (during the acrosome reaction) facilitate the penetration of an oocyte by a single spermatozoon.

ACTH *abbr* adrenocorticotrophic hormone.

actin *n* one of the contractile proteins in a muscle myofibril; it reacts with myosin to cause contraction.

acting out reducing distress by the release of disturbed or violent behaviour, which is unconsciously determined and reflects previous unresolved conflicts and attitudes.

actinic dermatoses skin conditions in which the integument is abnormally sensitive to ultraviolet radiation.

actinism *n* the chemical action of radiant energy, especially in the ultraviolet spectrum—**actinic** *adj*.

actinobiology *n* study of the effects of radiation on living organisms.

Actinomyces n a genus of branching micro-organisms. *Actinomyces israeli* causes disease in humans. ⇒ actinomycosis.

actinomycosis *n* a disease caused by *Actinomyces israeli*, the sites most affected being the face, neck, lung and abdomen. There is pus containing yellow 'sulphur granules', abscess formation with sinuses and necrosis—**actinomycotic** *adj*.

actinotherapy *n* treatment by use of infra-red or ultraviolet radiation.

action *n* the activity or function of any part of the body. *action potential* change in electrical potential and charge that occurs across excitable cell membranes during nerve impulse conduction or when muscles contract. *compulsive action* performed by an individual at the supposed instigation of another's dominant will, but against his own. *impulsive action* resulting from a sudden urge rather than the will. *reflex action* ⇒ reflex. *specific action* that brought about by certain remedial agents in a particular disease, e.g. antibiotics in infection.

activator *n* a substance which renders something else active, e.g. the hormone secretin, the enzyme enterokinase—**activate** *v*.

active *adj* energetic. ⇒ passive *opp*. *active hyperaemia* ⇒ hyperaemia. *active immunity* ⇒ immunity. *active principle* an ingredient which gives a complex drug its chief therapeutic value, e.g. atropine is the active principle in belladonna. *active range of motion* the movement of a joint without assistance through a range of motion. Those produced by patients using their own neuromuscular mechanisms.

activities of daily living (ADLs) tasks focusing on the occupational performance areas of self-care, work and play that enable individuals to consistently and competently perform their occupational roles in society. ⇒ DADL, IADL, PADL. *ADL assessment and training* a technique whereby formal and informal evaluation of a person's ability to perform activities of daily living is followed by a treatment programme designed to maintain or improve function.

activity *n* the execution of a series of linked, purposeful, productive, playful or creative tasks by an individual with the specific goal of changing objective reality or subjective experience. These may include physical and mental tasks at various levels of complexity.

activity analysis a cognitive process used to reduce an activity into its component tasks in order to understand the skills required for consistent and competent performance of activities of daily living (ADLs) in a specific environment.

activity limitations inability of an individual to perform activities of daily living as expected by his or her cultural and social environment.

activity theory a psychosocial theory of ageing. It supports the view that older people who develop different roles and are socially active into old age gain benefit and satisfaction. ⇒ disengagement theory.

actomyosin *n* the protein complex of actin and myosin formed during muscle fibre contraction.

acuity *n* clearness, sharpness, keenness. ⇒ auditory acuity, visual acuity.

acupuncture *n* a technique that involves the insertion of fine needles into specific parts of the body. There are approximately 365 points along meridians (channels through which energy known as *Qi* flows) at which needles can be inserted into the body to stimulate or depress the energy flow. Sometimes the herb moxa is also used to warm and stimulate certain points. This is known as moxibustion. Used for the treatment of disease, relief of pain or production of anaesthesia.

acute *adj* short and severe; not long drawn out or chronic. *acute abdomen* a pathological condition within the abdomen requiring immediate surgical intervention. *acute defibrination syndrome* ⇒ hypofibrinogenaemia. *acute dilatation of the stomach* sudden enlargement of this organ due to paralysis of the muscular wall ⇒ paralytic ileus. *acute heart failure* cessation or impairment of heart action, in previously undiagnosed heart disease, or in the course of another disease. *acute leukaemia* ⇒ leukaemia. *acute yellow atrophy* acute diffuse necrosis of the liver; icterus gravis; malignant jaundice.

acute coronary syndromes describes the spectrum of events ranging from the partial occlusion of a coronary artery resulting in unstable angina through to the complete occlusion of a coronary artery resulting in myocardial infarction.

acute injury an injury that presents with a rapid onset and has a short duration, due to a traumatic episode. Term used to describe the first 24–48 hours after onset of an injury such as that sustained during a sporting activity.

acute respiratory distress syndrome (ARDS) characterized by difficulty breathing, poor oxygenation, stiff lungs and typical changes on a chest X-ray, following a recognized cause of acute lung injury. Analysis of arterial blood gases reveals a fall in PaO_2 and eventually an increased $PaCO_2$ and a fall in pH.

acute tubular necrosis (ATN) rapid onset necrosis of the renal tubules. It is usually caused by renal ischaemia due to shock, but may be due to the nephrotoxic effects of bacterial or chemical toxins; ⇒ renal failure.

acyanosis *n* without cyanosis.

acyanotic *adj* without cyanosis; a word used to differentiate congenital cardiovascular defects.

acyesis *n* absence of pregnancy—**acyetic** *adj*.

acystia *n* congenital absence of the bladder—**acystic** *adj*.

Adam's apple the laryngeal prominence in front of the neck, especially in the adult male, formed by the junction of the two wings of the thyroid cartilage.

adaptability *n* the ability to adjust mentally and physically to circumstances in a flexible way.

adaptation *n* **1** a positive change in the function of an individual in order to meet the demands of the environment. **2** an alteration made to the environment in order to improve an individual's ability to consistently and competently perform activities of daily living. **3** in sports medicine describes the long-term physical changes that occur from the training effects produced as a result of overload. ⇒ aerobic adaptations, anaerobic adaptations.

adaptive behaviour advantageous or appropriate behaviour that follows a change.

addiction *n* craving for chemical substances such as drugs, alcohol and tobacco which the addicted person finds difficult to control.

Addison's disease deficient secretion of cortisol and aldosterone due to primary failure of the adrenal cortex, causing electrolyte imbalance, diminished blood volume, hypotension, weight loss, hypoglycaemia, muscular weakness, gastrointestinal upsets and pigmentation of skin.

adduct *vt* to draw towards the midline of the body. ⇒ abduct *opp*.

adduction *n* the act of adducting, drawing towards the midline of the body. ⇒ abduction *opp*.

adductor *n* any muscle which moves a part toward the median axis of the body. ⇒ abductor *opp*. *adductor longus* ⇒ Figure 4. *adductor magnus* ⇒ Figures 4, 5.

adenectomy *n* surgical removal of a gland.

adenitis *n* inflammation of a gland, or lymph node. *hilar adenitis* inflammation of bronchial lymph nodes.

adenocarcinoma *n* a malignant growth of glandular tissue—**adenocarcinomata** *pl*, **adenocarcinomatous** *adj*.

adenofibroma *n* ⇒ fibroadenoma.

adenoid *adj* resembling a gland. ⇒ adenoids.

adenoidectomy *n* surgical removal from the nasopharynx of enlarged pharyngeal tonsil (adenoid tissue).

adenoids *npl* abnormally enlarged pharyngeal tonsils. Lymphoid tissue situated in the nasopharynx which can obstruct breathing and impede hearing.

adenoma *n* a premalignant tumour of glandular epithelial tissue—**adenomata** *pl*, **adenomatous** *adj*.

adenomyoma *n* a non-malignant tumour composed of muscle and glandular elements, usually applied to benign growths of the uterus—**adenomyomata** *pl*, **adenomyomatous** *adj*.

adenopathy *n* any disease of a gland—**adenopathic** *adj*.

adenosine diphosphate (ADP) an important cellular metabolite involved in energy exchange within the cell. Chemical energy is conserved in the cell, by the phosphorylation of ADP to ATP primarily in the mitochondrion, as a high energy phosphate bond.

adenosine monophosphate (AMP) an important cellular metabolite involved in energy release for cell use. ⇒ cyclic adenosine monophosphate (cAMP).

adenosine triphosphate (ATP) an intermediate high energy compound which on hydrolysis to ADP releases chemically useful energy. ATP is generated during catabolism and utilized during anabolism.

adenotonsillectomy *n* surgical removal of the pharyngeal tonsil (adenoid tissue) and palatine tonsils.

adenovirus *n* a group of DNA-containing viruses. They cause upper respiratory and gastrointestinal infections and conjunctivitis.

ADH *abbr* antidiuretic hormone ⇒ vasopressin.

adhesion *n* abnormal union of two parts, occurring after inflammation; a band of fibrous tissue which joins such parts. In the abdomen such a band may cause intestinal obstruction; in joints it restricts movement; between two surfaces of pleura it prevents complete pneumothorax—**adherent** *adj*, **adherence** *n*, **adhere** *vi*.

adipose *n, adj* fat; of a fatty nature. The cells constituting adipose tissue contain either white or brown fat.

adiposity *n* excessive accumulation of fat in the body.

aditus *n* in anatomy, an entrance or opening.

adjustment *n* **1** stability within an individual and an acceptable relationship between the individual and his or her environment. **2** the mechanism used in focusing a microscope.

adjuvant *n* a substance included in a prescription to assist the action of other drugs. *adjuvant therapy* a treatment given together with another. It is usually applied to the treatment of cancer where cytotoxic drugs are used after removal of the tumour by surgery or radiotherapy. The purpose of treatment being to enhance the chance of cure and prevent recurrence. ⇒ neoadjuvant therapy.

ADLs *abbr* activities of daily living.

adnexa *npl* structures that are in close proximity to a part—**adnexal** *adj*. *adnexa oculi* the lacrimal apparatus. *adnexa uteri* the ovaries and uterine (fallopian) tubes.

adolescence *n* the period between the onset of puberty and full maturity; youth—**adolescent** *adj, n*.

adoption *n* the acquisition of legal responsibility for a child who is not a natural offspring of the adopter.

ADP *abbr* adenosine diphosphate.

ADPKD *abbr* adult dominant polycystic kidney disease.

adrenal *adj* near the kidney. *adrenal glands* endocrine glands, one situated on the upper pole of each kidney. (⇒ Figure 19). The *adrenal cortex* secretes glucocorticoids, mineralocorticoids and sex hormones which control metabolism, the chemical constitution of body fluids and secondary sexual characteristics. Under the control of the pituitary gland via the secretion of adrenocorticotrophic hormone. The *adrenal medulla* secretes noradrenaline (norepinephrine) and adrenaline (epinephrine). ⇒ adrenalectomy.

adrenalectomy *n* removal of an adrenal gland, usually for tumour. If both adrenal glands are removed, replacement administration of cortical hormones is required.

adrenal function tests tests to identify adrenocortical hypofunction or hyperfunction; random cortisol may identify gross abnormalities in function, but for the vast majority dynamic testing of the hypothalamo-pituitary-adrenal axis is needed ⇒ dexamethasone suppression tests, glucagon stimulation test, insulin tolerance test, tetracosactide (Synacthen) test.

adrenaline (epinephrine) *n* a catecholamine hormone, produced by the adrenal medulla. It enhances the effects of the sympathetic nervous system during times of physiological stress by preparing the body for 'fight or flight' responses. These include increased heart rate, bronchodilation and increased respiratory rate and glucose release. Adrenaline (epinephrine) is used therapeutically as a sympathomimetic in situations that include: acute allergic reactions, and in local anaesthetic to prolong the anaesthetic effects. ⇒ alpha (α)-adrenoceptor agonist, alpha (α)-adrenoceptor antagonist, beta (β)-adrenoceptor agonist, beta (β)-adrenoceptor antagonist, monoamine, noradrenaline (norepinephrine).

adrenergic *adj* describes nerves which liberate the catecholamine noradrenaline (norepinephrine) from their terminations. Most sympathetic nerves release noradrenaline as a neurotransmitter. ⇒ cholinergic *opp*.

adrenoceptor *n* (*syn* adrenergic receptor) receptor sites on the effector structures innervated by sympathetic nerves. Two main types: alpha (α) and beta (β). Both receptor types, which respond differently to neurotransmitters, have further subdivisions.

adrenocorticotrophic hormone (ACTH) (*syn* corticotrophin) secreted by the anterior lobe of the pituitary gland it stimulates the production of hormones by the adrenal cortex.

adrenogenital syndrome an endocrine disorder, usually congenital, resulting from abnormal activity of the adrenal cortex. A female child will show enlarged clitoris and possibly labial fusion, perhaps being confused with a male. The male child may show pubic hair and enlarged penis. In both male and female there is rapid growth, muscularity and advanced bone age.

adrenoleucodystrophy (ALD) a group of neurodegenerative disorders associated with adrenocortical insufficiency. X-linked inheritance. ⇒ Schilder's disease.

ADRs *abbr* adverse drug reactions.

adsorbents *npl* solids that bind dissolved substances or gases on their surfaces. Charcoal can be used to adsorb gases to act as a deodorant. Bacterial and other toxins are adsorbed by kaolin, which may be used in the treatment of food poisoning.

adsorption *n* the property of a substance to attract and to hold to its surface a gas, liquid or solid in solution or suspension—**adsorptive** *adj*, **adsorb** *vt*.

adult polycystic kidney diseases (APKD) ⇒ polycystic kidney disease.

advance directive also known as a 'living will'. A written declaration made by a mentally competent person setting out their wishes regarding life-prolonging medical interventions if they are incapacitated by an irreversible disease or are terminally ill, which prevents them making their wishes known to health professionals at the time. An advance directive is legally binding if it is in the form of an advanced refusal and the maker is competent at the time.

advanced life support (ALS) the use of drugs, artificial aids and advanced skills to save or preserve life during resuscitation procedures. ⇒ cardiopulmonary resuscitation. *paediatric advanced life support (PALS)* the special techniques, drug doses and equipment appropriate to the body weight and surface area of the child being resuscitated.

advancement *n* surgical detachment of a tendon or muscle followed by reattachment at an advanced point.

adventitia *n* the external coat, especially of an artery or vein—**adventitious** *adj*.

adverse drug reactions (ADRs) a term describing any unwanted effects of a drug. They range from very minor through to extremely unpleasant or life-threatening. They are classified into five types: A (augmented effects), B (bizarre effects), C (chronic effects), D (delayed effects) and E (ending effects, which occur when administration is stopped suddenly).

advocacy *n* process by which a person supports or argues for the needs of another. Healthcare professionals may act as advocate for their patients or clients, or assist individuals to develop the skills needed for self-advocacy.

Aedes *n* a genus of mosquitoes which includes *Aedes aegypti*, an important vector of dengue and yellow fever.

aerobe *n* a micro-organism that requires O_2 to maintain life—**aerobic** *adj*.

aerobic *adj* requiring free oxygen or air to support life or a specific process. *aerobic energy* the production of adenosine triphosphate (ATP) by oxidative phosphorylation.

aerobic adaptations long-term physical changes that result from aerobic exercise. They increase the body's ability to deal with endurance exercise.

aerobic exercise physical activity that requires the heart and lungs to work harder in order to obtain and supply increased oxygen to strenuously contracting skeletal muscles.

aerogenous *adj* gas producing.

aerophagia, aerophagy *n* excessive air swallowing.

aerosol *n* small particles finely dispersed in a gas phase. May be used: to deliver inhalation drug therapy, in insect control and for skin application. Aerosols such as those produced during sneezing can be responsible for the spread of infection.

aetiology *n* (etiology) the science of the causation of disease—**aetiological** *adj*, **aetiologically** *adv*.

AFB *abbr* acid-fast bacillus.

afebrile *adj* without fever.

affect *n* emotion or mood.

affection *n* the feeling or emotional aspects of mind; one of the three aspects. ⇒ cognition, conation.

affective *adj* pertaining to emotions or moods. *affective psychosis* mental illness characterized by mood disturbance together with psychotic symptoms. ⇒ psychosis.

afferent *adj* conducting inward to a part or organ; used to describe nerves, blood and lymphatic vessels ⇒ efferent *opp. afferent degeneration* that which spreads up sensory nerves.

affiliation *n* settling of the paternity of an illegitimate child on the putative father.

affinity *n* describes the chemical attraction between two substances, e.g. oxygen and haemoglobin.

afibrinogenaemia *n* a lack of fibrinogen resulting in a serious disorder of blood coagulation—**afibrinogenaemic** *adj*.

aflatoxin *n* carcinogenic metabolites of certain strains of *Aspergillus flavus* that can affect peanuts and carbohydrate foods stored in warm humid climates. Hepatic enzymes produce the metabolites of aflatoxins which predispose to liver cancer.

AFP *abbr* alphafetoprotein.

afterbirth *n* the placenta, cord and membranes which are expelled from the uterus after childbirth.

aftercare *n* a word denoting the care given during convalescence and rehabilitation. It may be within the remit of health professionals such as therapists or nurses, or may be provided by social care staff or family members.

aftereffect *n* a response occurring after the initial effect of a stimulus.

afterimage *n* a visual impression of an object persisting after the object has been removed. May be 'positive' when the image is seen in its natural bright colours or 'negative' if the dark parts are light and the bright parts become dark.

afterload the pressure of blood in the pulmonary artery and aorta that forms the resistance that ventricular contraction must overcome to pump blood into the circulation. ⇒ preload.

afterpains *n* the pains felt after childbirth, due to contraction and retraction of the uterine muscle fibres.

agalactia *n* non-secretion or imperfect secretion of milk after childbirth—**agalactic** *adj*.

agammaglobulinaemia *n* absence of gammaglobulin in the blood, with consequent inability to produce immunity to infection—**agammaglobulinaemic** *adj*. *Bruton's agammaglobulinaemia* a congenital condition in boys, in which B lymphocytes are absent but cellular immunity remains intact. ⇒ dysgammaglobulinaemia.

aganglionosis *n* absence of ganglia, as those of the distal bowel ⇒ Hirschsprung's disease, megacolon.

agar *n* a gelatinous substance obtained from certain seaweeds. It is used as a bulk-increasing laxative and for solidifying bacterial culture media.

age *n* ⇒ mental age. *age-associated memory impairment* an abnormal decline in memory (greater than one standard deviation from the normal) with age where there is no premorbid problem with IQ or the presence of dementia.

ageism *n* stereotyping people according to chronological age: overemphasizing negative aspects to the disadvantage of more positive points. Discriminatory attitudes in society disadvantage older people on the basis of age alone. However, ageist views can impact on people of any age.

agenesis *n* incomplete and imperfect development—**agenetic** *adj*.

agglutination *n* the clumping of bacteria, red blood cells or antigen-coated particles by antibodies called 'agglutinins', developed in the blood serum of a previously infected or sensitized person or animal. Agglutination forms the basis of many laboratory tests—**agglutinable, agglutinative**, *adj*, **agglutinate** *vt, vi*.

agglutinins *npl* antibodies that agglutinate or clump organisms or particles.

agility *n* the ability to control the direction of the body or body part during rapid movement.

aglossia *n* absence of the tongue—**aglossic** *adj*.

aglutition *n* dysphagia.

agnathia *n* absence or incomplete development of the jaw.

agnosia *n* inability to perceive the nature of sensory impressions. People and things are not recognized; usually classified by the sense or senses affected—**agnosic** *adj*. *spatial agnosia* loss of spatial appreciation.

agonist *n* a muscle that shortens to perform a movement. Also describes a drug or other chemical that imitates the response of the natural chemical at a receptor site. ⇒ antagonist *opp*.

agoraphobia *n* morbid fear of being alone in large open places—**agoraphobic** *adj*.

agranulocyte *n* a non-granular leucocyte.

agranulocytosis *n* marked reduction in or complete absence of granulocytes (polymorphonuclear leucocytes). Usually results from bone marrow depression caused by (a) hypersensitivity to drugs, (b) cytotoxic drugs or (c) irradiation. Symptoms include fever, ulceration of the mouth and throat. If untreated, prostration and death may ensue. ⇒ neutropenia—**agranulocytic** *adj*.

agraphia *n* loss of language facility. *motor agraphia* inability to express thoughts in writing, usually due to left precentral cerebral lesions. *sensory agraphia* inability to interpret the written word, due to lesions in the posterior part of the left parieto-occipital region—**agraphic** *adj*.

AHF *abbr* antihaemophilic factor.

AID *abbr* artificial insemination of a female with donor semen.

AIDS *abbr* acquired immune deficiency syndrome.

AIDS-defining illness CDC criteria for AIDS in a patient infected with HIV. Examples include candidiasis of bronchus, trachea, lungs or oesophagus, invasive cervical cancer, Kaposi's sarcoma, pulmonary tuberculosis or other mycobacterial infection, and *Peumocystis carinii* pneumonia.

AIH *abbr* artificial insemination of a female with her husband's semen.

air *n* the gaseous mixture which makes up the atmosphere surrounding the earth. It consists of approximately 78% nitrogen, 20% oxygen, 0.04% carbon dioxide, 1% argon, and traces of ozone, neon, helium, etc. and a variable amount of water vapour. *air embolism* results from an air bubble entering the circulation. *air hunger* a deep indrawing of breath which characterizes the late stages of uncontrolled haemorrhage. *air swallowing (aerophagia)* swallowing of excessive air particularly when eating: it may result in belching or the passage of flatus from the anus.

airway *n* used to describe the entry to the larynx from the pharynx. *Brook airway* oropharyngeal airway used in expired air resuscitation. *oropharyngeal airway* a flexible oval tube, such as a Guedel airway, which can be placed along the upper surface of the tongue to prevent a flaccid tongue from resting against the posterior pharyngeal wall, thereby obstructing the airway, and is commonly used during general anaesthesia. Also used during cardiopulmonary resuscitation.

akathisia *n* a subjective state of persistent motor restlessness: it can occur as a side-effect of antipsychotic (neuroleptic) drugs.

akinesia *n* impairment in initiation of movement or delay in reaction time—**akinetic** *adj*.

alactacid (alactic) anaerobic system a series of chemical reactions occurring within the cells whereby adenosine triphosphate for energy use is produced, without oxygen, from adenosine diphosphate (ADP) and creatine phosphate (phosphocreatine).

alactacid oxygen debt component the amount of oxygen required to replace the adenosine triphosphate (ATP) and creatine phosphate (phosphocreatine) stores in cells during the process of recovery from exercise.

alanine *n* a non-essential (dispensable) amino acid.

Albers-Schönberg disease ⇒ osteopetrosis.

albinism *n* a congenital hypopigmentation of the hair, skin and eyes. It is caused by a deficiency of melanin pigment in skin and/or the eye. Other associated eye and neurological defects can contribute to poor vision.

albino *n* a person affected with albinism—**albinotic** *adj*.

albumin *n* a protein found in animal and vegetable material. It is soluble in water and coagulates on heating. *serum albumin* the main protein of blood plasma. ⇒ lactalbumin—**albuminous, albuminoid** *adj*.

albuminuria *n* the presence of albumin in the urine. The condition may be temporary and clear up completely, as in many febrile states. May be indicative of serious kidney disease—**albuminuric** *adj*. ⇒ orthostatic albuminuria, proteinuria.

alcohol *n* a group of organic compounds. Absolute alcohol is occasionally used by injection for the relief of trigeminal neuralgia and other intractable pain. Ethyl alcohol (ethanol) is the intoxicating constituent of alcoholic drinks: wine, beer and spirits. It potentiates the effects of hypnotics and tranquillizers. ⇒ alcohol dependence, Korsakoff's syndrome, Wernicke's encephalopathy.

alcohol dependence a syndrome of physical, psychological and behavioural responses related to alcohol misuse. Characteristically there are withdrawal symptoms and drinking to relieve the same, tolerance to the effects of alcohol, compulsion to drink alcohol, narrowing of repertoire of drinking, etc.

alcohol-fast *adj* in bacteriology, describes a micro-organism which, when stained, is resistant to decolorization by alcohol.

Alcoholics Anonymous (AA) a fellowship of people who have had problems with alcohol dependence. Their aim is helping others with similar difficulties.

aldolase *n* an enzyme present in muscle tissue. *aldolase test* increased levels of aldolase and other enzymes in the blood are indicative of some muscle diseases, e.g. severe muscular dystrophy.

aldosterone *n* mineralocorticoid hormone secreted by the adrenal cortex. Secretion is regulated by the action of renin and angiotensin. It enhances the reabsorption of sodium accompanied by water and the excretion of potassium by the renal tubules.

aldosterone antagonist a drug that acts as an aldosterone antagonist. ⇒ potassium sparing diuretics, Appendix 5.

aldosteronism *n* ⇒ hyperaldosteronism.

Aleppo boil ⇒ leishmaniasis.

Alexander technique a series of techniques used to improve the functioning of mind and body in movement known as 'psychophysical' re-education. It is based on the belief that poor posture can lead to ill health, injury and chronic pain. The technique aims to promote postural improvement through self-awareness.

alexia *n* word blindness; an inability to interpret the significance of the printed or written word, but without loss of visual power. Can be due to a brain lesion or insufficient/inappropriate sensory experience during an 'ab initio' stage of learning—**alexic** *adj*.

ALG *abbr* antilymphocyte globulin.

algesimeter *n* an instrument that registers the degree of sensitivity to pain.

alginates *npl* seaweed derivatives used in some wound dressings. They have high absorbency, haemostatic properties and can be removed without damaging delicate tissues.

alienation *n* in psychology and sociology, estrangement from people.

alimentary *adj* pertaining to food. *alimentary tract* comprises the mouth, oesophagus, stomach, small intestine, ascending colon, transverse colon, descending colon, sigmoid colon, rectum and anal canal. ⇒ Figure 18b.

alimentation *n* the act of nourishing with food; feeding.

alkalaemia *n* low level of acid (hydrogen ions) in the blood resulting in an above normal pH >7.45 (hydrogen ion concentration <36 mmol/L). ⇒ alkalosis—**alkalaemic** *adj*.

alkali *n* also called a base. Substances that have an excess of hydroxyl ions over hydrogen ions, e.g. sodium bicarbonate. They have a pH greater than 7 and turn red litmus blue. Alkalis react with acids to produce salts plus water, and with fats to form soaps. *alkaline reserve* a biochemical term denoting the amount of buffered alkali (normally bicarbonate) available in the blood for buffering acids (normally dissolved CO_2) formed in or introduced into the body and limiting pH changes in the blood.

alkaline *adj* **1** relating to or possessing the properties of an alkali. **2** containing an excess of hydroxyl over hydrogen ions.

alkaline phosphatase an enzyme present in several tissues, e.g. bone, liver and kidney. An increase of this enzyme in the blood is indicative of obstructive jaundice and increased osteoblast activity associated with some bone disease.

alkalinuria *n* alkalinity of urine—**alkalinuric** *adj*.

alkaloid *n* similar to an alkali. Also describes a large group of organic bases present in plants and which have important physiological actions, e.g. morphine, atropine, quinine and caffeine—**alkaloidal** *adj*.

alkalosis *n* process leading to low levels of acid (excess of alkali) in the body. *metabolic alkalosis* due to loss of body acids (e.g. vomiting of gastric acid) or excess administration of alkali. *respiratory alkalosis* due to hyperventilation and lowering of carbon dioxide level.

alkaptonuria *n* the presence of alkaptone (homogentisic acid) in the urine, resulting from only partial oxidation of phenylalanine and tyrosine. Condition usually noticed because urine goes black in the nappies, or when left to stand. Apart from this, and a tendency to arthritis in later life, there are no ill-effects from alkaptonuria.

alkylating agents organic molecules that disrupt cell division by binding to the DNA in the nucleus. ⇒ cytotoxic. ⇒ Appendix 5.

allele *n* allelomorph. Describes the alternative forms of a gene at the same chromosomal location (locus). Previously used to denote inherited characteristics that are alternative and contrasting, such as normal colour vision contrasting with colour blindness, or the different ABO blood groups.

allelomorph ⇒ allele.

allergen *n* an antigen which produces an allergic, or immediate-type hypersensitivity response—**allergenic** *adj*, **allergenicity** *n*.

allergy *n* an immune response induced by exposure to an allergen causing a harmful hypersensitivity reaction on subsequent exposure—**allergic** *adj*. ⇒ anaphylaxis, sensitization.

allograft *n* grafting or transplanting an organ or tissue from one person to another who does not share the same transplantation antigens. Also known as a homograft.

allopathy *n* describes conventional medicine and health care—**allopathic** *adj*. ⇒ homoeopathy.

alopecia *n* baldness, which can be congenital, premature or senile. *alopecia areata* a patchy baldness, usually of a temporary nature. Cause unknown, probably autoimmune, but stress is a common precipitating factor. Exclamation mark hairs are diagnostic. *cicatricial alopecia* progressive alopecia of the scalp in which tufts of normal hair occur between scarred bald patches. Folliculitis decalvans is an alopecia of the scalp characterized by pustulation and scarring.

alpha (α)-adrenoceptor agonists (*syn* α stimulants) a group of drugs that stimulate α-adrenoceptors. ⇒ Appendix 5.

alpha (α)-adrenoceptor antagonists (*syn* α blockers) a group of drugs that block the stimulation of α-adrenoceptors. ⇒ Appendix 5.

alpha (α)-antitrypsin a liver protein that normally opposes trypsin. Reduced blood levels are linked with a genetic predisposition to emphysema and liver disease.

alphafetoprotein (AFP) *n* a protein produced by fetal gut and liver cells and by adult liver cancer cells. Raised levels are seen in maternal serum and amniotic fluid in fetal abnormalities including neural tube defects. May be used as a tumour marker for cancers of the liver and the testes affecting adults.

alpha (α)-glucosidase inhibitor an oral hypoglycaemic drug that slows the digestion and absorption of complex carbohydrates and sucrose from the intestine. ⇒ Appendix 5.

alpha (α) redistribution phase the point after an intravenous injection when the blood concentration of the drug begins to fall below the peak levels achieved.

ALS *abbr* 1 advanced life support. 2 amyotrophic lateral sclerosis.

ALT *abbr* alanine aminotransferase. ⇒ aminotransferases.

altitude training programme of exercise that aims to produce reversible physiological adaptations that increase a person's tolerance to the reduced PO_2 at altitude.

altitudinal *adj* when describing a visual field defect implies loss of vision in superior or inferior half of field.

alveolitis *n* inflammation of alveoli. When caused by inhalation of an allergen it is termed *extrinsic allergic alveolitis*.

alveolus *n* 1 an air sac of the lung. 2 in dentistry, a bony tooth socket within the jaw bone. 3 a gland follicle or acinus—**alveoli** *pl*, **alveolar** *adj*.

Alzheimer's disease a neurodegenerative disorder of the brain with distinct pathology causing a progressive loss of cognitive function (dementia). Usually occurs in older people for no obvious reason but can affect younger patients (i.e.<65 years of age), when it is often familial.

amalgam *n* any of a group of alloys containing mercury. ⇒ dental amalgam.

amastia *n* congenital absence of the breasts.

amaurosis *n* partial or total blindness. *amaurosis fugax* temporary loss of vision in an eye due to interruption of arterial supply.

ambidextrous *adj* able to use both hands equally well—**ambidexter** *adj*, **ambidexterity** *n*.

amblyopia *n* defective vision. Usually refers to failure of normal visual development (may be strabismic, refractive, deprivation). *toxic amblyopia* damage to the optic nerve by a noxious agent, usually related to heavy smoking—**amblyopic** *adj*.

ambulant *adj* able to walk.

ambulatory *adj* mobile, walking about. *ambulatory ECG* ⇒ electrocardiogram. *ambulatory surgery (day surgery)* surgery carried out on the day of admission and, in the absence of problems, the person is discharged the same day to the care of the primary care team. *ambulatory treatment* interventions, such as blood product transfusion or chemotherapy, provided for patients on a day care basis. ⇒ continuous ambulatory peritoneal dialysis.

amelia *n* congenital absence of a limb or limbs. *complete amelia* absence of both arms and legs.

amelioration *n* a reduction in the severity of symptoms.

amenorrhoea *n* absence of the menses. When menstruation has not been established at the time when it should have been, it is termed *primary amenorrhoea*; absence of the menses after they have once commenced is referred to as *secondary amenorrhoea*—**amenorrhoeal** *adj*.

ametria *n* congenital absence of the uterus.

ametropia *n* defective sight due to imperfect refractive power of the eye—**ametropic** *adj*, **ametrope** *n*.

amfetamine (amphetamine) *n* a sympathomimetic agent. A potent CNS stimulant. This stimulant effect has led to misuse and dependence. Clinical use is extremely limited.

amines *npl* group of organic molecules with amine (NH_2) groups. Many are important biochemical molecules, e.g. histamine, dopamine, etc.

aminoacidopathy *n* disease caused by imbalance of amino acids.

amino acids organic acids in which one or more of the hydrogen atoms are replaced by the amino group, NH_2. They are the end product of protein hydrolysis and from them the body synthesizes its own proteins. They are classified as either essential (indispensable) or non-essential (dispensable). Ten (eight in adults and a further two during childhood) cannot be synthesized in sufficient quantities in the body and are therefore essential (indispensable) in the diet—arginine, histidine, isoleucine, leucine, lysine, methionine, phenylalanine, threonine, tryptophan and valine. The remainder, which can be synthesized in the body if the diet contains sufficient amounts of the precursor amino acids, are designated non-essential (dispensable) amino acids. However, some of these are conditionally essential and depend upon adequate amounts of their precursor. ⇒ essential amino acids.

aminoaciduria *n* the abnormal presence of amino acids in the urine; it usually indicates an inborn error of metabolism as in cystinosis and Fanconi syndrome—**aminoaciduric** *adj*.

aminoglycosides *npl* a group of bactericidal antibiotic drugs. ⇒ Appendix 5.

aminopeptidases *npl* intestinal enzymes that act upon the amine end of the peptide chain during the digestion of protein.

aminotransferases *npl* transaminases. A group of enzymes that facilitate the transfer of amine (NH_2) groups between amino acids. *alanine aminotransferase (ALT)* formerly called serum glutamic pyruvic transaminase (SGPT). *aspartate aminotransferase (AST)* formerly called serum glutamic oxalacetic transaminase (SGOT). Aminotransferases are released by certain damaged cells and when blood levels are measured may be useful in the diagnosis of liver disease (ALT, AST) and heart disease (AST).

amitosis *n* division of a cell by direct fission—**amitotic** *adj*.

ammonia *n* a compound of nitrogen and hydrogen. Several inherited errors of ammonia metabolism can cause learning disability, seizures and other neurological manifestations.

ammonium bicarbonate sometimes used in expectorant cough mixtures but of doubtful value.

amnesia *n* complete loss of memory; can be divided into organic (true) amnesia (e.g. delirium, dementia, post ECT), and psychogenic amnesia (e.g. dissociative states, Ganser's syndrome). The term *anterograde amnesia* is used when there is impaired continuous recall for events following an accident or brain insult, and *retrograde amnesia* when the impairment is of events prior to the insult—**amnesic** *adj*.

amnesic syndrome chronic profound impairment of recent memory with preserved immediate recall. Often accompanied by disorientation for time and confabulation (the creation of false memory to fill the gaps in memory). Commonly caused by thiamin(e) deficiency, which can be secondary to chronic alcohol use, dietary deficiency, gastric cancer, etc. ⇒ Korsakoff's (Korsakov's) syndrome.

amniocentesis *n* a diagnostic procedure for detecting chromosomal, metabolic and haematological abnormalities of the fetus. It involves inserting a needle under ultrasound guidance through the abdominal wall into the amniotic sac to obtain a sample of amniotic fluid.

amniohook *n* an instrument for rupturing the fetal membranes. Also called an amniotome. ⇒ amniotomy.

amnion *n* membrane of embryonic origin lining the cavity of the uterus during pregnancy containing amniotic fluid and the fetus—**amnionic, amniotic** *adj*. ⇒ chorion.

amnionitis *n* inflammation of the amnion.

amnioscopy *n* amnioscope passed through the abdominal wall enables viewing of the fetus and amniotic fluid. Clear, colourless fluid is normal; yellow or green staining is due to meconium and occurs in cases of fetal hypoxia—**amnioscopic** *adj*, **amnioscopically** *adv*. *cervical amnioscopy* can be performed late in pregnancy. A different instrument is inserted via the vagina and cervix for the same reasons.

amniotic cavity the fluid-filled cavity between the fetus and the amnion.

amniotic fluid fluid produced by the inner fetal membrane (amnion) and the fetus, which surrounds the fetus throughout pregnancy. It protects the fetus from temperature variations and physical trauma, and permits fetal movement. It is secreted and reabsorbed by cells lining the amniotic cavity and is swallowed by the fetus and excreted as urine. ⇒ amniocentesis, amnioscopy. *amniotic fluid embolism* an embolus caused by amniotic fluid entering the maternal circulation. An extremely rare but very serious complication of pregnancy. ⇒ disseminated intravascular coagulation.

amniotome *n* ⇒ amniohook.

amniotomy *n* artificial rupture of the fetal membranes to induce or expedite labour.

amoeba *n* a unicellular (single cell) protozoon. Strains that are human parasites include *Entamoeba histolytica*, which causes amoebic dysentery (intestinal amoebiasis). ⇒ protozoon—**amoebae** *pl*, **amoebic** *adj*.

amoebiasis *n* infestation of large intestine by the protozoon *Entamoeba histolytica*, where it causes mucosal ulceration leading to pain, diarrhoea alternating with constipation and blood and mucus passed rectally, hence the term 'amoebic dysentery'. If the amoebae enter the hepatic portal circulation they may cause a liver abscess. Diagnosis is by isolating the amoeba in the stools. Cutaneous amoebiasis may cause perianal or genital ulceration in homosexual men.

amoebicide *n* an agent that kills amoebae—**amoebicidal** *adj*.

amoeboid *adj* resembling an amoeba in shape or in mode of movement such as leucocytes.

amoeboma *n* a tumour in the caecum or rectum caused by *Entamoeba histolytica*. Fibrosis may occur and obstruct the bowel.

amorph *n* a gene that is inactive, i.e. does not express a trait.

amorphous *adj* not having a regular shape.

AMP *abbr* adenosine monophosphate.

ampere (A) *n* one of the seven base units of the International System of Units (SI). A measurement of electrical current.

amphipathic *adj* describes a molecule that has parts with very different chemical properties. For example, possessing a non-polar (hydrophobic) end and a polar (hydrophilic) end.

ampoule *n* a hermetically sealed glass or plastic phial containing a single sterile dose of a drug.

ampulla *n* any flask-like dilatation such as that in the uterine (fallopian) tube ⇒ Figure 17—**ampullae** *pl*, **ampullar, ampullary, ampullate** *adj*. *ampulla of Vater* the enlargement formed by the union of the common bile duct with the pancreatic duct where they enter the duodenum.

amputation *n* removal of an appending part, e.g. limb.

amputee *n* a person who has had amputation of one or more limbs.

amylase *n* any enzyme that converts starches into sugars. Found in saliva and pancreatic juice; it converts starchy foods to maltose. The amount of amylase in the blood is increased in disorders of the pancreas such as pancreatitis.

amyloid *adj, n* resembling starch. A glycoprotein. ⇒ amyloidosis.

amyloidosis *n* formation and deposit of amyloid in any organ, notably the liver and kidney. *primary amyloidosis* has no apparent cause. *secondary amyloidosis* can occur in any prolonged toxic condition such as Hodgkin's disease, tuberculosis and leprosy. It is common in the genetic disease familial Mediterranean fever.

amylolysis *n* starch digestion—**amylolytic** *adj*.

amyotrophic lateral sclerosis (ALS) a form of motor neuron disease in which there is a loss of the upper motor neurons from the cortex to the brainstem and spinal cord as well as the loss of the lower motor neurons from the brainstem and spinal cord to the muscles.

ANA *abbr* antinuclear antibody.

anabolic steroids a group of androgens that stimulate anabolic effects such as the synthesis of body protein. They may be misused by body builders and athletes. ⇒ Appendix 5.

anabolism *n* the series of chemical reactions in the living body requiring energy to change simple substances into complex ones—**anabolic** *adj*. ⇒ adenosine triphosphate, catabolism, metabolism.

anacidity *n* lack of normal acidity, especially in the gastric juice. ⇒ achlorhydria.

anacrotic *adj* a wave in the ascending curve of an arterial tracing, indicating the opening of the aortic valve (that between the left ventricle and the aorta). An abnormality of this occurs in aortic stenosis. ⇒ dicrotic.

anaemia *n* a reduction in the haemoglobin content of the blood. Produces clinical manifestations arising from hypoxaemia, such as lassitude and breathlessness on exertion. There are very many possible causes. ⇒ haemolytic disease of the newborn, megaloblastic anaemia, thalassaemia—**anaemic** *adj*. *anaemia of chronic disease* anaemia associated with chronic inflammatory diseases, infection or cancer. *aplastic anaemia* is the result of complete bone marrow failure. *haemolytic anaemia* is caused by the premature destruction of red blood cells, as with some drugs and toxins, autoimmune processes, or inherited red cell disorders. *pernicious anaemia* results from the inability of the bone marrow to produce normal red cells because of the lack of a protein released by gastric parietal cells, called the intrinsic factor, which is necessary for the absorption of vitamin B_{12} from food. An autoimmune mechanism may be responsible. *sickle cell anaemia* ⇒ sickle cell disease.

anaerobe *n* a micro-organism that is unable to grow in the presence of molecular oxygen. When this is strictly so, it is called an *obligatory anaerobe*. Most pathogens are indifferent to atmospheric conditions and will grow whether oxygen is present or not and are therefore called *facultative anaerobes*—**anaerobic** *adj*.

anaerobic *adj* relating to the absence of oxygen. Describes processes that occur without oxygen, and certain micro-organisms that survive without free oxygen or air. *anaerobic energy* energy that is produced without using oxygen via two energy systems: alactacid and lactacid.

anaerobic adaptations long-term physical changes that result from anaerobic exercise. They increase the body's ability to deal with powerful dynamic exercise.

anaerobic exercise vigorous short-duration exercise where skeletal muscle oxygen supply is inadequate. Metabolic fuel molecules are broken down anaerobically to produce adenosine triphosphate (ATP) with the conversion of pyruvic acid to lactic acid. *anaerobic threshold* the point at which aerobic energy processes alone can no longer meet the musculoskeletal requirements for ATP.

anaesthesia *n* loss of sensation. ⇒ caudal anaesthesia, epidural anaesthesia. *general anaesthesia* loss of sensation with loss of consciousness. In *local anaesthesia* injection of a drug that inhibits peripheral nerve conduction so that painful stimuli fail to reach the brain. *spinal anaesthesia* loss of sensation by the injection of local anaesthetic into the cerebrospinal fluid between the vertebrae usually of the lower back, causing loss of sensation but no loss of consciousness. Also used to describe the loss of feeling produced by a spinal lesion.

anaesthesiology *n* the science dealing with anaesthetics, their administration and effect.

anaesthetic *n* **1** *n* a drug that induces general or local anaesthesia. **2** *adj* causing anaesthesia. **3** *adj* insensible to stimuli—**anaesthetize** *vt*. *general anaesthetic* a drug that produces general anaesthesia by inhalation or injection. *local anaesthetic* a drug that injected into the tissues or applied topically causes local insensibility to pain. *spinal anaesthetic* ⇒ spinal.

anaesthetic assistant trained operating department operative who provides support for the anaesthetist. Also called operating department assistant (ODA).

anaesthetist *n* a doctor with specialist training to administer general anaesthesia.

anaesthetize *vt* to administer drugs or gases to produce general anaesthesia.

analeptic *adj*, *n* restorative.

analgesia *n* loss of sensation of pain without loss of touch—**analgesic** *adj*. ⇒ patient controlled analgesia.

analgesic *n* a drug used to produce analgesia, i.e. relieves pain. ⇒ Appendix 5.

analogous *adj* similar in function but not in origin.

analysis *n* in chemistry the determination of the component parts of a compound substance. ⇒ psychoanalysis—**analyses** *pl*, **analytic** *adj*, **analytically** *adv*.

analysis of variance (ANOVA) a statistical method of comparing sample means.

anaphylactoid *adj* a systemic reaction, resembling anaphylaxis but not IgE-mediated.

anaphylaxis *n* a systemic reaction due to a type I, or immediate-type, hypersensitivity reaction caused by IgE-mediated release of inflammatory mediators (such as histamine) from mast cells on exposure to an allergen. Characterized by urticaria, pruritus, angioedema, respiratory distress, vascular collapse and shock ⇒ allergy, sensitization—**anaphylactic** *adj.*

anaplasia *n* loss of the distinctive characteristics of a cell, associated with proliferative activity as in cancer—**anaplastic** *adj.*

anarthria *n* a severe form of dysarthria. The affected person is unable to produce the motor movements required for speech. The muscle weakness is apparent in the phonatory, articulatory, respiratory and resonatory speech systems. ⇒ dysarthria.

anastomosis *n* **1** the anatomical intercommunication of the branches of two or more tubular structures, e.g. arteries or veins. **2** in surgery, the establishment of an intercommunication between two hollow organs, vessels or nerves—**anastomoses** *pl*, **anastomotic** *adj*, **anastomose** *vt.*

anatomical position for the purpose of accurate description the anterior view is of the upright body facing forward, hands by the sides with palms facing forwards. The posterior view is of the back of the upright body in that position.

anatomy *n* the science which deals with the structure of the body—**anatomical** *adj*, **anatomically** *adv.*

Ancylostoma *n* (*syn* human hookworm). *Ancylostoma duodenale* is mostly found in southern Europe and the Middle and Far East. *Necator americanus* is found in the New World and tropical Africa. Usually only significant when infestation is moderate or heavy. The worm lives in the duodenum and upper jejunum, eggs are passed in faeces, hatch in moist soil and produce larvae that can penetrate bare feet and reinfest individuals. Infestation is prevented by wearing shoes and using latrines.

ancylostomiasis *n* (*syn* hookworm disease, miners' anaemia) infestation of the human intestine with *Ancylostoma*, giving rise to malnutrition and severe anaemia.

androblastoma *n* (*syn* arrhenoblastoma) a tumour of the ovary; can produce male or female hormones and can cause masculinization in women or precocious puberty in girls.

androgens *npl* steroid hormones secreted by the testes (testosterone) and adrenal cortex in both sexes. They have widespread anabolic effects, produce the male secondary sex characteristics, e.g. male hair distribution and stimulate spermatogenesis—**androgenic, androgenous** *adj.*

anencephaly *n* absence of the brain. The condition is incompatible with life. It can be detected by raised levels of alphafetoprotein in the amniotic fluid—**anencephalous, anencephalic** *adj.*

aneuploidy *n* a chromosome number that is not a multiple of the normal haploid number (23). Includes; trisomy, e.g. Down's syndrome where the individual has 47 chromosomes, and monosomy where there are 45 chromosomes, e.g. Turner's syndrome. ⇒ polyploidy.

aneurysm *n* a sac formed by localized dilation of a blood vessel, usually an artery, due to a local fault in the wall through defect, disease or injury, producing a swelling, often pulsating, over which a murmur may be heard. True aneurysms may be saccular, fusiform, or dissecting where the blood flows between the layers of the arterial wall—**aneurysmal** *adj.*

angiectasis *n* abnormal dilatation of blood vessels. ⇒ telangiectasis—**angiectatic** *adj.*

angiitis *n* inflammation of a blood or lymph vessel. ⇒ vasculitis—**angiitic** *adj.*

angina *n* sense of constriction—**anginal** *adj. angina pectoris* severe but temporary attack of cardiac pain that may radiate to the arms, throat, lower jaw or the back. Results from myocardial ischaemia. Often the attack is induced by exercise (angina of effort).

angiocardiography *n* demonstration of the chambers of the heart and great vessels after injection of an opaque contrast medium—**angiocardiographic** *adj*, **angiocardiogram** *n*, **angiocardiograph** *n*, **angiocardiographically** *adv.*

angiodysplasia *n* vascular malformation initially involving the large bowel, which may cause lower gastrointestinal bleeding.

angiogenesis n the formation of new blood vessels (vascularization), e.g. during wound healing, or the development of new blood vessels supplying a tumour.

angiography n demonstration of the blood vessels of the arterial system after injection of an opaque contrast medium—**angiographic** adj, **angiogram** n, **angiograph** n, **angiographically** adv.

angiology n the science dealing with blood and lymphatic vessels—**angiological** adj, **angiologically** adv.

angio-oedema n (syn angioneurotic oedema) a severe form of urticaria which may involve the skin of the face, hands or genitalia and the mucous membrane of the mouth and throat: oedema of the glottis may be fatal. Immediately there is an abrupt local increase in vascular permeability, as a result of which fluid escapes from blood vessels into surrounding tissues. Swelling may be due to an allergic hypersensitivity reaction to drugs, pollens or other known allergens, but in many cases no cause can be found.

angioplasty n surgical reconstruction of blood vessels—**angioplastic** adj. percutaneous transluminal angioplasty a balloon is passed into a stenosed artery (e.g. coronary artery) and inflated with contrast medium; it presses the atheroma against the vessel wall, thereby increasing the diameter of the lumen.

angiosarcoma n a malignant tumour arising from blood vessels—**angiosarcomata** pl, **angiosarcomatous** adj.

angiospasm n spasm of blood vessels—**angiospastic** adj.

angiotensin n a substance formed by the action of renin on a precursor protein in the blood plasma. In the lungs angiotensin I is converted into angiotensin II, a highly active substance which constricts blood vessels and causes release of aldosterone from the adrenal cortex in the angiotensin-aldosterone response.

angiotensin-converting enzyme (ACE) inhibitor a group of drugs that block the angiotensin-aldosterone response. ⇒ Appendix 5.

Angleman syndrome an inherited condition that arises from mutations in the maternal chromosome 15 during formation of the gamete. Features include: 'puppet-like' gait, learning disability, brachycephaly (short, broad skull), inappropriate emotional outbursts, tongue protrusion and hooked nose. ⇒ Prader–Willi syndrome.

angular stomatitis ⇒ stomatitis.

anhedonia n a total inability to take pleasure in life. Associated with depressive disorder.

anhidrosis n deficient sweat secretion—**anhidrotic** adj.

anhidrotic n an agent that reduces perspiration.

anhydraemia n deficient fluid content of blood—**anhydraemic** adj.

anhydrous adj entirely without water, dry.

anicteric adj without jaundice.

anion n a negatively charged ion, e.g. chloride (Cl^-). They move towards the positive electrode (anode) during electrolysis. anion gap the difference between the amount of anions and cations in the blood. ⇒ cation.

aniridia n absence of the iris; usually congenital.

anisocoria n inequality in diameter of the pupils.

anisocytosis n inequality in size of red blood cells.

anisomelia n unequal length of limbs—**anisomelous** adj.

anisometropia n a difference in the refraction of the two eyes—**anisometropic** adj.

ankle n the joint formed between the talus, fibula and tibia.

ankle clonus a series of rapid muscular contractions of the calf muscle when the foot is dorsiflexed by pressure upon the sole.

ankle equinus a congenital or acquired condition or deformity, which is characterized by deficient dorsiflexion at the ankle joint. During the stance phase of normal gait a minimum 10° of ankle joint dorsiflexion is needed for normal walking. ⇒ talipes.

ankyloblepharon n adhesion of the eyelid margins, usually lateral, often secondary to chronic inflammation.

ankylosing spondylitis ⇒ spondylitis.

ankylosis n stiffness or fixation of a joint. ⇒ spondylitis—**ankylosed** adj, **ankylose** vt, vi.

annular adj ring-shaped. annular ligaments hold in proximity two long bones, as in the wrist and ankle joints.

anogenital *adj* pertaining to the anus and the genital region.

anomaly *n* that which is unusual or differs from the normal—**anomalous** *adj*.

anomia *n* a difficulty in word finding that affects many people with aphasia. Most frequently demonstrated when the person is required to perform a naming task but may also be recognized by the use of circumlocutions in spontaneous speech samples.

anomie *n* sociological term that describes a circumstance where the 'norms' that guide behaviour are absent. The 'norm-less' state that results from weak social controls and moral obligations leads to derangement in social behaviour.

anonychia *n* absence of nails.

anoperineal *adj* pertaining to the anus and perineum.

Anopheles *n* a genus of mosquito. The females of some species are the host of the malarial parasite, and their bite is the means of transmitting malaria to humans.

anoplasty *n* surgical repair or reconstruction of the anus—**anoplastic** *adj*.

anorchism *n* congenital absence of one or both testes—**anorchic** *adj*.

anorectal *adj* pertaining to the anus and rectum, e.g. a fissure.

anorexia *n* lack of appetite for food. *anorexia nervosa* a psychological illness, most common in female adolescents. There is avoidance of carbohydrate intake leading to weight loss. There is associated over-exercising, purging and disturbance of body image. Can lead to mortality by starvation in severe cases—**anorexic, anorectic** *adj*. ⇒ eating disorders.

anosmia *n* absence of the sense of smell—**anosmic** *adj*.

anovular *adj* relating to absence of ovulation. *anovular bleeding* occurs in dysfunctional uterine bleeding associated with hormone disturbance. *anovular menstruation* is the result of taking oral contraceptives.

anoxaemia *n* literally, no oxygen in the blood. Usually used to indicate hypoxaemia—**anoxaemic** *adj*.

anoxia *n* literally, no oxygen in the tissues. Usually used to signify hypoxia—**anoxic** *adj*.

antacid *n* a substance that neutralizes acidity. Often used in alkaline indigestion medicines. ⇒ Appendix 5.

antagonist *n* a muscle that reverses or opposes the action of an agonist muscle. Also describes a drug or chemical that blocks the action of another molecule at a cell receptor site, e.g. the narcotic antagonist naloxone reverses the action of opioid drugs. ⇒ agonist *opp*—**antagonism** *n*, **antagonistic** *adj*.

antagonistic action action performed by those muscles that limit the movement of an opposing group.

anteflexion *n* the bending forward of an organ, commonly applied to the position of the uterus. ⇒ retroflexion *opp*.

antemortem *adj* before death. ⇒ postmortem *opp*.

antenatal *adj* prenatal. ⇒ postnatal *opp*—**antenatally** *adj*.

antepartum *adj* before birth. From 24 weeks gestation to full term. ⇒ postpartum *opp*.

anterior *adj* in front of; the front surface of; ventral. ⇒ posterior *opp*—**anteriorly** *adv*. *anterior chamber of the eye* the space between the posterior surface of the cornea and the anterior surface of the iris. ⇒ aqueous. *anterior tibial syndrome* severe pain and inflammation over anterior tibial muscle group, with inability to dorsiflex the foot.

anterograde *adj* proceeding forward. ⇒ retrograde *opp*, amnesia.

anteversion *n* the normal forward tilting, or displacement forward, of an organ or part. ⇒ retroversion *opp*—**anteverted** *adj*, **antevert** *vt*.

anthelmintic *adj* describes a drug for the destruction or elimination of parasitic worms. ⇒ Appendix 5.

anthracosis *n* accumulation of carbon in the lungs due to inhalation of coal dust; may cause fibrotic reaction. A form of pneumoconiosis—**anthracotic** *adj*.

anthrax *n* a contagious disease of domestic animals such as cattle, which may be transmitted to humans by inoculation, inhalation and ingestion, causing malignant pustule (skin lesion) with septicaemia, inhalation anthrax or woolsorter's disease (haemorrhagic bronchopneumonia), meningitis and severe gastroenteritis. Causative organism is the bacterium *Bacillus anthracis*. Preventive measures include immunization of humans and animals, post-exposure prophylaxis with antibiotics, e.g. ciprofloxacin, and proper disposal of infected animals. Occupations at high risk include veterinary surgeons, livestock farmers, butchers, and those handling hides and wool.

anthropoid *adj* resembling man. The word is also used to describe a pelvis that is narrow from side to side, a form of contracted pelvis.

anthropology *n* the study of humankind. Subdivided into several specialties. ⇒ ethnology.

anthropometry *n* measurement of the human body and its parts for the purposes of comparison and establishing norms for sex, age, weight, race and so on—**anthropometric** *adj*.

antianabolic *adj* preventing the synthesis of body protein.

antiandrogens *npl* a group of drugs that block the activity of testosterone. ⇒ Appendix 5.

antiarrhythmic *adj* describes drugs and treatments used to treat a variety of cardiac arrhythmias. ⇒ Appendix 5.

antibacterial *adj* describes an agent that destroys bacteria or inhibits their growth. ⇒ antibiotics, antiseptics, bactericidal, bacteriostatic, disinfectants.

antiberi-beri *adj* against beri-beri, e.g. the thiamin portion of vitamin B complex.

antibilharzial *adj* against *Bilharzia*. ⇒ *Schistosoma*.

antibiosis *n* an association between organisms that is harmful to one of them. ⇒ symbiosis *opp*—**antibiotic** *adj*.

antibiotics *npl* antibacterial substances derived from fungi and bacteria, exemplified by penicillin. However, the term is generally used for all drugs that act against bacteria. Some have a narrow spectrum of activity whereas others act against a wide range of bacteria (broad spectrum). ⇒ aminoglycosides, antituberculosis drugs, bactericidal, bacteriostatic, β-lactam antibiotics, cephalosporins, glycopeptide antibiotics, macrolides, penicillins, fluoroquinolones, sulphonamides, tetracyclines. ⇒ Appendix 5.

antibodies *npl* (*syn* immunoglobulins) often used to indicate immunoglobulins with specific antigen-binding activity.

anticholinergic *adj* inhibitory to the action of a cholinergic nerve by interfering with the action of acetylcholine. ⇒ muscarinic antagonists (antimuscarinic).

anticholinesterase *n* any agent that inactivates cholinesterase.

anticoagulant *n* an agent that reduces the propensity of blood to clot. Uses: (a) to obtain specimens suitable for pathological examination and chemical analyses where whole blood or plasma is required instead of serum; (b) during the collection of blood for transfusion, the anticoagulant usually being sodium citrate; (c) as therapy in the prophylaxis and treatment of thromboembolic conditions. ⇒ Appendix 5, coumarins, heparin.

anticoagulation *n* the process of suppressing or reducing blood coagulation.

anticodon *n* genetics, the three bases (triplet) in transfer ribonucleic acid (tRNA) concerned with the synthesis of proteins (translation stage). ⇒ codon.

anticonvulsant *n* ⇒ antiepileptics—**anticonvulsive** *adj*.

anti-D *n* an antibody directed against the Rhesus D blood group antigen. Given to RhD-negative women who have RhD-positive babies to prevent subsequent immune mediated disease such as haemolytic disease of the newborn.

antidepressants *npl* drugs used to manage depression. There are three main groups: monoamine oxidase inhibitors (MAOIs), selective serotonin reuptake inhibitors (SSRIs) and tricyclic antidepressants (TCA). ⇒ Appendix 5.

antidiabetic *adj* literally 'against diabetes'. Used to describe therapeutic measures in diabetes mellitus to control blood glucose. ⇒ insulin, hypoglycaemic drugs.

antidiarrhoeals *npl* agents such as drugs used to reduce diarrhoea. ⇒ Appendix 5.

antidiuretic *adj* reducing the volume of urine. *antidiuretic hormone (ADH)* vasopressin.

antidote *n* a remedy that opposes, counteracts or neutralizes the action of a poison. For example, protamine sulphate is used to counteract the effects of an overdose of heparin.

antiembolic *adj* against embolism. Antiembolic stockings are worn to decrease the risk of deep vein thrombosis.

antiemetic *adj* against emesis. Any agent such as a drug that prevents or treats nausea and vomiting. ⇒ cannabinoids, D_2-receptor antagonists, H_1-receptor antagonists, 5-HT_3-receptor antagonists, muscarinic antagonists (antimuscarinic). ⇒ Appendix 5.

antienzyme *n* a substance that exerts a specific inhibiting action on an enzyme. Found in the digestive tract to prevent autodigestion of the mucosa, and in blood where they act as immunoglobulins.

antiepileptic *adj* (*syn* anticonvulsant) describes drugs which reduce the frequency of seizures. ⇒ Appendix 5.

antifebrile *adj* describes any agent which reduces or allays fever.

antifibrinolytic *adj* describes any agent which prevents fibrinolysis.

antifungal *adj* describes any agent which destroys fungi. ⇒ Appendix 5.

anti-GBM disease disease caused by specific antibodies to the glomerular basement membranes. It features rapidly progressive glomerulonephritis and pulmonary haemorrhage. Previously known as Goodpasture's disease.

antigen *n* substance inducing a specific immune response which interacts with the product of that immune response. This may be specific immunoglobulin or T cells bearing T cell receptors specific for that antigen—**antigenic** *adj*.

antigonococcal *adj* describes any measures used against infections caused by *Neisseria gonorrhoeae*.

antihaemophilic factor (AHF) factor VIII in the blood coagulation cascade, present in plasma. A deficiency causes haemophilia A (classical).

antihaemophilic factor B ⇒ Christmas factor.

antihaemorrhagic *adj* describes any agent which prevents haemorrhage.

antihistamines *npl* drugs which suppress some of the effects of histamine released in the body. ⇒ Appendix 5.

antihypertensive *adj* describes any agent that reduces high blood pressure. ⇒ (α)-adrenoceptor antagonists, angiotensin-converting enzyme inhibitors, (β)-adrenoceptor antagonists, calcium antagonists, diuretics. ⇒ Appendix 5.

anti-infective *adj* describes any agent which prevents infection.

anti-inflammatory *adj* tending to prevent or relieve inflammation. ⇒ non-steroidal anti-inflammatory drugs (NSAIDs). ⇒ Appendix 5.

antileprotic *adj* describing any agent which prevents or cures leprosy. ⇒ Appendix 5.

antilymphocyte globulin (ALG) an immunoglobulin which binds to antigens on T cells and inhibits T cell-dependent immune responses; occasionally used in preventing graft rejection during organ transplantation.

antimalarial *adj* against malaria. ⇒ Appendix 5.

antimetabolites *npl* molecules that prevent cell division. They are sufficiently similar to essential cell metabolites to be incorporated into the metabolic pathways, thereby preventing their use by the cell. ⇒ cytotoxic. ⇒ Appendix 5.

antimicrobial *adj* against microbes.

antimitochondrial antibody (AMA) autoantibodies against mitochondrial components. Certain types are a marker for primary biliary cirrhosis.

antimitotic *adj* preventing cell replication by mitosis. ⇒ cytotoxic.

antimutagen *n* a substance that cancels out the action of a mutagen—**antimutagenic** *adj*.

antimycotic *adj* ⇒ antifungal.

antineoplastic *adj* describes any substance or procedure that kills or slows the growth of cancerous/neoplastic cells, such as cytotoxic chemotherapy, radiotherapy, or hormonal or biological response modification therapy.

antineuritic *adj* describes any agent which prevents neuritis. Specially applied to vitamin B complex.

anti-neutrophil cytoplasmic antibody (ANCA) a group of autoantibodies directed against cytoplasmic components of neutrophils and associated with a range of pathological conditions such as polyarteritis.

antinuclear antibody (ANA) a family of many types of autoantibody directed against cell nuclei that are found in connective tissue disorders, particular systemic lupus erythematosus (SLE) and Sjögren syndrome. The many types recognized can be used to categorize rheumatological disorders.

antioestrogens *npl* antagonist drugs that block oestrogen receptors in various body sites. ⇒ selective (o)estrogen receptor modulators. ⇒ Appendix 5.

antioxidants *npl* substances that delay the process of oxidation. Some minerals, e.g. zinc, and vitamins A, C and E, contained in a balanced diet, function as antioxidants and help to minimize free radical oxidative damage to cells.

antiparasitic *adj* describes agents that prevent or destroy parasites.

antiparkinson(ism) drugs drugs used in the management of parkinsonism. ⇒ Appendix 5.

antipellagra *adj* against pellagra; a function of the nicotinic acid portion of vitamin B complex.

antiperistalsis *n* reversal of the normal peristaltic action—antiperistaltic *adj*.

antiplatelet drugs a group of drugs that reduce platelet aggregation. ⇒ Appendix 5.

antiprothrombin *n* stops blood coagulation by preventing conversion of prothrombin into thrombin. Anticoagulant.

antiprotozoal *n* a drug used to prevent or cure a protozoal disease. ⇒ Appendix 5.

antipruritic *adj* describes any agent which relieves or prevents itching.

antipsychotic *adj* against psychosis, such as drugs used to treat psychotic episodes. ⇒ neuroleptics.

antipyretic *adj* describes any agent which prevents or reduces fever. ⇒ Appendix 5.

antirachitic *adj* describes any agent which prevents or cures rickets, a function of vitamin D.

anti-Rhesus ⇒ anti-D.

antischistosomal *adj* describes any agent which destroys *Schistosoma*.

antiscorbutic *adj* describes any agent which prevents or cures scurvy, a function of vitamin C.

antisepsis *n* prevention of sepsis (tissue infection); introduced into surgical procedures in 1880 by Lord Lister—antiseptic *adj*.

antiseptics *npl* chemical substances that destroy or inhibit the growth of microorganisms. They can be applied to living tissues, e.g. chlorhexidine used for skin preparation before invasive procedures and hand decontamination.

antiserum *n* serum prepared from the blood of an animal immunized by the requisite antigen, containing a high concentration of polyclonal antibodies against that antigen.

antisocial *adj* against society. Used to describe a person who does not accept the responsibilities and constraints placed on a community by its members—anti-socialism *n*.

antispasmodic *adj* (*syn* spasmolytic) describes any measure or drugs used to relieve spasm in muscle. ⇒ Appendix 5.

antistatic *adj* preventing the accumulation of static electricity.

antistreptolysin *adj* against streptolysins. A raised antistreptolysin titre in the blood is indicative of recent streptococcal infection.

antisyphilitic *adj* describes any measures taken to combat syphilis.

antithrombin III *n* substance that inhibits blood coagulation. It is synthesized in the liver and is normally present in the blood, where it restricts coagulation to areas where it is needed. ⇒ thrombin.

antithrombotic *adj* describes any measures that prevent or cure thrombosis.

antithyroid *n* any agent used to decrease the activity of the thyroid gland. ⇒ Appendix 5.

antitoxin *n* an antibody which neutralizes a given toxin. Made in response to the invasion by toxin-producing bacteria, or the injection of toxoids—antitoxic *adj*.

antitreponemal *adj* describes any measures used against infections caused by *Treponema*.

antituberculosis drugs drugs used in the treatment of tuberculosis—antitubercular *adj*. ⇒ Appendix 5.

antitumour antibiotics cytotoxic antibiotics that act against tumour cells by disrupting cell membranes and DNA. ⇒ cytotoxic. ⇒ Appendix 5.

antitussive *adj* describes any measures which suppress cough.

antivenom *n* a serum prepared from animals injected with the venom of snakes; used as an antidote in cases of poisoning by snakebite.

antiviral *adj* acting against viruses. *antiviral drugs* ⇒ Appendix 5.

antivitamin *n* a substance interfering with the absorption or utilization of a vitamin, e.g. avidin.

antrectomy *n* surgical excision of the antrum of the stomach.

antro-oral *adj* pertaining to the maxillary antrum and the mouth.

antrostomy *n* surgical opening from nasal cavity to antrum of Highmore (maxillary sinus).

antrum *n* a cavity, especially in bone— **antral** *adj. antrum of Highmore* in the superior maxillary bone.

anuria *n* complete absence of urine output by the kidneys. ⇒ suppression—**anuric** *adj.*

anus *n* the end of the alimentary canal, at the extreme termination of the rectum. It is formed of a sphincter muscle which relaxes to allow faecal matter to pass through—**anal** *adj. artificial anus* ⇒ colostomy. *imperforate anus* ⇒ imperforate.

anxiety *n* feelings of fear, apprehension and dread. *anxiety disorder* a form of mental disorder characterized by recurrent acute anxiety attacks (panic) or by chronic anxiety. The attacks consist of both physical and psychological anxiety signs and symptoms.

anxiolytics *npl* agents that reduce anxiety. ⇒ Appendix 5.

aorta *n* the main artery arising out of the left ventricle of the heart. ⇒ Figure 8.

aortic *adj* pertaining to the aorta. *aortic murmur* abnormal heart sound heard over aortic area; a systolic murmur alone is the murmur of aortic stenosis, a diastolic murmur denotes aortic regurgitation. *aortic regurgitation (incompetence)* regurgitation of blood from aorta back into the left ventricle. *aortic stenosis* narrowing of aortic valve. This is usually due to rheumatic heart disease or a congenital bicuspid valve which predisposes to the deposit of calcium.

aortitis *n* inflammation of the aorta.

aortography *n* demonstration of the aorta after introduction of an opaque contrast medium, either via a catheter passed along the femoral or brachial artery or by direct translumbar injection—**aortographic** *adj,* **aortogram** *n,* **aortograph** *n,* **aortographically** *adv.*

apathy *n* **1** abnormal listlessness and deficiency of activity. **2** attitude of indifference—**apathetic** *adj.*

APD *abbr* automated peritoneal dialysis.

aperients *npl* ⇒ laxatives.

aperistalsis *n* absence of peristaltic movement in the bowel. Characterizes the condition of paralytic ileus—**aperistaltic** *adj.*

Apert's syndrome congenital craniosynostosis accompanied by deformities of the hands. ⇒ acrocephalosydactyly syndactyly.

apex *n* the summit or top of anything which is cone-shaped, e.g. the tip of a lung. ⇒ Figure 7—**apices** *pl,* **apical** *adj.* In a heart of normal size the *apex beat* (systolic impulse) can be seen or felt in the 5th left intercostal space in the mid-clavicular line. It is the lowest and most lateral point at which an impulse can be detected and provides a rough indication of the size of the heart.

Apgar score a measure used to evaluate the general condition of a newborn baby, developed by an American anaesthetist, Dr Virginia Apgar. A score of 0, 1 or 2 is given for the criteria of heart rate, respiratory effort, skin colour, muscle tone and response to stimulation. A score between 8 and 10 indicates a baby in good condition.

aphagia *n* inability to swallow—**aphagic** *adj.*

aphakia *n* absence of the lens. Describes the eye after removal of a cataract without artificial lens implantation—**aphakic** *adj.*

aphasia *n* a language disorder that follows brain damage, due primarily to an impaired linguistic system. The term does not describe language disorders that involve problems with expression or comprehension caused by mental health problems, including psychoses, confusion and dementia, or muscle weakness, or problems with hearing. There are several classifications but generally aphasia is described as being *expressive (motor) aphasia* or *receptive (sensory) aphasia.* However, many people exhibit problems with both language expression and comprehension—**aphasic** *adj.* ⇒ dysarthria.

aphonia *n* inability to make sound due to neurological, behavioural, psychogenic or organic causes. ⇒ dysarthria—**aphonic** *adj.*

aphrodisiac *n* an agent that stimulates sexual arousal.

aphthae *npl* small ulcers of the gastrointestinal mucosa surrounded by a ring of erythema—**aphtha** *sing,* **aphthous** *adj.*

aphthous stomatitis ⇒ stomatitis.

apicectomy *n* excision of the apex of the root of a tooth.

APKD *abbr* adult polycystic kidney disease.

aplasia *n* incomplete development of tissue; absence of growth.

aplastic *adj* **1** without structure or form. **2** incapable of forming new tissue. *aplastic anaemia* ⇒ anaemia.

apnoea *n* a transitory cessation of breathing as seen in Cheyne–Stokes respiration. It is due to lack of the necessary CO_2 tension in the blood for stimulation of the respiratory centre—**apnoeic** *adj. apnoea of the newborn* ⇒ periodic breathing.

apocrine glands modified sweat glands, especially in axillae, genital and perineal regions. Responsible after puberty for body odour. ⇒ eccrine.

apodia *n* congenital absence of the feet.

aponeurosis *n* a broad glistening sheet of tendon-like tissue which serves to invest and attach muscles, e.g. abdominal muscles, to each other, and also to the parts that they move—**aponeuroses** *pl*, **aponeurotic** *adj*.

aponeurositis *n* inflammation of an aponeurosis.

apophysis *n* a projection, protuberance or outgrowth. Usually used in connection with bone.

apoplexy *n* obsolete term for cerebrovascular accident (stroke)—**apoplectic, apoplectiform** *adj*.

apoprotein *n* a protein before it binds to the prosthetic group required for biological activity.

apoptosis *n* programmed cell death.

appendectomy *n* ⇒ appendicectomy.

appendicectomy *n* excision of the appendix vermiformis.

appendicitis *n* inflammation of the appendix vermiformis.

appendix *n* an appendage. *appendix vermiformis* a worm-like appendage of the caecum about the thickness of a pencil and usually measuring from 2.5 to 15 cm in length. It contains lymphoid tissue and its position is variable. (⇒ Figure 18b)—**appendices** *pl*, **appendicular** *adj*.

apperception *n* clear perception of a sensory stimulus, in particular where there is identification or recognition—**apperceptive** *adj*.

appetite *n* the desire for food, influenced by physical activity, metabolic, dietary, psychological and behavioural factors. It may be increased or decreased pharmacologically. Appetite is also influenced by health status. ⇒ anorexia, bulimia, eating disorders.

applicator *n* an instrument used for local application of remedies, e.g. vaginal medication applicator.

apposition *n* the approximation or bringing together of two surfaces or edges.

appraisal *n* making a valuation. *performance appraisal or review* a formal procedure whereby an appraiser (manager) systematically reviews the role performance of the appraisee and they jointly set goals for the future.

approved name the generic or non-proprietary name of a drug, such as salbutamol. Should be used in prescribing except in the case of drugs where bioavailability differs between brands. ⇒ Recommended International Non-proprietary Name.

approved social worker (ASW) a social worker appointed by the Local Health Authority with statutory duties under the Mental Health Act 1983 including: (a) making applications for compulsory or emergency admission to hospital and conveyance of patients there, (b) applications concerning guardianship, the functions of the nearest relative, or acting as a nearest relative if so appointed, (c) planning and providing aftercare of discharged mentally disordered patients.

apraxia *n* inability to perform a motor act or use an object normally, due typically to damage in the parietal lobe of the brain—**apraxic, apractic** *adj. constructional apraxia* inability to arrange objects to a plan.

apronectomy ⇒ abdominoplasty.

aptitude *n* natural ability and facility in performing tasks, either physical or mental.

apyrexia *n* absence of fever—**apyrexial** *adj*.

aqueduct *n* a canal. *aqueduct of Sylvius* the canal connecting the 3rd and 4th ventricles of the brain; aqueductus cerebri.

aqueous *adj* watery. *aqueous humour* the fluid contained in the anterior and posterior chambers of the eye. ⇒ Figure 15.

arachidonic acid a polyunsaturated fatty acid with four double bonds. Used in the body for the synthesis of important regulatory lipids that include: prostaglandins, prostacyclins and thromboxanes. A high concentration is found in brain and nervous tissue membranes. Arachidonic acid is important for brain development. The dietary intake of arachidonic acid is associated with birthweight, head circumference and placental weight. It can be synthesized from linoleic acid in the body, but may be considered to be an essential fatty acid (EFA) when linoleic acid is deficient in the diet.

arachis oil oil expressed from peanuts (groundnuts). Used for cooking, in the food industry and for some pharmaceutical products. Contains monounsaturated fatty acids. Should not be used by those with a peanut allergy.

arachnodactyly *n* congenital abnormality resulting in long, slender fingers. Said to resemble spider legs (hence 'spider fingers').

arachnoid *adj* resembling a spider's web. *arachnoid mater or membrane* a delicate membrane enveloping the brain and spinal cord, lying between the pia mater internally and the dura mater externally; the middle membrane of the meninges—**arachnoidal** *adj*.

arborization *n* an arrangement resembling the branching of a tree. Characterizes both ends of a neuron, i.e. the dendrites and the axon as it supplies each muscle fibre.

arboviruses *npl* abbreviation for ARthropod-BOrne viruses. Include various RNA viruses transmitted by arthropods: mosquitoes, ticks, sandflies, etc. They cause diseases such as yellow fever, dengue, sandfly fever and several types of encephalitis.

arch of aorta ⇒ Figure 9.

arcus senilis an opaque ring round the edge of the cornea, seen in old people.

ARDS *abbr* acute respiratory distress syndrome.

areola *n* the pigmented area round the nipple of the breast. A *secondary areola* surrounds the primary areola in pregnancy—**areolar** *adj*.

areolar tissue a loose connective tissue consisting of cells and fibres in a semisolid matrix.

ARF *abbr* **1** acute renal failure. ⇒ renal. **2** acute respiratory failure. ⇒ respiratory failure.

arginase *n* an enzyme present in the liver, kidney and spleen. It converts arginine into ornithine and urea.

arginine *n* one of the essential amino acids found in protein foods required for growth and recovery. It is hydrolysed by the enzyme arginase to urea and ornithine. Supplements have been shown to enhance immune function in high risk surgical patients.

argininosuccinuria *n* the presence of arginine and succinic acid in urine. Currently associated with learning disability. Also called argininosuccinic aciduria.

argon *n* an insert gas. Forms less than 0.1% of atmospheric air.

Argyll Robertson pupil small, irregular pupil that responds to accommodation but not to light, associated with neurosyphilis and chronic alcohol misuse.

argyria slate grey discoloration of the skin and conjunctivae resulting from chronic exposure to silver.

ariboflavinosis *n* a deficiency state caused by lack of riboflavin and other members of the vitamin B complex. Characterized by cheilosis, seborrhoea, angular stomatitis, glossitis and photophobia.

ARM *abbr* artificial rupture of the membranes. ⇒ amniotomy.

Arnold–Chiari malformation a group of disorders affecting the base of the brain. Commonly occurs in hydrocephalus associated with meningocele and myelomeningocele. There are degrees of severity but usually there is some 'kinking' or 'buckling' of the brainstem with cerebellar tissue herniating through the foramen magnum at the base of the skull.

aromatherapy *n* a complementary therapy that involves the use of fragrances derived from essential oils. These may be combined with a base oil, inhaled or massaged into intact skin.

arrectores pilorum internal, plain, involuntary muscles (⇒ Figure 12) attached to hair follicles, which, by contraction, erect the hair follicles, causing 'gooseflesh'—**arrector pili** *sing*.

arrhythmia *n* any deviation from the normal rhythm, usually referring to the heart beat. ⇒ asystole, extrasystole, fibrillation, heart, Stokes–Adams syndrome, supraventricular, tachycardia, Wolff–Parkinson–White syndrome.

arsenic *n* a poisonous metallic element present in preparations such as herbicides and pesticides. Vegetables, fruit and other foods may contain small amounts. Toxic effects include malaise, gastrointestinal symptoms, pigmentation of the skin, anaemia and nervous symptoms.

artefact *n* any artificial product resulting from a physical or chemical agent; an unnatural change in a structure or tissue.

arteralgia *n* pain in an artery.

arterial blood gases (ABGs) measurement of the oxygen (PaO_2), carbon dioxide ($PaCO_2$) and acid–base (pH or hydrogen ion concentration) content of the arterial blood.

arterial line a cannula placed in an artery to sample blood for gas analysis and for continuous blood pressure monitoring. Usually only used in specialist units (ITU, HDU and theatre) because of the potential risk of severe blood loss. They should always be attached to a pressure transducer and monitor, and have an alarm that indicates any disconnection. ⇒ arterial blood gases, blood pressure.

arterial ulcer a leg ulcer caused by a defect in arterial blood supply. They are found on the foot, usually between the toes or close to the ankle; the adjacent skin is discoloured, shiny and hairless; and the ulcer is small and deep with some exudate. They are often associated with a history of cardiovascular disease or diabetes mellitus. ⇒ claudication.

arteriography *n* demonstration of the arterial system after injection of an opaque contrast medium—**arteriographic** *adj*, **arteriogram** *n*, **arteriograph** *n*, **arteriographically** *adv*.

arteriole *n* a small artery, joining an artery to a capillary network. They control the amount of blood entering the capillary network. They are able to constrict and dilate to change peripheral resistance thereby influencing blood pressure.

arteriopathy *n* disease of any artery—**arteriopathic** *adj*.

arterioplasty *n* reconstructive surgery applied to an artery—**arterioplastic** *adj*.

arteriosclerosis *n* degenerative arterial change associated with advancing age. Primarily a thickening of the media (middle) layer and usually associated with some degree of atheroma—**arteriosclerotic** *adj*.

arteriotomy *n* incision or needle puncture of an artery.

arteriovenous *adj* pertaining to an artery and a vein. *arteriovenous fistula* the anastomosis of an artery to a vein to promote the enlargement of the latter, to facilitate the removal and replacement of blood during haemodialysis.

arteritis *n* an inflammatory disease affecting the media (middle) layer of arteries. It may be due to an infection such as syphilis or it may be part of a collagen disease. The arteries may become swollen and tender and the blood may clot in them. ⇒ temporal arteritis—**arteritic** *adj*.

artery *n* a vessel carrying blood from the heart to the various tissues. The internal endothelial lining provides a smooth surface to prevent clotting of blood. The middle layer of plain muscle and elastic fibres allows for distension as blood is pumped from the heart. The outer, mainly connective tissue layer prevents overdistension. The lumen is largest nearest to the heart; it gradually decreases in size—**arterial** *adj*. *artery forceps* forceps used to produce haemostasis.

arthralgia *n* (*syn* articular neuralgia, arthrodynia) pain in a joint, used especially when there is no inflammation—**arthralgic** *adj*. *intermittent* or *periodic arthralgia* is the term used when there is pain, usually accompanied by swelling of the knee at regular intervals.

arthritis *n* inflammation of one or more joints which swell, become warm to touch, and are tender and painful on movement. There are many causes and the treatment varies according to the cause—**arthritic** *adj*. ⇒ arthropathy, gout, osteoarthritis, rheumatoid arthritis, Still's disease.

arthroclasis *n* breaking down of adhesions within the joint cavity to produce a wider range of movement.

arthrodesis *n* the stiffening of a joint by operative means.

arthrodynia *n* ⇒ arthralgia—**arthrodynic** *adj*.

arthrography *n* a radiographic examination to determine the internal structure of a joint, outlined by contrast media—either a gas or a liquid contrast medium or both—**arthrographic** *adj*, **arthrogram** *n*, **arthrograph** *n*, **arthrographically** *adv*.

arthrology *n* the science that studies the structure and function of joints, their diseases and treatment.

arthropathy *n* any joint disease—**arthropathies** *pl*, **arthropathic** *adj*. The condition is currently classified as: *enteropathic arthropathies* resulting from chronic diarrhoeal disease; *psoriatic arthropathies* psoriasis; *seronegative arthropathies* include all other instances of inflammatory arthritis other than rheumatoid arthritis; *seropositive arthropathies* include all instances of rheumatoid arthritis.

arthroplasty *n* surgical remodelling of a joint—**arthroplastic** *adj*. *cup arthroplasty* articular surface is reconstructed and covered with a vitallium cup. *excision arthroplasty* gap is filled with fibrous tissue as in Keller's operation. *Girdlestone arthroplasty* excision arthroplasty of the hip. *replacement arthroplasty* insertion of an inert prosthesis of similar shape. *total replacement arthroplasty* replacement of the head of femur and the acetabulum, both being cemented into the bone.

arthroscope *n* an instrument used for the visualization of the interior of a joint cavity. ⇒ endoscope—**arthroscopic** *adj*.

arthroscopy *n* the act of visualizing the interior of a joint. Uses an intra-articular camera to assess, repair or reconstruct various tissues within and around joints—**arthroscopic** *adj*.

arthrosis *n* degeneration in a joint.

arthrotomy *n* incision into a joint.

articular *adj* pertaining to a joint or articulation. Applied to cartilage, surface, capsule, etc.

articulation 1 the junction of two or more bones; a joint. **2** enunciation of speech—**articular** *adj*.

artificial blood a fluid able to transport O_2.

artificial insemination ⇒ insemination.

artificial kidney ⇒ dialyser.

artificial limb ⇒ orthosis, prosthesis.

artificial lung ⇒ respirator.

artificial pacemaker cardiac pacemaker. ⇒ cardiac.

artificial pneumothorax ⇒ pneumothorax.

artificial respiration ⇒ cardiopulmonary resuscitation.

asbestos *n* a fibrous, mineral substance which does not conduct heat and is incombustible. It has many uses, including brake linings, asbestos textiles and asbestos-cement sheeting.

asbestosis *n* a form of pneumoconiosis from inhalation of asbestos dust and fibre. ⇒ mesothelioma.

ascariasis *n* infestation by nematodes (roundworms). The ova are ingested and hatch in the duodenum. The larvae pass to the lungs in the blood, from where they ascend to be swallowed and returned to the bowel. They may occasionally obstruct the intestine or the bile ducts.

ascaricide *n* a substance that kills ascarides—**ascaricidal** *adj*.

ascarides *npl* nematode worms of the family Ascaridae, e.g. the roundworm *Ascaris lumbricoides*. ⇒ ascariasis.

ascending colon ⇒ Figure 18b.

Aschoff's nodules nodules present in the myocardium in myocarditis caused by rheumatic fever.

ascites *n* (*syn* hydroperitoneum) free fluid in the peritoneal cavity—**ascitic** *adj*.

ascorbic acid vitamin C. A water-soluble antioxidant vitamin which is necessary for healthy connective tissue, particularly the collagen fibres and cell membranes. Also enhances absorption of dietary iron and is necessary for functioning of the immune system. It is present in fruits and vegetables. It is destroyed by cooking in the presence of air and by plant enzymes released when cutting and grating food: it is also lost by storage. Deficiency causes scurvy. Used as nutritional supplement in anaemia and to promote wound healing.

asepsis *n* the condition of being free from living pathogenic micro-organisms—**aseptic** *adj*.

aseptic technique describes procedures used to exclude pathogenic micro-organisms from an environment. It includes the use of sterile gloves and gowns in theatre, non-touch technique and the use of sterilized equipment. Used where there is a possibility of introducing micro-organisms into the patient's body.

ASO *abbr* antistreptolysin O.

asomatogosia *n* loss of awareness of parts of the body (soma) and their position in space, a perceptual sequela of cerebrovascular accident (stroke) affecting the right parietal lobe of the cerebrum, which may lead to lack of awareness, even denial, of the presence of disability.

asparaginase *n* an enzyme derived from micro-organisms. In the form of crisantaspase, used pharmacologically to treat cancers, e.g. acute lymphoblastic leukaemia. ⇒ cytotoxic.

asparagine *n* a conditionally essential (indispensable) amino acid.

aspartame *n* an artificial sweetener. It is converted to phenylalanine in the body and consequently should not be used by people with phenylketonuria.

aspartate (aspartic acid) *n* a non-essential (dispensable) amino acid.

Asperger's syndrome a pervasive developmental disorder sharing characteristics with autism, without delayed language or cognitive development. The relationship of Asperger's syndrome to autism remains unclear.

aspergillosis *n* opportunist infection, most frequently of lungs, caused by any species of *Aspergillus*. ⇒ bronchomycosis.

Aspergillus *n* a genus of fungi, found in soil, manure and on various grains. Some species are pathogenic.

aspermia *n* lack of secretion or expulsion of semen—**aspermic** *adj*.

asphyxia *n* lack of oxygen reaching the brain leading to unconsciousness and in the absence of effective treatment eventually death.

aspiration *n* (*syn* paracentesis, tapping) **1** the removal of fluids from a body cavity by means of suction or siphonage such as fluid from the peritoneal cavity, postoperative gastric aspiration, etc. **2** describes the entry of fluids or food into the airway. *aspiration pneumonia* inflammation of lung from inhalation of foreign body, most often food particles or fluids. ⇒ Heimlich's manoeuvre.

aspirator *n* a negative pressure device used for withdrawing fluids from body cavities.

aspirin ⇒ non-steroidal anti-inflammatory drugs.

assault *n* a threat of unlawful contact. Constitutes a trespass against the person. ⇒ battery.

assay *n* a quantitative test used to measure the amount of a substance present or its level of activity, e.g. hormones or drugs.

assertiveness training developing self-confidence in personal relationships. It concentrates on the honest expression of feelings, both negative and positive: learning occurs through role playing in a therapeutic setting followed by practice in real-life situations.

assimilation *n* the process whereby digested foodstuffs are absorbed and used by the cells and tissues—**assimilable** *adj*, **assimilate** *vt, vi*.

assisted conception techniques used when normal methods of conception have failed. They include in vitro fertilization (IVF) and transcervical embryo transfer or gamete intrafallopian tube transfer (GIFT), zygote intrafallopian transfer (ZIFT), preimplantation genetic diagnosis (PGD) and intracytoplasmic sperm injection (ICSI).

association *n* a term used in psychology. *association of ideas* the principle by which ideas, emotions and movements are connected so that their succession in the mind occurs. *controlled association* ideas called up in consciousness in response to words spoken by the examiner. *free association* ideas arising spontaneously when censorship is removed: an important feature of psychoanalysis.

AST *abbr* aspartate aminotransferase. ⇒ aminotransferases.

astereognosis *n* inability to recognize objects by touch and manipulation, especially inability to perceive the shape, texture and size of objects.

asteroid hyalosis a degenerative condition, usually asymptomatic, in which the vitreous of the eye contains numerous small opacities.

asthenia *n* lack of strength; weakness, debility—**asthenic** *adj*.

asthenopia *n* eye strain. Describes symptoms related to excessive effort of accommodation, e.g. headaches—**asthenopic** *adj*, **asthenope** *n*.

asthma *n* paroxysmal dyspnoea characterized by wheezing and difficulty in expiration because of muscular spasm in the bronchi. Recent immunological studies have implicated mast cells, lymphocytes and cytokines in an inflammatory cascade leading to bronchial wall hyperactivity and narrowing in response to a stimulus. Inhaled or oral corticosteroids damp down the acute immune reaction, while inhaled β_2 receptor-agonists relieve bronchial spasm. ⇒ Appendix 5. Newer anti-asthmatic drugs such as leukotriene inhibitors may offer more targeted therapy. ⇒ occupational asthma—**asthmatic** *adj.*

astigmatism *n* defective vision caused by refractive surfaces, usually corneal, focusing light onto more than one focal plane—**astigmatic, astigmic** *adj.*

astringent *adj* describes an agent which contracts organic tissue, thus lessening secretion. May be used in the management of heavily exuding wounds—**astringency, astringent** *n.*

astrocyte *n* a star-shaped neuroglial cell.

astrocytoma *n* a slowly growing tumour of astrocytes (neuroglial tissue) of the brain.

ASW *abbr* approved social worker.

asymmetry *n* lack of similarity of the organs or parts on each side.

asymptomatic *adj* symptomless.

asystole *n* absence of heart beat. One type of cardiac arrest.

ataractic *adj* describes drugs that tranquillize and relieve anxiety. ⇒ tranquillizers.

atavism *n* the reappearance of a hereditary characteristic that has missed one or more generations—**atavic, atavistic** *adj.*

ataxia, ataxy *n* ill-timed and incoordinate movements caused by hypotonia, dyssynergia and dysmetria—**ataxic** *adj. ataxic gait* ⇒ gait. *Friedreich's ataxia* ⇒ Friedreich's ataxia.

atelectasis *n* numbers of pulmonary alveoli do not contain air due to failure of expansion (congenital atelectasis) or resorption of air from the alveoli (collapse)—**atelectatic** *adj.*

atherogenic *adj* capable of producing atheroma—**atherogenesis** *n.*

atheroma *n* plaques of fatty (lipid) material in the intimal (inner) layer of the arteries. Starts as fatty streaks on the intima, deposition of low density lipoprotein and plaque formation. Eventually the lumen of the artery is reduced and ischaemia results. A thrombus may form if a plaque ruptures, which leads to further occlusion of the artery. Of great importance in the coronary arteries in predisposing to coronary thrombosis and myocardial infarction—**atheromatous** *adj.*

atherosclerosis *n* coexisting atheroma and arteriosclerosis—**atherosclerotic** *adj.*

athetosis *n* a largely obsolete word used to describe a slow writhing movement disorder typically in the context of cerebral palsy. Made worse by excitement and emotional stress—**athetoid, athetotic** *adj.*

athlete's foot tinea pedis. ⇒ tinea.

athletic trainer a term used in North America for an individual who is trained in the prevention, evaluation, treatment and rehabilitation of athletic injuries.

atlas *n* the first cervical vertebra.

ATN *abbr* acute tubular necrosis.

atom *n* the smallest particle of an element capable of existing individually, or in combination with one or more atoms of the same or another element—**atomic** *adj. atomic mass unit (amu) or Dalton* a relative weight used to measure atoms and subatomic particles. Protons and neutrons have both been designated as being 1 amu. *atomic number* the number of protons in the atomic nucleus or the number of electrons, such as hydrogen which, with one of each, has the atomic number 1. *atomic weight (mass)* or *relative atomic mass* the relative average mass of an atom based on the mass of an atom of carbon-12.

atomizer *n* nebulizer.

atonia *n* total flaccidity or no muscle tone caused by complete loss of motor supply to a muscle—**atonic** *adj.*

atopic syndrome a hereditary predisposition to develop hypersensitivity disorders, such as eczema, asthma, hay fever and allergic rhinitis. Associated with excess IgE production.

ATP *abbr* adenosine triphosphate.

atresia *n* imperforation or closure of a normal body opening, duct or canal such as the bowel or bile duct—**atresic, atretic** *adj.*

atrial fibrillation a cardiac arrhythmia. Chaotic irregularity of atrial rhythm with an irregular ventricular response. Commonly associated with mitral stenosis, hyperthyroidism (thyrotoxicosis) or heart failure.

atrial flutter a cardiac arrhythmia caused by irritable focus in atrial muscle and usually associated with coronary heart disease. Speed of atrial beats is between 260 and 340 per minute. The ventricular response is slower and may respond to every four atrial beats.

atrial septal defect a hole in the atrial septum. Most commonly due to a congenital defect. Types include: ostium secundum defect, which is most common and is situated around the site of the foramen ovale; and ostium primum defects situated lower down on the atrial septum.

atrioventricular (A-V) *adj* pertaining to the atria and the ventricles of the heart. Applied to a node, tract and valves. *atrioventricular bundle* also called the bundle of His. Part of the conducting system of the heart. Carries impulses from the atrioventricular node to the ventricles. Divides into right and left bundle branches that transmit the impulses to the apex of each ventricle. *atrioventricular node* part of the conducting system of the heart. Situated at the bottom of the right atrium, it transmits impulses from the sinus node to the atrioventricular bundle.

atrium *n* cavity, entrance or passage. One of the two upper receiving chambers of the heart ⇒ Figure 8—**atria** *pl*, **atrial** *adj*.

atrophic rhinitis (*syn* ozaena) chronic infective condition of the nasal mucous membrane with associated crusting and fetor.

atrophy *n* loss of substance of cells, tissues or organs. There is wasting and a decrease in size and function. The process may be physiological such as that occurring as part of normal ageing, or pathological, as in disuse atrophy when a limb is immobilized—**atrophied, atrophic** *adj*. *progressive muscular atrophy* ⇒ motor neuron disease.

atropine *n* the principal alkaloid of belladonna. ⇒ muscarinic antagonists.

attachment *n* in psychology a term describing the dependent relationship which one individual forms with another, emanating from the unique bonding between infant and parent figure.

attention *n* ability to select some stimuli for closer examination while discarding others considered less salient.

attention deficit hyperactivity disorder (ADHD) term used to describe children who have short attention spans and are easily distracted. They are frequently overactive, may be aggressive, and often have learning difficulties. ⇒ hyperkinetic syndrome.

attenuation *n* the process by which pathogenic micro-organisms are induced to develop or show less virulent characteristics. They can then be used in the preparation of vaccines—**attenuant, attenuated** *adj*, **attenuate** *vt, vi*.

attitudes *npl* reactions to and evaluations of individuals, situations and objects. They may be positive or negative.

attribution *n* in psychology, the theory that deals with the inferences that individuals make regarding the causes of their own and other individuals' behaviour.

atypical *adj* not typical; unusual, irregular; not conforming to type, e.g. atypical pneumonia.

audiogram *n* a graph of the acuity of hearing tested with an audiometer.

audiology *n* the scientific study of hearing—**audiological** *adj*, **audiologically** *adv*.

audiometer *n* an apparatus for the clinical testing of hearing. It generates pure tones over a wide range of pitch and intensity—**audiometric** *adj*, **audiometry** *n*.

audiometrist *n* a person qualified to carry out audiometry.

audit *n* investigative methods used to systematically measure outcomes and review performance. *audit trail* a way of working and record keeping that allows the processes to be transparent and clear. *medical audit* systematic and critical review of medical care, including diagnosis and treatment, outcomes and quality of life.

Audit Commission within the NHS the main role of the Audit Commission is to promote 'best practice' in terms of economy, effectiveness and efficiency.

auditory *adj* pertaining to the sense of hearing. *auditory acuity* ability to hear clearly and distinctly. Tests include the use of tuning fork, whispered voice and audiometer. Hearing can be tested in babies by otoacoustic emission testing (OAE). ⇒ neonatal hearing screening. *auditory area* that portion of the temporal lobe of the cerebral cortex which interprets sound. *external auditory meatus (auditory canal)* the canal between the pinna and eardrum. ⇒ Figure 13. *auditory nerves* the eighth pair of cranial nerves. Also called the vestibulocochlear nerve *auditory ossicles* three small bones—malleus, incus and stapes—located within the middle ear.

augmentation *n* enlargement. Commonly applied to plastic surgical procedures that increase breast size.

aura *n* a premonition; a peculiar sensation or warning of an impending attack, such as occurs in epilepsy or migraine.

aural *adj* pertaining to the ear.

auricle *n* **1** the pinna of the external ear. ⇒ Figure 13. **2** an appendage to the cardiac atrium. **3** obsolete term for atrium—**auricular** *adj*.

auriculoventricular *adj* obsolete term ⇒ atrioventricular.

auriscope ⇒ otoscope.

auscultation *n* a method of listening to the body sounds, particularly the heart, lungs and fetal circulation for diagnostic purposes. It may be: (a) immediate, by placing the ear directly against the body, (b) mediate, by the use of a stethoscope—**auscultatory** *adj*, **auscult**, **auscultate** *v*.

autism *n* a pervasive form of disordered child development characterized by difficulties with social interaction, communication and repetitive stereotyped behaviours.

autistic person a person who has autism.

autoantibody *n* an antibody which binds self-antigen expressed in normal tissue.

autoantigen *n* a self-antigen, expressed in normal tissue, which is the target of autoantibodies or self-reactive T cells.

autoclave 1 *n* an apparatus for high-pressure steam sterilization. **2** *vt* sterilize in an autoclave.

autodigestion *n* self-digestion of body tissue during life. ⇒ autolysis.

autoeroticism *n* self-gratification of the sex instinct. ⇒ masturbation—**autoerotic** *adj*.

autogenic *adj* describes a process or condition that originates from within the organism. *autogenic facilitation* reflex activation of a muscle through activation of its own sensory receptors; self-generated excitation of muscle, e.g. the stretch reflex. *autogenic inhibition* reflex inhibition of a muscle through activation of stretch receptors, the Golgi tendon organs, in its own tendons; self-generated relaxation of muscle that normally prevents build-up of too much, potentially injurious, tension in a muscle. *autogenic therapy* a complementary therapy that employs a combination of self-hypnosis and relaxation.

autograft *n* tissue grafted from one part of the body to another.

autoimmune disease an illness caused by, or associated with, the development of an immune response to normal body tissues.

autoinfection *n* ⇒ infection.

autointoxication *n* poisoning from abnormal or excessive metabolic products produced in the body. Some of which may originate from infected or necrotic tissue.

autologous *adj* when a patient acts as the source of cells. This may include a patient donating blood or blood products prior to elective surgery to be transfused postoperatively. Cross-matching and compatibility problems are avoided, as is the risk of blood-borne infections. *autologous bone marrow transplant* reinfusion of bone marrow cells originating from the recipient. May be performed for patients with leukaemia. Their bone marrow is harvested, stored and replaced after leukaemic cells have been destroyed with cytotoxic chemotherapy or radiotherapy.

autolysis *n* autodigestion which occurs if digestive enzymes escape into surrounding tissues. Occurs as a physiological process, e.g. of the uterus during the puerperium—**autolytic** *adj*.

automated peritoneal dialysis (APD) a type of peritoneal dialysis where the fluid exchanges are performed at night by the use of a mechanical device.

automatic *adj* occurring without the influence of the will; spontaneous; without volition; involuntary acts.

automatism *n* organized behaviour which occurs without subsequent awareness of it. For example somnambulism, hysterical and epileptic states.

autonomic *adj* independent; self-governing. *autonomic nervous system (ANS)* is divided into parasympathetic and sympathetic portions. They are made up of nerve cells and fibres which cannot be controlled at will. They are concerned with the control of glandular secretion and involuntary muscle.

autopsy *n* the examination of a dead body (cadaver) for diagnostic purposes.

autosome *n* in humans one of 44 (22 pairs) of non-sex chromosomes. The full chromosome complement of 46 (23 pairs) found in somatic cells comprises 44 autosomes and 2 sex chromosomes—**autosomal** *adj* relating to autosomes. *autosomal inheritance* is determined by the expression or not of genes on the autosomes. It may be dominant or recessive.

autosuggestion *n* self-suggestion; uncritical acceptance of ideas arising in the individual's own mind. Occurs in hysteria.

avascular *adj* bloodless; not vascular, i.e. without blood supply. *avascular necrosis* death of tissue due to complete depletion of its blood supply. Usually applied to that of bone tissue following injury or possibly through disease. Commonly seen with fractures of the femoral neck, leading to death of the femoral head. Also seen in scaphoid and head of humerus fractures. Often a precursor of osteoarthritis—**avascularity** *n*, **avascularize** *vt*, *vi*.

aversion therapy a method of treatment by deconditioning. Effective in some forms of addiction and abnormal behaviour.

avian *adj* relating to birds. *Avian tuberculosis* is caused by *Mycobacterium avium complex (MAC)* or *M. avium-intracellulare (MAI)*, which also cause atypical tuberculosis in humans, especially in immunocompromised individuals.

avidin *n* a high molecular weight protein with a high affinity for biotin which can interfere with the absorption of biotin. Found in raw egg white.

avitaminosis *n* any disease resulting from a deficiency of vitamins.

avulsion *n* a forcible wrenching away of a structure or part of the body.

axilla *n* the armpit.

axillary *adj* applied to nerves, blood and lymphatic vessels, of the axilla. *axillary artery* ⇒ Figure 9. *axillary vein* ⇒ Figure 10.

axis *n* **1** the second cervical vertebra. **2** an imaginary line passing through the centre; the median line of the body—**axial** *adj*.

axon *n* the long process of a nerve cell conveying impulses away from the cell body—**axonal** *adj*.

axonotmesis *n* (*syn* neuronotmesis, neurotmesis) peripheral degeneration as a result of damage to the axons of a nerve, through pinching, crushing or prolonged pressure. The internal architecture is preserved and recovery depends upon regeneration of the axons, and may take many months.

axon reflex reflex dilatation of the arterioles occurring when sensory nerves in the skin are stimulated by massage manipulations or trauma.

azoospermia *n* sterility of the male through non-production of spermatozoa.

azygos *adj* occurring singly, not paired. *azygos veins* three unpaired veins of the abdomen and thorax which empty into the inferior vena cava—**azygous** *adj*.

B

Babinski's reflex or sign movement of the great toe upwards (dorsiflexion) instead of downwards (plantar flexion) on stroking the sole of the foot. It is indicative of disease or injury to upper motor neurons. Babies exhibit dorsiflexion, but after learning to walk they show the normal plantar flexion response.

bacillaemia *n* the presence of bacilli in the blood—**bacillaemic** *adj*.

bacille Calmette–Guérin ⇒ BCG.

bacilluria *n* the presence of bacilli in the urine—**bacilluric** *adj*.

Bacillus *n* (colloquial term for any rod-shaped micro-organism). A genus of bacteria consisting of aerobic, Gram-positive, rod-shaped cells that produce endospores. The majority have flagella and are motile. The spores are common in soil and dust. *Bacillus anthracis* causes anthrax in humans and domestic animals. *Bacillus cereus* produces exotoxins and causes food poisoning. It can occur after eating cooked food, e.g. rice, that has been stored prior to reheating.

bacteraemia *n* the presence of bacteria in the blood—**bacteraemic** *adj*.

bacteria *n* microscopic unicellular organisms widely distributed in the environment. They may be free-living, sacrophytic or parasitic. Bacteria can be pathogenic to humans, other animals and plants, or non-pathogenic. Pathogens may be virulent and always cause infection, whereas others, known as opportunists, usually only cause infection when the host defences are impaired, such as during cancer chemotherapy. Non-pathogenic bacteria may become pathogenic if they move from their normal site, e.g. intestinal bacteria causing a wound infection. Reproduction is generally by simple binary fission when environmental conditions are suitable. Many bacteria have developed adaptations that allow them to exploit environments and survive unfriendly conditions, e.g. flagella, pili, waxy outer capsules, spore formation and enzymes that destroy antibiotics. Bacteria are classified and identified by features that include: shape and staining characteristics with Gram stain (positive or negative). Bacteria may be: (a) round (cocci), paired (diplococci), in bunches (staphylococci) or in chains (streptococci); (b) rod-shaped (bacilli); or (c) curved or spiral (vibrios, spirilla and spirochaetes)—**bacterium** *sing*.

bacterial *adj* pertaining to bacteria. *bacterial vaginosis* ⇒ vaginosis.

bactericidal *adj* describes agents that kill bacteria, e.g. some antibiotics—**bactericide** *n*, **bactericidally** *adv*.

bactericidin *n* antibody that kills bacteria.

bacteriologist *n* an expert in bacteriology.

bacteriology *n* the scientific study of bacteria—**bacteriological** *adj*, **bacteriologically** *adv*.

bacteriolysin *n* a specific antibody formed in the blood that causes bacteria to break up.

bacteriolysis *n* the disintegration and dissolution of bacteria—**bacteriolytic** *adj*.

bacteriophage *n* a virus parasitic on bacteria. Some of these are used in phagetyping staphylococci, etc.

bacteriostatic *adj* describes an agent that inhibits bacterial growth, e.g. some antibiotics—**bacteriostasis** *n*.

bacteriuria *n* the presence of bacteria in the urine (100 000 or more pathogenic microorganisms per millilitre). Acute cystitis may be preceded by, and active pyelonephritis may be associated with, asymptomatic bacteriuria.

Bainbridge reflex stretch receptors in the heart (right atrium) can increase heart rate through sympathetic stimulation when venous return increases.

baker's itch 1 contact dermatitis resulting from flour or sugar. **2** itchy papules from the bite of the flour mite *Pyemotes*.

BAL *abbr* bronchial alveolar lavage.

balance *n* the ability to maintain body equilibrium by controlling the body's centre of gravity over its base of support.

balance of probabilities the standard of proof required in civil proceedings.

balanced diet a diet that contains the correct amount of all nutrients from a wide range of foods. Should also contain the correct proportions of food types, for example, not too many fatty foods and plenty of fruit and vegetables.

balanitis *n* inflammation of the glans penis. *balanitis xerotica obliterans (BXO)* inflammatory condition involving the glans and prepuce.

balanoposthitis *n* inflammation of the glans penis and prepuce.

balanus *n* the glans of the penis or clitoris.

baldness *n* ⇒ alopecia.

ballistic stretching the use of a rapid stretch or repetitive bouncing motions at the end of the available range of movement to increase soft tissue flexibility.

ballottement *n* testing for a floating object, especially used to diagnose pregnancy—**ballottable** *adj*.

bandage *n* material applied to a wound or used to bind an injured part of the body. May be used to: (a) retain a dressing or splint; (b) support, compress, immobilize; (c) prevent or correct deformity. Available in strips or circular form in a range of different materials and applying varying levels of pressure. Compression bandages are widely used in the management of venous leg ulceration.

Bankart's operation for recurrent dislocation of the shoulder joint: the defect of the glenoid cavity is repaired.

Barbados leg (*syn* elephant leg) ⇒ elephantiasis.

barbiturates *npl* a group of sedative/ hypnotic drugs. They are associated with serious problems of dependence and tolerance, and sudden withdrawal may cause a serious withdrawal syndrome that includes anxiety, convulsions and even death. They have been replaced by safer drugs and their use is limited to anaesthesia and sometimes for epilepsy.

barbotage *n* a method of extending the spread of spinal anaesthesia whereby local anaesthetic is directly mixed with aspirated cerebrospinal fluid and reinjected into the subarachnoid space.

barium enema a radiographic examination of the large bowel using barium sulphate as the contrast medium. Barium sulphate liquid, plus a quantity of air, is introduced into the large bowel by means of a rectal tube, during fluoroscopy. It is used for diagnostic purposes, e.g. for colon cancers, in conjunction with endoscopy. ⇒ barium sulphate, colonoscopy.

barium meal, swallow a radiographic examination of the upper gastrointestinal tract (oesophagus and stomach) and the small intestine with follow-through X-rays, using barium sulphate as the contrast medium. The barium sulphate suspension is swallowed and X-rays are taken of the gastrointestinal tract. Pre-examination fasting is required and medicines, e.g. some antacids, that may interfere with the examination should be stopped. Further fasting may be required until follow-through X-rays are completed.

barium sulphate a heavy insoluble powder used, in an aqueous suspension, as a contrast agent in X-ray visualization of the alimentary tract.

Barlow's test a manoeuvre designed to test for congenitally dislocatable hips in the neonate. Often used in association with the Ortolani test. ⇒ developmental dysplasia of the hip.

baroreceptors *npl* sensory nerve endings which respond to pressure changes. They are present in the cardiac atria, aortic arch, venae cavae, carotid sinus and the internal ear.

barotrauma *n* injury due to unequalized changes in atmospheric or water pressure, e.g. ruptured eardrum.

Barr body ⇒ sex chromatin.

Barrett's oesophagus columnar lined oesophagus replacing normal squamous mucosa. Related to chronic gastric acid reflux. Predisposes to oesophageal cancer.

barrier nursing a method of preventing the spread of infection from an infectious individual to other people. It is achieved by isolation techniques. ⇒ containment isolation, isolation, protective isolation, source isolation.

Bartholin's glands (greater vestibular glands) two small glands situated at each side of the external orifice of the vagina. Their ducts open into the vestibule. They produce lubricating mucus that facilitates coitus.

bartholinitis *n* inflammation of Bartholin's (greater vestibular) glands.

basal ganglia ⇒ basal nuclei.

basal metabolic rate (BMR) the energy consumed at complete rest for essential physiological functions. It is influenced by nutritional status, age, gender, physiological status, disease, certain drugs and ambient temperature. It is determined by measuring the oxygen consumption when the energy output has been reduced to a basal minimum, that is the person is fasting and is physically and mentally at rest, and is expressed per kilogram body weight. In clinical practice it is usually estimated by prediction equations and used to estimate energy requirements.

basal narcosis the preanaesthetic administration of narcotic drugs which reduce fear and anxiety and induce sleep.

basal nuclei a collection of interconnected structures (grey cells) deep within the cerebral hemispheres concerned with cognition, and modifying and coordinating voluntary muscle movement. Their proper functioning requires the release of the neurotransmitter dopamine. Sometimes erroneously referred to as ganglia, which more properly describes structures in the peripheral nervous system. Site of degeneration in Parkinson's disease. ⇒ dopamine.

base *n* **1** the lowest part such as the lung. ⇒ Figure 7. **2** the major part of a compound. **3** an alkali—**basal, basic** *adj*.

baseline measurements in sports medicine the initial physical findings which are usually performed while the athlete is in a healthy state.

basic life support (BLS) a term that describes the application of artificial respiration (usually by mouth-to-mouth breathing) and external cardiac massage to save life without the use of artificial aids or equipment.

basilic *adj* prominent. *basilic vein* on the inner side of the arm (⇒ Figure 10).

basophil *n* **1** a cell which has an affinity for basic dyes. **2** a polymorphonuclear granulocyte (white blood cell) which takes up a particular dye: it is phagocytic and has granules containing heparin and histamine.

basophilia *n* **1** increase in the number of basophils in the blood. **2** basophilic staining of red blood cells.

Batchelor plaster a type of double abduction plaster, with the legs encased from groins to ankles, in full abduction and medial rotation. The feet are then attached to a wooden pole or 'broomstick'. Alternative to frog plaster, but the hips are free. ⇒ developmental dysplasia of the hip.

bath *n* **1** the apparatus used for bathing. **2** the immersion of the body or any part of it in water or any fluid; or the application of spray, jet or vapour of such a fluid to the body. The term is modified according to (a) temperature, e.g. cold, contrast, hot, tepid; (b) medium used, e.g. mud, water, wax; (c) medicament added, e.g. potassium permanganate; (d) function of medicament, e.g. astringent, antiseptic. ⇒ hydrotherapy.

battery *n* legal term. An unlawful touching. Constitutes a trespass against the person. ⇒ assault.

Battle's sign ecchymosis over the mastoid process indicative of a skull fracture.

Bazin's disease (*syn* erythema induratum) a chronic recurrent disorder, involving the skin of the legs of women. There are deep-seated nodules which later ulcerate.

BBA *abbr* born before arrival (at hospital).

BBV *abbr* blood-borne virus.

B cells ⇒ lymphocytes.

BCG *abbr* bacille Calmette–Guérin. An attenuated form of tubercle bacilli: it has lost its power to cause tuberculosis, but retains its antigenic function; it is the base of a vaccine used for immunization against tuberculosis. Also used in urology for the treatment of high risk superficial bladder cancer.

beam *n* metal pole attached to a hospital bed to facilitate the use of traction. For example, a Thomas' splint can be slung up, with pulleys and weights attached, to allow movement and provide counter-balance to the weight of the splint and leg.

bearing-down *n* **1** a pseudonym for the expulsive pains in the second stage of labour. **2** a feeling of weight and descent in the pelvis associated with uterine prolapse or pelvic tumours.

beat *n* pulsation of the blood in the heart and blood vessels. *apex beat* ⇒ apex. *dropped beat* refers to the loss of an occasional ventricular beat as occurs in extrasystoles. *premature beat* an extrasystole.

Beau's lines transverse ridges or grooves which reflect a temporary retardation of the normal nail growth following a debilitating illness. They first appear towards the proximal nail fold and move towards the free edge as the nail grows. The distance the groove has moved indicates quite accurately the length of time since the illness or trauma (nail growth being about 1 mm per week).

becquerel (Bq) *n* the derived SI unit (International System of Units) for radioactivity. Equals the amount of a radioactive substance undergoing one nuclear disintegration per second. Has replaced the curie.

bedbug *n* a blood-sucking insect belonging to the genus *Cimex*. The commonest species are *Cimex lectularius* in temperate zones and *C. hemipterus* in tropical zones. They live and lay eggs in cracks and crevices of furniture and walls. They are active at night and their bites provide a route for secondary infection.

bedsore *n* obsolete term. ⇒ pressure ulcer.

bedwetting *n* ⇒ enuresis.

Beevor's sign movement of the umbilicus as an athlete performs a half sit-up. It indicates an interruption to the nerve supply (innervation) of the abdominal muscles.

behaviour *n* the observable behavioural response of a person to an internal or external stimulus. *behaviour modification* in a general sense, an inevitable part of living, resulting from the consistent rewarding or punishing of response to a stimulus, whether that response is negative or positive. Some education systems deliberately employ a modification approach to maximize learning. *behaviour therapy* a kind of psychotherapy to modify observable, maladjusted patterns of behaviour by the substitution of a learned response or set of responses to a stimulus. The treatment is designed for a particular patient and not for the particular diagnostic label which has been attached to that patient. Such treatment includes assertiveness training, aversion therapy, conditioning and desensitization.

behaviour change psychological concept generally applied to lifestyle in relation to health. An approach used in health education, whereby individuals are encouraged to make lifestyle changes by providing information, looking at existing health beliefs and values and increasing self-confidence. The change may be the adoption of health-protective behaviour (e.g. healthy eating, regular exercise) or changing health-threatening behaviour (e.g. excessive alcohol intake, smoking).

behaviourism *n* in psychology describes an approach which studies and interprets behaviour by objective observation of that behaviour without regard to any subjective mental processes such as ideas, emotions and will. Behaviour is considered to be a series of conditioned reflexes.

Behçet syndrome a form of systemic vasculitis. There is stomatitis, genital ulceration and uveitis. There may also be skin nodules, thrombophlebitis and arthritis of one or more of the large joints. Gastrointestinal and neurological complications may occur. The syndrome is associated with the presence of a certain HLA. Treatment is with NSAIDs, corticosteroids and immunosuppressant drugs.

bejel *n* a non-venereal form of syphilis mainly affecting children in the Middle East and sub-Saharan Africa. The causative organism is *Treponema pallidum*. It usually starts in the mouth and affects mucosae, skin and bones. ⇒ pinta, yaws.

beliefs *npl* a set of ideas and thoughts that a person uses to construct attitudes, views and behaviour. They are formed by culture, family, experiences and many other factors.

belladonna *n* deadly nightshade. The poisonous alkaloid (*Atropa belladonna*) contains atropine and other muscarinic antagonists.

'belle indifference' the incongruous lack of appropriate affect in the presence of incapacitating symptoms commonly shown by patients with dissociative disorders.

Bell's palsy usually non-permanent facial hemiparesis due to idiopathic (cause unknown) lesion of the seventh (facial) cranial nerve.

Bence Jones protein protein that is excreted in the urine of some patients with multiple myeloma, composed of fragments of immunoglobulin molecules.

benchmarking *n* part of quality assurance. Involves the identification of examples of best practice from others engaged in similar practice. From this, best practice benchmark scores in agreed areas of care are identified, against which individual units can compare their own performance.

bends *npl* (*syn* caisson disease) ⇒ decompression illness.

beneficence *n* the principle of doing good that also includes avoiding, removing and preventing harm and promoting good. Ethical dilemmas and problems may arise when the common good is at odds with that for individuals. ⇒ non-maleficence.

benign *adj* **1** non-malignant (of a growth), non-invasive (no capacity to metastasize), non-cancerous (of a growth). **2** describes a condition or illness which is not serious and does not usually have harmful consequences. *benign myalgic encephalomyelitis (BME)* a flu-like illness with varied symptoms including dizziness, muscle fatigue and spasm, headaches and other neurological pain. A high percentage of BME sufferers have a higher level of coxsackie B antibodies in their blood than the rest of the population.

benign hypotonia describes infants who are initially floppy but otherwise healthy. Improvement occurs and the infant regains normal tone and motor development.

benign intracranial hypertension (BIH) a condition in which there is raised intracranial pressure with papilloedema and which can lead to the loss of vision, typically in young, obese women. Often associated with thrombosis in the sagittal sinus.

Bennett's fracture fracture of proximal end of first metacarpal involving the articular surface.

benzene *n* a colourless inflammable liquid obtained from coal tar. Extensively used as a solvent. Continued occupational exposure to it results in aplastic anaemia and, rarely, leukaemia.

benzodiazepines *npl* a group of anxiolytic/hypnotic drugs. Dependence and withdrawal problems may occur. They may be misused. ⇒ Appendix 5.

benzoic acid an antiseptic and antifungal agent used sometimes in an ointment for ringworm.

benzoin *n* (*syn* Friar's balsam) a resin of balsam used traditionally in inhalations but of doubtful value.

bereavement *n* a response to a life event involving loss. Includes that which happens to a person after the death of another person who has been important in his or her life. It also occurs in other situations of loss, such as redundancy, loss of home, divorce or loss of a body part, e.g. mastectomy, amputation. ⇒ grieving process.

beri-beri *n* a deficiency disease caused by lack of vitamin B_1 (thiamin). It occurs mainly in those countries where the staple diet is polished rice. Beri-beri is usually described as either 'wet' (cardiac) or 'dry' (neurological) depending on the symptoms. The symptoms are pain from neuritis, paralysis, muscular wasting, progressive oedema, mental deterioration and, finally, heart failure.

berylliosis *n* an industrial disease: there is impaired lung function because of interstitial fibrosis from inhalation of beryllium. Corticosteroids are used in treatment.

beta (β)-adrenoceptor agonists (*syn* beta stimulants, sympathomimetics) a group of drugs that stimulate β-adrenoceptors. ⇒ Appendix 5.

beta (β)-adrenoceptor antagonists (*syn* beta blockers) a group of drugs that block the stimulation of β-adrenoceptors in the myocardium and other locations. ⇒ Appendix 5.

beta blockers *npl* ⇒ beta (β)-adrenoceptor antagonists.

beta (β)-lactam antibiotics antibiotics containing a β-lactam ring in their structure. They include the cephalosporins and penicillins. Many bacteria produce enzymes (β-lactamases) that destroy the β-lactam ring, which renders the antibiotic ineffective.

beta (β)-lactamases previously known as penicillinases. The enzymes, produced by certain bacteria, e.g. most staphylococci and *Escherichia coli*, that destroy β-lactam antibiotics.

beta (β) oxidation metabolic process whereby fatty acids are converted to acetyl CoA prior to the production of energy (ATP).

beta (β) phase the period after the alpha redistribution phase of drug administration. There is a slow decrease in drug blood levels during its metabolism and excretion.

bibliographical databases details of papers, etc., but sometimes abstracts and full articles, are available electronically via CD-ROM or the internet, e.g. Medline.

bicarbonate *n* also called hydrogen carbonate. A salt of carbonic acid. *serum (plasma) bicarbonate* that in the blood. Represents the alkali reserve.

bicellular *adj* composed of two cells.

biceps *n* two-headed muscle of the upper arm ⇒ Figure 4. *biceps femoris* ⇒ Figure 5.

biconcave *adj* concave or hollow on both surfaces.

biconvex *adj* convex on both surfaces.

bicornuate *adj* having two horns; generally applied to a double uterus or a single uterus possessing two horns.

bicuspid *adj* having two cusps or points. *bicuspid teeth* the premolars. *bicuspid valve* the mitral valve between the left atrium and ventricle of the heart.

BID *abbr* brought in (to hospital) dead.

bifid *adj* divided into two parts. Cleft or forked.

bifurcation *n* division into two branches— bifurcate *adj, vt, vi*.

biguanides *npl* a group of oral hypoglycaemic drugs. ⇒ Appendix 5.

bilateral *adj* pertaining to both sides— bilaterally *adv*.

bile *n* a bitter, alkaline, viscid, greenish-yellow fluid secreted by the liver and stored in the gallbladder. 500–1000 mL is produced each day. It contains water, mucin, lecithin, cholesterol, bile salts, bile acids, the pigments bilirubin and biliverdin and substances for excretion. Bile is needed for the absorption of fat-soluble vitamins, stimulates peristalsis and deodorizes faeces. *bile acids* organic acids; cholic and chenodeoxycholic, present in bile. *bile ducts* the hepatic and cystic, which join to form the common bile duct that empties into the duodenum (⇒ Figure 18b). *bile pigments* ⇒ bilirubin, biliverdin. *bile salts* emulsifying agents, sodium glycocholate and taurocholate. Conjugated bile acids (with taurine and glycine) form these sodium salts—**bilious, biliary** *adj*.

Bilharzia n ⇒ *Schistosoma*.

bilharziasis n ⇒ schistosomiasis.

biliary *adj* pertaining to bile. *biliary colic* pain in the right upper quadrant of abdomen, due to obstruction of the gallbladder or common bile duct, usually by a stone; it may last several hours and is usually steady, which differentiates it from other forms of colic. Vomiting may occur. *biliary fistula* an abnormal track conveying bile to the surface or to some other organ.

bilious *adj* **1** a word usually used to signify vomit containing bile. **2** a non-medical term, usually meaning 'suffering from indigestion'.

bilirubin n a red pigment mostly derived from haemoglobin during red blood cell breakdown. Unconjugated fat-soluble bilirubin, which gives an indirect reaction with Van den Bergh's test, is potentially toxic to metabolically active tissues, particularly the basal nuclei of the immature brain. Unconjugated bile is transported to the blood attached to albumen to make it less likely to enter and damage brain cells. In the liver the enzyme glucuronyl transferase conjugates fat-soluble bilirubin with glucuronic acid to make it water-soluble, in which state it is relatively non-toxic (reacts directly with Van den Bergh's test) and can be excreted in the bile. ⇒ haemolytic disease of the newborn, jaundice, phototherapy.

bilirubinaemia n the presence of bilirubin in the blood. Sometimes used (incorrectly) for an excess of bilirubin in the blood. ⇒ hyperbilirubinaemia.

bilirubinuria n the presence of the bile pigment bilirubin in the urine.

biliverdin n the green pigment formed by oxidation of bilirubin.

Billroth's operation ⇒ gastrectomy.

bilobate *adj* having two lobes.

bilobular *adj* having two little lobes or lobules.

bimanual *adj* performed with both hands. A method of examination sometimes used in gynaecology whereby the internal genital organs are examined between one hand on the abdomen and the other hand or finger within the vagina.

binary fission a method of reproduction common among the bacteria and protozoa. The cell divides into two equal 'daughter' cells.

binaural *adj* pertaining to, or having two ears. Applied to a type of stethoscope.

binge–purge syndrome ⇒ bulimia.

binocular vision the focusing of both eyes on one object at the same time, in such a way that only one image of the object is seen.

binovular *adj* derived from two separate ova. Binovular twins may be of different sexes. ⇒ uniovular *opp*.

bioavailability n the amount of a drug (or nutrient) that enters the circulation in the active form. It is dependent on the route of administration and the degree to which the drug is metabolized before it reaches the bloodstream. Drugs administered intravenously will have 100% bioavailability, whereas those given orally may not be fully absorbed and are subject to first-pass metabolism in the liver. Some drugs are totally metabolized in the liver, so other routes of administration must be used such as sublingually.

biochemistry n the chemistry of life and organic molecules—**biochemical** *adj*.

bioethics n the application of ethical principles to biological problems.

biofeedback n presentation of immediate visual or auditory information about usually unconscious body functions such as blood pressure, heart rate and muscle tension. Either by trial and error or by operant conditioning a person can learn to repeat behaviour which results in a satisfactory level of body functions.

biofilm n collection of micro-organisms and their products that stick to a surface, e.g. a urinary catheter.

bioflavonoids *npl* a large group of coloured substances that occur naturally in many vegetables and fruit (e.g. tomatoes, broccoli, cherries, plums, etc.). Bioflavonoids are also present in tea and wine. Many are antibacterial and some may offer protection against heart disease and cancer.

biohazard n anything that presents a hazard to life. Some specimens for the pathological laboratory are so labelled.

biological engineering designing micro-electronic or mechanical equipment for external use by patients: for attachment to patients, or placement inside patients.

biological response modifier (BRM) cancer treatment that manipulates the patient's immune response in order to destroy cancer cells. They include colony stimulating factors, interleukins and interferons.

biology *n* the science of life, concerned with the structure, function and organization of all living organisms—**biological** *adj*, **biologically** *adv*.

biomechanics *n* the study of the structure and function of biological systems relative to the methods of mechanics.

biopsy *n* excision of tissue to provide a sample for microscopic examination to establish a precise diagnosis.

biopsychosocial *adj* relating to biological, psychological and social perspectives.

biorhythm *n* the cyclical patterns of biological functions unique to each person, e.g. sleep–wake cycles, body temperature, etc.—**biorhythmic** *adj*.

biosensors *npl* non-invasive devices that measure the result of biological processes, e.g. skin temperature or blood oxygen saturation.

biotechnology *n* the use of biology in the scientific study of technology and vice versa—**biotechnical** *adj*, **biotechnically** *adv*.

biotin *n* a member of vitamin B complex. Dietary sources are liver, soya flour, egg yolk, cereals and yeast. It is synthesized by colonic bacteria. Deficiency is rare in humans; symptoms include fatigue, anorexia, muscle pains and dermatitis.

BIPAP *abbr* biphasic positive airways pressure.

biparous *adj* producing two offspring at one birth.

biphasic positive airways pressure (BIPAP) mode of ventilatory (respiratory) support in which the airway pressure alternates between two levels. The higher pressure ventilates the patient or provides pressure support, whilst the lower pressure acts as positive end expiratory pressure/continuous positive airway pressure. Can be delivered non-invasively (without intubation) by mask to patients with chronic lung disease or as an aid to weaning from ventilatory support.

bipolar *adj* having two poles.

bipolar affective disorder (*syn* manic-depressive illness) repeated episodes of mood disturbance with mania/hypomania and depression.

birth *n* the act of expelling the young from the mother's body; delivery; being born. *birth canal* the cavity or canal of the pelvis through which the baby passes during labour. *birth certificate* in the UK a legal document given on registration, within 42 days of a birth. *birth control* prevention or regulation of conception by any means; contraception. *birth injury* any injury occurring during parturition, e.g. fracture of a bone, subluxation of a joint, injury to peripheral nerve, intracranial haemorrhage. *birth mark* naevus. *premature birth* one occurring between 24 and 37 weeks of pregnancy.

bisexual *adj* **1** having some of the physical genital characteristics of both sexes; a hermaphrodite. When there is gonadal tissue of both sexes in the same person, that person is a true hermaphrodite. **2** describes a person who is sexually attracted to both men and women.

Bishop's score an assessment of the cervix used in induction of labour. The score is made up of the sum of individual scores of 0, 1 or 2 assigned for cervical length, consistency, dilatation and position along with a score for the station of the presenting part. A score of 4 or less suggests that induction may be difficult.

bisphosphonates *npl* drugs that reduce bone turnover. Used in the management of bone diseases and the hypercalcaemia associated with cancer. ⇒ Appendix 5.

Bitot's spots (*syn* xerosis conjunctivae) localized area of thickened, keratinized epithelium, with micro-organisms, at the limbus of the cornea. A manifestation of vitamin A deficiency.

bivalve *adj* having two blades such as in the vaginal speculum. In orthopaedics, the division of a plaster of Paris splint into two portions—an anterior and posterior half.

bivariate statistics descriptive statistics that compare the relationship between two variables, such as correlations. Can be used to decide whether multivariate statistics are needed.

blackhead *n* ⇒ comedone.

blackwater fever a serious complication of some forms of malaria where there is red blood cell haemolysis. The resultant haemoglobinuria causes dark coloured urine, jaundice and renal failure.

bladder *n* a membranous sac containing fluid or gas. A hollow organ for receiving fluid. ⇒ gallbladder, urinary bladder.

bladder outflow obstruction pathophysiological obstruction to the lower urinary tract commonly due to benign prostatic hyperplasia in older males.

Blalock–Taussig procedure a temporary measure to improve pulmonary blood flow in congenital heart abnormalities, such as tetralogy of Fallot. A shunt is constructed by anastomosing the subclavian artery to the pulmonary artery to divert blood from the systemic circulation to the lungs.

blastocyst (blastula) *n* stage in early embryonic development that follows the morula, which becomes cystic and enfolds. Comprises a fluid-filled cavity and inner cell mass surrounded by trophoblast cells. ⇒ gastrula.

blastoderm *n* a cell layer of the blastocyst. Eventually becomes the three primary germ layers, ectoderm, endoderm and mesoderm, from which the embryo will form.

Blastomyces *n* a genus of pathogenic fungi—**blastomycetic** *adj.*

blastomycosis *n* granulomatous condition caused by *Blastomyces dermatitidis*; infection starts in the lungs and lymph nodes. May affect the skin, viscera, bones and joints—**blastomycotic** *adj.*

blastula *n* ⇒ blastocyst.

bleb *n* a large blister. ⇒ bulla, vesicle.

'bleeding time' the time required for the spontaneous arrest of bleeding from a skin puncture: under controlled conditions this forms a clinical test.

blepharitis *n* inflammation of the eyelids, particularly the lid margins—**blepharitic** *adj.*

blepharon *n* the eyelid; palpebra—**blephara** *pl.*

blepharoplasty *n* plastic surgery of the eyelid. An operation in which excess skin is removed from the eyelid.

blepharospasm *n* spasm of the muscles in the eyelid. Excessive winking. A condition in which there is involuntary shutting of the eye, which can occur in isolation or be due either to local irritative lesions in the eye or to a movement disorder.

blind loop syndrome a condition resulting from stasis in the small intestine leading to bacterial growth, thus producing diarrhoea and malabsorption (e.g. due to surgical anastomosis or dysmotility).

blind spot the spot at which the optic nerve leaves the retina. Without any cones or rods it is insensitive to light.

blister *n* an elevated lesion of the skin containing fluid, usually serum. ⇒ bulla.

blood *n* the red viscid fluid filling the heart and blood vessels. It consists of a colourless fluid, plasma, in which are suspended the red blood cells (erythrocytes), the white cells (leucocytes), and the platelets (thrombocytes). The plasma contains a great many substances in solution including factors which enable the blood to clot.

blood bank the area or department of a hospital responsible for the selection and storage of blood for later transfusion to patients.

blood-borne viruses (BBV) viruses transmitted via blood to cause infection. Include: HIV and several hepatitis viruses.

blood–brain barrier (BBB) the protective arrangement that prevents many substances crossing from the blood to the brain. It consists of capillary endothelial cells and astrocytes that ensure that the capillary wall is relatively impermeable. The barrier allows the passage of nutrients and metabolic waste. However, some drugs, alcohol and other toxic substances, e.g. lead in young children, can pass from the blood through this barrier to the cerebrospinal fluid.

blood coagulation ⇒ coagulation.

blood count calculation of the number of red or white cells per cubic millimetre of blood, using a haemocytometer. *differential blood count* the estimation of the relative proportions of the different leucocyte cells in the blood. The normal differential count is: polymorphonuclear 65–70%, lymphocytes 20–25%, monocytes 5%, eosinophils 0–3%, basophils 0–0.5%. In childhood the proportion of lymphocytes is higher.

blood culture a sample of venous blood is incubated in a suitable medium at an optimum temperature, so that any microorganisms can multiply and so be isolated and identified microscopically. ⇒ septicaemia.

blood doping a prohibited ergogenic aid, which is used illicitly by some athletes to increase aerobic performance. It involves the removal and subsequent reinfusion of blood, which in the short term increases the number of red blood cells and hence the oxygen-carrying capacity of the blood.

blood film the result of spreading a droplet of blood very thinly on a microscope slide. The blood can then be stained with dyes and examined for abnormalities under a microscope.

blood formation haemopoiesis.

blood gases ⇒ arterial blood gases.

blood glucose profiles ⇒ continuous glucose monitoring (CGM), self-monitoring blood glucose (SMBG).

blood groups ABO system. There are four groups, A, B, AB and O. The red cells of these groups contain the corresponding antigens (agglutinogens): group A has A; group B has B; group AB has both antigens; and group O has neither. In the plasma there are antibodies (agglutinins) which will cause agglutination (clumping) of any cell carrying the corresponding antigen. Group A plasma contains anti-B; group B plasma contains anti-A; group O plasma contains both anti-A and anti-B; and group AB plasma contains no agglutinins. This grouping is determined by (a) testing a suspension of red cells with anti-A and anti-B serum or (b) testing serum with known cells. Transfusion with an incompatible ABO group will cause a severe haemolytic reaction and death may occur unless the transfusion is promptly stopped. For most transfusion purposes, group A can receive groups A and O; group B can receive groups B and O; group AB can have blood of any group; and group O can only have group O. The terms universal donor and recipient are outdated and confusing because many other blood groups exist. *Rhesus blood group* a further three pairs of antigens coded for by genes designated the letters Cc, Dd and Ee are present on the red cells. The letters denote allelomorphic genes which are present in all cells except the gametes where a chromosome can carry C or c, but not both. In this way the Rhesus genes and blood groups are derived equally from each parent. When the cells contain only the cde

groups, then the blood is Rhesus negative (Rh−); when the cells contain C, D or E singly or in combination with cde, then the blood is Rhesus positive (Rh+). For general purposes, only the Dd antigens are of clinical significance. About 85% of the Caucasian population have the D antigen. In contrast to the ABO system, there are no preformed antibodies to the D antigen but these groups are antigenic and can, under suitable conditions, produce the corresponding antibody in the serum. Antibodies are formed if there is (a) transfusion of Rhesus positive blood to a Rhesus negative person, (b) immunization during pregnancy by Rhesus positive fetal red cells, with the D antigen, entering the maternal circulation where the women is Rhesus negative. This can cause haemolytic disease of the newborn (erythroblastosis fetalis). ⇒ anti-D, Rhesus incompatibility.

blood-letting venesection.

blood plasma ⇒ plasma.

blood pressure the pressure exerted by the blood on the blood vessel walls. Usually refers to the pressure within the arteries, which may be measured in millimetres of mercury (mmHg) using a sphygmomanometer. The arterial blood pressure fluctuates with each heart beat, having a maximum value (the systolic pressure) which is related to the ejection of blood from the heart into the arteries and a minimum value (diastolic pressure) when the aortic and pulmonary valves are closed and the heart is relaxed. Usually values for both systolic and diastolic pressures are recorded (e.g. 120/70). Arterial blood pressure may also be recorded directly using an arterial pressure transducer. ⇒ hypertension, hypotension, Korotkoff sounds.

blood sugar the amount of glucose in the blood; varies within the normal range. It is regulated by hormones, e.g. insulin. ⇒ hyperglycaemia, hypoglycaemia.

blood transfusion ⇒ transfusion.

blood urea the amount of urea (the end product of protein metabolism) in the blood; varies within the normal range. This is virtually unaffected by the amount of protein in the diet when the kidneys, which are the main organs of urea excretion, are functioning normally.

When they are diseased the blood urea quickly rises. ⇒ uraemia.

blow-out fracture fracture of the orbital wall due to blunt trauma.

BLS *abbr* basic life support.

'blue baby' cyanotic appearance at birth, often attributed to congenital cyanotic heart defects.

blue pus bluish/green discharge from a wound infected with *Pseudomonas aeruginosa*.

BME *abbr* benign myalgic encephalomyelitis.

BMI *abbr* body mass index.

BMR *abbr* basal metabolic rate.

BMT *abbr* bone marrow transplantation/transplant.

BNF *abbr* British National Formulary. ⇒ formulary.

Boari flap method of extending one side of the bladder to compensate for a shortened/pathological distal ureter.

Bobath concept the concept of treatment of abnormal muscle tone and movement disorder, seen in children with cerebral palsy and adults after a stroke, and now widely applied to similar dysfunction caused by multiple sclerosis and other neurological conditions.

body image the image present in an individual's mind of his or her own body. Distortions of this occur in anorexia nervosa. ⇒ mutilation.

body language non-verbal symbols that express a person's current physical, emotional and mental state. They include body movements, postures, gestures, facial expressions, spatial positions, clothes and other bodily adornments.

body mass index (BMI) used as an index of adiposity. It is calculated by dividing an individual's weight (kg) by their height (m) squared. Separate charts are available for adults and children, adult charts should not be used for children. The WHO (1998) classification for BMI is: less than 18.5 underweight, 18.6–24.9 normal weight, 25–29.9 pre-obese, 30–34.9 obese class 1, 35–39.9 obese class 2 and greater than 40 obese class 3.

body temperature the balance between heat produced and heat lost in the body. It is maintained around 37°C throughout the 24 h, but varies between 0.5 and 1.0°C during that period. Most heat is produced by metabolism, voluntary and involuntary muscular activities, and heat loss occurs through convection, conduction and evaporation of sweat; small amounts are lost during expiration, urination and defecation. *core body temperature* that in the organs of the central cavities of the body (cranium, thorax and abdomen). *shell body temperature* that outside the body core. Varies between sites, e.g. 35°C at the forehead and 20°C in the feet.

Boeck's disease a form of sarcoidosis.

Bohn's nodules tiny white nodules on the palate of the newly born.

boil *n* (*syn* furuncle) an acute inflammatory condition, surrounding a hair follicle; often caused by *Staphylococcus aureus*. Usually attended by suppuration; it has one opening for drainage in contrast to a carbuncle.

Bolam test the test laid down in the case of Bolam v. Friern HMC on the standard of care expected of a professional in cases of alleged negligence.

bolus *n* **1** a soft, pulpy mass of masticated food. **2** a large dose of a drug given at the beginning of a treatment regimen to raise the blood concentration rapidly to a therapeutic level.

bonding *n* the emotional tie one person forms with another, making an enduring and special emotional relationship. There is a fundamental biological need for this to occur between an infant and its parents, particularly the mother. When newborn babies are cared for in an intensive care setting, special arrangements have to be made to encourage bonding between the parents and their new baby.

bone *n* connective tissue in which salts, such as calcium carbonate and calcium phosphate, are deposited in an organic matrix to make it hard and dense. Bone tissue is of two types, hard dense compact bone and spongy cancellous bone. The separate bones make up the skeleton.

bone density a description of bone mass. It is decreased in osteoporosis. ⇒ peak bone density.

bone graft the transplantation of a piece of bone from one part of the body to another, or from one person to another. Used to repair bone defects or to supply osteogenic tissue.

bone marrow the substance contained within bone cavities. At birth the cavities are filled with blood-forming *red marrow* but later in life, deposition of fat in the long bones converts the red into *yellow bone marrow*. *bone marrow biopsy (sampling)* an investigation of blood cell production whereby a sample of marrow is obtained by aspiration or trephine. Usually the site used is the iliac crest or sometimes the sternum. *bone marrow transplantation (BMT)* (*syn* stem cell transplant) the infusion of bone marrow into a patient's vein. The bone marrow may be obtained either on an earlier occasion from the patient (autologous transplantation) or from a suitable donor (allogeneic transplantation). Usually follows myeloablative doses of chemotherapy or radiotherapy as therapy for (most commonly) haematological cancers although also used therapeutically and experimentally for some solid tumours.

Bonnevie–Ullrich syndrome ⇒ Noonan syndrome.

borborygmi *n* rumbling noises caused by the movement of gas in the intestines.

Bordetella n a genus of Brucellaceae bacteria. *B. pertussis* causes whooping cough (pertussis).

Bornholm disease (*syn* epidemic myalgia) an epidemic pleurodynia usually associated with B group of coxsackie viruses. 2–14 days incubation. There is sudden onset of severe pain in lower chest and/or abdominal and/or lumbar muscles. Breathing may be difficult, because of the pain, and fever is common. May last up to one week. There is no specific treatment.

Borrelia a genus of spirochaetes. Lyme disease is caused by the bacterium *Borrelia burgdorferi*.

botulism *n* an intoxication with the preformed exotoxin of *Clostridium botulinum*. Vomiting, respiratory, ocular and pharyngeal paralysis occur within 24–72 h of eating food contaminated with the spores, which require anaerobic conditions to produce the toxin. Associated with home preserving of vegetables and meat and improperly treated tinned food.

bougie *n* a cylindrical instrument made of gum elastic, metal or other material. Used in varying sizes for dilating strictures, e.g. oesophageal or urethral.

bovine *adj* relating to the cow or ox. *bovine spongiform encephalopathy (BSE)* a fatal, infective (prion) neurological disease of cattle. ⇒ Creutzfeldt–Jakob disease. *bovine tuberculosis* ⇒ tuberculosis.

bowel *n* the large intestine. ⇒ intestine.

bowleg *n* varum genu.

bowler's finger in sports medicine a colloquial term used to describe compression of the digital nerve on the medial aspect of the thumb leading to paraesthesia of the thumb.

boxer's fracture in sports medicine a colloquial term used to describe a fracture of the fifth metacarpal bone secondary to a compressive force when the head of the metacarpal rotates over the neck leading to a flexion deformity.

Boyle's anaesthetic machine apparatus for delivering anaesthetic agents mixed with oxygen and nitrous oxide or air. ⇒ pin index.

brachial *adj* pertaining to the arm. Applied to vessels in this region and a nerve plexus at the root of the neck. *brachial artery* ⇒ Figure 9. *brachial vein* ⇒ Figure 10.

brachialis *n* a muscle of the upper arm. ⇒ Figure 4.

brachiocephalic *adj* pertaining to the arm and head. *brachiocephalic (innominate) artery* large artery branching from the aortic arch which forms the right common carotid and right subclavian arteries. ⇒ Figure 9. *brachiocephalic (innominate) veins* two large veins derived from the internal jugular and subclavian veins. Convey blood to the heart via the superior vena cava. ⇒ Figure 10.

brachioradialis *n* a muscle of the forearm. ⇒ Figure 4.

brachium *n* the arm (especially from shoulder to elbow), or any arm-like appendage—**brachia** *pl*, **brachial** *adj*.

brachytherapy *n* radiotherapy delivered from a small radioactive source or sources which are implanted in or close to the tumour. The technique may be used to treat cancers of the anus, breast, cervix, lung, oesophagus and the tongue.

Bradford frame a stretcher type of bed used for: (a) immobilizing the spine; (b) resting trunk and back muscles; (c) preventing deformity. It is a tubular steel frame fitted with two canvas slings allowing a

100–150 mm gap to facilitate personal care and elimination.

bradycardia *n* slow rate of heart contraction, resulting in a pulse rate less than 60 beats per minute.

bradykinesia abnormally slow or retarded movement associated with difficulty initiating and then stopping a movement; typically seen in Parkinson's disease.

brain *n* the encephalon; the largest part of the central nervous system: it is contained in the cranial cavity and is surrounded by three membranes called meninges. It comprises the cerebral hemispheres, brainstem (midbrain, pons varolii and medulla oblongata) and the cerebellum. The brainstem connects the cerebral hemispheres to the cerebellum and the spinal cord. The cerebrospinal fluid inside the brain is contained in the ventricles, and outside in the subarachnoid space acts as a shock absorber to the delicate nerve tissue. ⇒ Figure 1. *brain death* a situation where the brainstem is fatally and irreversibly damaged. The brainstem is responsible for maintaining vital functions including breathing. Strict criteria must be met before the patient is declared dead. These include testing certain reflexes, e.g. gag and pupillary, and the absence of factors that could depress brainstem activity. Suitable patients may become organ donors if this coincides with the wishes of the family and those of the patient if known. ⇒ death.

bran *n* the husk of grain. The coarse outer part of cereals, especially wheat, high in non-starch polysaccharide (NSP) and the vitamin B complex.

branchial *adj* relating to the gills. Embryonic clefts or fissures either side of the neck from which the nose, ears and mouth will eventually develop. *branchial cyst* a cyst in the neck resulting from a developmental abnormality of the branchial clefts.

Braun's frame a metal frame, bandaged for use, and equally useful for drying a lower leg plaster and for applying skeletal traction (Steinmann's pin or Kirschner wire inserted through the calcaneus) to a fractured tibia, after reduction.

break-bone fever ⇒ dengue.

break test an isometric contraction against manual resistance (provided by the examiner) with the joint in its mid-range position; used to determine the athlete's ability to generate a static force within a muscle or muscle group.

breast *n* **1** the anterior upper part of the thorax. **2** the mammary gland. *breast bone* the sternum.

breech *n* the buttocks. ⇒ buttock.

breech/birth presentation refers to the position of a baby in the uterus such that the buttocks would be born first: the normal position is head first.

bregma *n* the anterior fontanelle. ⇒ fontanelle.

bridge *n* in dentistry, restoration to replace one or more teeth using artificial crowns connected to natural teeth.

British sign language (BSL) a type of sign language (signing) used in the UK.

broad ligaments lateral ligaments; double fold of parietal peritoneum which hangs over the uterus and outstretched uterine (fallopian) tubes, forming a lateral partition across the pelvic cavity. ⇒ Figure 17.

broad thumb syndrome Rubinstein–Taybi syndrome.

Broca's area the motor speech area, situated in the dominant cerebral hemisphere (usually the left). Injury to this centre can result in an inability to speak.

Brodie's abscess chronic abscess in bone.

bromidrosis *n* a profuse, fetid perspiration, especially associated with the feet—**bromidrotic** *adj*.

bromism *n* chronic poisoning due to continued or excessive use of bromides.

bronchi *npl* the two tubes into which the trachea divides at its lower end. ⇒ Figures 6, 7—**bronchus** *sing*.

bronchial *adj* pertaining to the bronchi. *bronchial alveolar lavage (BAL)* irrigation of the lungs with small volumes of saline which are then aspirated and examined for infection; occasionally large volume lavage may be therapeutic. *bronchial cancer* ⇒ non-small cell carcinoma, oat cell carcinoma. *bronchial tree* network of bronchi as they subdivide within the lungs.

bronchial asthma ⇒ asthma.

bronchiectasis *n* abnormal dilatation of the bronchi which, when localized, is usually the result of pneumonia or lobar collapse in childhood, but when generalized is due to some inherent disorder of the bronchial mucous membrane as in cystic fibrosis.

Characterized by recurrent respiratory infections with profuse purulent sputum and digital clubbing. Eventually leads to respiratory failure. Mainstay of treatment is prompt treatment with appropriate antibiotics and regular physiotherapy to optimize sputum clearance—**bronchiectatic** *adj*.

bronchiole *n* one of the minute subdivisions of the bronchi which terminate in the alveoli (air sacs) of the lungs—**bronchiolar** *adj*.

bronchiolitis *n* inflammation of the bronchioles, usually due to viral infection in children in the first year of life—**bronchiolitic** *adj*.

bronchiolitis obliterans syndrome (BOS) progressive scarring and loss of function seen in the lungs, in part as a result of chronic rejection of a transplanted lung over time.

bronchitis *n* inflammation of the bronchi *acute bronchitis* as an isolated incident is usually a primary viral infection occurring in children as a complication of the common cold, influenza, whooping cough, measles or rubella. Secondary infection occurs with bacteria, commonly *Streptococcus pneumoniae* or *Haemophilus influenzae*. Acute bronchitis in adults is usually an acute exacerbation of chronic bronchitis precipitated by a viral infection but sometimes by a sudden increase in atmospheric pollution. *chronic bronchitis* is defined as a cough productive of sputum for at least three consecutive months in two consecutive years. The bronchial mucus-secreting glands are hypertrophied with an increase in goblet cells and loss of ciliated cells due to irritation from tobacco smoke, or atmospheric pollutants. ⇒ chronic obstructive pulmonary disease (COPD), pulmonary emphysema—**bronchitic** *adj*.

bronchoconstrictor *n* any agent which constricts the bronchi.

bronchodilator *n* any agent which dilates the bronchi. ⇒ beta (β)-adrenoceptor agonists, muscarinic antagonists. ⇒ Appendix 5.

bronchogenic *adj* arising from one of the bronchi.

bronchography *n* obsolete radiological demonstration of the bronchial tree.

bronchomycosis *n* general term describing a variety of fungal infections of the bronchi and lungs, e.g. pulmonary candidiasis—**bronchomycotic** *adj*.

bronchophony *n* abnormal transmission of voice sounds heard over consolidated lung or over a thin layer of pleural fluid.

bronchopleural fistula pathological communication between the pleural cavity and one of the bronchi.

bronchopneumonia *n* describes a type of pneumonia in which areas of consolidation are distributed widely around bronchi and not in a lobar pattern. Generally affects patients at the extremes of age, those who are debilitated or secondary to existing condition—**bronchopneumonic** *adj*.

bronchopulmonary *adj* pertaining to the bronchi and the lungs—**bronchopulmonic** *adj*.

bronchorrhoea *n* an excessive discharge of mucus from the bronchial mucosa—**bronchorrhoeal** *adj*.

bronchoscope *n* an endoscope used for examining and taking biopsies from the interior of the bronchi. Also used for removal of inhaled foreign bodies. Bronchoscopes are either flexible fibreoptic instruments or rigid tubes—**bronchoscopic** *adj*, **bronchoscopically** *adv*.

bronchoscopy *n* endoscopic examination of the tracheobronchial tree.

bronchospasm *n* sudden constriction of the bronchial tubes due to contraction of involuntary smooth muscle in their walls—**bronchospastic** *adj*.

bronchostenosis *n* narrowing of one of the bronchi—**bronchostenotic** *adj*.

bronchotracheal *adj* pertaining to the bronchi and trachea.

bronchus *n* ⇒ bronchi.

brought in dead (BID) describes a situation where the person has died prior to arriving at the hospital.

brow *n* the forehead; the region above the supraorbital ridge.

brown fat present in infant tissue. Enzymes allow the rapid production of energy and heat—a form of non-shivering thermogenesis.

Brucella *n* a genus of bacteria causing brucellosis (undulant fever in humans; contagious abortion in cattle). *Brucella abortus* is the bovine strain. *Brucella* *melitensis* the sheep/goat strain, both transmissible via infected milk.

brucellosis *n* (*syn* melitensis) a generalized infection in humans resulting from one of the species of *Brucella*: *B. abortus* in cattle, *B. suis* in pigs and *B. melitensis* in sheep and goats. It is transmitted by contaminated milk or contact with the carcass of an infected animal. High risk groups include farmers, abattoir workers and veterinary surgeons. There are recurrent attacks of continuous or undulating fever and mental depression. It may last for months with relapses. The condition is also known as 'Malta fever', 'abortus fever', 'Mediterranean fever' and 'undulant fever'.

Brudzinski's sign immediate flexion of knees and hips on raising head from pillow. Seen in meningitis.

bruise *n* (*syn* contusion, ecchymosis) a discoloration of the skin due to an extravasation of blood into the underlying tissues; there is no break of the skin.

bruit *n* ⇒ murmur.

bruxism *n* abnormal grinding of teeth, often producing attrition.

Bryant's 'gallows' traction skin traction applied to the lower limbs; the legs are then suspended vertically (from an overhead beam), so that the buttocks are lifted just clear of the bed. Used for fractures of the femur in children up to 4 years. Now largely replaced with hoop traction.

BSE *abbr* **1** bovine spongiform encephalopathy. **2** breast self-examination.

bubo *n* enlargement of lymph nodes, especially in the groin. A feature of chancroid, lymphogranuloma venereum and bubonic plague—**bubonic** *adj*.

bubonic plague ⇒ plague.

buccal *adj* relating to the cheek or mouth.

bucket handle tear a description given to a type of tear of the meniscus of the knee joint that extends along the length of the meniscus.

Buerger's disease (*syn* thromboangiitis obliterans) a chronic obliterative vascular disease of peripheral vessels that results in ischaemia, intermittent claudication, skin changes and gangrene. The incidence is associated with the presence of HLA-A9 and HLA-B5. It affects young and middle-aged men. *Buerger's exercises* were designed to treat this condition. The legs

are placed alternately in elevation and dependence to assist perfusion of the extremities with blood.

buffer *n* **1** substances that limit pH change by their ability to accept or donate hydrogen ions as appropriate. In biological systems they limit pH changes that would inhibit cell functioning. The important buffer systems in the body include: bicarbonate (hydrogen carbonate) system, hydrogen phosphates and proteins, e.g. haemoglobin. **2** any agent that reduces shock or jarring due to contact.

bulbar *adj* pertaining to the medulla oblongata. *bulbar palsy or paralysis* paralysis which involves the labioglossopharyngeal (lips, tongue and pharynx) region and results from degeneration of the motor nuclei in the medulla oblongata. There are problems with swallowing and speech. Individuals are at risk of inhaling fluids and food, with the development of pneumonia.

bulbourethral (Cowper's) glands two mucus-secreting glands which open into the bulb of the male urethra. Their secretion is part of seminal fluid.

bulimia *n* an eating disorder involving repeated uncontrolled consumption of large quantities of food. Many anorectics have a history of such episodes. *bulimia nervosa* (*syn* binge–purge syndrome) self-induced vomiting after binge eating. ⇒ anorexia, eating disorders.

bulk-forming laxatives ⇒ laxatives. ⇒ Appendix 5.

bulla *n* (*syn* blister) a large watery blister. In dermatology, multiple bullae may suggest pemphigoid or pemphigus, but they occur sometimes in other diseases of the skin, e.g. in impetigo, in dermatitis herpetiformis, etc.—**bullae** *pl*, **bullate**, **bullous** *adj*.

bunion *n* ⇒ hallux valgus.

buphthalmos *n* (ox eye) enlarged eye, usually secondary to congenital glaucoma.

Burch colposuspension operation the vagina is suspended from the iliopectineal ligament. Carried out for severe stress incontinence of urine.

Burkitt's lymphoma a highly malignant lymphoma frequently of the jaw but other sites as well. Most commonly diagnosed in areas of Africa and New Guinea where malaria is endemic.

burn *n* tissue damage (necrosis) due to chemicals, moist heat, dry heat, electricity, flame, friction or radiation; classified as partial or full thickness according to the depth of skin destroyed: the latter usually requiring skin graft(s). Analgesia and the prevention of shock, infection and malnutrition are important aspects of treatment.

burnout syndrome a condition resulting from exposure to stressors. The stressors are often chronic and work-related, but burnout may occur after exposure to an acute stressor and may also result from stressful family roles such as caring for a relative, or a combination. Health professionals are at particular risk of burnout because of their prolonged contact with ill people. It has been described as emotional exhaustion, isolation, becoming indifferent to others, and a lack of ability to deal with problems. The adverse effects may be physical, emotional, intellectual, social and spiritual, and may include anxiety, poor coping strategies, insomnia, inability to make decisions, appetite and weight changes, excessive tiredness, apathy, lack of motivation, relationship difficulties and possible misuse of alcohol and drugs. ⇒ general adaptation syndrome, stress, stressor.

burr *n* an attachment for a surgical drill which is used for cutting into tooth or bone.

burrow *n* a tunnel in the skin that may house an ectoparasite, e.g. acarus of scabies.

bursa *n* a fibrous sac lined with synovial membrane and containing a small quantity of synovial fluid. Bursae are found between (a) tendon and bone, (b) skin and bone, (c) muscle and muscle. Their function is to facilitate movement by reducing friction between these surfaces—**bursae** *pl*.

bursitis *n* inflammation of a bursa. *olecranon bursitis* inflammation of the bursa over the point of the elbow. *prepatellar bursitis* (*syn* housemaid's knee) a fluid-filled swelling of the bursa in front of the knee cap (patella). It is frequently associated with excessive kneeling. A blow can result in bleeding into the bursa and there can be infection with pyogenic pathogens. *retrocalcaneal bursitis* inflammation of an anatomical bursa located between the posterior angle of the calcaneus and the Achilles tendon near to its insertion. There is a fluctuant soft tissue swelling both sides of the tendon.

buttock *n* one of the two projections posterior to the hip joints. Formed mainly of the gluteal muscles.

byssinosis *n* a form of pneumoconiosis caused by inhalation of cotton or linen dust.

C

CA-125 may be used as a tumour marker for ovarian cancers.

cachexia *n* a state of constitutional disorder, malnutrition and general ill health. There is debility, muscle weakness and anaemia. The chief signs of this condition are emaciation, sallow unhealthy skin and heavy lustreless eyes. A feature of advanced disease such as cancer—**cachectic** *adj*.

cadaver *n* a corpse. In a medical context it implies a dead body which is dissected in a medical school, or in a mortuary at a postmortem examination.

caecostomy *n* a surgically established fistula between the caecum and anterior abdominal wall, usually to achieve drainage and/or decompression of the caecum. It is usually created by inserting a widebore tube into the caecum at operation.

caecum *n* the blind, pouch-like commencement of the colon in the right iliac fossa. To it is attached the vermiform appendix; it is separated from the ileum by the ileocaecal valve—**caecal** *adj*.

caesarean section delivery of the fetus through an abdominal incision. It is said to be named after Caesar, who is supposed to have been born in this way.

caesium-137 (¹³⁷Cs) *n* a radioactive substance which, when sealed in needles or tubes, can be used for interstitial and surface applications. It can also be employed as a source for treatment by Selectron. Historically has been used for external beam therapy.

caffeine *n* the central nervous system stimulant that is present in tea, coffee, chocolate and cola drinks. It has been given as a diuretic, but its main use is in analgesic preparations.

caisson disease ⇒ decompression illness.

calamine *n* zinc carbonate with ferric oxide. Used in lotions and creams for the relief of itching; however, it is not generally effective.

calcaneus (*syn* calcaneum, os calcis) the heel bone.

calcareous *adj* chalky. Relating to lime or calcium.

calciferol ⇒ ergocalciferol.

calcification *n* the hardening of an organic substance by a deposit of calcium salts within it. May be physiological, as in bone, or pathological, as in arteries.

calcitonin *n* (*syn* thyrocalcitonin) hormone secreted by the thyroid gland. It has a fine-tuning role in calcium homeostasis. It opposes the action of parathyroid hormone and reduces levels of calcium and phosphate in the serum by its action on the kidneys and bone. It inhibits calcium reabsorption from bone and stimulates the excretion of calcium and phosphate in the urine. Calcitonin is released when the serum calcium level rises. Synthetic calcitonin is used in the management of metastatic bone cancer, Paget's disease and osteoporosis.

calcitriol *n* 1,25-dehydroxycholecalciferol. The active form of vitamin D concerned with calcium homeostasis.

calcium (Ca) *n* a metallic element. Needed by the body for neuromuscular conduction and blood coagulation and as an important component of the skeleton and teeth. An essential nutrient. *calcium carbonate* a calcium salt used in many antacid medicines. *calcium gluconate* a calcium salt used to treat calcium deficiencies and disorders such as rickets.

calcium channel blockers (antagonists) a group of drugs that block the flow of calcium ions in smooth muscle. They are negatively inotropic. ⇒ inotropes. ⇒ Appendix 5.

calculus *n* a stone. An abnormal concretion composed chiefly of mineral substances and formed in the passages which transmit secretions, or in the cavities which act as reservoirs for them. Examples include gallstones and renal calculi. *dental calculus*

a hard calcified deposit that forms on the surface of the teeth. Also known as tartar—**calculi** *pl*, **calculous** *adj*.

Caldwell–Luc operation (*syn* radical antrostomy) a radical operation previously used for sinusitis.

caliper *n* **1** a two-pronged instrument for measuring the diameter of a round body. Used chiefly in pelvimetry. **2** a two-pronged instrument with sharp points which are inserted into the lower end of a fractured long bone. A weight is attached to the other end of the caliper, which maintains a steady pull on the distal end of the bone. **3** *Thomas' walking caliper* is similar to the Thomas' splint, but the W-shaped junction at the lower end is replaced by two small iron rods which slot into holes made in the heel of the boot. The ring should fit the groin perfectly, and all weight is then borne by the ischial tuberosity.

callosity *n* a local hardening of the skin. ⇒ callus.

callus *n* **1** the partly calcified tissue which forms about the ends of a broken bone and ultimately accomplishes repair of the fracture. When this is complete the bony thickening is known as *permanent callus*—**callous** *adj*. **2** (*syn* callosity, corn, keratoma, mechanically induced hyperkeratosis) a yellowish plaque of hard skin caused by pressure or friction. The stratum corneum becomes hypertrophied. Most commonly seen on the feet and palms of the hands. A painful, cone-shaped overgrowth and hardening of the epidermis, with the point of the cone in the deeper layers. Corns on the sole of the foot and over joints are often described as hard corns, and those occurring between the toes are described as soft corns.

calor *n* heat: one of the five classic local signs and symptoms of inflammation—the others are dolor, loss of function, rubor and tumor.

caloric test irrigation of the external ear canal with water at 30°C and then at 44°C to assess vestibular function by stimulating the lateral semicircular canals. Each ear is tested separately. When the ear is normal the test produces nystagmus, whereas nystagmus may not be produced if the ear is diseased.

calorie *n* a unit of heat. In practice the calorie is too small a unit to be useful and the kilocalorie (kcal) is the preferred unit in studies in metabolism. A kcal is the amount of heat required to raise the temperature of 1 kg of water by 1°C. In medicine, science and technology generally, the calorie has been replaced by the joule (derived SI unit) as a unit of energy, work and heat. For approximate conversion 4.2 kJ = 1 kcal.

calorific *adj* describes any phenomena that relate to heat production.

cAMP *abbr* cyclic adenosine monophosphate.

Campylobacter *n* a genus of Gram-negative motile bacteria. *Campylobacter jejuni* is a common cause of bacterial food poisoning. It causes abdominal pain and bloodstained diarrhoea that may last for 10–14 days. The micro-organism is associated with raw meat and poultry, the fur of infected pet animals and unpasteurized milk. No reported person-to-person spread.

canaliculus *n* a minute capillary passage. Any small canal, such as the passage leading from the edge of the eyelid to the lacrimal sac or one of the numerous small canals leading from the Haversian canals and terminating in the lacunae of bone—**canaliculi** *pl*, **canalicular** *adj*, **canaliculization** *n*.

canal of Schlemm a canal in the inner part of the sclera, close to its junction with the cornea, which it encircles. It drains excess aqueous humour to maintain normal intraocular pressure. Impaired drainage results in raised intraocular pressure. ⇒ Figure 15. ⇒ glaucoma.

cancellous *adj* resembling latticework; light and spongy; like a honeycomb. Describes a type of bone tissue.

cancer *n* a general term which covers any malignant growth in any part of the body. The growth is purposeless, parasitic, and flourishes at the expense of the human host. Characteristics are the tendency to cause local destruction, to invade adjacent tissues and to spread by metastasis. Frequently recurs after removal. Carcinoma refers to malignant tumours of epithelial tissue, sarcoma to malignant tumours of connective tissue—**cancerous** *adj*.

cancerophobia *n* obsessive fear of cancer—**cancerophobic** *adj*.

cancrum oris gangrenous stomatitis of cheek in debilitated children. Often called 'noma'. Associated with measles in malnourished African children.

candela (cd) one of the seven base units of the International System of Units (SI). Measures luminous intensity.

Candida *n* (*syn Monilia*) a genus of fungi. They are widespread in nature. *Candida albicans* is a commensal of the gastrointestinal tract of humans.

candidiasis *n* (*syn* candidosis, moniliasis, thrush) infections caused by a species of *Candida*, usually *Candida albicans*. Infection may involve the mouth, gastrointestinal tract, skin, nails, respiratory tract or genitourinary tract (vulvovaginitis, balanitis), especially in individuals who are debilitated, e.g. by cancer or diabetes mellitus, or immunosuppressed and after long-term or extensive treatment with antibiotics, which upsets the microbial flora, and other drugs, e.g. corticosteroids. Oral infection can be caused by poor oral hygiene, including carious teeth and ill-fitting dentures.

canicola fever leptospirosis.

canine *adj* of or resembling a dog. *canine tooth* pointed tooth with a single cusp (cuspid), placed third from the midline in both primary and secondary dentitions. A lay term for the upper permanent canine is 'eye tooth'. There are four in all.

cannabinoids *npl* a group of antiemetic drugs derived from cannabis. ⇒ Appendix 5.

cannabis (*syn* marihuana, pot, hashish, etc.) a psychoactive drug that produces euphoria and hallucinations. It is usually smoked. In the UK the cultivation, possession and supply of cannabis are criminal offences (⇒ Appendix 5). There is, however, considerable interest in possible medicinal uses and trials are ongoing.

cannula *n* a hollow tube, usually plastic, for the introduction or withdrawal of fluid from the body. In some types the lumen is fitted with a sharp-pointed trocar to facilitate insertion, which is withdrawn when the cannula is in situ—**cannulae** *pl*.

cannulation *n* insertion of a cannula, such as into a vein to facilitate the administration of intravenous fluids.

canthus *n* the angle formed by the junction of the eyelids. The inner one is known as the *nasal canthus* and the outer as the *temporal canthus*—**canthi** *pl*, **canthal** *adj*.

CAPD *abbr* continuous ambulatory peritoneal dialysis.

CAPE *abbr* Clifton Assessment Procedures for the Elderly.

capelline bandage (divergent spica) a bandage applied in a circular fashion to the head or an amputated limb.

capillarization *n* a long-term adaptation to endurance exercise where the number and usage of blood capillaries in muscle tissue increases to meet the need for oxygenated blood. ⇒ aerobic adaptations.

capillary *n* (literally, hair-like) any tiny thin-walled vessel forming part of a network which facilitates rapid exchange of substances between the contained fluid and the surrounding tissues. *bile capillary* begins in a space in the liver and joins others, eventually forming a bile duct. *blood capillary* unites an arteriole and a venule. *capillary fragility* an expression of the ease with which blood capillaries may rupture. *lymph capillary* begins in the tissue spaces throughout the body and joins others, eventually forming a lymphatic vessel.

capital budget financial allocation for the purchase of items, such as equipment, that will last longer than 12 months, or items that cost more than an agreed level. ⇒ revenue budget.

capitation funding method of allocating money and other resources based on the number of people living in a geographical area. *weighted capitation* the allocation of resource based on the number of people in an area but adjusted for the age profile or the relative economic and social conditions, e.g. areas with a high level of social deprivation would be allocated extra resource.

capsaicin *n* a chemical present in sweet peppers. It prevents the transmission of pain impulses. Used topically to relieve pain following shingles.

capsule *n* **1** the ligaments which surround a joint. **2** a gelatinous or rice paper container for a drug. **3** the outer membranous covering of certain organs, such as the kidney, liver—**capsular** *adj*.

capsulectomy *n* the surgical excision of a capsule. Refers to a joint or lens; less often to the kidney.

capsulitis *n* inflammation of a capsule. Sometimes used as a synonym for frozen shoulder.

capsulotomy *n* incision of a capsule, usually referring to that surrounding the crystalline lens of the eye, which remains after modern cataract surgery. Usually created by a laser.

caput *n* the head. *caput medusae* dilated knot of veins around the umbilicus, associated with portal hypertension. *caput succedaneum* an oedematous swelling covering the fetal scalp at birth. Occurs as a result of pressure during labour. The swelling is diffuse, not delineated by skull suture lines and resolves spontaneously after delivery.

carbaminohaemoglobin *n* a compound formed between carbon dioxide and haemoglobin. Some carbon dioxide in the blood is carried in this form.

carbapenems *npl* a group of β-lactam antibiotics. ⇒ Appendix 5.

carbohydrate *n* an organic compound containing carbon, hydrogen and oxygen. Formed in nature by photosynthesis in plants. Carbohydrates are the major source of energy in most diets, on average 1 g of carbohydrate is metabolized to produce 16 kJ heat. They include starches, sugars and non-starch polysaccharides (NSP), and are classified in three groups—monosaccharides, disaccharides and polysaccharides.

carbohydrate loading (carbo-loading) a term used in sports medicine to describe the dietary regimens intended to increase the glycogen stores in the liver and muscles before major endurance activity such as running a marathon.

carbolic acid ⇒ phenol.

carbon *n* a non-metallic element found in all organic molecules and living matter. Carbon can bond with four other atoms and is able to form a huge number of complex molecules. *carbon dioxide* a gas; a waste product of many forms of combustion and metabolism, excreted via the lungs. Builds up in respiratory insufficiency or failure and carbon dioxide tension in arterial blood ($PaCO_2$) rises above normal levels. ⇒ hypercapnia.

carbon monoxide a poisonous gas that combines with haemoglobin to form a stable compound. This blocks the normal reversible oxygen-carrying function and leads to hypoxia. The onset of hypoxia may be insidious but it is associated with confusion, headache, increasing respiratory rate, flushed appearance, changes in conscious level, seizures and cardiac arrhythmias. *carbon tetrachloride* colourless volatile liquid used in dry cleaning and some types of antifreeze. Exposure may result in toxicity and liver damage.

carbonic anhydrase an enzyme that assists the transfer of carbon dioxide from tissues to blood and to alveolar air by reversibly catalysing the decomposition of carbonic acid into carbon dioxide and water.

carbonic anhydrase inhibitors drugs that reduce the production of aqueous humour, thereby reducing intraocular pressure. They also have diuretic effects. ⇒ Appendix 5.

carboxyhaemoglobin *n* a stable compound formed by the union of carbon monoxide and haemoglobin; the red blood cells thus lose their respiratory function.

carboxyhaemoglobinaemia *n* carboxyhaemoglobin in the blood—**carboxyhaemoglobinaemic** *adj.*

carboxyhaemoglobinuria *n* carboxyhaemoglobin in the urine—**carboxyhaemoglobinuric** *adj.*

carbuncle *n* an acute inflammation (usually caused by *Staphylococcus*). There is a collection of boils causing necrosis in the skin and subcutaneous tissue.

carcinoembryonic antigen (CEA) increased amounts in the serum of adults can be a tumour marker for colorectal cancers and for non-malignant conditions, such as liver cirrhosis caused by alcohol misuse.

carcinogen *n* agent, substance or environment causing cancer—**carcinogenic** *adj*, **carcinogenicity** *n.*

carcinogenesis *n* the production of cancer—**carcinogenetic** *adj.*

carcinoid syndrome cluster of symptoms including flushing, palpitation, diarrhoea and bronchospasm from histological (usually low grade) malignancy; often originates in the appendix.

carcinoma *n* a cancerous growth of epithelial tissue (e.g. mucous membrane) and derivatives such as glands. *carcinoma in situ* condition with cells closely resembling cancer cells. A very early cancer. Well described in uterus and prostate. Previously called preinvasive carcinoma—**carcinomata** *pl*, **carcinomatous** *adj.*

carcinomatosis *n* widespread malignancy affecting many organs.

cardia *n* the oesophageal opening into the stomach.

cardiac *adj* **1** pertaining to the heart **2** pertaining to the cardia of the stomach. *cardiac arrest* complete cessation of effective output (of blood) from heart activity. Failure of the heart action to maintain an adequate circulation. The clinical picture of cessation of circulation in a patient who was not expected to die at the time. There are several forms: asystole, electromechanical dissociation, pulseless ventricular tachycardia or ventricular fibrillation. *cardiac bed* one which can be manipulated so that the patient is supported in a sitting position. *cardiac bypass operation* the bypassing of atheromatous vessels supplying heart muscle (myocardium). *cardiac catheterization* ⇒ catheterization. *cardiac cycle* the series of movements through which the heart passes in performing one heart beat, which corresponds to one pulse beat and takes about one second ⇒ diastole, systole. *cardiac enzymes* released from damaged myocardial cells. Abnormal levels found in the blood are suggestive of a diagnosis of myocardial infarction. Used to confirm or refute the diagnosis of myocardial infarction. The enzymes usually measured are troponins and creatine kinase (CK) but aspartate aminotransferase (AST) and lactate dehydrogenase (LDH) may also be measured. *cardiac massage* performed during cardiac arrest. With the person lying on his or her back on a firm surface, the lower part of the sternum (breastbone) is depressed to compress the heart and force blood into the circulation. ⇒ cardiopulmonary resuscitation (CPR). *cardiac oedema* gravitational oedema. Such patients secrete excessive aldosterone which increases excretion of potassium and conserves sodium and chloride. Antialdosterone (aldosterone antagonists) drugs useful, e.g. spironolactone. ⇒ oedema. *cardiac output (CO)* the volume of blood ejected by the heart per minute, typically 4–5 L/min at rest. It can be expressed as the cardiac index (CI), cardiac output divided by body surface area. *cardiac pacemaker* an electrical device for maintaining myocardial contraction by stimulating the heart muscle. A pacemaker may be permanent or temporary. They are programmed in a variety of modes. Nowadays pacemakers can be programmed to alter their rate in response to physical activity. *cardiac tamponade* excessive fluid surrounding the heart, usually blood when the cause is traumatic. Can occur in surgery and penetrating wounds or cardiac rupture. Causes compression of the heart leading to heart failure from haemopericardium.

cardialgia *n* literally, pain in the heart. Often used to mean heartburn (pyrosis).

cardiogenic *adj* of cardiac origin, such as the shock that may occur following a myocardial infarction.

cardiograph *n* an instrument for recording graphically the force and form of the heart beat—**cardiographic** *adj*, **cardiogram** *n*, **cardiographically** *adv*.

cardiologist *n* a medically qualified person who specializes in diagnosing and treating diseases of the heart.

cardiology *n* study of the structure, function and diseases of the heart.

cardiomegaly *n* enlargement of the heart.

cardiomyopathy *n* a disease of the myocardium associated with cardiac dysfunction. It is classified as dilated cardiomyopathy, hypertrophic cardiomyopathy, arrhythmogenic right ventricular cardiomyopathy or restrictive cardiomyopathy. Management includes treatment of the cause (if possible), treatment of heart failure and sometimes heart transplantation—**cardiomyopathic** *adj*.

cardiomyotomy *n* cutting or dissection of the muscular tissue at the gastro-oesophageal junction for achalasia.

cardiophone *n* a microphone strapped to a patient which allows audible and visual signal of heart sounds. By channelling pulses through an electrocardiograph, a graphic record can be made. Can be used for the fetus.

cardioplegia *n* the use of an electrolyte solution to induce electromechanical cardiac arrest. *cold cardioplegia* cardioplegia

combined with hypothermia to reduce the oxygen consumption of the myocardium during open heart surgery.

cardiopulmonary *adj* pertaining to the heart and lungs. *cardiopulmonary bypass* used in open heart surgery. The heart and lungs are excluded from the circulation and replaced by a pump oxygenator—**cardiopulmonic** *adj*.

cardiopulmonary resuscitation (CPR) the techniques used to maintain circulation and respiration following cardiopulmonary arrest. It involves (a) the maintenance of a clear airway, (b) artificial respiration using mouth-to-mouth or mouth-to-nose respiration, or by a bag and face mask, or by an endotracheal tube, and (c) maintenance of the circulation by external cardiac massage. ⇒ resuscitation.

cardiorenal *adj* pertaining to the heart and kidney.

cardiorespiratory *adj* pertaining to the heart and the respiratory system.

cardiorrhaphy *n* stitching of the heart wall: usually reserved for traumatic surgery.

cardiothoracic *adj* pertaining to the heart and thoracic cavity. A specialized branch of surgery.

cardiotocograph *n* the instrument used in cardiotocography.

cardiotocography (CTG) *n* a procedure whereby the fetal heart rate is measured either by an external microphone or by the application of an electrode to the fetal scalp, recording the fetal ECG and from it the fetal heart rate. An external transducer placed on the mother's abdomen measures the uterine contractions.

cardiotomy syndrome pyrexia, pericarditis and pleural effusion following heart surgery. It may develop weeks or months after the operation and is thought to be an autoimmune reaction.

cardiotoxic *adj* describes any agent that has an injurious effect on the heart.

cardiovascular *adj* pertaining to the heart and blood vessels. *cardiovascular endurance* the ability to sustain exercise without undue fatigue, cardiac distress or respiratory distress.

cardioversion *n* use of electrical countershock for restoring the heart rhythm to normal.

carditis *n* inflammation of the heart. A word seldom used without the appropriate prefix, e.g. endo-, myo-, peri-.

care pathway an integrated plan or pathway agreed locally by the multidisciplinary team for specific patient/client groups. The agreed pathway is based on available evidence and guidelines.

caries *n* inflammatory decay of bone, usually associated with pus formation— **carious** *adj.* ⇒ dental caries.

carina *n* a keel-like structure exemplified by the keel-shaped cartilage at the bifurcation of the trachea into two bronchi— **carinal** *adj.*

cariogenic *adj* causing caries, by convention referring to dental caries.

carminative *adj, n* having the power to relieve flatulence and associated colic. They include cinnamon, nutmeg, peppermint.

carneous mole a fleshy mass in the uterus comprising blood clot and a dead fetus or parts thereof that have not been expelled with miscarriage.

carotenes *npl* a group of naturally occurring pigments within the larger group of carotenoids. They are fat-soluble and have antioxidant properties. Carotene occurs in three forms—alpha (α), beta (β) and gamma (γ). The β form is converted in the body to vitamin A; it is therefore a provitamin.

carotenoids *npl* a group of about 100 naturally occurring yellow to red pigments found mostly in plants, some of which are carotenes. Heating of foods before eating usually improves carotenoid availability.

carotid *n* the principal artery on each side of the neck. ⇒ Figure 9. At the bifurcation of the common carotid into the internal and external carotids there are: (a) the *carotid bodies* a collection of chemoreceptors which, being sensitive to chemical changes in the blood, protect the body against lack of O_2; (b) the *carotid sinus* a collection of baroreceptors; increased pressure causes slowing of the heart beat and lowering of blood pressure.

carpal *adj* pertaining to the wrist. *carpal tunnel syndrome* nocturnal pain, numbness, weakness of the thumb and tingling in the area of distribution of the median nerve in the hand. Due to compression as the nerve passes under the fascial band. Most common in middle-aged women.

carphology *n* involuntary picking at the bedclothes, as seen in exhaustive or febrile delirium.

carpometacarpal *adj* pertaining to the carpal and metacarpal bones.

carpopedal *adj* pertaining to the hands and feet. *carpopedal spasm* painful spasm of hands and feet in tetany. ⇒ Chvostek's sign, hypocalcaemia, Trousseau's sign.

carpus *n* the wrist. ⇒ Figure 2.

carrier *n* **1** a person who, without manifesting an infection, harbours the microorganism which can cause the overt infection, and who can transmit infection to others. **2** a person who carries a recessive gene at a specific chromosome location (locus).

carrier molecule a cell membrane protein that assists the transfer of drugs, ions and nutrients into the cell.

cartilage *n* a dense connective tissue capable of withstanding pressure. There are several types according to the function it has to fulfil. There is relatively more cartilage in a child's skeleton but much of it has been converted into bone by adulthood—**cartilaginous** *adj.*

caruncle *n* a red fleshy projection. Hymenal caruncles surround the entrance to the vagina after rupture of the hymen. The lacrimal caruncle is the fleshy prominence at the inner angle of the eye.

case control study a retrospective research study that compares outcomes for a group with a particular condition with those of a control group who do not have the condition.

case study research that studies data from one case, or a small group of cases.

caseation *n* the formation of a soft, cheese-like mass, as occurs in tuberculosis— **caseous** *adj.*

casein *n* a protein produced when milk enters the stomach. Coagulation occurs and is due to the action of rennin upon the caseinogen in the milk, splitting it into two proteins, one being casein. The casein combines with calcium and a clot is formed. Casein is known as paracasein in the United States. *casein hydrolysate* predigested protein food derived from casein; can be added to other foods to increase the protein content.

caseinogen *n* the principal protein in milk. It is not soluble in water but is kept in solution in milk by inorganic salts. The proportion to lactalbumin is much higher in cows' milk than in human milk. In the presence of rennin it is converted into insoluble casein. Caseinogen is known as casein in the United States.

caseous degeneration cheese-like tissue resulting from atrophy in a tuberculoma or gumma.

Casoni test intradermal injection of fresh, sterile hydatid fluid. A white papule indicates a hydatid cyst.

cast *n* **1** material or exudate that has been moulded to the form of the cavity or tube in which it has collected. **2** a rigid casing often made with plaster of Paris and applied to immobilize a part of the body.

castor oil a vegetable oil previously used as a stimulant laxative. ⇒ laxatives. Used with zinc ointment as a barrier cream for napkin and urinary rash.

castration *n* surgical removal of the testes in the male, or of the ovaries in the female. Castration can be part of the treatment for a hormone-dependent cancer—**castrated** *adj*, **castrate** *n*, *vt*.

CAT *acron* computed axial tomography.

catabolism (or katabolism) *n* the series of chemical reactions in the living body whereby complex substances are broken down into simpler ones accompanied by the release of energy. This energy is needed for anabolism and the other activities of the body. ⇒ adenosine diphosphate, adenosine triphosphate, anabolism, hypercatabolism, metabolism—**catabolic** *adj*.

catalase *n* an enzyme that catalyses the breakdown of hydrogen peroxide.

catalysis *n* an increase in the rate at which a chemical reaction proceeds to equilibrium through the medium of a catalyst or catalyser. Reaction retardation is termed negative catalysis—**catalytic** *adj*.

catalyst *n* any substance that regulates or accelerates the rate of a chemical reaction without itself undergoing a permanent change.

cataplexy *n* a condition of muscular rigidity induced by severe mental shock or fear. The patient remains conscious—**cataplectic** *adj*.

cataract *n* an opacity of the crystalline lens. Usually age-related, but many causes including congenital, traumatic or metabolic such as diabetes mellitus—**cataractous** *adj*.

catarrh *n* chronic inflammation of a mucous membrane with constant flow of a thick sticky mucus—**catarrhal** *adj*.

catatonic schizophrenia a form of schizophrenia characterized by psychomotor disturbances (e.g. stupor, posturing, negativism, hyperkinesis). ⇒ schizophrenia.

cat cry syndrome ⇒ 'cri du chat' syndrome.

catecholamines *npl* a group of important physiological amines, such as adrenaline (epinephrine), noradrenaline (norepinephrine) and dopamine. They act as hormones and neurotransmitters and affect blood pressure, heart rate, respiratory rate and blood sugar. Abnormally high levels are secreted by adrenal and other tumours and can be detected in the urine. ⇒ phaeochromocytoma.

categorical data data that can be categorized, e.g. hair colour. ⇒ nominal data, ordinal data.

catgut *n* a form of ligature and suture of varying thickness, strength and absorbability, prepared from animal tissue. The plain variety is usually absorbed in 5–10 days, whereas chromic catgut takes 10–21 days to be absorbed.

cat scratch fever a virus infection resulting from a cat scratch or bite. There is fever and lymph node swelling about a week after the incident. Recovery is usually complete, although an abscess may develop.

catharsis *n* in psychology, it describes the purging or outpouring of emotion through experiencing it deeply—**cathartic** *adj*.

catheter *n* a hollow tube of variable length and bore, usually having one fluted end and a tip of varying size and shape according to function. Catheters are made of many substances including soft and hard rubber, gum elastic, glass, silver, other metals and plastic materials, some of which are radiopaque. They have many uses including: insufflation of hollow tubes, cardiac catheterization, introduction of contrast medium for angiography, withdrawal of fluid from body cavities, e.g. urinary catheter and the administration of drugs, fluids and nutrients.

catheterization *n* insertion of a catheter, most usually into the urinary bladder. *cardiac catheterization* a long plastic catheter or tubing is inserted into an artery or vein and moved under X-ray guidance until it reaches the heart. A catheter inserted into the brachial or femoral artery gives access to the left side of the heart and those inserted into the brachial or femoral vein can be guided into the right atrium, ventricle and the pulmonary artery. Cardiac catheterization can be used for: (a) recording pressures and cardiac output, ⇒ pulmonary artery occlusion pressure; (b) the introduction of radiopaque contrast medium for angiography; (c) treatments, such as angioplasty and stent insertion, ⇒ angioplasty—**catheterize** *vt*.

cathetron *n* a high rate dose, remotely controlled, afterloading device for radiotherapy. Hollow steel catheters are placed in the desired position. They are then connected to a protective safe by hollow cables. The radioactive cobalt moves from the safe into the catheters. After delivery of the required dose, the cobalt returns to the safe, thus avoiding radiation hazard to staff. Currently superseded by units such as the Selectron.

cauda *n* a tail or tail-like appendage. *cauda equina* lower part of the spinal cord where the nerves for the legs and bladder originate—**caudal, caudate** *adj*.

caudal anaesthesia injection of local anaesthetic into the epidural space at the level of the sacrum causing loss of sensation in the lower abdomen and pelvis.

caul *n* the amnion, instead of rupturing as is usual to allow the baby through, persists and covers the baby's head at birth.

cauliflower ear in sports medicine a colloquial term used to describe deformity of the pinna that may follow auricular haematoma (collection of blood between the perichondrium and cartilage of the outer ear) caused by repeated trauma sustained during contact sports.

causalgia *n* excruciating neuralgic pain, resulting from physical trauma to a cutaneous nerve. Also known as reflex sympathetic dystrophy.

caustic *adj, n* corrosive or destructive to organic tissue; the agents which produce such results. Usually a strong alkali or acid, they are used to destroy overabundant granulation tissue, warts or polyps. Carbolic acid, carbon dioxide snow and silver nitrate are most commonly employed.

cauterize *vt* to cause tissue destruction by applying a heated instrument, a cautery—**cauterization** *n*.

cautery *n* an agent or device, e.g. electricity, chemicals or extremes of temperature, which destroys cells and tissues. Uses include the prevention of blood loss during surgery, or to remove abnormal tissue.

cavernous *adj* having hollow spaces. *cavernous sinus* a channel for venous blood, on either side of the sphenoid bone. It drains blood from the cerebral hemispheres, orbits and the bones of the skull. Sepsis around the eyes or nose can cause cavernous sinus thrombosis.

cavitation *n* the formation of a cavity, as in pulmonary tuberculosis.

cavity *n* a hollow; an enclosed area. *abdominal cavity* that below the diaphragm; the abdomen. *buccal cavity* the mouth. *cerebral cavity* the ventricles of the brain. *cranial cavity* the brain box formed by the bones of the cranium. *medullary cavity* the hollow centre of a long bone, containing yellow bone marrow or medulla. *nasal cavity* that in the nose, separated into right and left halves by the nasal septum. *oral cavity* buccal cavity. *pelvic cavity* that formed by the pelvic bones, more particularly the part below the iliopectineal line. *peritoneal cavity* a potential space between the parietal and visceral layers of the peritoneum. Similarly, the *pleural cavity* is the potential space between the visceral and parietal pleurae which in health are in contact in all phases of respiration. *synovial cavity* the potential space in a synovial joint. *uterine cavity* that of the uterus, the base extending between the orifices of the uterine tubes.

CBA *abbr* cost-benefit analysis.

CCK *abbr* cholecystokinin.

CCPNS *abbr* cell cycle phase non-specific.

CCPS *abbr* cell cycle phase specific.

CCU *abbr* coronary care unit. ⇒ high dependency unit, intensive care/therapy unit.

CD *abbr* controlled drug.

CDC *abbr* Centers for Disease Control and Prevention.

CDH *abbr* congenital dislocation of the hip. ⇒ developmental dysplasia of the hip.

CEA *abbr* carcinoembryonic antigen.

cell *n* basic structural unit of living organisms. A mass of protoplasm (cytoplasm) and usually a nucleus within a plasma or cell membrane. Some cells, e.g. erythrocytes, are non-nucleated whereas others, such as voluntary muscle, may be multinucleated. The cytoplasm contains various subcellular organelles—mitochondria, ribosomes, etc.—that undertake the metabolic processes of the cell—**cellular** *adj*. *cell cycle* the events occurring within a cell from one mitotic division to the next. Comprises the dynamic course of division of normal and cancer cells incorporating phases of DNA synthesis (S-phase), growth phases (GI and GII), mitosis (M) and 'rest phase' (G0).

cell cycle phase non-specific describes a cytotoxic drug that acts at any time in the cell cycle.

cell cycle phase specific describes a cytotoxic drug that acts during a specific phase of the cell cycle.

cell mediated immunity ⇒ immunity.

cellulitis *n* a diffuse inflammation of the skin and connective tissue, especially the loose subcutaneous tissue. When it involves the pelvic tissues in the female it is called parametritis. When it occurs in the floor of the mouth it is called Ludwig's angina.

cellulose *n* a carbohydrate forming the outer walls of plant and vegetable cells. A polysaccharide which cannot be digested by humans but supplies non-starch polysaccharides (NSP) for stimulation of peristalsis.

Celsius the derived SI unit (International System of Units) for temperature. Named after Anders Celsius (1701–1744) who constructed the first centigrade thermometer. ⇒ centigrade.

cementum *n* calcified organic hard tissue forming on the surface of a root of a tooth,

and providing attachment for the periodontal ligament.

censor *n* term used by Freud to describe the resistance that prevents repressed material from easily re-entering the conscious mind from the subconscious (unconscious) mind.

Centers for Disease Control and Prevention (CDC) a federal agency in the US (Atlanta). Its functions include the investigation, identification, prevention and control of disease.

centigrade *n* a scale with one hundred divisions or degrees. Most often refers to the thermometric scale in which the freezing point of water is fixed at $0°$ and the boiling point at $100°$. It is usually called Celsius for medical and scientific purposes. ⇒ Celsius.

central cyanosis ⇒ cyanosis.

central limit theorem in research. Sampling distribution becomes more normal the more samples that are taken.

central sterile supplies department (CSSD) designated an area where packets are prepared containing the equipment and/ or swabs and dressings necessary to perform activities requiring aseptic technique. ⇒ hospital sterilization and disinfection unit (HSDU).

central tendency statistic averages. The tendency for observations to centre around a specific value rather than across the entire range. ⇒ mean, median, mode.

central venous catheter/line specialized intravenous cannula placed in a large vein (jugular, subclavian or femoral). ⇒ Figure 10. Used for the measurement of central venous pressure, and fluids and drugs. Also allows long-term vascular access for the administration of drugs, blood products or nutritional support.

central venous pressure (CVP) the pressure of the blood within the right atrium. It is measured using a central venous catheter attached to a manometer or pressure transducer.

centrifugal *adj* efferent. Having a tendency to move outwards from the centre, as the nerve impulses from the brain to the peripheral structures.

centrifuge *n* an apparatus which subjects solutions to centrifugal forces by high-speed rotation, thereby separating substances of different densities into discrete bands within the liquid phase. It is usually used to separate ('spin down') particulate material (e.g. subcellular particles) from a suspending liquid.

centriole *n* a subcellular organelle that aids spindle formation during nuclear division. ⇒ meiosis, mitosis.

centripetal *adj* afferent. Having a tendency to move towards the centre, as the rash in chickenpox.

centromere *n* the structure that joins the double chromosome (2 chromatids) and eventually attaches to the spindle during nuclear division. ⇒ meiosis, mitosis.

centrosome *n* a region adjacent to the cell nucleus that contains the centrioles.

cephalalgia *n* pain in the head; headache.

cephalhaematoma *n* a collection of blood in the subperiosteal tissues of the scalp of an infant. It is usually caused by pressure on the scalp during a long labour. ⇒ caput succedaneum.

cephalic *adj* pertaining to the head; near the head. *cephalic vein* ⇒ Figure 10. *cephalic version* ⇒ version.

cephalocele *n* hernia of the brain; protrusion of part of the brain through the skull.

cephalohaematoma *n* cephalhaematoma.

cephalometry *n* measurement of the living human head.

cephalosporins *npl* a large group of beta-lactam antibiotics, closely related to the penicillins. ⇒ Appendix 5.

cerebellar gait a staggering, unsteady, wide based walk seen in patients with damage to the cerebellum or its connections. ⇒ gait.

cerebellum *n* that part of the brain which lies behind and below the cerebrum (⇒ Figures 1, 11). Its chief functions are the coordination of fine voluntary movements and the control of posture—**cerebellar** *adj*.

cerebral *adj* pertaining to the cerebrum. *cerebral compression* arises from any space-occupying intracranial lesion. *cerebral cortex* the outer layer of cells (grey matter) in the cerebral hemispheres. *cerebral hemisphere* one side of the cerebrum, right or left. *cerebral palsy* non-progressive brain damage that typically occurs at, or shortly after, birth resulting in a range of mainly motor conditions ranging from clumsiness to severe spasticity.

cerebral function monitor (CFM) equipment for continuous monitoring of brain wave activity, e.g. to detect seizures in sedated and paralysed patients.

cerebral perfusion pressure (CPP) the pressure which drives blood through the brain. It is the difference between the arterial blood pressure and the intracranial pressure. If CPP is too low the blood flow to the brain may be inadequate and the brain deprived of oxygen.

cerebration *n* mental activity.

cerebrospinal *adj* pertaining to the brain and spinal cord. *cerebrospinal fluid* the clear fluid found within the ventricles (cavities) of the brain, central canal of the spinal cord and beneath the cranial and spinal meninges in the subarachnoid space. Protects and nourishes the brain and spinal cord. It is formed by the choroid plexus in the ventricles and circulates around the brain and spinal cord before it is reabsorbed on the outside of the brain.

cerebrovascular *adj* pertaining to the blood vessels of the brain. *cerebrovascular accident (stroke)(CVA)* interference with the cerebral blood flow due to embolism, haemorrhage or thrombosis. Signs and symptoms vary according to the duration, extent and site of tissue damage; there may be only a passing, even momentary inability to move a hand or foot; weakness or tingling in a limb; stertorous breathing; incontinence of urine and faeces; coma; paralysis of a limb or limbs; and speech deficiency (aphasia). ⇒ transient ischaemic attack.

cerebrum *n* the largest and uppermost part of the brain (⇒ Figures 1, 11). The longitudinal fissure divides it into two hemispheres, each containing a lateral ventricle. A mass of nerve fibres (white matter) is covered by a thin layer of nerve cells (grey matter). It controls the higher functions and contains major motor and sensory areas. The outer surface is convoluted—**cerebral** *adj*.

certified *adj* a redundant term. In the UK patients detained under current mental health legislation are said to be formally detained or 'sectioned'.

ceruloplasmin *n* plasma protein involved in copper transport.

cerumen *n* ear wax, sticky brown secretion from glands in the external auditory canal. Traps dust and other particles entering the ear—**ceruminous** *adj*.

cervical *adj* **1** pertaining to the neck **2** pertaining to the cervix (neck) of an organ. *cervical amnioscopy* ⇒ amnioscopy. *cervical canal* the lumen of the cervix uteri, from the internal to the external os. *cervical nerve roots* (⇒ Figure 11). *cervical rib* ⇒ thoracic inlet syndrome. *cervical smear* ⇒ cervical intraepithelial neoplasia, Papanicolaou test. *cervical vertebrae* ⇒ Figure 3.

cervical intraepithelial neoplasia (CIN) staging of cellular changes in the cervix uteri that occur prior to the development of carcinoma in-situ and invasive cancer. Abnormal cells are detected by a smear test and the diagnosis is confirmed by colposcopy and biopsy. CIN1, mild dysplasia; CIN2, moderate dysplasia; CIN3, severe dysplasia, carcinoma in-situ. ⇒ conization.

cervicectomy *n* amputation of the uterine cervix.

cervicitis *n* inflammation of the uterine cervix.

cervix *n* a neck. *cervix uteri, uterine cervix* the neck of the uterus (⇒ Figure 17)—**cervical** *adj*.

cestode *n* tapeworm ⇒ *Taenia*.

cetrimide *n* a disinfectant with detergent properties. Used for wound cleansing and skin preparation.

CF *abbr* cystic fibrosis.

CFM *abbr* cerebral function monitor.

CFT *abbr* complement fixation test.

CGM *abbr* continuous glucose monitoring.

Chagas' disease ⇒ trypanosomiasis.

chalazion *n* a cyst in the eyelid caused by chronic inflammation of retained secretion of a meibomian gland.

chalone *n* a substance that inhibits rather than stimulates, e.g. enterogastrone inhibits gastric secretions and motility.

chancre *n* the primary syphilitic ulcer developing at the site of infection with *Treponema pallidum*. It is associated with swelling of local lymph nodes. The chancre is painless, indurated, solitary and highly infectious.

chancroid *n* (*syn* soft sore) a type of sexually transmitted infection prevalent in warmer climates. Caused by *Haemophilus ducreyi*.

Causes multiple, painful, ragged ulcers on the genitalia, often with bubo formation.

character *n* the sum total of the known and predictable mental characteristics of an individual, particularly his or her conduct. *character change* denotes change in the form of conduct, to one foreign to the patient's natural disposition, e.g. violent or indecent behaviour.

charcoal *n* used therapeutically for its adsorptive and deodorant properties. Activated charcoal incorporated into dressings is used to reduce odour in malodorous discharging wounds.

Charcot's joint complete disorganization of a joint associated with syringomyelia, diabetes mellitus, or advanced cases of tabes dorsalis (locomotor ataxia). The condition is painless. *Charcot's triad* manifestation of multiple sclerosis—nystagmus, intention tremor and staccato speech.

CHART *acron* continuous hyperfractionated accelerated radiotherapy.

CHD *abbr* coronary heart disease.

cheilitis *n* inflammation of the lip.

cheiloplasty *n* any plastic operation on the lip.

cheilosis *n* maceration at the angles of the mouth; fissures occur later. May be due to riboflavin deficiency.

cheiropompholyx *n* symmetrical eruption of skin of hands (especially fingers) characterized by the formation of tiny vesicles and associated with itching or burning. On the feet the condition is called podopompholyx.

chelating agents soluble organic compounds that combine with certain metallic ions, such as iron, to form complexes that are safely excreted in the urine. ⇒ haemochromatosis, thalassaemia. ⇒ Appendix 5.

chemonucleolysis *n* injection of an enzyme, usually into an intervertebral disc, for dissolution of same—**chemonucleolytic** *adj*.

chemopallidectomy *n* the destruction of a predetermined section of globus pallidus by chemicals.

chemoprophylaxis *n* the prevention of disease (or recurrent attack) by administration of drugs such as antibiotics for people exposed to infection and antimalarial drugs—**chemoprophylactic** *adj*.

chemoreceptor *n* a sensory nerve ending or a cell having an affinity for, and capable of reacting to, a chemical stimuli, e.g. taste, oxygen levels in the blood.

chemoresistant *adj* describes a tumour that does not usually shrink with chemotherapy.

chemosensitive *adj* describes a tumour that shrinks following chemotherapy administration.

chemosis *n* oedema or swelling of the bulbar conjunctiva—**chemotic** *adj*.

chemotaxis *n* movements of a cell (e.g. leucocyte) or a micro-organism in response to chemical stimuli; attraction is termed *positive chemotaxis*, repulsion is *negative chemotaxis*—**chemotactic** *adj*.

chemotherapy *n* chemical agents of various types; prescribed to delay or arrest growth of cancer cells through interruption/inhibition of cell cycle; usually given in combination rather than as single agents. They are non-selective and non-specific and therefore affect all cycling cells whether benign or malignant. Administration is by oral, intramuscular, intravenous, intracavitary, or intra-arterial routes. ⇒ alkylating agents, antimetabolites, antitumour antibiotics, vinca alkaloids. ⇒ Appendix 5.

chenodeoxycholic acid a bile acid. It can be taken orally to dissolve certain types of gallstones.

Cheyne–Stokes respiration cyclical waxing and waning of breathing, characterized at one extreme by deep fast breaths and at the other by apnoea: it generally has an ominous prognosis.

CHF *abbr* congestive heart failure.

chi ⇒ Qi energy.

CHI *abbr* Commission for Health Improvement.

chiasma *n* an X-shaped crossing or decussation. *optic chiasma* the meeting of the two optic nerves; where the fibres from the medial or nasal half of each retina (supplying half the visual field in either eye) cross the middle line to join the optic tract of the opposite side—**chiasmata** *pl*.

chickenpox *n* (*syn* varicella) a mild, specific infection with varicella-zoster virus (VZV). The incubation is 12–21 days. Successive crops of vesicles appear first on the trunk; they scab and usually heal without scars.

chikungunya *n* a mosquito-transmitted haemorrhagic fever occurring in Africa.

chilblain *n* (*syn* erythema pernio) seasonal vasospasm (spasm of blood vessels) caused by cold. It mainly affects children and older people, and leads to congestion and swelling of the feet or hands. In the short, acute stage there is redness with severe itching and burning sensation. The chronic stage is characterized by dull redness and congestion in the affected area. The affected skin is easily damaged and healing is prolonged. ⇒ perniosis.

child abuse physical, sexual or emotional abuse or neglect of children by relatives or health and social care staff. ⇒ non-accidental injuries.

Chinese restaurant syndrome (Kwok's syndrome) postprandial disturbance due to eating the flavour enhancer monosodium glutamate, which is used as a food additive and to enhance flavours in Chinese cooking. The symptoms include flushing, headache and abdominal symptoms.

chiropodist *n* ⇒ podiatrist.

chiropody *n* ⇒ podiatry.

chiropractic *n* a technique of spinal manipulation, based on the principle that defects in vertebral alignment may result in various problems caused by functional changes in the nervous system.

chiropractor *n* a person who uses chiropractic techniques.

chi-square statistic (χ^2) a technique used to analyse the relationship between expected frequency and the actual frequency of data obtained. A test of statistical significance used to determine the probability of results occurring by chance. ⇒ non-parametric tests.

chlamydiae *npl* micro-organisms of the genus *Chlamydia*. They are intracellular parasites and have features common to both bacteria and viruses. *Chlamydia psittaci* infects birds and causes psittacosis in humans. ⇒ ornithosis. Subgroups of *Chlamydia trachomatis* cause genital tract infection in adults, and are sexually transmitted. In men, may be associated with urethritis, but infection is often symptomless; epididymitis may be a complication. In women, most infections are symptomless; about 20% of untreated women develop pelvic inflammatory disease with subsequent scarring of the uterine (fallopian) tubes with risk of infertility or of ectopic pregnancy. Reactive arthritis is an uncommon complication. Autoinoculation from the genital tract can cause conjunctivitis in adults. Chlamydial conjunctivitis and pneumonia in infants can result from infection during birth. Lymphogranuloma venereum is caused by a different subgroup of *Chlamydia trachomatis*. The micro-organism also causes trachoma.

chloasma *n* patchy brown discoloration of the skin, especially the face. Can appear during pregnancy and during use of the oral contraceptive. ⇒ melasma.

chlorhexidine *n* a disinfectant solution which is effective against a wide range of bacteria. Used for general skin cleansing and disinfection, and hand decontamination, etc.

chloride *n* a salt of hydrochloric acid. A major anion in extracellular fluid.

chlorine *n* a greenish-yellow, irritating gaseous element. Powerful disinfectant, bleaching and deodorizing agent in the presence of moisture when nascent oxygen is liberated. Mainly used as hypochlorites, or other compounds which slowly liberate active chlorine.

chloroform *n* a heavy liquid, once used extensively as a general anaesthetic. Used as chloroform water as a flavouring and preservative in aqueous mixtures.

choanae *npl* funnel-shaped openings. ⇒ nares—**choana** *sing*, **choanal** *adj*.

chocolate cyst an endometrial cyst containing altered blood. The ovaries are the most usual site.

cholagogue *n* a drug which increases the flow of bile into the intestine.

cholangiography *n* rarely performed radiographic examination of hepatic, cystic and bile ducts. Can be performed: (a) after oral or intravenous administration of radiopaque substance, (b) by direct injection at operation to detect any further stones in the ducts, (c) during or after operation by way of a T-tube in the common bile duct, (d) by means of an injection via the skin on the anterior abdominal wall and the liver, when it is called percutaneous transhepatic cholangiography (PTC).

⇒ endoscopic retrograde cholangiopancreatography.

cholangitis *n* inflammation of the bile ducts.

cholecalciferol *n* vitamin D$_3$. An essential precursor of the active forms of vitamin D.

cholecystectomy *n* surgical removal of the gallbladder. *laparoscopic cholecystectomy* removal of the gallbladder using minimally invasive surgical techniques.

cholecystenterostomy *n* literally, the establishment of an artificial opening (anastomosis) between the gallbladder and the small intestine. Specific terminology more frequently used.

cholecystitis *n* inflammation of the gallbladder.

cholecystoduodenal *adj* pertaining to the gallbladder and duodenum as an anastomosis between them.

cholecystoduodenostomy *n* the establishment of an anastomosis between the gallbladder and the duodenum.

cholecystography *n* rarely performed radiographic examination of the gallbladder after administration of opaque contrast medium. Superseded by CT and MRI.

cholecystojejunostomy *n* an anastomosis between the gallbladder and the jejunum.

cholecystokinin (CCK) *n* a hormone that contracts the gallbladder and relaxes the sphincter of Oddi thus allowing bile into the duodenum, and stimulates the secretion of pancreatic enzymes. Secreted by the duodenal mucosa.

cholecystolithiasis *n* the presence of stone or stones in the gallbladder.

cholecystostomy *n* a surgically established fistula between the gallbladder and the abdominal surface; used to provide drainage, in empyema of the gallbladder.

cholecystotomy *n* incision into the gallbladder.

choledochoduodenal *adj* pertaining to the bile ducts and duodenum, e.g. *choledochoduodenal fistula*.

choledochography *n* cholangiography.

choledochojejunostomy *n* an anastomosis between the bile duct and the jejunum.

choledocholithiasis *n* the presence of a gallstone or gallstones in the extrahepatic bile ducts.

choledocholithotomy *n* surgical removal of a stone from the common bile duct.

choledochoscope *n* endoscopic instrument used to examine the lumen of the biliary tree (bile ducts).

choledochoscopy *n* endoscopic examination of the biliary tree.

choledochostomy *n* drainage of the common bile duct using a T-tube, usually after exploration for a stone.

choledochotomy *n* incision into the common bile duct.

cholelithiasis *n* the presence or formation of gallstones in the gallbladder or bile ducts.

cholera *n* acute enteritis occurring in Africa and Asia, where it is endemic and epidemic. It is caused by the bacterium *Vibrio cholerae* and is associated with faecal contamination of water, overcrowding and insanitary conditions. There is diarrhoea (rice-water stools) accompanied by agonizing cramp and vomiting, resulting in dehydration, electrolyte imbalance and severe collapse. High mortality rates without adequate fluid and electrolyte replacement.

choleric temperament one of the four classical types of temperament, hasty and with a propensity to emotional outbursts.

cholestasis *n* an obstruction to the flow of bile. It produces jaundice, dark urine, pale stools, metallic taste and pruritus. *extrahepatic cholestasis* caused by a blockage to a large duct, e.g. the common bile duct, by a gallstone or cancer of the pancreas. *intrahepatic cholestasis* caused by blockage of the small bile ducts within the liver, such as in hepatitis or cirrhosis—**cholestatic** *adj*.

cholesteatoma *n* a benign encysted tumour containing squamous epithelial debris. Mainly occurs in the middle ear—**cholesteatomatous** *adj*.

cholesterol *n* a sterol found in many tissues. It is an important component of cell membranes and is the precursor of many biological molecules, such as steroid hormones. High levels in the blood are linked with the development of arterial disease and some types of gallstones. ⇒ hypercholesterolaemia.

cholesterosis *n* abnormal deposition of cholesterol.

cholic acid a bile acid.

choline *n* a chemical found in animal tissues as a component of phospholipids; has an important influence on the production of the neurotransmitter acetylcholine. Experimental choline deficiency affects memory.

cholinergic *adj* applied to nerves that release acetylcholine as their neurotransmitter. They include those innervating voluntary skeletal muscle, all parasympathetic nerves and a few postganglionic sympathetic nerves. ⇒ adrenergic. *cholinergic crisis* severe muscle weakness and respiratory failure resulting from overtreatment with anticholinesterase drugs. *cholinergic receptors* receptor sites on the effector structures innervated by parasympathetic and voluntary motor nerves. The receptors may be muscarinic or nicotinic depending on their response to acetylcholine. They may be excitatory or inhibitory depending on their location. Both muscarinic and nicotinic receptors are further subdivided. ⇒ edrophonium test.

cholinesterase *n* an enzyme that inactivates acetylcholine at nerve endings.

chondritis *n* inflammation of cartilage.

chondrocostal *adj* pertaining to the costal cartilages and ribs.

chondrodynia *n* pain in a cartilage.

chondrolysis *n* dissolution of cartilage—**chondrolytic** *adj*.

chondroma *n* a benign tumour of cartilage.

chondromalacia *n* softening of cartilage.

chondrosarcoma *n* malignant tumour of cartilage—**chondrosarcomata** *pl*, **chondrosarcomatous** *adj*.

chondrosternal *adj* pertaining to the costal cartilages and sternum.

chordee *n* angulation of the penis associated with hypospadias.

chordotomy ⇒ cordotomy.

chorea *n* describes irregular and jerky dance-like movements, beyond the patient's control. Chorea may follow childhood rheumatic fever *Sydenham's chorea*, but usually results from a disorder or drug affecting the basal nuclei. In adults, chorea is a feature of the inherited condition Huntington's disease and the administration of drugs including the phenothiazines and L-dopa used in parkinsonism—**choreal, choreic** *adj*.

choreiform *adj* resembling chorea.

choriocarcinoma *n* (*syn* chorionepithelioma) a malignant tumour of chorionic cells; develops following normal pregnancy (rarely), miscarriage or evacuation of a hydatidiform mole. A sensitive (though not specific) tumour marker is human chorionic gonadotrophin (HCG). Choriocarcinoma is usually chemosensitive and curable.

chorion *n* the outer membrane forming the sac that contains the amniotic fluid and the fetus—**chorial, chorionic** *adj. chorion biopsy* ⇒ amnion, chorionic villus sampling.

chorionepithelioma ⇒ choriocarcinoma.

chorionic *adj* pertaining to the chorion. *chorionic gonadotrophin* ⇒ human chorionic gonadotrophin. *chorionic villi* vascular projections from the chorion from which the fetal part of the placenta is formed. Through which substances such as nutrients and waste diffuse between maternal and fetal blood and vice versa.

chorionic villus sampling (CVS) also known as chorion or chorionic villus biopsy. A prenatal screening test for chromosomal and other inherited disorders. Samples of fetal tissue are obtained via the cervix for the detection of genetic abnormalities during early pregnancy (around 11 weeks).

chorioretinal *adj* pertaining to the choroid and the retina.

chorioretinitis *n* (*syn* retinochoroiditis) inflammation of the choroid and retina.

choroid *n* the middle pigmented, vascular coat of the posterior five-sixths of the eyeball, continuous with the iris in front (⇒ Figure 15). It lies between the sclera externally and the retina internally, and prevents the passage of light rays—**choroidal** *adj.*

choroiditis *n* inflammation of the choroid.

choroid plexus specialized capillaries in the cerebral ventricles that produce cerebrospinal fluid.

Christmas disease ⇒ haemophilias.

Christmas factor factor IX (or antihaemophiliac factor B) in the coagulation cascade.

chromatid *n* one of the strands that result from the duplication of chromosomes during nuclear division.

chromatin *n* the threads of DNA and protein that form the substance of chromosomes.

chromatography *n* analytical methods used to separate and identify substances in a complex mixture based on their differential movement through a two-phase system. Include: gel filtration chromatography, gas chromatography and ion exchange chromatography.

chromium (Cr) *n* an essential element required in very small amounts in the diet. It potentiates the action of insulin in carbohydrate, lipid and protein metabolism. Symptoms of chromium deficiency include impaired glucose tolerance.

chromosome *n* the genetic material present in the nucleus of the cell. During the preparation for cell division chromosomes appear as microscopic threads. They contain strands of DNA molecules or genes. Each species has a constant number; humans have 23 pairs (46) in each somatic cell: 22 pairs of autosomes and 1 pair of sex chromosomes (males have XY and females have XX). Mature gametes, however, have half the usual number (haploid) which results from the reduction division during meiosis. The 23 unpaired chromosomes inherited from each parent unite to produce an embryo with 46 chromosomes (diploid). Genetic sex is determined by the male gamete and depends on whether the oocyte is fertilized by a sperm that contributes a Y chromosome (genetic male) or an X chromosome (genetic female). Some genetic material is also present in organelles, such as the mitochondria—**chromosomal** *adj.* ⇒ meiosis, mitosis.

chronic *adj* lingering, lasting, opposed to acute. The word does not imply anything about the severity of the condition. *chronic fatigue syndrome* ⇒ benign myalgic encephalomyelitis. *chronic heart failure* ⇒ congestive heart failure. *chronic leukaemia* ⇒ leukaemia. ⇒ chronic obstructive pulmonary disease—**chronicity** *n,* **chronically** *adv.*

chronic injury an injury with long onset and duration.

chronic obstructive pulmonary disease (COPD) group of obstructive lung diseases where airway resistance is increased with impaired airflow, e.g. pulmonary emphysema and chronic bronchitis. Defined on spirometric grounds as an FEV_1 <80% and an FEV_1:FVC ratio <70%. Usually seen as a long-term sequela of smoking. Genetic factors include α1-antitrypsin deficiency, and more recently, family clustering studies suggest other genetic susceptibility factors.

chronological age a person's age in years.

chronotherapy *n* the administration of treatment modalities, such as chemotherapy or radiotherapy, at the most effective time.

chunking *n* the organization and coding of 'chunks' of data/information that facilitates an increase in the effective capacity of short-term memory, which can only store around seven items of information.

Chvostek's sign excessive twitching of the face on tapping the facial nerve: a sign of tetany.

chyle *n* fatty, milky fluid formed from chylomicrons within the lymphatic lacteals of the intestinal villi—**chylous** *adj*.

chylomicron *n* tiny particles formed from triglycerides, lipoproteins and cholesterol and lipoproteins within the intestinal mucosa following the absorption of digested fat. They form chyle within the lacteals.

chylothorax *n* leakage of chyle from the thoracic duct into the pleural cavity.

chyluria *n* chyle in the urine, which can occur in some nematode infestations, either when a fistulous communication is established between a lymphatic vessel and the urinary tract or when the distension of the urinary lymphatics causes them to rupture—**chyluric** *adj*.

chyme *n* partially digested food which is acidic passes from the stomach to the duodenum. Its acidity controls the pylorus to regulate the amount entering the duodenum.

chymotrypsin *n* an inactive proteolytic enzyme secreted by the pancreas: it is activated by trypsin.

cicatrix *n* ⇒ scar.

cilia *npl* **1** the eyelashes. **2** microscopic hair-like projections from certain epithelial cells. Membranes containing such cells, e.g. those lining the trachea and uterine (fallopian) tubes, are known as ciliated membranes—**cilium** *sing*, **ciliary, ciliated, cilial** *adj*.

ciliary *adj* hair-like, *ciliary body* a specialized structure in the eye connecting the anterior choroid to the iris (⇒ Figure 15); it is composed of the ciliary muscles and processes. *ciliary muscles* fine muscle fibres arranged in a circular manner. They control accommodation. *ciliary processes* about 70 in number, they secrete aqueous humour.

Cimex *n* a genus of insects of the family Cimicidae. *Cimex lectularius* is the common bedbug.

CIN *abbr* cervical intraepithelial neoplasia.

cinchona *n* the bark from which quinine is obtained.

cinchonism *n* quininism.

C1 inhibitor (C1 INH) an essential regulator of the classical complement pathway.

circadian rhythm any rhythm with a periodicity of 24 h.

circinata *n* ⇒ tinea.

circinate *adj* in the form of a circle or segment of a circle, e.g. the skin eruptions of late syphilis, ringworm, etc.

circulation *n* passage in a circle. Usually means circulation of the blood—**circulatory** *adj*, **circulate** *vi, vt*. *circulation of bile* ⇒ enterohepatic circulation; *circulation of blood* the passage of blood from heart to arteries to capillaries to veins and back to heart; *circulation of cerebrospinal fluid* takes place from the ventricles of the brain to the cisterna magna, whence the fluid bathes the surface of the brain and the spinal cord, including its central canal. It is absorbed into the blood in the cerebral venous sinuses. *circulation of lymph* lymph is collected from the tissue spaces and passed in the lymphatic capillaries, vessels, nodes and ducts to be returned to the bloodstream. *pulmonary circulation* circulation of deoxygenated blood from right ventricle to pulmonary artery, to lungs and back to left atrium of heart. *systemic circulation* circulation of oxygenated blood from left ventricle to aorta, to tissues and back to right atrium of heart.

circumcision *n* excision of the prepuce or foreskin of the penis, usually for religious or cultural reasons. The operation is sometimes required for phimosis or paraphimosis. *female circumcision* excision of the clitoris, labia minora and labia majora. The extent of cutting varies from country to country. The simplest form is clitoridectomy; the next form entails excision of the prepuce, clitoris and all or part of the labia minora. The most extensive form, infibulation, involves excision of clitoris, labia minora and labia majora. The vulval lips are sutured together but total obliteration of the vaginal introitus is prevented by inserting a piece of wood or reed to preserve a small passage for urine and menstrual fluid.

circumcorneal *adj* (*syn* limbal) around the cornea.

circumoral *adj* surrounding the mouth. *circumoral pallor* a pale appearance of the skin around the mouth, in contrast to the flushed cheeks. A characteristic of scarlet fever—**circumorally** *adv.*

circumvallate *adj* surrounded by a raised ring, as the large circumvallate papillae at the base of the tongue.

cirrhosis *n* hardening of an organ. There are degenerative changes in the tissues with resulting fibrosis. *cirrhosis of liver* increasing in prosperous countries. Damage to liver cells can be from viruses, other micro-organisms or toxic substances and dietary deficiencies interfering with the nutrition of liver cells—often the result of alcohol misuse. Associated developments include ascites, obstruction of the circulation through the hepatic portal vein with haematemesis, jaundice and enlargement of the spleen—**cirrhotic** *adj.*

cisterna *n* any closed space serving as a reservoir for a body fluid. *cisterna chyli* the pear-shaped commencement of the thoracic duct. It receives lymph. *cisterna magna* is a subarachnoid space in the cleft between the cerebellum and medulla oblongata—**cisternal** *adj.*

cisternal puncture insertion of a special hollow needle with stylet between the occiput and atlas, into the cisterna magna. One method of obtaining cerebrospinal fluid but rarely used. ⇒ lumbar puncture.

citric acid an organic acid present in citrus fruit such as oranges and in soft fruit. *citric acid cycle* ⇒ Krebs cycle.

civil law law relating to non-criminal matters. *civil action* proceedings brought in the civil courts. *civil wrong* act or omission which can be pursued in the civil courts by the person who has suffered the wrong.

CJD *abbr* Creutzfeldt–Jakob disease.

clap *n* a slang term for gonorrhoea.

clasp-knife phenomenon a pathological manifestation of the stretch reflex in which great resistance at the beginning of passive movement suddenly collapses; characteristic of spasticity.

class *n* the socioeconomic diversity between groups that explains the differences in their level of wealth and influence. ⇒ social class.

claudication *n* limping caused by interference with the blood supply to the legs. The cause may be spasm or disease of the vessels themselves. In *intermittent claudication* the patient experiences severe pain in the legs (calves or thighs) when walking; after a short rest the patient is able to continue.

claustrophobia *n* a fear of enclosed spaces—**claustrophobic** *adj.*

clavicle *n* the collar bone (⇒ Figure 2)—**clavicular** *adj.*

clavus *n* a corn. ⇒ callus.

claw-foot *adj*, *n* ⇒ pes cavus.

claw-hand *n* the hand is flexed and contracted giving a claw-like appearance; the condition may be due to injury or disease.

cleanser *n*, *adj* (describes) agents that have cleansing properties. Drugs such as cetrimide are both disinfectant and cleansing. Used to remove dirt, grease, etc., from the skin or wounds, and for removing crusts and other debris from skin lesions.

clearance *n* the ability of the kidney to remove a specific substance from the blood. *renal clearance* used to measure glomerular filtration rate and kidney function by calculating the volume of blood cleared of a substance such as creatinine, in a given time, usually one minute.

cleft lip a congenital defect in the lip; a fissure extending from the margin of the lip to the nostril; may be single or double, and is often associated with cleft palate.

cleft palate congenital failure of fusion between the right and left palatal processes. Often associated with cleft lip.

Clifton Assessment Procedures for the Elderly a series of tests which measure cognitive function as well as behaviour.

climacteric *n* a period of time during which ovarian activity declines and eventually ceases. In most women it occurs between the mid forties to mid fifties. The stopping of menstruation is a single event during the climacteric. ⇒ menopause.

clinical *adj* pertaining to a clinic. Describes the practical observation and treatment of sick persons as opposed to theoretical study.

clinical audit critical and systematic analysis of the quality of clinical care and treatment. It includes diagnostic procedures, treatment, resource use and outputs including quality of life.

clinical governance the framework within which all NHS organizations are accountable for their services, and are required to operate an active programme of continuous quality improvement within an overall, coherent framework of cost-effective service delivery.

clinical guidelines systematically developed statements that help the practitioner and patient in making decisions about care. ⇒ evidence-based practice.

clinical thermometer previously, glass and mercury thermometers of various types were used. These have mostly been replaced by safer alternatives, such as electronic probes, e.g. tympanic membrane thermometers, and single-use thermometers.

clitoridectomy *n* the surgical removal of the clitoris.

clitoriditis *n* inflammation of the clitoris.

clitoris *n* a small erectile organ situated at anterior junction of the labia minora. Involved in the female sexual response.

cloaca *n* in osteomyelitis, the opening through the involucrum which discharges pus—**cloacal** *adj*.

clone *n* a group of genetically identical cells or organisms derived from a single cell or common ancestor.

clonic *adj* ⇒ clonus.

clonus *n* a series of intermittent muscular contractions and relaxations. ⇒ tonic *opp*, ankle clonus—**clonic** *adj*, **clonicity** *n*. ⇒ myoclonus.

closed chain exercise ⇒ closed kinetic chain.

closed fracture ⇒ fracture.

closed kinetic chain in sports medicines describes a motion during which the distal segment of the extremity is weight bearing or otherwise fixed, e.g. a squat (lower limb) or a press up (upper limb). ⇒ open kinetic chain.

Clostridium *n* a genus of bacteria. They are large Gram-positive, spore-forming anaerobic bacilli found as commensals of the gut of animals and humans and as saprophytes in the soil. Many species are pathogenic due to the production of exotoxins, e.g. *Clostridium botulinum* (botulism); *C. difficile* (pseudomembranous colitis); *C. perfringens (welchii)* (gas gangrene); *C. tetani* (tetanus).

clubbed fingers a thickening and broadening of the bulbous fleshy portion of the fingers under the nails. The cause is not known but it occurs in people who have chronic heart and/or lung disease.

clue cell epithelial cell to whose surface Gram-variable, Gram-negative and Gram-positive bacteria adhere. A microscopical feature of bacterial vaginosis.

club foot *n* a congenital malformation, either unilateral or bilateral. ⇒ talipes.

clumping *n* agglutination.

Clutton's joints joints which show symmetrical swelling usually painless, the knees often being involved. Associated with congenital syphilis.

CMV *abbr* **1** cytomegalovirus. **2** controlled mandatory ventilation.

CNS *abbr* central nervous system.

CO (CI) *abbr* cardiac output (cardiac index).

coach's finger in sports medicine a colloquial term used to describe the dislocation of the proximal interphalangeal joint leading to a fixed flexion deformity of the finger.

coagulase *n* an enzyme produced by some staphylococci: it coagulates plasma and is used to classify staphylococci as coagulase-negative or coagulase-positive.

coagulation the third of four overlapping processes involved in haemostasis. Coagulation (clotting) occurs through a series of complex reactions that use enzyme cascade amplification to start the formation of a fibrin clot to stop bleeding.

There are two pathways/systems, intrinsic and extrinsic, which converge to follow a common final pathway. Coagulation starts when platelets break down, tissue is damaged and thromboplastins are released. Various factors are involved in coagulation: I, fibrinogen; II, prothrombin; III, tissue thromboplastin; IV, calcium ions; V, labile factor (proaccelerin); VII, stable factor (proconvertin); VIII, antihaemophilic factor (AHF); IX, Christmas factor; X, Stuart–Prower factor; XI, plasma thromboplastin antecedent; XII, Hageman factor; and XIII, fibrin-stabilizing factor. During the final common pathway, inactive prothrombin is converted to thrombin, the active enzyme. Thrombin converts soluble fibrinogen to insoluble fibrin, which forms a network of fibres in which blood cells are caught to form the clot. ⇒ fibrinolysis, haemostasis, platelet plug.

coalesce *vi* to grow together; to unite into a mass. Often used to describe the development of a skin eruption, when discrete areas of affected skin coalesce to form sheets of a similar appearance—**coalescence** *n*, **coalescent** *adj*.

coal tar obtained by the distillation of coal. Used in topical preparations for the treatment of psoriasis and eczema.

coarctation *n* contraction, stricture, narrowing; applied to a vessel or canal. *coarctation of the aorta* congenital narrowing of the aorta, commonly affecting the area just after the origin of the left subclavian artery. ⇒ Figure 9.

coarse tremor violent trembling.

cobalamins *npl* a group of molecules containing a cobalt atom and four pyrrole units. A constituent of substances having vitamin B_{12} activity. ⇒ cyanocobalamin.

cobalt (Co) *n* an essential trace element, utilized as a constituent of vitamin B_{12} (cobalamins). Required for healthy red blood cell production and proper neurological function. *cobalt-60* a radioactive isotope of cobalt which is used as a source of radiation in teletherapy.

COC *abbr* combined oral contraceptive.

cocaine *n* a powerful local anaesthetic obtained from the leaves of the coca plant. It is a controlled drug which is highly addictive and subject to considerable criminal misuse. ⇒ Appendix 5. Toxic, especially to the brain; may cause agitation, disorientation and convulsions. *crack cocaine* a highly potent and addictive form.

coccidioidomycosis *n* infection caused by the fungus *Coccidioides immitis*. Occurs in Central and South America, and the southern United States.

coccus *n* a spherical bacterium—**cocci** *pl*, **coccal, coccoid** *adj*.

coccydynia *n* pain in the region of the coccyx.

coccygeal nerve ⇒ Figure 11.

coccygectomy *n* surgical removal of the coccyx.

coccyx *n* the last bone of the vertebral column (⇒ Figure 3). It is composed of four or five rudimentary vertebrae, cartilaginous at birth, ossification being completed at about the 30th year—**coccygeal** *adj*.

cochlea *n* a spiral canal resembling the interior of a snail shell, in the anterior part of the bony labyrinth of the ear (⇒ Figure 13)—**cochlear** *adj*.

code of practice the guidelines setting out how healthcare professionals should fulfil their roles, duties, obligations and responsibilities, such as those produced by the statutory bodies whose functions are to regulate the registration and practice of healthcare professionals, e.g. General Medical Council.

codon *n* in genetics, the three complementary bases carried by messenger RNA (mRNA) involved in protein synthesis (transcription stage). ⇒ anticodon.

coeliac *adj* relating to the abdominal cavity; applied to arteries and a nerve plexus. *coeliac disease* (*syn* gluten-induced enteropathy) due to intolerance to the protein gluten in wheat and rye, the gliadin fraction being harmful. This results in subtotal villous atrophy of the mucosa of the small intestine and the malabsorption syndrome. Symptoms may become apparent at any age or patients may be asymptomatic. Treatment is with gluten-free diet.

coenzyme *n* an enzyme activator, e.g. substances formed from the B vitamins.

coffee ground vomit vomit containing blood, which in its partially digested state resembles coffee grounds. Indicative of slow upper gastrointestinal bleeding ⇒ haematemesis.

cognition *n* awareness; one of the three aspects of mind. A general term that describes all the psychological processes by which individuals gain awareness and knowledge about their environment—**cognitive** *adj*. ⇒ affection, conation.

cognitive therapy an approach to the psychological treatment of some mental health problems such as anxiety-related disorders. It concentrates on, and is effective through, correcting the individual's cognitive dysfunctions, such as errors in thinking and poor problem-solving.

cogwheel rigidity a pathological pattern of resistance to passive movement of a limb which yields in a series of jerks, observed in Parkinson's patients, thought to be due to tremor superimposed on lead pipe rigidity.

cohort *n* a group of people who have some common feature or characteristic, e.g. year group at university. *cohort study* research that studies a population that shares a common feature, such as occupation.

coitus *n* insertion of the erect penis into the vagina; the act of sexual intercourse or copulation. *coitus interruptus* removal from the vagina of the penis before ejaculation of semen as a means of contraception. The method is considered unsatisfactory as it is not only unreliable but can lead to sexual disharmony—**coital** *adj*.

cold abscess ⇒ abscess.

cold flow *n* ⇒ creep.

cold sore *n* oral herpes simplex.

colectomy *n* excision of part or the whole of the colon.

colic *n* severe pain resulting from periodic spasm in an abdominal organ. *biliary colic* ⇒ biliary. *intestinal colic* abnormal peristaltic movement of an irritated gut. *renal colic* spasm of ureter due to the presence of a stone. *uterine colic* dysmenorrhoea—**colicky** *adj*.

coliform *adj* describes any of the enterobacteria (intestinal bacteria) such as *Escherichia coli*.

colitis *n* inflammation of the colon. May be acute or chronic, and may be accompanied by ulcerative lesions. ⇒ inflammatory bowel disease, ulcerative colitis.

collagen *n* the main protein constituent of white fibrous tissue of skin, tendon, bone, cartilage and all connective tissue. *collagen diseases* there is inflammation of unknown aetiology affecting collagen and small blood vessels. They involve autoimmune responses and include dermatomyositis, polyarteritis nodosa, rheumatoid arthritis, scleroderma and systemic lupus erythematosus (SLE).

collapse 1 the 'falling in' of a hollow organ or vessel, e.g. collapse of lung from change of air pressure inside or outside the organ. **2** a vague term describing physical or nervous prostration.

collapsing pulse also known as Corrigan's pulse. The water-hammer pulse of aortic regurgitation with high initial upthrust which quickly falls away.

collar-bone *n* the clavicle.

collateral circulation an alternative route provided for the blood by secondary blood vessels when a primary vessel is blocked.

Colles' fracture a break at the lower end of the radius following a fall on the outstretched hand. The backward displacement of the hand produces the 'dinner fork' deformity. A common fracture in older women and associated with osteoporosis.

collision sport individual or team sports during which the participants use their bodies to deter or block opponents, thereby relying on the physical dominance of one athlete over another.

collodion *n* a solution forming a flexible film on the skin. Previously used as a protective dressing.

colloid *n* glue-like. A non-crystalline chemical; diffusible but not soluble in water; unable to pass through a semipermeable membrane. Some drugs can be prepared in their colloidal form. *colloid degeneration* that which results in the formation of gelatinous material, as in tumours. *colloid goitre* enlargement of the thyroid gland caused by the presence of viscid, iodine-containing colloid within the gland.

colloid solutions ones containing large molecules used intravenously in the treatment of shock.

coloboma *n* a developmental discontinuity in a layer of the eyeball caused by failure of closure of the optic fissure. Can also occur in the eyelids—**colobomata** *pl*.

colon *n* the large bowel extending from the caecum to the rectum (⇒ Figure 18b). Comprises the ascending, transverse, descending and sigmoid colon. ⇒ flexure; *spasmodic colon* ⇒ megacolon—**colonic** *adj.*

colonization *n* the installation of micro-organisms in a specific environment, such as a body site with only minimal or no response. There is no disease or symptoms, but colonization leads to the formation of a reservoir of micro-organisms that may be a source of infection—**colonize** *vt.*

colonoscopy *n* use of an endoscope to view the colonic mucosa—**colonoscopic** *adj*, **colonoscopically** *adv.*

colony *n* a mass of bacteria resulting from the multiplication of one or more micro-organisms. Containing many millions of individual micro-organisms it may be visible to the unaided eye; its physical features are often characteristic of the species.

colony stimulating factors (CSF) growth factors that cause blood stem cells to produce a specific cell line.

colorectal *adj* pertaining to the colon and the rectum.

colostomy *n* a surgically established fistula between the colon and the surface of the abdomen; a type of stoma that discharges faeces.

colostrum *n* fluid secreted by the breasts during late pregnancy and in the 3 days following parturition. It is a source of maternal antibodies, and has a different composition to true milk, i.e. more protein, but less fat and lactose.

colotomy *n* incision into the colon.

colour blindness dysfunction in or absence of a photoreceptor subtype (cones) stimulated by red, green or blue light, leading to difficulty distinguishing between certain colours. ⇒ achromatopsia.

colpitis *n* inflammation of the vagina.

colpocele *n* protrusion or prolapse of either the bladder or rectum so that it presses on the vaginal wall.

colpocentesis *n* withdrawal of fluid from the vagina, as in haematocolpos.

colpohysterectomy *n* removal of the uterus through the vagina. ⇒ hysterectomy.

colpoperineorrhaphy *n* the surgical repair of vaginal injury and deficient perineum.

colpophotography *n* filming the cervix using a camera and colposcope.

colporrhaphy *n* surgical repair of the vagina. An anterior colporrhaphy repairs a cystocele and a posterior colporrhaphy repairs a rectocele.

colposcope *n* a binocular instrument used to obtain a high power view of the cervix in cases of abnormal cervical smears. Used for diagnostic procedures and local treatments to the cervix—**colposcopy** *n*, **colposcopically** *adv.*

colposuspension *n* surgical procedure involving placement of sutures between the vaginal fornices and the pectineal ligaments for genuine stress incontinence.

colpotomy *n* incision of the vaginal wall. A posterior colpotomy drains an abscess in the pouch of Douglas through the vagina.

coma *n* a state of unrousable unconsciousness, the severity of which can be assessed by corneal and pupillary reflexes and withdrawal responses to painful stimuli. ⇒ Glasgow Coma Scale—**comatose** *adj.*

comedone, comedo *n* a worm-like cast formed of sebum which occupies the outlet of a hair follicle in the skin, a feature of acne vulgaris. Open comedones have a black colour because of pigmentation (blackheads). Closed comedones are closed cysts (whiteheads)—**comedones** *pl.*

commensals *npl* parasitic micro-organisms adapted to grow on the skin and mucous surfaces of the host, forming part of the normal flora. Some commensals are potentially pathogenic, e.g. bowel commensals that cause urinary tract infection.

comminuted fracture ⇒ fracture.

Commission for Health Improvement (CHI) a body with statutory powers to inspect and support the implementation of clinical governance arrangements in Health Authorities and NHS Trusts. Their remit also includes targeted support when requested by organizations with a specific problem, and in more serious situations they may intervene by direction of the Secretary of State or at the request of Health Authorities, NHS Trusts or Primary Care Trusts.

commissioning *n* a complex process that aims to ensure that a specific population has an appropriate level of service provision. The stages include a needs assessment that is used to determine priorities, taking into account the overall national policy guidance from government. On completion of this process, an appropriate range of services are purchased from relevant providers. The final stage is evaluation.

Committee on Safety of Medicines (CSM) in the UK the body that monitors drug safety and advises the licensing authority regarding the safety, efficacy and quality of medicines. ⇒ yellow card reporting.

common variable immunodeficiency (CVID) one of the primary antibody deficiency syndromes, presenting in children or adulthood and associated with recurrent infections, autoimmunity, and an increased risk of malignancy.

communicable *adj* transmissible directly or indirectly from one person to another.

communicating *n* the exchange of information between at least two individuals. Most often accomplished by the use of language: verbal, which can be spoken, hand written, word processed/typed, printed or displayed on a screen; or nonverbal, which allows the transmission of attitudes, values and beliefs that are appropriate and relevant to the information exchanged.

community *n* a social group defined by geographical boundaries and/or common values and interests. Also implies shared relationships, lifestyles, and a greater frequency and intimacy of contact among those who live in a community.

community care the care and support of individuals in community settings. Such care is delivered by health and social care professionals and unpaid carers such as family and neighbours. The community or primary care setting is increasingly important in the development and delivery of health services. ⇒ Primary Care Trust.

community development whole-community initiatives that enable individual communities to assess their particular needs, such as for health care, and decide on what action should be taken by the community. In the broadest sense, community care services could be provided by the 'community' on a voluntary basis, or by statutory organizations in residential settings or by professionals working in the community. For example,

the development of adequate provision of (community) care services such as the treatment of long-term sick and frail people in their own homes. This can be interpreted to cover personal, domiciliary and social care as well as medical or nursing care. The community includes family, friends and community self-help.

community occupational therapist an occupational therapist who works in the community to carry out home visits and home assessments and to provide services, including the provision of adaptive equipment and adaptations to the environment.

comorbidity *n* coexistence of two or more diseases.

comparative study research study that compares two separate populations.

compartment syndrome 1 swelling of the muscles in one of the limb compartments leading to ischaemia and necrosis of muscle tissue. Treatment is fasciotomy. **2** in sports medicine a term used to describe a condition where increased intramuscular pressure brought on by activity impedes blood flow and function of the tissues within that intermuscular compartment.

compatibility *n* suitability; congruity. The ability of a substance to mix with another without unfavourable results, e.g. two medicines, blood plasma and cells—**compatible** *adj*.

compensation *n* **1** a mental mechanism, employed by a person to cover up a weakness, by exaggerating a more socially acceptable behaviour trait. **2** the state of counterbalancing a functional or structural defect, e.g. cardiac compensation, where the heart muscle enlarges by hypertrophy to maintain cardiac output in chronic heart failure.

compensatory techniques adaptive techniques using relatively intact skills to compensate for physical or cognitive deficits in performance. This might include the provision of adaptive equipment, adaptations to the environment, or new methods of performing tasks.

complement *n* a system of over 20 serum proteins involved in cytolysis, opsonization, phagocytosis and anaphylaxis. Several cascading systems, including the classical pathway (antibody mediated), alternate pathway and a third pathway, converge resulting in the formation of a multimeric (composed of multiple parts) membrane attack complex capable of lysing cells. The system is regulated by numerous proteins and cell surface receptors. *complement fixation test* a test in which complement fixation is found. It indicates the presence of a particular specific antigen.

complemental air the extra air that can be drawn into the lungs by deep inspiration.

complementary feed a bottle feed of infant formula milk given to an infant to complement breast feeding.

complementary medicine a range of therapies currently regarded as adjuncts to conventional medicine. These include: acupuncture, aromatherapy, homeopathy, osteopathy and yoga. ⇒ integrated medicine.

complete abortion ⇒ miscarriage.

complex *n* a psychodynamic term meaning a series of emotionally charged ideas repressed because they conflict with ideas acceptable to the individual. ⇒ Electra complex, Oedipus complex.

compliance *n* the acceptance (understanding and remembering) of and following health (medical) advice or specific regimens of treatment. Two main models are proposed for health professionals to increase compliance when giving health (medical) advice: (a) the adherence model suggesting that there are patient centred factors that affect the process of following advice, such as locus of control, social support and disruption of life style; (b) the cognitive model where compliance is influenced by the level of understanding, satisfaction with and recall of the advice given.

complicated fracture ⇒ fracture.

complication *n* in medicine, an accident or second disease arising in the course of a primary disease; it can be fatal.

compos mentis of sound mind. Mentally competent is now the preferred term.

compound *n* a substance composed of two or more elements, chemically combined in a definitive proportion to form a new substance which displays new properties.

compound (open) fracture ⇒ fracture.

comprehension *n* mental grasp of ideas, their meaning and relationships.

compress *n* usually refers to a folded pad of lint, gauze or other material used to arrest haemorrhage or apply pressure, cold, heat, moisture or medication. Used to reduce swelling or pain, such as a cold compress to ease a headache.

compression *n* the state of being compressed. Pressing or squeezing together. ⇒ intermittent pneumatic compression. *compression bandage/therapy* used in the management of venous leg ulcers to increase venous return and reduce venous hypertension. Compression stockings are used to prevent venous leg ulcers occurring where there is venous insufficiency, or to reduce the risk of deep vein thrombosis following surgery or immobility. ⇒ antiembolic hose. *compression fracture* ⇒ fracture.

compressive force a force applied along the length of a structure, causing the tissues to approximate one another. This force can be caused by muscular activity, weight bearing, gravity or external loading down the length of the bone. It is necessary for the development and growth of bone. If a large compressive force, which surpasses the stress limits of the structure, is applied, a fracture will occur.

compromise *n* in psychoanalysis, a mental mechanism whereby a conflict is evaded by disguising the repressed wish to make it acceptable in consciousness.

compulsion *n* an urge to carry out an act, recognized to be irrational. Resisting the urge leads to increasing tension which is only relieved by carrying out the act.

computed axial tomography ⇒ computed tomography.

computed tomography (CT) computer-constructed imaging technique of a thin slice through the body, derived from X-ray absorption data collected during a circular scanning motion.

conation *n* the will, desire or volition. The conscious tendency to action. One of the three aspects of mind. ⇒ affection, cognition.

concentric *adj* having a common centre or point. *concentric muscle work* the shortening of a muscle to pull its attachments closer together and produce movement at a joint. For example, the quadriceps muscles of the anterior thigh work concentrically to straighten the knee. ⇒ eccentric muscle work.

concept *n* the abstract idea or image of the properties of a class of objects. Results from the mental process of abstracting and recombining certain qualities or characteristics of a number of ideas.

conception *n* **1** the creation of a state of pregnancy: impregnation of the oocyte by the spermatozoon. **2** an abstract mental idea of anything—**conceptive** *adj*.

concha *n* ⇒ Figure 14.

concretion *n* a deposit of hard material; a calculus.

concussion *n* a condition resulting from a blow to the head characterized by headache, amnesia, memory loss and visual symptoms. ⇒ Glasgow Coma Scale.

condensation *n* the process of becoming more compact, e.g. the changing of a gas to a liquid.

conditioned reflex a reflex in which the response occurs, not to the sensory stimulus which caused it originally, but to another stimulus which the subject has learned to associate with the original stimulus: it can be acquired by training and repetition. In Pavlov's classic experiments, dogs learned to associate the sound of a bell with the sight and smell of food: even when food was not presented, salivation occurred at the sound of a bell.

conditioning *n* the encouragement of new (desirable) behaviour by modification of the stimulus/response associations. *classical conditioning* where the conditioned reflex occurs in response to a neutral stimulus, i.e. a conditioned reflex. *operant conditioning* the term used when there is a programme to reward (or withhold the reward) a response each time it occurs, so that given time, it occurs more (or less) frequently. ⇒ deconditioning.

condom *n* a latex sheath used as a male contraceptive. It protects both partners against sexually transmitted infections. *female condom* a polyurethane tube that fits inside the vagina to provide contraception and protection against STIs.

conduction *n* the transmission of heat, light, or sound waves through suitable media; also the passage of electrical currents and nerve impulses through body tissues—**conductivity** *n*.

conductor *n* a substance or medium which transmits heat, light, sound, electric current, etc. The degree of conductivity varies, some substances being good conductors, whereas others are non-conductors.

condyle *n* a rounded projection situated at the end of some bones, e.g. tibia.

condyloma *n* papilloma. *condylomata acuminata* fleshy, viral warts affecting the genital or anal areas. *condylomata lata* wart-like lesions found in moist areas of the body during the secondary stage of syphilis—**condylomata** *pl*, **condylomatous** *adj*.

cones *npl* photoreceptors in the retina, responsible for high definition colour vision in good light. ⇒ rods.

confabulation *n* a symptom common in delirium when there is impairment of memory for recent events. The gaps in the patient's memory are filled in with fabrications. ⇒ amnesic syndrome, Korsakoff's (Korsakov's) syndrome.

confidence interval in statistics, a level, e.g. 95%, that indicates the level of confidence that the test result, such as a mean, will occur within a specified range.

confidentiality *n* a legal and professional requirement to protect all confidential information concerning patients/clients obtained in the course of professional practice, and make disclosures only with consent, where required by specific legislation, or a court order, or where disclosure in the wider public interest is justified.

conflict *n* in psychoanalysis, the presence of two incompatible and contrasting wishes or emotions. When the conflict becomes intolerable, repression of the wishes may occur. Mental conflict and repression form the basic causes of many 'neuroses' especially hysteria.

confluence *n* becoming merged; flowing together; a uniting, as of adjacent lesions of a rash.

conformal therapy a system that allows the radiotherapy treatment volume to be shaped to conform to the shape of the tumour, permitting a high dose to be given to the tumour and a lesser dose to surrounding tissue than with conventional radiotherapy. Employs the use of a multi-leaf collimator.

conformity *n* a propensity to alter views and/or behaviour to better match the prevailing social norms in response to social pressure.

confounding factors extraneous factors, apart from the variables already allowed for, that distort research findings.

confusion *n* being out of touch with reality—associated with a clouding of consciousness. Occurs in a wide variety of mental illnesses, particularly organic disorders. Acute confusional states may have an acute medical cause, such as infection, anaemia, inappropriate medication, etc. Chronic confusion may have an insidious onset and be caused by an unnoticed chronic condition, e.g. hypothyroidism.

congenital *adj* of abnormal conditions, present at birth, often genetically determined ⇒ genetic. Existing before or at birth, usually associated with a defect or disease, e.g. developmental dysplasia of the hip (DDH) (previously known as congenital dislocation of the hip). *congenital heart disease* developmental abnormalities in the anatomy of the heart, resulting postnatally in imperfect circulation of blood and often manifested by murmurs, cyanosis, breathlessness and sweating. ⇒ 'blue baby'. *congenital syphilis* ⇒ syphilis.

congestion *n* hyperaemia. Passive congestion results from obstruction or slowing down of venous return, as in the lower limbs or the lungs—**congestive** *adj*, **congest** *vi, vt. congestive dysmenorrhoea* ⇒ dysmenorrhoea.

congestive heart failure a chronic inability of the heart to maintain an adequate output of blood from one or both ventricles, resulting in pulmonary congestion and overdistension of certain veins and organs with blood, and in an inadequate blood supply to the body tissues.

congruent *adj* when describing a visual field defect implies the defect affects the same area of the field in both eyes.

conization *n* removal of a cone-shaped part of the cervix by knife or cautery.

conjugate *n* a measurement of the bony pelvis. *diagonal conjugate* the clinical measurement taken in pelvic assessment, from the lower border of the symphysis pubis to the sacral promontory = 111–126 mm. It is 18.5 mm greater than *obstetrical conjugate*, the available space for the fetal head, i.e. the distance from the sacral promontory to the posterior surface of the top of the symphysis pubis = 108–114 mm. *true conjugate* the distance from the sacral promontory to the summit of the symphysis pubis = 110.5 mm.

conjunctiva *n* the delicate transparent membrane which lines the inner surface of the eyelids (palpebral conjunctiva) and reflects over the eyeball (bulbar or ocular conjunctiva)—**conjunctival** *adj*.

conjunctivitis *n* inflammation of the conjunctiva. Usually infective or allergic. Follicular and papillary types may indicate cause.

connective tissue the diverse group of tissue that includes adipose, areolar, bone, cartilage, blood and blood producing tissue, elastic, fibrous and reticular. *connective tissue massage* manipulations that stretch the superficial and deep connective tissue in order to stimulate the circulation.

Conn syndrome primary hyperaldosteronism. ⇒ hyperaldosteronism.

Conradi–Hünermann syndrome a skeletal dysplasia which is inherited as an autosomal dominant trait. Skeletal abnormalities are variable; they are present at birth. After the first few weeks, life expectancy is normal.

consanguinity *n* blood relationship. May be close (as between parent and child) or less so (as between cousins)—**consanguineous** *adj*.

conscientious objection a legal recognition that an individual is not bound to take part in some specific activities such as termination of pregnancy. It may also apply to other strongly held beliefs that are not acknowledged by law.

consciousness *n* a complex concept which implies that a person is consciously perceiving the environment through the five sensory organs, and responding to the perceptions. ⇒ anaesthesia, sleep.

consent *n* patients are legally required to consent to treatment, surgery and any intervention that requires physical contact. Consent may be verbal, written, or implied, i.e. by non-verbal communication.

However, where there are likely to be risks or disputes, written consent is advisable. It is the responsibility of the healthcare professional undertaking the procedure to provide a full explanation to the patient prior to treatment or surgery about what is involved and any additional measures that may be required and to obtain written consent. Previously this was the doctor concerned, but increasingly other healthcare professionals are undertaking treatments, e.g. endoscopy by nurses. If the patient is a minor, or incapable of giving informed consent, the next-of-kin must sign the consent form.

conservative treatment aims at preventing a condition from becoming worse without using radical measures. For example, the use of drug therapy rather than surgery.

consolidation *n* becoming solid, as, for instance, the state of the lung due to exudation and organization in lobar pneumonia.

constipation *n* an implied chronic condition of infrequent and often difficult evacuation of faeces due to insufficient high fibre food or fluid intake, immobility, or to sluggish or disordered action of the bowel musculature or nerve supply, or to habitual failure to empty the rectum. Other causes include pain on defaecation, inability to respond to the urge to defaecate, hypokalaemia, drugs such as iron preparations, pregnancy (hormonal), depression, colorectal cancer (alternating with diarrhoea) and some systemic diseases. *Acute constipation* signifies obstruction or paralysis of the gut of sudden onset.

consumption *n* **1** act of consuming or using up. **2** a once popular term for pulmonary tuberculosis, which 'consumed' the body—**consumptive** *adj.*

contact *n* **1** direct or indirect exposure to infection. **2** a person who has been so exposed. *contact lens* of glass or plastic, worn under the eyelids in direct contact with conjunctiva (in place of spectacles) for therapeutic or cosmetic purposes. *contact tracer* ⇒ health adviser.

contact sports individual or team sports in which contact between two players, although not an integral part of the game, is unavoidable.

contagious *adj* capable of transmitting infection or of being transmitted.

containment isolation separation of a patient with any sort of infection to prevent spread of the condition to others. ⇒ protective isolation, source isolation.

continent diversion surgical technique of bladder reconstruction by creation of a catheterizable pouch.

contingency fund an amount of money included in the costings of a project that would be used for some unplanned or unpredictable expense.

continuous ambulatory peritoneal dialysis (CAPD) peritoneal dialysis carried out every day, by patients needing renal replacement therapy, at home.

continuous glucose monitoring (CGM) use of a subcutaneous probe to monitor tissue glucose concentrations giving a continuous profile over 48 to 72 hours; useful for adjustment of insulin doses.

continuous passive motion (CPM) form of passive mobilization, used to help the recovery of cartilage after knee surgery.

continuous positive airways pressure (CPAP) the application of gas at a constant positive pressure, to the airway of a spontaneously breathing patient, via an endotracheal tube or tightly fitting face mask. It reduces alveolar collapse at the end of expiration and reduces the work of breathing; used at night in patients with sleep apnoea.

continuous subcutaneous insulin infusion (CSII) the use of a pump to deliver insulin continuously, either with a fixed or variable basal rate, and with a facility for bolus dosing, to achieve almost physiological control of diabetes mellitus.

contraceptive *n, adj* (describes) an agent used to prevent conception, e.g. condom, spermicidal vaginal pessary or cream, rubber cervical cap, intrauterine device. ⇒ combined oral contraceptive, intrauterine device—**contraception** *n.*

contract *v* **1** draw together; shorten; decrease in size. **2** acquire by contagion or infection.

contractile *adj* having the ability to shorten—usually following stimulation; a property of muscle tissue—**contractility** *n.*

contraction *n* shortening, e.g. in muscle fibres.

contracture *n* shortening of scar or muscle tissue, causing deformity ⇒ Dupuytren's contracture, Volkmann's ischaemic contracture.

contraindication *n* any factor or condition indicating that a certain type of treatment (usually used for that condition) should be discontinued or not used.

contralateral *adj* on the opposite side—**contralaterally** *adv.*

contrecoup *n* injury or damage at a point opposite the impact, resulting from transmitted force. It can occur in an organ or part containing fluid, as the skull.

control group in research, the group that is not exposed to the independent variable, such as a therapeutic intervention or experimental drug. ⇒ experimental group, variable.

controlled-dose transdermal absorption of drugs application of a drug patch to the skin: gradual absorption gives a constant level in the blood. Examples include hormone replacement, and nicotine for smoking cessation.

controlled drugs (CD) drugs that are subject to statutory control, e.g. barbiturates, cocaine, morphine. ⇒ Appendix 5.

Control of Substances Hazardous to Health (COSHH) regulations relating to obligatory risk assessment and action to be taken, such as during the use of certain anaesthetic agents.

contusion *n* ⇒ bruise—**contuse** *vt.*

convection *n* transfer of heat from the hotter to the colder part; the heated substance (air or fluid), being less dense, tends to rise. The colder portion, flowing in to be heated, rises in its turn; thus *convection currents* are set in motion.

conversion *n* a mental defence mechanism. A psychological conflict being expressed as a physical symptom. *conversion disorder* an old term for dissociative disorders.

convolutions *npl* folds, twists or coils as found in the intestine, renal tubules and the surface of the brain—**convoluted** *adj.*

convulsions *npl* involuntary contractions of muscles resulting from abnormal electrical activity in the brain: there are many causes. They occur with or without loss of consciousness. ⇒ epilepsy. *clonic convulsions* show alternating contraction and relaxation of muscle groups. *tonic convulsions* reveal sustained rigidity—**convulsive** *adj.*

Cooley's anaemia thalassaemia.

Coombs' test a highly sensitive test designed to detect antibodies to red blood cells, such as those found in Rhesus incompatibility or haemolytic anaemia. The indirect method detects unbound antibodies in the serum, whereas the direct method detects those bound to the red cells.

coordination *n* moving in harmony. The body's ability to execute smooth, fluid, accurate and controlled movements.

COPD *abbr* chronic obstructive pulmonary disease.

coping *n* the way in which a person deals with a circumstance which can be either negative or positive. The coping response can be negative, e.g. reducing social activities because of failing sight; or it can be positive, e.g. increasing participation in sport although confined to a wheelchair.

copper (Cu) *n* essential trace element widely distributed in the body tissues; an important component of metalloenzymes involved in protein synthesis. Copper deficiency can develop in preterm infants and term infants who have been fed cows' milk instead of infant formula milk.

coprolalia *n* obscene speech. Occurs as a sign most commonly in cerebral deterioration or trauma affecting frontal lobes of the brain. ⇒ Tourette's syndrome.

coprolith *n* faecalith.

coproporphyrin *n* a porphyrin normally excreted in the faeces.

copulation *n* coitus.

coracobrachialis muscle a muscle of the upper arm. ⇒ Figure 4.

cord *n* a thread-like structure. *spermatic cord* that which suspends the testes in the scrotum. *spinal cord* a structure which lies in the spinal column, reaching from the foramen magnum to the first or second lumbar vertebra. It is a direct continuation of the medulla oblongata. *umbilical cord* attaching the fetus to the placenta. It contains two arteries and a vein. *vocal cord* the membranous bands in the larynx, vibrations of which produce the voice.

cordectomy *n* surgical excision of a cord, usually reserved for a vocal cord.

cordotomy *n* (*syn* chordotomy) division of the anterolateral nerves in the spinal cord to relieve intractable pain in the pelvis or lower limbs.

core *n* central portion, usually applied to the slough in the centre of a boil.

corn *n* ⇒ callus.

cornea *n* the outwardly convex transparent membrane forming part of the anterior outer coat of the eye. It is situated in front of the iris and pupil and merges backwards into the sclera (⇒ Figure 15)— **corneal** *adj*.

corneal graft (*syn* keratoplasty) replacement of the cornea with a healthy cornea from a human donor.

corneoscleral *adj* pertaining to the cornea and sclera, as the circular junction of these structures.

coronal *adj* in dentistry relating to a crown.

coronal plane ⇒ frontal plane.

coronary *adj* crown-like; encircling, as of a vessel or nerve. *coronary arteries* those supplying the myocardium, the first pair to be given off by the aorta as it leaves the left ventricle. Spasm, narrowing or blockage of these vessels causes angina pectoris or myocardial infarction (heart attack). Diseased vessels may be cleared by balloon angioplasty, lasers or replaced with veins taken from the legs. ⇒ angioplasty. *coronary sinus* channel receiving most venous blood from the myocardium and opening into the right atrium. *coronary thrombosis* occlusion of a coronary vessel by a thrombus. The area deprived of blood becomes necrotic and is called an infarct. ⇒ ischaemic heart disease, myocardial infarction.

coronary care unit (CCU) high dependency area in a hospital specialized in the care of patients with heart problems, particularly after a heart attack.

coronary heart disease (CHD) also known as ischaemic heart disease. It includes angina pectoris and myocardial infarction. A deficient supply of oxygenated blood to the myocardium, causing central chest pain of varying intensity that may radiate to arms and jaws. The lumen of the blood vessels is usually narrowed by atheromatous plaques. If treatment with drug therapy is unsuccessful, percutaneous transluminal angioplasty, or surgery, may be considered. ⇒ angina pectoris, angioplasty, myocardial infarction.

coronaviruses *npl* a group of RNA viruses responsible for acute respiratory infections such as the common cold.

coroner *n* in England and Wales, an officer of the Crown, usually a solicitor, barrister or doctor, who presides over the Coroner's Court responsible for establishing the cause of death in cases where violence may be a possibility or suspected. Where doubts exist about the cause of death the doctor should consult the coroner and act on his or her advice. The coroner must be notified if a patient dies within 24 hours of admission to hospital. In addition all theatre/anaesthetic deaths must also be reported. Any death where the deceased has not been seen by a doctor recently requires that a coroner's postmortem is undertaken. In Scotland, reports about such deaths are submitted to the Procurator Fiscal but a postmortem is normally only ordered if foul play is suspected. The Scottish equivalent of the Coroner's Inquest is the Fatal Accident Enquiry, presided over by the Sheriff.

cor pulmonale heart disease resulting from disease of the lung (emphysema, silicosis, etc.) which strains the right ventricle.

corpus *n* any mass of tissue which is easily distinguishable from its surroundings— **corpora** *pl*. *corpus callosum* white matter joining the two cerebral hemispheres. *corpus cavernosum* ⇒ Figure 16. *corpus luteum* a yellow mass which forms in the ovary after ovulation. It secretes progesterone and persists to maintain pregnancy should it occur. *corpus spongiosum* ⇒ Figure 16.

corpuscle *n* outdated term for blood cells— **corpuscular** *adj*. ⇒ erythrocytes, leucocytes.

corrective *adj, n* something which changes, counteracts or modifies something harmful.

Corrigan's pulse ⇒ collapsing pulse.

cortex *n* the outer layer of an organ or structure beneath its capsule or membrane such as the cerebral cortex or renal cortex—**cortices** *pl*, **cortical** *adj*.

corticosteroids *npl* hormones produced by the adrenal cortex. The word is also used for synthetic steroids such as prednisolone and dexamethasone. ⇒ Appendix 5.

corticotrophin *n* ⇒ adrenocorticotrophic hormone.

cortisol *n* hydrocortisone, one of the principal adrenal cortical steroids. It is essential to life. There is decreased secretion in Addison's disease and increased amounts in Cushing's disease and syndrome.

cortisone *n* one of the hormones of the adrenal gland. It is converted into cortisol before use by the body. Used therapeutically as replacement in conditions that include Addison's disease. *cortisone suppression test* differentiates primary from secondary hypercalcaemia.

Corynebacterium *n* a bacterial genus of Gram-positive, rod-shaped bacteria. Many strains colonize the upper respiratory tract, and some are pathogenic and produce exotoxins such as *Corynebacterium diphtheriae* that causes diphtheria.

coryza *n* the 'common cold'. Rhinoviruses, coronaviruses and adenoviruses cause an acute upper respiratory infection of short duration; highly contagious.

COSHH *abbr* Control of Substances Hazardous to Health.

cosmetic *adj, n* or aesthetic. (That which is) performed to improve the appearance or prevent disfigurement. ⇒ plastic surgery.

costal *adj* pertaining to the ribs. *costal cartilages* those which attach the ribs to the sternum and each other.

cost-benefit analysis (CBA) method of analysis used in the economic evaluation of healthcare interventions (programmes or procedures). Health outcomes are measured in monetary terms to enable comparisons between interventions from a variety of disciplines. There are problems with valuing life and health in monetary terms. So this method is not widely used.

cost centre a department, for example physiotherapy or catering, for which a budget covering staff and other resources has been set.

cost effectiveness analytical technique used in the economic evaluation of healthcare interventions (programmes and procedures). A cost effectiveness analysis is used when the outcomes of the procedures are not necessarily the same, but can be measured in the same natural units. For example, the outcomes may be measured in death rates, healthy years of life gained, symptom free days, or even blood pressures. The output of this type of analysis is 'cost per unit increase'. For example, cost of intervention against cost per life year gained. Health benefits are measured in natural units (e.g. mortality rates, survival rates) or final clinical outcomes (e.g. cost per life years gained, cost per days off sick reduced). Intermediate clinical outcomes are sometimes used (e.g. number of cancers detected in a screening programme) but this is not valid if a clear association between cancer detected and survival or quality of life cannot be demonstrated.

costive *adj* lay term for constipated. ⇒ constipation—**costiveness** *n*.

cost minimization analytic technique used in economic evaluation of healthcare interventions (programmes or procedures). A cost minimization analysis is used when the outcomes or consequences of the procedures are the same. A prerequisite for such a study is that there is evidence (preferably from a randomized clinical trial) that the different procedures are equally effective. A cost minimization analysis therefore consists solely of the analyses of costs. Common examples include comparisons of home and hospital care for chronic and terminal conditions.

costochondral *adj* pertaining to a rib and its cartilage.

costochondritis *n* inflammation of the costochondral cartilage. ⇒ Tietze syndrome.

costoclavicular *adj* pertaining to the ribs and the clavicle. *costoclavicular syndrome* is a synonym for cervical rib syndrome. ⇒ cervical.

cost utility analytic technique used in economic evaluation of healthcare interventions (programmes or procedures). A cost utility analysis is used when the outcomes cannot be measured in natural units, so a utility or value scale has to be employed. This may be because the important outcomes of the procedures are not directly comparable or they are multi-faceted, e.g. a comparison of amputation against waiting for the treatment of a gangrenous foot—outcomes could be pain, mobility and/or survival. The commonly used utility scale is quality-adjusted life years (QALYs), which use survey tools such as the Nottingham Health Profile to allocate 'relative qualities' to different health states. However, different people value their health differently; therefore utility ratings are not unique. Research has provided 'average' utility. Cost utility analyses report results as 'costs per QALY (gained)'.

cot death ⇒ sudden infant death syndrome.

cotton wool spot white swelling in the nerve fibre layer of the retina caused by microinfarction.

cotyledon *n* one of the subdivisions of the uterine surface of the placenta.

cough *n* explosive expulsion of air from the lungs. It may be voluntary, or as protective reflex that expels a foreign body such as food or sputum. Cough may be a feature of numerous respiratory and cardiac conditions. ⇒ postural drainage.

coumarins *npl* a group of anticoagulant drugs, e.g. warfarin. ⇒ Appendix 5.

counselling *n* a professional helping relationship with a client who is experiencing psychological problems. The counsellor listens actively and helps the client to identify and clarify the problems and supports the client in making a positive attempt to overcome the problems.

counterirritant *n* an agent which, when applied to the skin, initiates a mild inflammatory response (hyperaemia) and relief of pain and congestion associated with deep-seated inflammation—**counterirritation** *n*.

countertraction *n* traction upon the proximal extremity of a fractured limb opposing the pull of the traction apparatus on the distal extremity.

couvade *n* exhibiting of the symptoms of pregnancy and childbirth by the father. Common in some cultures.

Cowper's glands ⇒ bulbourethral glands.

coxa *n* the hip joint—**coxae** *pl. coxa valga* an increase in the normal angle between neck

and shaft of femur. *coxa vara* a decrease in the normal angle plus torsion of the neck, e.g. slipped femoral epiphysis.

coxalgia *n* pain in the hip joint.

Coxiella *n* a microbial genus closely related to *Rickettsia* including *Coxiella burnetii* which causes Q fever.

coxitis *n* inflammation of the hip joint.

coxsackievirus *n* one of the three groups of viruses included in the family of enteroviruses. Divided into groups A and B. Cause conditions that include: aseptic meningitis, herpangina, Bornholm disease, gastroenteritis and myocarditis.

CPAP *abbr* continuous positive airways pressure.

CPK *abbr* creatine phosphokinase ⇒ creatine kinase.

CPR *abbr* cardiopulmonary resuscitation.

crab louse phthirus pubis.

cradle cap *n* scaling of the scalp of infants, often due to atopic dermatitis or seborrhoeic dermatitis.

cramp *n* spasmodic contraction of a muscle or group of muscles; involuntary and painful: may result from fatigue.

cranial *adj* pertaining to the cranium.

craniofacial *adj* pertaining to the cranium and the face.

craniometry *n* the science which deals with the measurement of skulls.

craniopharyngioma *n* a tumour which develops between the brain and the pituitary gland.

cranioplasty *n* operative repair of a skull defect—**cranioplastic** *adj*.

craniosacral *adj* pertaining to the skull and sacrum. Applied to the outflow of the parasympathetic nervous system.

craniostenosis *n* a condition in which the skull sutures fuse too early and the fontanelles close. It may cause increased intracranial pressure requiring surgery.

craniosynostosis *n* premature fusion of cranial sutures resulting in abnormal skull shape and craniostenosis. Deformities depend on which sutures are affected.

craniotabes *n* a thinning or wasting of the cranial bones occurring in infancy and usually due to rickets—**craniotabetic** *adj*.

craniotomy *n* a surgical opening of the skull in order to remove a growth, relieve pressure, evacuate blood clot or arrest haemorrhage.

cranium *n* the part of the skull enclosing the brain. It is composed of eight bones: the occipital, two parietals, frontal, two temporals, sphenoid and ethmoid—**cranial** *adj*.

craquelé *adj* describes cracked skin resembling crazy paving. A term used in association with a certain type of eczema seen in older people.

C-reactive protein (CRP) test an acute phase protein. Elevated amounts are present in the plasma in response to inflammation and tissue damage. It is a very sensitive progress indicator of many inflammatory conditions, such as infective endocarditis.

creatinase *n* ⇒ creatine kinase.

creatine *n* a nitrogenous compound produced in the body. *creatine kinase* (*syn* ATP: creatine phosphotransferase) occurs as three isoenzymes. It is found in brain tissue, skeletal muscle, blood and in myocardial tissue. *creatine kinase test* increased levels of the myocardial isoenzyme in serum is indicative of acute myocardial infarction. *phosphorylated creatine* the important storage form of high-energy phosphate.

creatinine *n* a waste product of protein (endogenous) and nucleic acid metabolism found in muscle and blood and excreted in normal urine. Serum creatinine is raised in hyperthyroidism, muscle wasting disorders and in renal failure.

creep *n* (*syn* cold flow) the continued change in the size of the lumen of plastic tubing in intravenous giving sets after release of the clamp. It can change the rate of the fluid passing along the tube.

crepitus *n* **1** (crepitation) grinding noise or sensation within a joint, as in osteoarthritis. A feature of fracture in overuse injury. **2** crackling sound heard via stethoscope. **3** crackling sound elicited by pressure on tissue containing air (surgical emphysema).

cresol *n* chemically related to phenol. Used in many general environmental disinfectants.

CREST syndrome *acron* calcinosis, Raynaud's phenomenon, (o)esophageal dysfunction, sclerodactyly and telangiectasis. A form of systemic sclerosis.

cretinism *n* obsolete term. ⇒ hypothyroidism.

Creutzfeldt–Jakob disease (CJD) a progressive dementia transmissible through prion protein. New variant CJD, mainly affecting young adults, is possibly linked with the prion causing bovine spongiform encephalopathy (BSE). CJD follows a rapid degenerative course often with myoclonus and is usually fatal.

CRF *abbr* chronic renal failure. ⇒ renal.

cribriform *adj* perforated, like a sieve. *cribriform plate* that portion of the ethmoid bone allowing passage of fibres of olfactory nerve.

cricoid *adj* ring-shaped. Applied to the cartilage forming the inferior posterior part of larynx. ⇒ Figure 6. *cricoid pressure* a practical manoeuvre in which manual pressure is applied over the cricoid cartilage to occlude the oesophagus to prevent regurgitation and aspiration of gastric contents during induction of anaesthesia.

cricothyroidotomy *n* (*syn* cricothyrotomy) incision through the skin and cricothyroid membrane to secure a patent airway for emergency relief of upper airway obstruction. ⇒ tracheostomy.

'cri du chat' syndrome produced by partial loss of one of the number 5 chromosomes leading to learning disability. There are certain physical abnormalities and a curious flat, toneless cat-like cry in infancy.

criminal abortion ⇒ abortion.

criminal law the law that creates offences heard in the criminal courts such as theft. *criminal wrong* an act or omission that can be pursued in the criminal courts.

crisis 1 *n* the turning point of a disease—as the point of defervescence in fever. ⇒ lysis *opp*. **2** muscular spasm in tabes dorsalis referred to as visceral crisis (gastric, vesical, rectal, etc.)—**crises** *pl*.

critical appraisal the process of making an objective judgement regarding a research study. Includes research design, methodology, analysis, interpretation of results and the applicability of the study findings to a particular area of health care.

Crohn's disease a chronic recurrent granulomatous inflammation affecting any part of the bowel from mouth to anus. Inflammation may be discontinuous ('skip lesions') with normal bowel in between. May be complicated by fistulae and strictures. ⇒ inflammatory bowel disease.

Crosby capsule a special tube which is passed through the mouth to the small intestine. Allows biopsy of jejunal mucosa. Endoscopic biopsy is often used in preference to this time-consuming investigation.

cross infection ⇒ infection.

cross-over studies a research study where the participants are exposed to both the experimental intervention and the placebo one after another.

croup *n* viral infection leading to laryngeal narrowing. The child has 'croupy', stridulous (noisy or harsh-sounding) breathing. Narrowing of the airway which gives rise to the typical attack with crowing inspiration may be the result of oedema or spasm, or both.

crown *n* the top part of a structure. *artificial crown* in dentistry, restoration used to cover the part of the tooth that projects above the gum line, usually made of metal, porcelain, or a combination of both. *crown of a tooth* that part of the tooth covered with enamel.

CRP *abbr* ⇒ C-reactive protein test.

cruciate *adj* shaped like a cross such as the ligaments stabilizing the knee joint.

crus *n* a structure which is leg-like or root-like. Applied to various parts of the body, e.g. crus of the diaphragm—**crura** *pl*, **crural** *adj*.

'crush' syndrome traumatic uraemia. Following extensive trauma to muscle, there is a period of delay before the effects of renal damage manifest themselves. There is an increase of non-protein nitrogen in the blood, with oliguria, proteinuria and urinary excretion of myohaemoglobin. Loss of blood plasma to damaged area is marked. Where hypotension has occurred the renal failure will be exacerbated by tubular necrosis.

crutch palsy paralysis of extensor muscles of wrist, fingers and thumb from repeated pressure of a crutch upon the radial nerve in the axilla.

cryaesthesia *n* **1** the sensation of coldness. **2** exceptional sensitivity to a low temperature.

cryoanalgesia *n* the relief of pain symptoms by blocking peripheral nerve conduction with extreme cold.

cryogenic *adj, n* produced by low temperature. Also used to describe any means or apparatus involved in the production of low temperature.

cryoglobulin *n* an immunoglobulin that precipitates on cooling, and redissolves on warming; associated with numerous pathological conditions including occlusion of peripheral blood vessels, ulceration and gangrene. Type 1 cryoglobulins are monoclonal and are associated with lymphoproliferative disorders. Type 2 cryoglobulins are monoclonal with reactivity against polyclonal immunoglobulins, i.e. they are rheumatoid factors. Type 3 are polyclonal with rheumatoid factor activity.

cryokinetics *n* use of cold treatments prior to activity.

cryopexy *n* surgical fixation by freezing, of a detached retina.

cryoprobe *n* freezing probe which can be used to destroy tumours.

cryosurgery *n* the use of intense, controlled cold to remove or destroy diseased tissue.

cryothalamectomy *n* freezing applied to destroy groups of neurons within the thalamus in the treatment of Parkinson's disease and other hyperkinetic conditions.

cryotherapy *n* the use of cold for the treatment of disease.

cryptococcosis *n* the disease resulting from infection with the yeast *Cryptococcus neoformans*, which is present in soil and pigeon excreta. It most commonly causes meningitis but may also affect the lungs, skin and bones. Immunocompromised individuals, such as those with AIDS, are at increased risk.

Cryptococcus *n* a genus of fungi. *Cryptococcus neoformans* occasionally causes disease in humans.

cryptogenic *adj* of unknown or obscure cause.

cryptogenic fibrosing alveolitis interstitial lung disease characterized by cellular infiltration and thickening of the alveolar walls. Pulmonary macrophages are implicated in fibrosis, and in recruiting other cell types such as neutrophils to the lung.

cryptomenorrhoea *n* retention of the menses due to a congenital obstruction, such as an imperforate hymen or atresia of the vagina. ⇒ haematocolpos.

cryptorchism *n* a developmental defect whereby the testes do not descend into the scrotum; they are retained within the abdomen or inguinal canal—**cryptorchid, cryptorchis** *n*.

cryptosporidiosis *n* infection caused by cryptosporidium species (protozoa). The organisms are present in the faeces of both domestic and farm animals, and transmission to humans occurs through contaminated water and food. Infection may be symptomless or result in profuse watery diarrhoea. Immunocompromised individuals may be seriously affected.

crystalline *adj* like a crystal. *crystalline lens* a biconvex body, oval in shape, which is suspended just behind the iris of the eye, and separates the aqueous from the vitreous humour. It is slightly less convex on its anterior surface and it contributes to refraction of light rays so that they focus directly on to the retina.

crystallins *npl* proteins forming the lens of the eye.

crystalloids *npl* substances in solution that will diffuse through a semipermeable membrane.

crystalloid solutions ones containing small molecules used intravenously for hydration.

crystalluria *n* excretion of crystals in the urine—**crystalluric** *adj*.

crystal violet (*syn* gentian violet) a brilliant, violet-coloured, antiseptic aniline dye, used as 0.5% solution as a stain. It is only licensed for application to intact skin, the exception being marking the skin before surgery.

CSF *abbr* **1** cerebrospinal fluid. **2** colony stimulating factor.

CSII *abbr* continuous subcutaneous insulin infusion.

CSM *abbr* Committee on Safety of Medicines.

CSSD *abbr* central sterile supplies department.

CSSU *abbr* central sterile supply unit.

CT *abbr* computed tomography.

CTG *abbr* cardiotocography.

cubital tunnel external compression syndrome ulnar paralysis resulting from compression of the ulnar nerve within the cubital tunnel situated on the inner and posterior aspect of the elbow—sometimes referred to as the 'funny bone'.

cubital vein situated in the arm. ⇒ Figure 10.

cubitus *n* the forearm; elbow—**cubital** *adj*.

cuboid *adj* shaped like a cube.

cue *n* during communication, a verbal or non-verbal signal from another individual that is perceived by the observer to require sensitive exploration (by prompting or reflection) as to its meaning for the individual exhibiting it.

culdocentesis *n* aspiration of the pouch of Douglas via the posterior vaginal wall.

culdoscope *n* an endoscope used via the vaginal route.

culdoscopy *n* a form of peritoneoscopy or laparoscopy. Passage of a culdoscope through the posterior vaginal fornix, behind the uterus to enter the peritoneal cavity, for viewing same—**culdoscopic** *adj*, **culdoscopically** *adv*.

culture *n* the growth of micro-organisms on artificial media under ideal conditions.

cumulative action when a dose of a slowly excreted drug is repeated too frequently, an increasing action occurs. This may lead to an accumulation of the drug in the system and toxic symptoms, such as with digoxin.

Cumulative Index to Nursing and Allied Health Literature (CINAHL) computerized database of literature relevant to nursing and allied health.

cupping *n* space within the optic nerve head due to absence of nerve fibres, often due to glaucoma.

curettage *n* the scraping of unhealthy or exuberant tissue from a cavity. This may be treatment or may be done to establish a diagnosis after laboratory analysis of the scrapings.

curette *n* a spoon-shaped instrument or a metal loop which may have sharp and/or blunt edges for scraping out (curetting) cavities.

curettings *npl* the material obtained by scraping or curetting and usually sent for histological examination.

Curling's ulcer acute peptic ulceration which occurs either in the stomach or duodenum as a response to the physiological stress of extensive burns or scalds.

Cuscoe's speculum a bivalve speculum used for inspection of the cervix and vagina and for holding the vaginal walls apart while taking high vaginal swabs and cervical smears.

cushingoid a description of the moon face, central obesity and facial plethora common in people with elevated levels of plasma glucocorticoids from whatever cause.

Cushing's disease a rare disorder, mainly of females, characterized principally by a cushingoid appearance, proximal myopathy, hyperglycaemia, hypertension and osteoporosis; due to excessive cortisol production by hyperplastic adrenal glands as a result of increased adrenocorticotrophin (ACTH) secretion by a tumour or hyperplasia of the anterior pituitary gland.

Cushing's reflex a rise in blood pressure and a fall in pulse rate; occurs in cerebral space-occupying lesions.

Cushing's syndrome clinically similar to Cushing's disease but including all causes: (a) adrenocortical hyperplasia, adenoma or carcinoma, which can be associated with hirsutism and hypokalaemia due to excess of other adrenal steroids; (b) ectopic ACTH secretion by tumours, e.g. small cell lung cancer, often associated with hyperpigmentation; (c) iatrogenic due to treatment with glucocorticoids.

cusp *n* a projecting point, such as the edge of a tooth or the segment of a heart valve. The cardiac tricuspid valve has three, the mitral (bicuspid) valve two cusps.

cutaneous *adj* relating to the skin. *cutaneous nerve* ⇒ Figure 12. *cutaneous ureterostomy* the ureters are transplanted so that they open on to the skin of the abdominal wall.

cuticle *n* the epidermis or dead epidermis, as that which surrounds a nail—**cuticular** *adj*.

CVA *abbr* cerebrovascular accident.

CVP *abbr* central venous pressure.

CVS *abbr* chorionic villus sampling.

CVVH *abbr* continuous veno-venous haemofiltration. ⇒ haemofiltration.

CVVHD *abbr* continuous veno-venous haemodiafiltration (haemodialysis). ⇒ haemodiafiltration.

cyanocobalamin *n* the most stable form of vitamin B_{12}, which is produced commercially by bacterial fermentation. This synthetic form must be converted in the body to a naturally occurring form before it can be utilized by the body. ⇒ cobalamins.

cyanosis *n* a bluish tinge manifested by hypoxic tissue, observed most frequently under the nails, lips and skin. It is always due to lack of oxygen, and the causes of this are legion—**cyanosed, cyanotic** *adj*. *central cyanosis* blueness seen on the warm surfaces such as the oral mucosa and tongue. It increases with exertion. *peripheral cyanosis* blueness of the limb extremities, the nose and the ear lobes.

cycle *n* a regular series of movements or events; a sequence which recurs. ⇒ cardiac, menstrual—**cyclical** *adj*.

cyclic adenosine monophosphate (cAMP) a metabolic molecule that acts as a 'second messenger' for many hormones and in processes where many reactions are occurring simultaneously (enzyme cascade).

cyclical syndrome an alternative term preferred by some people to that of premenstrual syndrome.

cyclical vomiting periodic attacks of vomiting in children, usually associated with ketosis and usually with no demonstrable pathological cause. Occurs mainly in highly strung children.

cyclist's nipples a colloquial expression used in sports medicine to describe the irritation of the nipple due to the combined effects of perspiration and windchill.

cyclist's palsy a colloquial expression used in sports medicine to describe the paraesthesia of the ulnar nerve distribution of the forearm and hand due to prolonged leaning on the handlebars when cycling.

cyclitis *n* inflammation of the ciliary body of the eye. ⇒ iridocyclitis.

cyclodestruction *n* destruction of the ciliary body by heat (usually laser induced) or freezing.

cyclodialysis *n* a communication between anterior chamber and suprachoroidal space.

cycloplegia *n* paralysis of the ciliary muscle of the eye—**cycloplegic** *adj.*

cycloplegics *npl* drugs which paralyse the ciliary muscle of the eye, e.g. atropine, cyclopentolate. ⇒ mydriatics.

cyclothymia *n* a tendency to alternating but relatively mild mood swings between elation and depression—**cyclothymic** *adj.*

cyclotron *n* an apparatus that produces high energy positive ion beams used to bombard a suitable target resulting in the production of radionuclides. These can then be used as a source of neutrons or protons for therapeutic purposes.

cyesis *n* pregnancy. When there are signs and symptoms of pregnancy in a woman who believes she is pregnant, and this is not so, it is called pseudocyesis. ⇒ phantom pregnancy.

cylindroma *n* a tumour of the endothelial element of apocrine tissue such as a sweat gland or a salivary gland. The supporting stroma is hyalinized.

cyst *n* a closed cavity or sac usually with an epithelial lining, enclosing fluid or semisolid matter—**cystic** *adj.*

cystadenoma *n* an innocent cystic new growth of glandular tissue. Liable to occur in the female breast.

cystathioninuria *n* inherited disorder of cystathionine metabolism marked by excessive excretion of cystathionine in the urine, an intermediate product in conversion of methionine to cysteine. Sometimes associated with learning disability.

cystectomy *n* usually refers to the removal of part or the whole of the urinary bladder. This necessitates urinary diversion.

cysteine *n* a sulphur-containing conditionally essential (indispensable) amino acid. The amino acids methionine and serine are precursors for its synthesis.

cysticercosis *n* infection of humans with cysticercus, the larval stage of the pork tapeworm (*Taenia solium*). After ingestion, the ova do not develop further, but form 'cysts' in subcutaneous tissues, voluntary muscle and the brain, where they cause seizures.

cysticercus *n* the larval form of *Taenia solium*.

cystic fibrosis (*syn* fibrocystic disease of the pancreas, mucoviscidosis) the commonest genetically determined disease in Caucasian populations; there is abnormality of secretion of the exocrine glands. Thick mucus can block the intestinal glands and cause meconium ileus in a baby; later it can cause steatorrhoea and malabsorption. Thick mucus in the respiratory glands predisposes to repeated infections and bronchiectasis. Abnormality of the sweat glands increases the chloride content of sweat, which is a diagnostic tool. ⇒ sweat test.

cystine *n* a sulphur-containing amino acid, produced by the breakdown of proteins during the digestive process. It is readily reduced to two molecules of cysteine.

cystinosis *n* a recessively inherited metabolic disorder in which crystalline cystine is deposited in the body. Cystine and other amino acids are excreted in the urine.

cystinuria *n* metabolic disorder in which cystine and other amino acids appear in the urine. A cause of renal stones—**cystinuric** *adj.*

cystitis *n* inflammation of the urinary bladder; the cause is usually bacterial. The condition may be acute or chronic, primary or secondary to stones, etc. More frequent in females, as the urethra is short.

cystocele *n* prolapse of the posterior wall of the urinary bladder into the anterior vaginal wall. ⇒ colporrhaphy.

cystodiathermy *n* the application of a cauterizing electrical current to the walls of the urinary bladder through a cystoscope, or by open operation.

cystography *n* radiographic examination of the urinary bladder, after it has been filled with a contrast medium—**cystographic** *adj*, **cystograph** *n*, **cystogram** *n*, **cystographically** *adv.*

cystolithiasis *n* the presence of a stone or stones in the urinary bladder.

cystometer *n* an apparatus for measuring the pressure under various conditions in the urinary bladder.

cystometrogram *n* a record of the changes in pressure within the urinary bladder under various conditions; used in the study of voiding disorders.

cystometry *n* the study of pressure changes within the urinary bladder—**cystometric** *adj.*

cystoplasty *n* surgical repair or augmentation of the urinary bladder.

cystoscope *n* an endoscope used to visualize the inner aspect of the bladder—**cystoscopic** *adj*, **cystoscopically** *adv*.

cystoscopy *n* use of a cystoscope to view the internal surface of the urinary bladder.

cystostomy *n* (*syn* vesicostomy) an operation whereby a fistulous opening is made into the urinary bladder via the abdominal wall. Usually the fistula can be allowed to heal when it is no longer needed.

cystotomy *n* incision into the urinary bladder via the abdominal wall.

cystourethritis *n* inflammation of the urinary bladder and urethra.

cystourethrogram *n* radiographic examination of the urinary bladder and urethra. *micturating cystourethrogram* a dynamic X-ray performed during micturition, often to assess the degree of ureteric reflux—**cystourethrographic** *adj*, **cystourethrograph** *n*, **cystourethrographically** *adv*.

cystourethropexy *n* operation used for some types of urinary incontinence. The bladder and upper urethra are fixed in a forward position. ⇒ Marshall–Marchetti–Krantz operation.

cytochrome *n* a series of proteins containing iron or copper. They have a similar structure to haemoglobin and are involved in mitochondrial oxidation-reduction reactions (electron transport chain) that produce ATP. *cytochrome* P_{450} liver enzyme important in the oxidation and clearance of lipid-soluble drugs.

cytodiagnosis *n* diagnosis by the microscopic study of cells—**cytodiagnostic** *adj*.

cytogenetics *n* the scientific study of cells; particularly of chromosomes, genes and their behaviour. Chromosomes can be studied by culture techniques, using either tissue such as skin or lymphocytes, or fetal cells obtained by chorionic villus sampling or amniocentesis—**cytogenesis** *n*.

cytokines *npl* proteins which act either on the cytokine-producing cell, or on other cells, via cell-surface receptors. The term is usually applied to proteins which act on immune cells (T cells, B cells, monocytes, etc.). Cytokines have many diverse effects on many different cell types. Examples include interleukins (e.g. IL-1, IL-2), tumour necrosis factor, interferon-alpha and interferon-gamma.

cytology *n* the microscopic study of cells. The term *exfoliative cytology* is used when the cells studied have been shed, or sampled, from the surface of an organ or lesion—**cytological** *adj*.

cytolysis *n* the degeneration, destruction, disintegration or dissolution of cells—**cytolytic** *adj*.

cytomegalovirus (CMV) *n* a herpesvirus. Can cause latent and symptomless infection. The virus is excreted in urine and saliva. It can be passed to the fetus in utero and may cause miscarriage, stillbirth or serious neonatal disease characterized by hepatosplenomegaly, purpura, encephalitis and microcephaly with learning disability, or death. In adults it causes an illness similar to infectious mononucleosis and pneumonia. The virus is a serious threat to immunocompromised individuals.

cytoplasm *n* (*syn* protoplasm) the complex chemical compound constituting the main part of the living substance of the cell, other than the contents of the nucleus—**cytoplasmic** *adj*.

cytoscreening *n* the process of carefully evaluating cells on a cytological preparation for the detection of malignancy.

cytospin *n* process of centrifuging fluid in order to separate the cells for cytological evaluation.

cytostasis *n* arrest or hindrance of cell development—**cytostatic** *adj*.

cytotoxic *n*, *adj* any substance which kills cells. *cytotoxic drugs* drugs used mainly for the treatment of malignant diseases, but sometimes for other conditions. They work in different ways, but they all eventually cause cancer cell death by either disrupting DNA or causing apoptosis. Some are cell cycle phase specific and others work at any point in the cell cycle. They also harm some normal cells and some have longer-term side-effects. ⇒ chemotherapy. There are five groups: (a) alkylating agents that disrupt DNA, e.g. busulfan, cyclophosphamide; (b) antimetabolites that disrupt DNA by blocking enzymes required for its synthesis, e.g. 5-fluorouracil; (c) antitumour antibiotics that disrupt DNA and the cell membrane, e.g. bleomycin; (d) vinca alkaloids and other plant extracts that disrupt microtubules during cell division, e.g.

vincristine; (e) miscellaneous group that work in a variety of ways, e.g. asparaginase.

cytotoxins *npl* antibodies which are toxic to cells.

D

Da Costa syndrome cardiac neurosis. An anxiety state in which palpitations and left-sided chest pain are the most prominent symptoms.

dacr(y)oadenitis *n* inflammation of a lacrimal gland. May occur in mumps.

dacryocystectomy *n* excision of any part of the lacrimal sac.

dacryocystitis *n* infective inflammation of the lacrimal sac.

dacryocystography *n* rarely used radiographic examination of the tear drainage apparatus after it has been rendered radiopaque. Superseded by CT and MRI.

dacryocystorhinostomy (DCR) *n* an operation to establish drainage from the lacrimal sac into the nose when there is obstruction of the nasolacrimal duct.

dacryolith *n* a concretion in the lacrimal passages.

dactyl *n* a digit, finger or toe—**dactylar, dactylate** *adj*.

dactylitis *n* inflammation of finger or toe. The digit becomes swollen due to periostitis. Associated with congenital syphilis, tuberculosis, sarcoid.

dactylology *n* finger spelling. Used in conjunction with British sign language to communicate with hearing impaired people. ⇒ Makaton.

DADL *abbr* domestic activities of daily living.

D and C *abbr* dilatation and curettage.

D and E *abbr* dilatation and evacuation.

dandruff *n* (*syn* scurf) the common scaly condition of the scalp. May be the forerunner of skin diseases of the seborrhoeic type, such as seborrhoeic dermatitis, or psoriasis.

dandy fever dengue.

Dane particle the complete hepatitis B virus particle.

dark adaptation adjustments made by the eye in reduced light or darkness. The pupils dilate, cones function ceases, rhodopsin is formed and the rod activity increases. ⇒ light adaptation.

data *npl* items of information, usually collected for a specific purpose—**datum** *sing*. *data analysis* describes statistical analyses on data. *data processing* storage, sorting and analysis of data, usually electronically with computers. *data protection* rules relating to information held about individuals, such as in Data Protection Act 1998. *data set* the data relating to a specific group such as a particular age group.

Davier's disease (*syn* keratosis follicularis) an autosomal dominant condition characterized by greasy scaled papules on the flexures, trunk and face.

day case surgery ⇒ ambulatory surgery.

day hospital a centre which patients attend daily. Recreational and occupational therapy and physiotherapy often provided. Greatest use is in the services for older people and those with mental health problems.

deafness *n* a partial or complete loss of hearing. *conductive deafness* is due to interruption of the conduction of sound waves from the atmosphere to the inner ear. *congenital deafness* present at birth, e.g. caused by maternal rubella in early pregnancy. *sensorineural (perceptive)* or *nerve deafness* is due to a lesion in the inner ear, the auditory nerve or the auditory centres in the brain. ⇒ hearing impairment.

deamination *n* removal of an amino group (NH$_2$) from organic compounds such as excess amino acids.

death *n* irreversible cessation of vital functions usually assessed by the absence of heart beat and breathing. Mechanical ventilation may maintain vital functions despite the fact that the brainstem is fatally and irreversibly damaged. Consequently stringent tests are necessary to diagnose death. ⇒ brainstem death, coroner. *death certificate* official document, issued by the registrar of deaths to relatives or other authorized person, that allows for the disposal of the body. It is issued after a notification of probable cause of death is completed by the doctor in attendance upon the deceased or the appropriate documentation from the coroner.

debility *n* a condition of weakness with lack of muscle tone.

débridement *n* the removal of foreign matter and contaminated or devitalized tissue from or adjacent to a wound. *chemical/medical débridement* is accomplished by the external application of a substance to the wound, such as a specific wound dressing. *surgical débridement* is accomplished by using surgical instruments and aseptic technique.

debulking *n* removal of a significant proportion of a pathological mass.

decalcification *n* the removal of mineral salts, as from teeth in dental caries, bone in disorders of calcium metabolism.

decannulation *n* the removal of a cannula such as an intravenous cannula.

decapsulation *n* the surgical removal of a capsule.

decay *n* a psychological term that describes the loss of information from the memory that occurs spontaneously over time.

decerebrate *adj* without cerebral function; a state of deep unconsciousness. *decerebrate posture* a condition of the unconscious patient in which all four limbs are spastic and which indicates severe damage to the cerebrum. *decerebrate rigidity* hypertonus of the physiological extensor muscles following severe decerebrating brain injury. ⇒ opisthotonos.

decibel (dB) a unit of sound intensity (loudness).

decidua *n* the endometrial lining of the uterus thickened and altered for the reception of the fertilized ovum. It is shed at the end of pregnancy. *decidua basalis* that part which lies under the embedded ovum and forms the maternal part of the placenta. *decidua capsularis* that part that lies over the developing ovum. *decidua vera* the decidua lining the rest of the uterus—**decidual** *adj*.

deciduous *adj* by convention refers to the teeth of the primary dentition.

decompensation *n* a failure of compensation usually referring to heart failure.

decompression *n* removal of pressure or a compressing force. *decompression of brain* achieved by trephining the skull in order to evacuate clot; *decompression of bladder* in cases of chronic urinary retention, by continuous or intermittent drainage via catheter inserted per urethra.

decompression illness results from sudden reduction in atmospheric pressure, as experienced by divers on return to surface, aircrew ascending to great heights. Caused by bubbles of nitrogen which are released from solution in the blood; symptoms vary according to the site of these. The condition is largely preventable by proper and gradual decompression technique. Variously described as 'bends, chokes and creeps' depending on the symptomatology. Originally called caisson disease when identified as a hazard for divers. Later recognized as a complication of high altitude.

deconditioning *n* eliminating an unwanted particular response to a particular stimulus ⇒ aversion therapy, conditioning.

decongestants *npl* agents which decrease congestion, usually referring to nasal congestion. Administered orally, or locally as drops or sprays. ⇒ Appendix 5.

decongestion *n* relief of congestion— **decongestive** *adj*.

decortication *n* surgical removal of cortex or outer covering of an organ such as the lung or kidney.

decubitus *n* the recumbent position; lying down. *decubitus ulcer* ⇒ pressure ulcer— **decubiti** *pl*, **decubital** *adj*.

decussation *n* intersection; crossing of nerve fibres at a point beyond their origin, as in the optic and pyramidal tracts.

deep vein thrombosis (DVT) thrombus forming in a deep vein such as those in the legs or pelvis. It is associated with slowing of blood flow, abnormal or inappropriate clotting processes, or damage to veins. A thrombus may break off to form an embolus that travels in the venous circulation, through the heart to the lungs. ⇒ pulmonary embolus.

defaecation *n* voiding of faeces per anus— **defaecate** *vi*.

deferent duct (*syn* vas deferens) ⇒ Figure 16.

defervescence *n* the time during which a fever is declining. If the body temperature falls rapidly it is spoken of as crisis; if it falls slowly the term lysis is used.

defibrillation *n* the application of a direct current (DC) electric shock to arrest ventricular fibrillation of the heart and restore normal cardiac rhythm—**defibrillate** *vt*.

defibrillator *n* equipment for the application of DC electric shock to the heart. ⇒ implantable defibrillator.

defibrinated *adj* rendered free from fibrin. A necessary process in the preparation of serum from whole blood. ⇒ blood—**defibrinate** *v*.

deficiency disease disease resulting from deficiency of any essential nutrient. Can be caused by a diet that is deficient in a particular nutrient or because the nutrient present in the diet cannot be absorbed and metabolized by that individual.

degeneration *n* deterioration in quality or function. Regression from more specialized to less specialized type of tissue—**degenerative** *adj*, **degenerate** *vi*.

deglutition *n* swallowing, a complex process that is partly voluntary, partly involuntary.

dehiscence *n* the process of splitting or bursting open, as of a wound.

dehydration *n* loss or removal of fluid. In the body this condition arises when the fluid intake fails to replace fluid loss. This is liable to occur when there is bleeding, diarrhoea, excessive exudation from a raw area as in burns, excessive sweating, polyuria or vomiting, and usually upsets the body's electrolyte balance. If suitable fluid replacement cannot be achieved orally, then parenteral administration must be instituted—**dehydrate** *vt, vi*.

7-dehydrocholesterol *n* a sterol found in the skin. It is converted to a form of vitamin D by the action of ultraviolet radiation.

déjà vu phenomenon occurs in epilepsy involving temporal lobes of the brain and in certain epileptic dream states. An intense feeling of familiarity as if everything had happened before.

delayed onset muscle soreness (DOMS) appears 24–48 hours after exercise; may be caused by severe, unaccustomed exercise, particularly that involving eccentric muscle contractions.

delayed union longer than expected healing of a fracture.

Delhi boil ⇒ oriental sore.

deliberate self-harm (DSH) wilful non-fatal act(s) carried out in the knowledge that it was potentially harmful. Examples include self-poisoning (overdose), self-cutting and self-mutilation.

deliquescent *adj* capable of absorption, thus becoming fluid.

delirium *n* abnormal mental condition based on hallucinations or illusion. May occur in high fever, in mental health problems, or be toxic in origin. *delirium tremens* results from alcoholic intoxication and is represented by a picture of confusion, terror, restlessness and hallucinations—**delirious** *adj*.

Delphi technique a research method where a consensus of expert opinion is obtained during a multiple-step process where the contributors are asked to rate a number of items, e.g. research priorities, in order of importance.

deltoid *adj* triangular. *deltoid muscle* muscle acting at the shoulder (⇒ Figures 4, 5).

delusion *n* a fixed, usually false belief, inconsistent with an individual's culture and intelligence, which cannot be altered by argument or reasoning. A type of psychotic symptom.

demarcation *n* an outlining of the junction of diseased and healthy tissue, often used when referring to gangrene.

dementia *n* (*syn* organic brain syndrome—OBS) an irreversible organic brain disease causing disturbance of memory and personality, deterioration in personal care, impaired cognitive ability and disorientation. ⇒ Creutzfeldt–Jakob disease. *presenile dementia* occurring in people between 50 and 60 years of age. ⇒ Alzheimer's disease, multi-infarct dementia, Pick's disease.

demographic indices such as age distribution, birth and mortality rates, occupation and geographical distribution. They are used to obtain a profile of a given population, compare different areas and plan services.

demography *n* the study of population—**demographic** *adj*.

demulcent *n* a slippery, mucilaginous fluid that alleviates irritation and inflammation, especially of mucous membranes.

demyelination *n* destruction of the myelin sheaths surrounding nerve fibres. Can occur in the peripheral nerves (e.g.

Guillain–Barré syndrome), or in the central nervous system (e.g. multiple sclerosis).

dendrite *n* (*syn* dendron) one of the branched filaments which are given off from the body of a nerve cell. That part of a neuron which transmits an impulse to the nerve cell—**dendritic** *adj*.

dendritic cell an antigen-presenting cell that presents a processed antigen to B and T lymphocytes bearing antigen-specific receptors. They are thought to be the cells important in determining the type of immune response generated against an antigen.

dendritic ulcer a linear corneal ulcer that sends out tree-like branches. Usually caused by herpes simplex virus.

dendron *n* ⇒ dendrite.

denervation *n* the means by which a nerve supply is cut off. Usually refers to incision, excision or blocking of a nerve.

dengue *n* (*syn* 'break-bone fever') a mosquito-transmitted viral haemorrhagic fever occurring in tropical regions. The severity varies but may cause fever, headache, limb pains, vomiting and a rash. Mortality is high in cases where disseminated intravascular coagulation and acute circulatory collapse occurs.

denial *n* a complex unconscious mental defence mechanism in which difficult situations, or unacceptable or distressing facts, are not acknowledged, so as to avoid distress, anxiety and emotional conflict. It may occur in response to drastically changed circumstances, e.g. sudden incapacitating illness, or terminal illness.

Dennis Browne splints splints used to correct congenital talipes equinovarus (club foot).

dental *adj* relating to teeth.

dental amalgam a compound of a basal alloy of silver and tin with mercury, used for restoring teeth. ⇒ amalgam.

dental attrition non-carious, mechanical wearing of teeth, either through normal mastication or as a result of parafunctional habits, e.g. bruxism.

dental caries a microbial disease of the calcified tissues of the teeth, characterized by demineralization of the inorganic portion and destruction of their organic substance.

dental enamel hard, acellular calcified tissue covering the crown of a tooth.

dental erosion non-carious wearing away of the surfaces of the teeth due to chemical causes.

dental hygienist dental auxiliary trained to scale and clean teeth, carry out certain preventive procedures and give oral hygiene instruction to the prescription of a dentist.

dental plaque soft deposit of bacteria and cellular debris that rapidly forms on the surface of a tooth in the absence of oral hygiene.

dental pulp tissue consisting of blood vessels, nerves and connective tissue that occupies the core of the crown and the root canal(s) of a tooth.

dental restoration the process of replacing part or all of a tooth by artificial means; also the term given to the type of replacement used, e.g. filling, crown, bridge.

dental scaling the removal of calculus, using special instruments, from the surfaces of the teeth.

dental therapist dental auxiliary who is trained to carry out certain dental operative procedures to the prescription of a dentist.

dentate *adj* having natural teeth present.

dentine *n* calcified organic hard tissue forming the bulk of the crown and roots of teeth. ⇒ tooth.

dentist *n* any person who practises dentistry, and is qualified and licensed to do so.

dentistry *n* profession concerned with the diagnosis, prevention and treatment of diseases of the teeth and their supporting tissues, including their restoration and replacement. *conservative dentistry* the diagnosis, treatment and restoration of diseased or injured teeth. *cosmetic dentistry* the restoration or enhancement of dental aesthetics. *forensic dentistry* the examination, interpretation and presentation of dentally related evidence in a legal context. *paediatric dentistry* the diagnosis, prevention and treatment of dental and related diseases in children. *preventive dentistry* the prevention of, and preventive treatment for, dental disease and the promotion of good oral health. *prosthetic dentistry* the restoration of the function and aesthetics of missing teeth using artificial dentures.

dentition the natural teeth collectively in an individual.

dento-alveolar abscess localized collection of pus within the alveolar bone, of dental origin.

denture *n* a removable dental prosthesis. May be partial or full (replacing some, or all, of the teeth in either jaw respectively).

deodorant *n, adj* a substance which destroys or masks an (unpleasant) odour. Deodorants are used for personal hygiene and within the environment. Topical antibiotics and charcoal dressings can be used to deodorize malodorous infected wounds—**deodorize** *vt*.

deontological *adj* ethical theory based on the science of deontology that supports the view that there is a duty to act within certain universal rules of morality. A theory associated with the work of Immanuel Kant. ⇒ utilitarianism.

deoxygenation *n* the removal of oxygen—**deoxygenated** *adj*.

deoxyribonucleic acid (DNA) a double-strand nucleic acid molecule found in the chromosomes of all organisms (except some viruses). DNA (as genes) carries the coded instructions for passing on hereditary characteristics. DNA is a polymer formed from many nucleotides. These consist of the sugar deoxyribose, phosphate groups and four nitrogenous bases: adenine (A), guanine (G), thymine (T) and cytosine (C). Adenine and guanine are purine bases, and thymine and cytosine are pyrimidine bases. The nucleotide units are bound together to form a double helix with the adenine of one strand opposite the thymine of the other and the same for guanine and cytosine.

dependency culture a sociological term that describes the opinion that unlimited state welfare provision may reduce individuals' ability to be assertive and support themselves.

depersonalization *n* a subjective feeling that one no longer feels that one is real or exists. Occurs in a wide range of disorders including depressive states, anxiety disorder, with psychoactive substance misuse, etc.

depilate *vt* to remove hair from—**depilatory** *adj, n*, **depilation** *n*.

depilatories *npl* substances usually made in pastes (e.g. barium sulphide) which remove excess hair only temporarily; they do not act on the papillae, consequently the hair grows again. ⇒ epilation—**depilatory** *sing*. *Preoperative depilation* lessens the risk of wound infection because it is non-abrasive.

depolarization *n* in excitable cells the inside of the membrane becomes electrically positive with respect to the outside. Occurs during the transmission of a nerve impulse. ⇒ polarized.

depot *n* a body area where a drug is deposited or stored, and from where it can be released and distributed, such as hormone therapy. *depot injection* drugs, usually psychotropic, that are given by deep intramuscular injections. Used when clients are unable to take their drugs on a regular basis.

depressed fracture ⇒ fracture.

depression *n* **1** a hollow place or indentation. **2** a downward or inward movement or displacement. **3** diminution of power or activity. **4** an emotional disorder characterized by feelings of profound sadness. May be classified by severity (mild/moderate/severe), by the presence of somatic symptoms (anorexia, weight loss, impaired libido, sleep disturbance, etc.) and by the presence or absence of psychotic symptoms. Recognized cognitive symptoms include hopelessness, helplessness, guilt, low self-esteem and suicidal thoughts. The previous description of reactive versus endogenous depression is outdated and not thought to be relevant to treatment or prognosis.

deprivation indices a set of census variables and weightings used to assess levels of deprivation within a specific community or population. They include: levels of unemployment, single-parent households, pensioners living alone and households without a car. ⇒ Jarman index, Townsend index.

De Quervain's thyroiditis *n* an inflammatory condition of the thyroid gland. Often follows a viral infection of the upper respiratory tract. It is characterized by tenderness and swelling of the thyroid gland, pyrexia, neck pain and dysphagia.

Derbyshire neck goitre.

derealization *n* feelings that people, events or surroundings have changed and are unreal. These sensations may occur in normal people during dreams, in states of fatigue or after sensory deprivation. May sometimes occur in schizophrenia and depressive states.

dereistic *adj* of thinking, not adapted to reality. Describes autistic thinking.

dermabrasion *n* removal of superficial layers of the skin by abrasive methods.

dermatitis *n* inflammation of the skin (by custom limited to an eczematous reaction). ⇒ eczema. *atopic dermatitis* that variety of infantile eczema that may be associated with asthma or hay fever. *dermatitis herpetiformis* (*syn* hydroa) an intensely itchy skin eruption of unknown cause, most commonly characterized by papules and vesicles, which remit and relapse. Associated with coeliac disease (gluten-induced enteropathy). *industrial dermatitis* a term used in the National Insurance (Industrial Injuries) Act to cover occupational skin conditions.

dermatoglyphics *n* study of the ridge patterns of the skin of the fingertips, palms and soles to discover developmental anomalies.

dermatographia *n* ⇒ dermographia.

dermatologist *n* medically qualified individual who studies skin diseases and is skilled in their treatment. A skin specialist.

dermatology *n* the science which deals with the skin, its structure, functions, diseases and their treatment—**dermatological** *adj*, **dermatologically** *adv*.

dermatome *n* **1** an instrument for cutting slices of skin of varying thickness, usually for grafting. **2** the area of skin supplied by a single spinal nerve.

dermatomycosis *n* a fungal infection of the skin—**dermatomycotic** *adj*.

dermatomyositis *n* an autoimmune connective tissue disease mainly affecting the skin and muscles. Presents with a characteristic skin rash and muscle weakness. Can be associated with an underlying malignancy in more elderly people. ⇒ collagen.

dermatophytes *npl* a group of fungi that cause superficial infections of skin, hair and nails.

dermatophytosis *n* infection of the skin with dermatophyte species.

dermatosis *n* generic term for skin disease—**dermatoses** *pl*.

dermis *n* the true skin; the cutis vera; the layer below the epidermis ⇒ Figure 12—**dermal** *adj*.

dermographia *n* (*syn* dermatographia, factitial urticaria) a condition in which weals occur on the skin after a blunt instrument or fingernail has been lightly drawn over it. Seen in vasomotor instability and urticaria—**dermographic** *adj*.

dermoid *adj* pertaining to or resembling skin. *dermoid cyst* a cyst which is congenital in origin and usually occurs in the ovary. It contains elements of hair, nails, skin, teeth, etc.

descending colon ⇒ Figure 18b.

descriptive statistics that which describes or summarizes the observations of a sample. ⇒ inferential statistics.

desensitization *n* **1** process of reducing subsequent immediate-type hypersensitivity reactions to venoms and other allergens by repeated injection of minute quantities of allergen in order to modulate the immune response away from the harmful allergic type reaction to a less pathological response. **2** a behavioural therapy used for phobias where people are helped to overcome their irrational fear. There is a gradual introduction to the object or situation through imagining the object, looking at pictures or by eventually confronting the real thing—**desensitize** *vt*.

desiccation *n* drying out. There can be desiccation of the nucleus pulposus, thus diminishing the cushioning effect of a healthy intervertebral disc.

desloughing the process of removing slough from a wound.

desquamation *n* shedding; flaking off; casting off—**desquamate** *vi*, *vt*.

detached retina separation of the neurosensory retina from the pigment epithelium. May be caused by retinal tears or holes, fibrous traction on the retina, or by exudation of fluid under the neurosensory retina.

detained patient a person with a mental disorder who has been detained under the relevant legislation such as the Mental Health Act. ⇒ informal patient.

detergent *n, adj* (describes) a cleansing agent. ⇒ cetrimide.

deterioration *n* progressive impairment of function: worsening of the patient's condition.

determinants of health factors that may influence the health of an individual, or differences in health between individuals, apart form age, sex and constitution (physiological, genetic factors). These could be social and economic, environmental or psychological factors that increase the risk of ill health or disease (e.g. heart disease, cancers, diabetes). These determinants, or indicators, are associated with better or worse health of populations as measured by mortality (standardized mortality ratios), valid measures of morbidity or self-reported health status (e.g. health surveys, census, standardized illness ratios). For example, higher infant mortality may be associated with environmental factors, healthcare provision, social and community support, maternal deprivation and poverty. There may also be a cultural and behavioural perspective. ⇒ morbidity, mortality.

detoxication *n* the removal of the poisonous property of a substance—**detoxicant** *adj, n*, **detoxicate** *vt*.

detritus *n* matter produced by detrition; waste matter from disintegration.

detrusor *n* an expelling muscle such as that of the urinary bladder. *detrusor instability* failure to inhibit reflex detrusor contraction. ⇒ incontinence.

detumescence *n* subsidence of a swelling.

developmental dysplasia of the hip (DDH) also known as congenital dislocation of the hip. The term DDH is useful in describing the varying causes and severity of the condition. There is poor development of the acetabulum which allows the head of the femur to dislocate.

deviance *n* a variation from normal. A sociological term that describes a change from the accepted social norm.

dexamethasone suppression tests tests using different doses and duration of dexamethasone treatment to identify patients producing excess glucocorticoid, Cushing's syndrome, and the source.

dextran *n* a colloid solution obtained by the action of a specific bacterium on sugar solutions. Previously used for replacing fluids in hypovolaemia. It is no longer routinely used as a colloid. Dextran may cause allergic reactions. It also affects clotting and interferes with blood cross-matching.

dextrin *n* a soluble polysaccharide resulting from the hydrolysis of starch.

dextrocardia *n* transposition of the heart to the right side of the thorax—**dextrocardial** *adj*.

dextrose *n* (*syn* glucose) a soluble carbohydrate (monosaccharide) widely used in intravenous infusion solutions. Also given orally as a readily absorbed sugar in rehydration fluids for fluid and electrolyte replacement, and for hypoglycaemia.

dhobie itch tinea cruris.

diabetes *n* a disease characterized by polyuria, with consequent polydipsia; used without qualification implies diabetes mellitus—**diabetic** *adj, n*.

diabetes insipidus diabetes caused by disordered water homeostasis. It may be *cranial* due to deficiency of vasopressin (AVP), either idiopathic or due to trauma, tumour or inflammation affecting posterior pituitary function, or *nephrogenic* due to renal tubular resistance to AVP action.

diabetes mellitus diabetes due to glycosuria and osmotic diuresis resulting from hyperglycaemia; defined as fasting blood glucose >7.0 mmol/L, 2 hour glucose following 75 g glucose load (oral glucose tolerance test) equal to or greater than 11.1 mmol/L. Diabetes mellitus may classified as: *type 1* due to autoimmune destruction of insulin producing cells in the pancreatic islets, if uncontrolled leading to ketoacidosis; *type 2* due to varying degrees of insulin resistance, often due to obesity, and impaired insulin secretion, if uncontrolled leading to hyperosmolar non-ketotic coma (HONK, HHNK); may also be *secondary* to other diseases, e.g. pancreatitis, Cushing's syndrome, haemochromatosis; or *genetic* e.g. maturity onset diabetes of the young (MODY), mitochondrial diabetes; or *gestational diabetes* diagnosed in pregnancy, usually resolving afterwards, when it reflects the increased burden placed on the pancreatic beta cells by hormone changes in later pregnancy.

diabetic nephropathy a glomerulosclerosis caused by damage to the glomerular capillaries. There is microalbuminuria, hypertension, and eventually loss of glomeruli and renal failure.

diagnosis *n* the art or act of distinguishing one disease from another. *differential diagnosis* is the term used when making a correct decision between diseases presenting a similar clinical picture—**diagnoses** *pl*, **diagnose** *vt*.

diagnostic *adj* **1** pertaining to diagnosis. **2** serving as evidence in diagnosis—**diagnostician** *n*.

dialysate *n* exogenous fluid used in dialysis to promote diffusion and removal of waste products.

dialyser *n* (*syn* artificial kidney) used in haemodialysis; consists of blood and dialysate compartments separated by a semipermeable membrane.

dialysis process by which solutes are removed from solution by diffusion across a porous membrane; requires the presence of a favourable solute gradient. ⇒ haemodialysis, peritoneal dialysis—**dialyses** *pl*, **dialyse** *vt*.

diapedesis *n* the passage of cells from within blood vessels through the vessel walls into the tissues—**diapedetic** *adj*.

diaphoresis *n* perspiration.

diaphoretic *adj*, *n* (*syn* sudorific) an agent which induces diaphoresis (sweating).

diaphragm *n* **1** the dome-shaped muscular partition between the thorax above and the abdomen below. **2** any partitioning membrane or septum. **3** a cap which encircles the cervix to act as a barrier contraceptive. Reliable when fitted correctly and used correctly with a spermicidal chemical—**diaphragmatic** *adj*.

diaphysis *n* the shaft of a long bone—**diaphyses** *pl*, **diaphyseal** *adj*.

diarrhoea *n* deviation from established bowel rhythm characterized by an increase in frequency and fluidity of the stools. May cause dehydration, hypokalaemia, acidosis (metabolic), malabsorption of nutrients and perianal soreness. Causes include, infection, food sensitivity, laxative misuse, drugs such as antibiotics, dietary change or indiscretion, anxiety, colorectal cancer (alternating with constipation) and some systemic diseases. ⇒ spurious diarrhoea.

diarthrosis *n* a synovial, freely movable joint—**diarthroses** *pl*, **diarthrodial** *adj*.

diastasis *n* a separation of bones without fracture.

diastema *n* a naturally occurring space between two teeth.

diastole *n* the relaxation filling period of the cardiac cycle—**diastolic** *adj*. ⇒ systole.

diathermy *n* the passage of a high frequency electric current through the tissues whereby heat is produced. When both electrodes are large, the heat is diffused over a wide area according to the electrical resistance of the tissues. In this form it is widely used in the treatment of inflammation, especially when deeply seated (e.g. sinusitis, pelvic cellulitis). When one electrode is very small the heat is concentrated in this area and becomes great enough to destroy tissue. In this form (surgical diathermy) it is used to stop bleeding at operation by coagulation of blood, or to cut through tissue.

dibenzodiazepines *npl* a group of atypical neuroleptics. ⇒ Appendix 5.

DIC *abbr* disseminated intravascular coagulation.

dicephalous *adj* two-headed.

dicrotic *adj*, *n* (pertaining to, or having) a double beat, as indicated by a second expansion of the artery during diastole. *dicrotic notch* the second rise in the arterial tracing caused by the closure of the aortic valve (that between the left ventricle and the aorta). ⇒ anacrotic.

dietary fibre ⇒ non-starch polysaccharides.

dietary reference values (DRVs) in the UK a set of tables that estimate a range of nutritional requirements for different groups of the population (healthy individuals). Usually three values are given—estimated average requirement, lower reference nutrient intake and reference nutrient intake.

dietary supplementation a term in sports medicine used to describe the food supplements (above what is required to ensure the intake of nutrients for a balanced diet) taken as an ergogenic aid. For example carbohydrate loading, creatine supplements and isotonic sports drinks.

dietetics *n* the interpretation and application of the scientific principles of nutrition to feeding in health and disease.

dietitian *n* one who applies the principles of nutrition to the feeding of an individual or a group of individuals. Dietitians are employed in a range of hospital and community settings, the food industry, by local authorities and by national and international agencies, e.g. WHO.

differential blood count ⇒ blood count.

differential diagnosis ⇒ diagnosis.

differentiation *n* the process during which cells and tissues expand the ability to perform specialized functions that distinguish them from other cell types. Cancer cells are graded by their degree of differentiation.

diffusion *n* **1** the process whereby gases and liquids of different concentrations mix when brought into contact, until their concentration is equal throughout. **2** dialysis.

digestion *n* the process by which food is rendered absorbable—**digestible, digestive** *adj*, **digestibility** *n*, **digest** *vt*.

digestive system ⇒ Figure 18b.

digit *n* a finger or toe—**digital** *adj*.

digital compression pressure applied by the fingers, usually to an artery to stop bleeding.

digitalis *n* leaf of the common foxglove containing glycosides, such as digoxin. ⇒ glycosides.

digitalization *n* physiological saturation with digitalis to obtain optimum therapeutic effect.

digiti minimi quinti varus (*syn* congenital overlapping fifth toe) the smallest toe lies on the dorsum of the base of the fourth toe in a medially deviated position. It may be bilateral or unilateral.

dilatation *n* stretching or enlargement. May occur physiologically, pathologically or be induced artificially.

dilatation and curettage (D and C) by custom refers to dilating the uterine cervix to obtain an endometrial sample by curettage. ⇒ hysteroscopy.

dilatation and evacuation (D and E) dilatation of the cervix and evacuation of a fetus under anaesthetic for therapeutic termination of pregnancy or for the removal of a dead fetus in the second trimester of pregnancy.

dimercaprol (BAL) *n* an organic compound used as an antidote for poisoning by heavy metals such as arsenic, bismuth, gold and mercury. It forms soluble but stable compounds with the metals, which are then rapidly excreted by the kidneys.

Diogenes syndrome gross self-neglect. Most often seen in older people who are living in appalling conditions of squalor. The person concerned usually rejects offers of help, and strenuously resists any measures to change the situation.

dioptre *n* a unit of measurement in refraction. A lens of one dioptre has a focal length of 1 metre.

dioxide *n* oxide containing two atoms of oxygen in each molecule, e.g. CO_2.

dipeptidases *npl* digestive enzymes that split dipeptides (paired amino acids) into individual amino acids.

2,3-diphosphoglycerate (2,3-DPG) *n* substance present in red blood cells that decreases the affinity of haemoglobin for oxygen, thus allowing oxygen to be released to the tissues.

diphtheria *n* an acute, specific, infectious notifiable disease caused by *Corynebacterium diphtheriae*. Characterized by a grey, adherent, false membrane growing on a mucous surface, usually that of the upper respiratory tract. Locally there is pain and swelling, and there may be airway obstruction. Bacterial exotoxins may cause serious damage to nerves and heart muscle. Immunization is available as part of routine programmes during childhood. Close contacts with infected people are immunized and given antibiotic prophylaxis—**diphtheritic** *adj*.

diplegia *n* symmetrical paralysis of legs, usually associated with cerebral damage—**diplegic** *adj*.

diplococcus *n* a coccal bacterium that occurs in pairs. *Diplococcus* may be used in a binomial to describe a characteristically paired coccus, e.g. *Diplococcus pneumoniae* (*Streptococcus pneumoniae* or pneumococcus).

diploid (2n) *adj* describes a cell with a full set of paired chromosomes. In humans the diploid number is 46 chromosomes (44 autosomes and 2 sex chromosomes) arranged in 23 pairs in all cells except the gametes.

diplopia *n* the seeing of two objects when only one exists (double vision).

direct cost a cost that can be directly attributed to the budget of a specific department, for example pharmacy costs in a given department.

disaccharide *n* a carbohydrate made up of two monosaccharide molecules, e.g. lactose, maltose, sucrose, which yields two molecules of monosaccharide on hydrolysis.

disarticulation *n* amputation at a joint.

discectomy *n* surgical removal of a disc, usually an intervertebral disc.

discogenic *adj* arising in or produced by a disc, usually an intervertebral disc.

discrete *adj* distinct, separate, not merging. For example used to describe some types of skin lesions.

disease *n* any deviation from or interruption of the normal structure and function of any part of the body. It is manifested by a characteristic set of signs and symptoms and in most instances the aetiology, pathology and prognosis is known.

disease prevention reducing the risk of a disease process, illness, injury or disability. Includes preventive services, e.g. immunization and screening, preventive health education, e.g. advice about sensible drinking, and preventive health protection, e.g. taxing tobacco and fluoridating water. Preventive activities are classified as primary, secondary or tertiary prevention. *primary prevention* (1°) includes all activities to eradicate the cause of disease or decrease the susceptibility of the individual to the causative agent. Examples include smoking cessation advice, immunization programmes. *secondary prevention* (2°) is the detection and treatment of disease before symptoms or disordered function develops, i.e. before irreversible damage occurs, generally achieved through screening. Examples include cervical cytology screening, hypertension screening. *tertiary prevention* (3°) is the monitoring and management of established disease in order to prevent the complications of the disease process, disability or handicap. For example monitoring of patients with diabetes in order to detect and treat early complications.

disengagement theory a psychosocial theory of ageing. It describes a process whereby older people gradually disengage from social life and physical activity as they become older. ⇒ activity theory.

disimpaction *n* separation of the broken ends of a bone that have been driven into each other during the impact which caused the fracture. Traction may then be applied to maintain the bone ends in good alignment and separate.

disinfectants *npl* the term usually reserved for chemical germicides that are too corrosive or toxic to be applied to tissues, but which are suitable for application to inanimate objects.

disinfection *n* the removal or destruction of harmful microbes but not usually bacterial spores. It is commonly achieved by using heat or chemicals.

disinfestation *n* eradication of an infestation, especially of lice (delousing).

dislocation *n* displacement of organs, or the articular surfaces of joints, so that all apposition between them is lost. The disruption of the joint is such that the bony components no longer form a working joint. It may be congenital, spontaneous, traumatic or recurrent. Treatment may include reduction under anaesthetic—**dislocated** *adj*, **dislocate** *vt*.

disobliteration *n* rebore. Removal of that which blocks a vessel, most often intimal plaques in an artery, when it is called endarterectomy.

disorientation *n* loss of orientation.

displacement *n* **1** a mental defence mechanism whereby a painful emotion is transferred to a another person or object. **2** describes the loss of pieces of information from short-term memory as new information is added.

disposable soma theory a theory of ageing attributed to Tom Kirkwood that posits that reproductive potential in early years is maximized at the expense of ageing in later years.

dissection *n* separation of tissues by cutting. When a group of lymph nodes are totally excised it is referred to as a *block dissection of nodes*: it is usually part of the treatment for cancer.

disseminated widely spread or scattered. *disseminated intravascular coagulation (DIC)* an abnormal overstimulation of coagulation processes characterized by a rapid consumption of clotting factors which leads to microvascular thrombi and bleeding. It is associated with conditions leading to inadequate organ perfusion, such as hypovolaemia and or sepsis. ⇒ multiple organ dysfunction syndrome, systemic inflammatory response syndrome.

dissociation *n* 1 separation of complex substances into their components. 2 ionization; when ionic compounds dissolve in water they dissociate or ionize into their ions.

dissociative disorder formerly known as conversion/hysteria disorders. Loss of conscious integration between control of body movement, sensory perceptions, self-identity and memory. Generally considered to be of 'psychogenic' aetiology. Usually of sudden onset/termination and short duration. Often associated with striking denial.

distal *adj* farthest from the head or source. ⇒ proximal *opp*—**distally** *adv*.

distichiasis *n* extra eyelashes at the posterior lid margin, which turn inwards against the eye.

distractibility *n* a psychiatric disorder of the power of attention when it can only be applied momentarily.

distress ⇒ stress.

diuresis *n* increased production/secretion of urine. *forced diuresis* drugs may be used in some cases of poisoning in order to increase elimination of the poison.

diuretics *npl* substances that increase the secretion of urine by the kidney. ⇒ caffeine, carbonic anhydrase inhibitors, loop diuretics, osmotic diuretics, potassium sparing diuretics, thiazide diuretics. ⇒ Appendix 5.

divarication *n* separation of two points on a straight line.

divers' paralysis ⇒ decompression illness.

diverticulitis *n* inflammation of a diverticulum.

diverticulosis *n* a condition in which there are many diverticula, especially in the intestines. Colonic diverticula increase in frequency with age. May be asymptomatic, bleed, become infected or perforate.

diverticulum *n* a pouch or sac protruding from the wall of a tube or hollow organ. May be congenital or acquired—**diverticula** *pl*.

dizygotic relating to two zygotes. Describes non-identical twins that develop from two separate zygotes. ⇒ monozygotic *opp*.

dizziness *n* a feeling of unsteadiness, usually accompanied by anxiety.

DNA *abbr* deoxyribonucleic acid.

Döderlein's bacillus a non-pathogenic Gram-positive rod normally part of the vaginal flora in women of reproductive age. It contributes to the protective acidic environment by the production of lactic acid. ⇒ lactobacillus.

dolor *n* pain; usually used in the context of being one of the five classical signs and symptoms of inflammation—the others being calor, loss of function, rubor and tumor.

domestic activities of daily living (DADL) include activities such as cooking and cleaning.

dominant *adj* describes a gene with the ability to override the expression of other recessive genes. Dominant genes are expressed in both the homozygous state and the heterozygous state. Examples of dominant gene expression include: normal skin and hair pigmentation and Huntington's disease. ⇒ Mendel's law, recessive.

dominant hemisphere on the opposite side of the brain to that of the preferred hand. The dominant hemisphere for language is the left in most right-handed and around a third of left-handed people.

DOMS *abbr* delayed onset muscle soreness.

donor *n* a person who gives blood for transfusion, or semen for AID, or donates tissue for transplantation.

Donovan bodies Leishman–Donovan bodies.

donovanosis *n* chronic granulomatous ulceration of the genitalia or anal region, caused by *Klebsiella granulomatis*. Prevalent in warmer climates.

dopa *n* a compound formed in an intermediate stage during the synthesis of catecholamines, e.g. adrenaline, from tyrosine.

dopamine *n* a monoamine neurotransmitter. It functions in the central nervous system, especially the basal nuclei. Reduced levels are associated with Parkinson's disease. Used intravenously in some types of shock to increase cardiac output and blood flow to the kidneys.

Doppler technique can be used to measure the velocity of blood flow through a vessel to determine the degree of occlusion or stenosis. *Doppler scanning* combines ultrasonography with pulse echo. *Doppler ultrasound technique* can be used to calculate cardiac output and stroke volume by measuring blood flow in the aorta via a probe passed into the oesophagus. Used to monitor haemodynamic status and response to treatment.

dorsal *adj* pertaining to the back, or the posterior part of an organ.

dorsiflexion *n* bending backwards. In the case of the great toe—upwards. ⇒ Babinski's reflex.

dorsocentral *adj* at the back and in the centre.

dorsolumbar *adj* pertaining to the lumbar region of the back.

dosimeter, dosemeter *n* a device worn by personnel or placed within equipment to measure incident X-rays or gamma rays. Thermoluminescent dosimeters, using lithium fluoride powder impregnated into plastic discs, are used in personnel monitoring. Previously, photographic film in a special filter holder was used.

double vision ⇒ diplopia.

doubling time time over which a tumour will double in size. A mark of tumour virulence and occasionally an indicator of chemoresponsiveness (faster doubling time often associated with high growth fraction and occasionally with higher chemoresponsiveness).

douche *n* a stream of fluid directed against the body externally or into a body cavity.

Down's syndrome a congenital condition in which there is learning disability and facial characteristics that include: oval tilted eyes, squint and a flattened occiput. The chromosome abnormality is of two types: (a) Primary trisomy, caused by abnormal division of chromosome 21 (at meiosis). This results in an extra chromosome instead of the normal pair: the infant has 47 chromosomes and is often born of an older mother. (b) Structural abnormality involving chromosome 21, with a total number of 46 chromosomes, one of which has an abnormal structure as the result of a special translocation. Such

infants are usually born of younger mothers and there is a higher risk of recurrence in subsequent pregnancies.

dracontiasis *n* infestation with *Dracunculus medinensis* common in Africa, Middle East and Asia. It is transmitted through contaminated drinking water. The female worm moves from the intestine to emerge through the skin surface in order to deposit larvae. There is inflammation, thickening and ulceration.

Dracunculus medinensis (*syn* Guinea worm) a nematode parasite (tissue-dwelling) that infests humans.

drain *n* ⇒ wound drains.

dreaming altered state of consciousness where fantasies and remembered events are confused with reality.

D_2-receptor antagonists a group of antiemetic drugs that act by blocking the dopamine receptors. ⇒ Appendix 5.

dressings *npl* ⇒ wound dressings.

Dressler's syndrome ⇒ postmyocardial infarction syndrome.

drop attacks periodic falling because of sudden loss of postural control of the lower limbs, without vertigo or loss of consciousness. Usually followed by sudden return of normal muscle tone, allowing the person to rise, if uninjured. ⇒ vertebrobasilar insufficiency.

droplet infection pathogen transmission in droplets of moisture such as during coughing or talking.

dropsy *n* ⇒ oedema—**dropsical** *adj*.

drug *n* the generic name for any substance used for the prevention, diagnosis and treatment of diagnosed disease and also for the relief of symptoms. The term 'prescribed drug' describes such usage. ⇒ prescription only medicine (POM). The word medicine is usually preferred for therapeutic drugs to distinguish them from the addictive drugs which are used illegally. For alleviating unpleasant symptoms of self-limiting illnesses, any remedy which does not require a medical prescription is termed an 'over-the-counter (OTC)' medicine. ⇒ general sales list (GSL). *drug clearance* ⇒ clearance. *drug dependence* a state arising from repeated administration of a drug on a periodic or continuous basis (WHO, 1964). Now a preferable term to drug addiction and drug habituation. *drug interaction* occurs when the action of one drug is affected by another drug, beverage or food taken previously or simultaneously. *drug misuse* term increasingly used to describe the illegal use of drugs. Substance misuse includes solvents and alcohol, as well as drugs. *drug reaction* ⇒ adverse drug reactions. *drug tolerance* a situation where the therapeutic effects of a drug lessen over time, which necessitates the administration of a larger dose to achieve the same benefit.

drug errors are described as preventable prescribing, dispensing or administration mistakes.

drug resistance the increasing problem caused by the ability of some microorganisms to develop resistance to certain antibiotics, e.g. vancomycin-resistant enterococci and methicillin-resistant *Staphylococcus aureus*.

drug trials several levels of testing occurring during the development of new drugs. (a) Phase I trials where small numbers of healthy volunteers (usually male) are given small doses and monitored for adverse reactions. Blood samples are tested to determine drug distribution and excretion. (b) Phase II trials involve patients, and the new drug's efficacy is compared with existing treatments. (c) Phase III trials involve large multiple centre studies carried out before the drug is approved and licensed for use by the appropriate bodies. ⇒ Committee on Safety of Medicines, Medical Control Agency. (d) Phase IV trials take place after the drug has been approved for clinical use. Aim to monitor and report adverse and idiosyncratic reactions not seen earlier.

drusen *npl* yellow or white spots present beneath the neurosensory retina, usually in the macula.

DRVs *abbr* dietary reference values.

dry eye syndrome ⇒ Sjögren syndrome.

DSH *abbr* deliberate self-harm.

dualism *n* in psychology, a view that mind and body are separate.

Dubowitz score assesses gestational age.

Duchenne muscular dystrophy an X-linked recessive disorder affecting only boys. The disorder usually begins to show between 3 and 5 years and is characterized by progressive muscle weakness and

loss of locomotor skills. Death usually occurs during the teens or early twenties from respiratory or cardiac failure.

Ducrey's bacillus *Haemophilus ducreyi*.

duct *n* a tube for carrying away the secretions from a gland.

ductless glands endocrine glands.

ductus arteriosus a fetal blood vessel connecting the left pulmonary artery to the aorta, to bypass the lungs in the fetus. At birth the duct closes, but if it remains open it is called *persistent or patent ductus arteriosus*, a congenital heart defect.

ductus venosus connection between the umbilical vein and inferior vena cava in the fetal circulation. Closes at birth.

Dukes' staging a system for the staging of colorectal cancer. It has four categories A–D, and is based on the degree of tissue invasion and metastasis.

dumbness *n* ⇒ mutism.

'dumping syndrome' the name given to the symptoms of epigastric fullness and a feeling of faintness and sweating after meals that sometimes follow partial gastrectomy. Rapid movement of hypertonic gastric contents into the duodenum causes fluid to move from the blood to the bowel lumen. Rapid absorption of glucose leads to rebound insulin secretion and hypoglycaemia.

duodenal intubation ⇒ intubation.

duodenal ulcer a peptic ulcer occurring in the duodenal mucosa. The majority are associated with the presence of the bacterium *Helicobacter pylori* in the stomach. Other factors include NSAIDs, smoking and genetic factors. Epigastric pain may occur some time after meals or during the night. The pain may be relieved by food, antacids and vomiting. The ulcer can bleed, leading to haematemesis and/or melaena, or it can perforate. Severe scarring following chronic ulceration may produce pyloric stenosis and gastric outlet obstruction. Management includes: (a) general measures; smoking cessation, avoiding foods that cause pain, avoiding aspirin and NSAIDs; (b) antibiotic drugs to eradicate *H. pylori*; (c) drugs to reduce gastric acid; H_2 receptor antagonists, e.g. ranitidine, proton pump inhibitors, e.g. omeprazole, antacids based on calcium, magnesium or aluminium salts; (d) rarely surgical treatment, e.g. after perforation.

duodenitis *n* inflammation of the duodenum.

duodenojejunal *adj* pertaining to the duodenum and jejunum.

duodenopancreatectomy *n* ⇒ pancreaticoduodenectomy.

duodenoscope *n* a side-viewing flexible fibreoptic endoscope—**duodenoscopic** *adj*, **duodenoscopy** *n*.

duodenostomy *n* a surgically made fistula between the duodenum and another cavity, e.g. cholecystoduodenostomy.

duodenum *n* the fixed, curved, first portion of the small intestine, connecting the stomach above to the jejunum below (⇒ Figure 18b)—**duodenal** *adj*.

Dupuytren's contracture painless, chronic flexion of the digits of the hand, especially the third and fourth, towards the palm. The aetiology is uncertain but some cases are associated with hepatic cirrhosis.

dura mater the outer meningeal membrane. ⇒ falx cerebri, meninges, tentorium cerebelli.

duty of care the legal responsibility in the law of negligence that a person must take reasonable care to avoid causing harm.

DVT *abbr* deep vein thrombosis.

dwarf *n* person of stunted growth. May be due to growth hormone deficiency. Also occurs in untreated congenital hypothyroidism and juvenile hypothyroidism, achondroplasia and other conditions.

dwarfism *n* arrested growth and development as occurs in congenital hypothyroidism, and in some chronic diseases such as intestinal malabsorption, renal failure and rickets.

dynamic flexibility active range of motion exercises used to increase flexibility.

dynamic psychology a psychological approach which stresses the importance of (typically unconscious) energy or motives, as in Freudian or psychoanalytic theory.

dynamometer *n* a device used to measure strength.

dysaesthesia *n* impairment of touch sensation.

dysarthria *n* a speech disorder that results from a problem in muscular control of the mechanisms of speech. It is caused by damage to either the central or the peripheral nervous system, or both. Loss of muscular control may involve incoordination and/or slowness and weakness. The problem may affect articulation, phonation, prosody, resonance and respiration—**dysarthric** *adj*.

dyschondroplasia *n* a disorder of bone growth resulting in normal trunk, short arms and legs.

dyscrasia *n* an abnormality in the cellular composition of the blood.

dysdiadochokinesia *n* impairment of the ability to perform alternating movements, such as pronation and supination, in rapid, smooth and rhythmical succession; a sign of cerebellar disease but also seen in the so-called 'clumsy child' with minimal brain damage.

dysentery *n* inflammation of the bowel with evacuation of blood and mucus, accompanied by tenesmus and colic—**dysenteric** *adj*. *amoebic dysentery* is caused by the protozoon *Entamoeba histolytica* ⇒ amoebiasis. *bacillary dysentery* is caused by bacilli of the genus *Shigella*: *S. dysenteriae*, *S. flexneri*, *S. boydii* or *S. sonnei* (the commonest cause in the UK). The organism is excreted by cases and carriers in their faeces, and contaminates hands, food and water, from which new hosts are infected.

dysfunction *n* **1** a temporary, or permanent, inability to adapt to the demands of a normal situation in a normal environment. **2** abnormal functioning of a body part or organ.

dysgammaglobulinaemia *n* impaired immunoglobulin production in terms of quantitative or qualitative humoral immunity. There are numerous primary and secondary causes including common variable immunodeficiency, X-linked agammaglobulinaemia, X-linked hyper-IgM syndrome, myeloma and transient hypogammaglobulinaemia of infancy.

dysgenesis *n* malformation during embryonic development—**dysgenetic** *adj*, **dysgenetically** *adv*.

dysgerminoma *n* ovarian tumour, benign or of low grade malignancy. It originates from primitive/undifferentiated gonadal cells.

dysgeusia *n* impaired or abnormal sense of taste.

dysgraphia *n* an acquired problem of written language caused by brain damage. The affected person's ability to spell familiar and/or unfamiliar words is altered in one or many modes, e.g. word-processing or handwriting. Several different types of dysgraphia are described—**dysgraphic** *adj.*

dyshidrosis *n* a vesicular skin eruption on the palms and soles, formerly thought to be caused by blockage of the sweat ducts at their orifice, histologically an eczematous process.

dyskaryosis *n* abnormality of nuclear chromatin, indicating a malignant or premalignant condition.

dyskeratosis abnormal keratin production by epithelial cells; may indicate malignancy.

dyskinesia *n* **1** (clumsy child syndrome) impairment of voluntary movement—**dyskinetic** *adj.* **2** involuntary purposeless movement. ⇒ tardive dyskinesia.

dyslexia *n* a disorder affecting the ability to read. There are a number of different types of dyslexia, for example, *deep dyslexia* and *surface dyslexia*. Many individuals with dyslexia may also exhibit dysgraphia—**dyslexic** *adj.*

dysmaturity *n* signs and symptoms of growth retardation at birth. ⇒ low birthweight.

dysmelia *n* limb malformation, including deficiency.

dysmenorrhoea *n* painful menstruation. It may be *spasmodic or primary dysmenorrhoea*, most often affecting young women once ovulation has become established, or *congestive or secondary dysmenorrhoea* usually affecting women in their late twenties and may be associated with pelvic pathology, such as fibroids or endometriosis.

dysmetria *n* difficulty in assessing and achieving the correct distance and range of movement causing undershooting or overshooting of a target and the appearance of homing in on it.

dysmorphogenic ⇒ teratogen.

dysmotility *n* abnormality of intestinal peristalsis.

dyspareunia *n* painful or difficult coitus, experienced by the woman.

dyspepsia *n* indigestion—**dyspeptic** *adj.*

dysphagia *n* difficulty in swallowing. Dysphagia can occur in a variety of medical conditions including oesophageal cancer, cerebral palsy, motor neuron disease, cerebrovascular accident, dementia and head and neck cancer. The difficulty in swallowing may be experienced with fluids and/or solid food. The extent of difficulty can range from a mild to a very severe problem. Assessment and management of dysphagia is best conducted by a multidisciplinary team that may include a gastroenterologist, specialist nutrition nurse, dietitian, speech and language therapist. The composition of the team will be determined by the needs of the patient, the medical condition underlying the swallowing problem, whether surgery is indicated, the clinical setting and the aim of treatment (curative or palliative)—**dysphagic** *adj.*

dysphasia *n* also sometimes known as aphasia. Dysphasia is a disorder of language and has nothing to do with intelligence level or an intellectual disorder. It is most commonly associated with cerebrovascular accident affecting the left side of the brain, but can occur after a head injury or brain surgery. Dysphasia can affect the ability to understand language and also the use of language for expression. The presentation of dysphasia varies greatly and those affected have very different skills and difficulties. It is important that detailed, individual consideration is given to their difficulties. The understanding of language includes understanding both what is said and what is written. Likewise, expression includes both verbal expression and written expression. Discrepancies between the level of understanding and expression of language are common. Most often, people with dysphasia have problems both in comprehension and in expression although the degree of impairment in each may vary. Assessment and treatment of dysphasia needs a detailed understanding and breakdown of language. Speech and language therapists can provide therapy to assist individuals and their carers to improve their communication. Dysphasia has a considerable impact on most areas of life such as relationships, work and leisure activities.

Rehabilitation takes time and may last many months. People affected by dysphasia can become very withdrawn and isolated if they do not receive sufficient support. ⇒ aphasia.

dysplasia *n* developmental abnormality, often referring to a premalignant condition and graded according to severity—**dysplastic** *adj.*

dysphonia *n* a voice disorder. It may have a neurological, behavioural, organic or psychogenic cause.

dyspnoea *n* difficulty in, or laboured, breathing; can be mainly of an inspiratory or expiratory nature—**dysponoeic** *adj.*

dyspraxia *n* lack of voluntary control over muscles, particularly the orofacial ones—**dyspraxic** *adj.*

dysrhythmia *n* ⇒ arrhythmia.

dyssynergia loss of fluency of movement; poor sequencing and timing of movements; loss of coordination of muscles that normally act in unison, particularly the abnormal state of muscle activity due to cerebellar disease.

dystaxia *n* difficulty in controlling voluntary movements—**dystaxic** *adj.*

dystocia *n* difficult or slow labour.

dystonia *n* a movement disorder in which there is the abnormal posturing of a part of the body, examples of which are spasmodic torticollis and writer's cramp.

dystrophy *n* defective nutrition of an organ or tissue, usually muscle. The word is applied to several unrelated conditions. ⇒ muscular dystrophy, Duchenne muscular dystrophy.

dysuria *n* painful micturition—**dysuric** *adj.*

E

ear *n* the sensory organ concerned with hearing and balance. It has three parts, the outer (external), middle (tympanic cavity) and inner (internal) ear. The outer ear comprises the auricle (pinna) and the external auditory canal along which sound waves pass to vibrate the tympanic membrane which separates it from the middle ear. The middle ear cavity is air-filled and contains three tiny bones or ossicles: malleus, incus and stapes. The ossicles transmit the sound waves to the inner ear via the oval window. The middle ear communicates with the nasopharynx via the eustachian tube (pharyngotympanic tube). The fluid-filled inner ear comprises the cochlea (organ of hearing) and the semicircular canals which are concerned with balance. The cochlea and semicircular canals contain the nerve endings of the cochlear and vestibular branches of the vestibulocochlear or auditory nerve (eighth cranial). ⇒ cerumen, cochlea. ⇒ Figure 13.

EAR *acron* estimated average requirement.

eardrum *n* the tympanic membrane at the end of the external auditory canal. The first auditory ossicle is attached to the inner surface. ⇒ Figure 13.

eating disorders a term used to describe the range of conditions in which an individual's eating behaviour and nutrient intake is inappropriate for their needs. Anorexia nervosa is characterized by distorted body image and a deliberate restriction of food intake, resulting in severe weight loss, malnutrition, endocrine disorders and electrolyte disturbances. Bulimia nervosa—body weight is controlled by periods of restricted eating, purging and binge eating. Weight usually remains stable and within normal range. Binge eating disorder—periods of binge eating without periods of food restriction or purging which result in the development of obesity. A complex mixture of social and psychological factors and life events predispose to and precipitate the development of eating disorders. Consequently they are best treated by a multidisciplinary team.

EBM *abbr* **1** evidence-based medicine. **2** expressed breast milk.

ebola *n* one of the viral haemorrhagic fevers, usually transmitted by ticks.

EBV *abbr* Epstein–Barr virus.

ecbolic *adj* describes any agent that causes contraction of the gravid uterus and accelerates expulsion of its contents. ⇒ oxytocic.

eccentric *adj* positioned off centre. *eccentric muscle work* paying out of a muscle, allowing attachments to be moved further apart. For example when going downstairs, the hamstring muscles of the posterior thigh work eccentrically to control straightening of the knee. ⇒ concentric muscle work.

ecchondroma *n* a benign tumour composed of cartilage which protrudes from the surface of the bone in which it arises—**ecchondromata** *pl.*

ecchymosis *n* ⇒ bruise—**ecchymoses** *pl.*

eccrine *adj* the most abundant type of sweat gland. ⇒ apocrine glands.

ECG *abbr* electrocardiogram ⇒ electrocardiograph.

Echinococcus *n* a genus of cestodes, tapeworms, e.g. *Echinococcus granulosa*; the adults infest dogs and other canines (primary host). The larval stage can infect humans through contaminated drinking water or handling affected dogs. The encysted larvae cause hydatid disease in humans and animals such as cattle and sheep who are secondary hosts. ⇒ hydatid cyst.

echocardiography *n* the use of ultrasound as a diagnostic tool for studying the structure and motion of the heart.

echoencephalography *n* passage of ultrasound waves across the head. Can detect abscess, blood clot, injury or tumour within the brain.

echolalia *n* repetition, almost automatically, of words or phrases heard. Occurs most commonly in schizophrenia and dementia and sometimes in delirium—**echolalic** *adj.*

echoviruses *npl* name originates from Enteric Cytopathic Human Orphan. They are enteroviruses that cause conditions that include: gastroenteritis, respiratory infection, meningitis, encephalitis and rashes.

echoxia *n* involuntary mimicking of another's movements.

eclampsia *n* **1** occurrence of convulsions in a pregnant woman with signs of pre-eclampsia. **2** a sudden convulsive attack—**eclamptic** *adj.*

ecmnesia *n* impaired memory for recent events with normal memory of remote ones. Common in old age and in early cerebral deterioration.

ecological study a research study where a particular group of individuals rather than an individual, e.g. schools, towns, etc., form the unit being observed.

economy *n* describes spending or using as little as possible whilst still maintaining quality.

ecstasy *n* colloquial term for an amphetamine derivative methylenedioxymethamphetamine (MDMA) that causes euphoria and hallucinations. Use is widespread at 'raves' and clubs. It is considered by many users to be safe, but serious effects from excessive physical activity and dehydration which leads to hyperpyrexia and possibly death have occurred.

ECT *abbr* electroconvulsive therapy.

ecthyma *n* a crusted eruption of pyogenic infection, usually on the legs, producing necrosis of the skin, which heals with scarring.

ectoderm *n* the outer of the three primary germ layers of the early embryo. It gives rise to some epithelial and nervous tissues, e.g. skin structures, inner ear, mammary glands, pituitary gland, the central nervous system, cranial, spinal and autonomic nerves, adrenal medulla and the lens and retina—**ectodermal** *adj.* ⇒ endoderm, mesoderm.

ectogenesis *n* the growth of the embryo outside the uterus (in vitro fertilization).

ectoparasite *n* a parasite that lives on the exterior surface of its host—**ectoparasitic** *adj.*

ectopia *n* malposition of an organ or structure, usually congenital. *ectopia vesicae* an abnormally placed urinary bladder which protrudes through or opens on to the abdominal wall—**ectopic** *adj.*

ectopic beat ⇒ extrasystole.

ectopic pregnancy (*syn* tubal pregnancy) extrauterine gestation, the uterine (fallopian) tube being the most common site.

ectrodactyly, ectrodactylia *n* congenital absence of one or more fingers or toes or parts of them.

ectropion *n* an eversion or turning outward, especially of the lower eyelid or of the pupil margin—*ectropion uveae*.

ECV *abbr* external cephalic version.

eczema *n* an inflammatory skin reaction that may begin with erythema, then vesicles appear. These rupture, forming exudative areas that may crust. Scaling may occur. In chronic forms the skin becomes thickened. Some authorities limit the word 'eczema' to the cases with internal (endogenous) causes while those caused by external (exogenous) contact factors are called dermatitis. The skin of patients with eczema may be colonized or infected with *Staphylococcus aureus.* ⇒ dermatitis—**eczematous** *adj.*

EDD *abbr* expected date of delivery.

edentulous *adj* without natural teeth.

edrophonium test in patients with myasthenia gravis, a small intramuscular dose of edrophonium chloride will immediately relieve symptoms, albeit temporarily, while quinine sulphate will increase the muscular weakness.

Edward syndrome an autosomal trisomy of number 18 chromosome associated with abnormal facial appearance, growth retardation and learning disability. The cells have 47 chromosomes.

EEG *abbr* electroencephalogram ⇒ electroencephalograph.

EFAs *abbr* essential fatty acids.

effective dose the amount of a drug that can be expected to initiate a specific intensity of effect in people taking the drug.

effectiveness *n* describes using resources to achieve the required outcomes.

effector *n* a motor or secretory nerve ending in a muscle, gland or organ.

efferent *adj* carrying, conveying, conducting away from a centre. ⇒ afferent *opp.*

efficiency *n* describes the use of minimum resources to achieve the maximum outcomes.

effleurage *n* a massage manipulation, using long, whole-hand strokes in the direction of venous and lymphatic drainage, that aims to help venous return to the heart and the reduction of oedema. Deep effleurage causes dilatation of the arterioles by stimulating the axon reflex.

effort syndrome a form of anxiety disorder, manifesting itself in a variety of cardiac symptoms including chest pain, for which no pathological explanation can be discovered.

effusion *n* extravasation of fluid into body tissues or cavities, such as a pleural effusion, or into joints where it causes swelling.

ego *n* one of the three main aspects of the personality (the others being the id and superego); refers to the conscious self, the 'I', which according to Freud, deals with reality; is influenced by social forces and controls unconscious instinctual urges.

EHEC *abbr* enterohaemorrhagic *Escherichia coli.*

EIA *abbr* exercise induced asthma. ⇒ asthma.

EIEC *abbr* enteroinvasive *Escherichia coli.*

ejaculation *n* sudden emission of semen from the penis at the moment of male orgasm. *retrograde ejaculation* a situation where semen is discharged backwards into the bladder. It may follow prostate surgery or be associated with diabetic neuropathy.

ejaculatory duct ⇒ Figure 16.

elder abuse physical (including neglect), sexual, psychological, pharmacological or financial abuse of older people. May be carried out by family and other carers, neighbours, or by health and social care staff.

Electra complex excessive emotional attachment of daughter to father. The name is derived from Greek mythology.

electrocardiogram (ECG) *n* a recording of the electrical activity of the heart muscle during the cardiac cycle made by an electrocardiograph. The normal heart produces a typical waveform, sinus rhythm, which consists of five deflection waves, known universally as PQRST. ⇒ PQRST complex. *ambulatory ECG (Holter monitoring)* recording heart rhythm and rate over a 24 hour period to detect transient ischaemia or arrhythmias. The person continues with their normal activities and keeps a record of times and activities. *exercise (stress) ECG* performed during increasing levels of exertion, such as on a treadmill, to detect arrhythmias or ischaemic changes caused by physical stress. Frequently used for the diagnosis or prognosis of heart disease or to guide cardiac rehabilitation.

electrocardiograph *n* an instrument that records the electrical activity of the heart from electrodes on the limbs and chest—**electrocardiographic** *adj*, **electrocardiography** *n*, **electrocardiographically** *adv*.

electrocoagulation *n* technique of surgical diathermy. Coagulation, especially of bleeding points, by means of electrodes.

electrocochleography (ECoG) *n* direct recording of the action potential generated following stimulation of the cochlear nerve. ⇒ vestibulocochlear nerve.

electroconvulsive therapy (ECT) a physical treatment used in psychiatry, mainly in the treatment of severe/life-threatening depression or psychotic states. A device is used that delivers a definite electrical voltage for a precise fraction of a second to electrodes placed on the head, producing a convulsion. The convulsion is modified by use of an intravenous anaesthetic and a muscle relaxant prior to treatment. *unilateral ECT* avoids the sequela of amnesia for recent events. The mechanism for memory of recent events is probably in the dominant cerebral hemisphere. ECT is therefore applied to the right hemisphere to reduce memory disturbance.

electrode *n* in medicine or therapy, a conductor in the form of a pad or plate, whereby electricity enters or leaves the body.

electrodesiccation *n* a technique of surgical diathermy. There is drying and subsequent removal of tissue.

electroencephalogram (EEG) *n* a recording of the electrical activity of the brain, made by an electroencephalograph.

electroencephalograph *n* an instrument by which electrical impulses derived from the brain can be amplified and recorded, in a fashion similar to that of the electrocardiograph—electroencephalographic *adj*, electroencephalography *n*, electroencephalographically *adv*.

electrolysis *n* 1 chemical decomposition by electricity, with ion movement shown by changes at the electrodes. 2 term used for the destruction of individual hairs (epilation), removal of moles, spider naevi, etc., using electricity.

electrolyte *n* a solution of a substance, such as sodium chloride, which dissociates into ions with an electrical charge (anions, cations). In medicine it describes the individual ion, e.g. potassium and bicarbonate ions in the body. *electrolyte balance* the balance of relative amounts of electrolytes, e.g. potassium, sodium, magnesium, calcium, chloride, bicarbonate (hydrogen carbonate) and phosphate in blood, other fluids and tissues. The balance between ions with a positive charge and those with a negative charge ensures overall electrical neutrality in the body. Many conditions and diseases cause electrolyte imbalance, which is often associated with loss of fluid and pH homeostasis—electrolytic *adj*.

electromechanical dissociation (EMD) a type of cardiac arrest where there is a normal or nearly normal electrical activity without an effective cardiac output. ⇒ cardiac arrest.

electromotive force (EMF) measures the force needed for an electric current to flow between two points. A derived SI unit (International System of Units), the volt (V), is used.

electromyography (EMG) *n* the use of an instrument which records electric currents generated in contracting muscle—electromyographical *adj*, electromyogram *n*, electromyograph *n*, electromyographically *adv*.

electron *n* a negatively charged subatomic particle. *electron microscopy* the use of a beam of electrons to visualize very small structures, such as virus particles. *electron transfer chain* a series of mitochondrial oxidation-reduction reactions that generate cellular energy as ATP.

electro-oculography *n* the use of an instrument which records eye position and movement, and potential difference between front and back of the eyeball using electrodes placed on skin near the eye. Can be used as a diagnostic test of retinal function—electro-oculogram (EOG) *n*.

electrophoresis *n* a technique where charged particles are separated in a liquid medium by their characteristic speed and direction of migration in an electrical field. Used for measuring serum proteins.

electroretinography *n* the use of an instrument to measure electrical currents generated in the retina stimulated by light—electroretinogram (ERG) *n*.

element *n* one of the constituents of a compound. The elements are the primary substances which in pure form, or in combinations as compounds, constitute all matter.

elephantiasis *n* the swelling of a limb, usually a leg, as a result of lymphatic obstruction (lymphoedema), followed by thickening of the skin (pachyderma) and subcutaneous tissues. A complication of filariasis in tropical countries. ⇒ *Filaria*, filariasis, lymphoedema.

elevation *n* an upward movement such as the scapulae when the shoulders are lifted.

elimination *n* the passage of waste from the body—urine and faeces—**eliminate** *vt*.

ELISA *abbr* enzyme-linked immunosorbent assay.

elixir *n* a sweetened, aromatic solution of a drug, often containing alcohol.

elliptocytosis *n* hereditary disorder of red blood cells, which results in them appearing as ellipses when viewed under a light microscope.

emaciation *n* excessive leanness, or wasting of body tissue—**emaciate** *vt*.

emasculation *n* castration.

embolectomy *n* surgical removal of an embolus. Usually a fine balloon (Fogarty) catheter is used to extract the embolus.

embolic *adj* pertaining to an embolism or an embolus.

embolism *n* obstruction of a blood vessel by a body of undissolved material. Usually caused by a thrombus, but other causes include cancer cells, fat, amniotic fluid, gases, bacteria and parasites. Rarer emboli, such as fat, may follow long bone fractures, air may enter the circulation via a penetrating chest wound or during surgery, and amniotic fluid during labour. *arterial embolism*, originating from the left side of the heart or arterial disease, may travel to various sites including brain, bowel or limb; the effects dependent on the size of vessel affected and site, e.g. gangrene of a limb or a portion of bowel. ⇒ cerebrovascular accident, deep vein thrombosis, pulmonary embolism.

embolization *n* therapeutic occlusion of a blood vessel using a foreign substance.

embologenic *adj* capable of producing an embolus.

embolus *n* solid body or gas bubble transported in the circulation. ⇒ embolism—**emboli** *pl*.

embrocation *n* a liquid applied topically by rubbing.

embryo *n* developmental stage starting two weeks after fertilization until the end of week eight of gestation—**embryonic** *adj*.

embryology *n* study of embryonic development—**embryological** *adj*, **embryologically** *adv*.

embryoma *n* ⇒ teratoma.

embryopathy *n* abnormality or disease of the embryo—**embryopathic** *adj*.

embryotomy *n* a procedure that involves the destruction of the fetus to facilitate delivery.

emesis *n* vomiting.

emetic *n* any agent used to produce vomiting.

emetogenic *adj* term that describes substances that cause vomiting or may do so, e.g. cancer chemotherapy.

emission *n* an ejaculation or sending forth, especially an involuntary ejaculation of semen.

emmetropia *n* normal refractive power of the eye, such that light from a distant object forms a clear image on the retina without accommodative effort—**emmetropic** *adj*.

emollient *adj*, *n* (an agent) which moisturizes and soothes skin or mucous membrane.

emotion *n* the tone of feeling recognized in ourselves by certain physiological changes, and in others by tendencies to certain characteristic behaviour. Aroused usually by ideas or concepts.

emotional *adj* characteristic of or caused by emotion. *emotional bias* tendency of emotional attitude to affect logical judgement. *emotional lability* ⇒ lability. *emotional state* effect of emotions on normal mood, e.g. agitation.

empathy *n* identifying oneself with another person or the actions of another person. Described as having awareness of and insight into the biopsychosocial experiences of another person—**empathic** *adj*.

emphysema *n* gaseous distension of the tissues. ⇒ crepitation, pulmonary emphysema, surgical emphysema—**emphysematous** *adj*.

empirical *adj* based on observation rather than on scientific reasoning.

empyema *n* pus in the pleural cavity.

EMRSA *abbr* epidemic methicillin-resistant *Staphylococcus aureus*.

emulsion *n* a uniform suspension of fat or oil particles in an aqueous continuous phase (*O/W emulsion*) or aqueous droplets in an oily continuous phase (*W/O emulsion*).

enamel *n* ⇒ dental enamel.

encapsulation *n* enclosure within a capsule.

encephalins *npl* ⇒ enkephalins.

encephalitis *n* inflammation of the brain.

encephalocele *n* protrusion of brain substance through the skull. Often associated with hydrocephalus when the protrusion occurs at a suture line.

encephalography *n* a general term for techniques used to examine the brain. ⇒ echoencephalography, electroencephalography, pneumoencephalography—**encephalogram** *n*.

encephalomalacia *n* softening of the brain.

encephalomyelitis *n* inflammation of the brain and spinal cord.

encephalomyelopathy *n* disease affecting both brain and spinal cord—**encephalomyelopathic** *adj*.

encephalon *n* the brain.

encephalopathy *n* any disease of the brain causing reduced levels of arousal and cognitive function—**encephalopathic** *adj*.

enchondroma *n* a cartilaginous tumour—**enchondromata** *pl*.

encopresis *n* involuntary passage of faeces; the term is usually reserved for faecal incontinence associated with mental health problems—**encopretic** *adj, n*.

encounter group a form of psychotherapy. Small groups of individuals focus on becoming aware of their feelings and developing the ability to express them openly, honestly and with clarity. The objectives are to increase self-awareness, promote personal growth and improve interpersonal skills.

endarterectomy *n* the surgical removal of an atheromatous core from an artery, sometimes called disobliteration or 'rebore'. Carbon dioxide gas can be used to separate the occlusive core.

endarteritis *n* inflammation of the intima or inner lining coat of an artery. *endarteritis obliterans* the new intimal connective tissue obliterates the lumen.

endemic *adj* recurring in an area, particularly a disease that is always present in an area, e.g. a particular communicable disease. ⇒ epidemic *opp*.

endemic syphilis usually found in children, the infection is spread by skin-to-skin contact or from contaminated drinking vessels. Features similar to those of syphilis.

endemic treponematoses the non-venereal treponemal diseases—yaws and pinta. They tend to exist among people living in rural communities in underdeveloped countries. Transmission occurs by skin contact in childhood.

endemiology *n* the special study of endemic diseases.

end feel the quality of the feel or sensation felt by the examiner when pressure is applied to the joint at the end of its range of movement.

endobronchial tube plastic double-lumen tube introduced via the mouth into either of the two main bronchi in thoracic anaesthesia.

endocardial mapping the recording of electrical potentials from various sites on the endocardium to determine the origin of cardiac arrhythmias.

endocarditis *n* inflammation of the inner lining of the heart (endocardium) due to infection by micro-organisms (bacteria, fungi or *Rickettsia*), or to rheumatic fever. There may be temporary or permanent damage to the heart valves.

endocardium *n* the smooth endothelium that lines the heart and covers the valves.

endocervical *adj* pertaining to the inside of the cervix uteri.

endocervicitis *n* inflammation of the mucous membrane lining the cervix uteri.

endocrine *adj* secreting internally. ⇒ exocrine *opp*—**endocrinal** *adj. endocrine glands* the ductless glands that produce a hormone which passes directly into the blood or lymph. They include the hypothalamus, pineal body, pituitary, thyroid, parathyroids, adrenals, ovaries, testes and pancreas. Other structures also produce hormones, e.g. placenta, gastrointestinal tract, kidneys and the heart.

endocrinology *n* the study of the endocrine structures (ductless glands) and their internal secretions.

endocrinopathy *n* abnormality of one or more of the endocrine glands or their secretions.

endoderm *n* inner layer of the three primary germ layers of the early embryo. It gives rise to some epithelial tissue, e.g. that of the pharynx, middle ear, respiratory tract, gastrointestinal tract and bladder. ⇒ ectoderm, mesoderm.

endodontics *n* branch of dentistry concerned with the diagnosis and treatment of diseases of the dental pulp and periapical tissues.

endogenous *adj* originating within the organism. ⇒ ectogenous, exogenous *opp.*

endolymph *n* the fluid within the membranous labyrinth of the internal ear.

endometrial *adj* pertaining to the endometrium. *endometrial destruction* transcervical destruction of the basal layer of the endometrium by transcervical resection, laser ablation or by using heat. Used in suitable cases as an alternative to hysterectomy in the treatment of menorrhagia.

endometrioma *n* a tumour of misplaced endometrium ⇒ chocolate cyst—**endometriomata** *pl.*

endometriosis *n* the presence of endometrium in abnormal sites, i.e. outside the uterus. ⇒ chocolate cyst.

endometritis *n* inflammation of the endometrium.

endometrium *n* the specialized lining mucosa of the uterus—**endometrial** *adj.*

endomyocardial *adj* relating to the endocardium and myocardium—**endomyocardium** *n.*

endomysium *n* thin, inner connective tissue surrounding the muscle fibres.

endoneurium *n* the delicate, inner connective tissue surrounding the nerve fibres.

endoparasite *n* any parasite living within the host—**endoparasitic** *adj.*

endophthalmitis *n* inflammation of the eye involving the anterior chamber and vitreous humour and one or more layers of the wall of the eye. Commonly infective cause.

endorphins *npl* a group of opioid-like neuropeptides. They are active in both central and peripheral nervous functions where they modulate pain interpretation and induce feelings of euphoria. ⇒ enkephalins.

endoscope *n* an instrument for visualization of the interior of hollow tubular structures such as the urinary and gastrointestinal tracts, or body cavities, e.g. joints. The older ones were rigid, tubular and made of metal. Those in general use are of the fibreoptic variety: light is transmitted by means of very fine glass fibres along a flexible tube. It permits examination, photography, biopsy and treatment of the cavities or organs of a relaxed (sedated) conscious person—**endoscopic** *adj,* **endoscopy** *n.*

endoscopic retrograde cholangiopancreatography (ERCP) introduction of an opaque medium into the pancreatic and bile ducts via a catheter from an endoscope located in the duodenum.

endospore *n* a bacterial spore that has a solely vegetative function. It forms during adverse environmental conditions, such as drying. Its metabolism is minimal, thus allowing the micro-organism to resist heat, desiccation and disinfectants. Endospores can remain dormant for long periods and can become active when environmental conditions are suitable. The only genera which include spore-forming pathogenic species are *Bacillus* and *Clostridium.*

endothelioid *adj* resembling endothelium.

endothelioma *n* a tumour derived from endothelial cells.

endothelium *n* the lining membrane of serous cavities, heart, blood and lymph vessels—**endothelial** *adj.*

endotoxin *n* a toxin found within the cell wall of certain bacteria, e.g. *Neisseria meningitidis*. It is only released if the cell wall is destroyed. ⇒ exotoxin—**endotoxic** *adj.*

endotracheal *adj* within the trachea. *endotracheal anaesthesia* the administration of an anaesthetic through an endotracheal tube. *endotracheal tube* a plastic tube introduced via the nose or mouth into the trachea to maintain an airway during general anaesthesia and intermittent positive pressure ventilation.

endovascular *adj* intraluminal (within the lumen) surgical approach to correction of vascular abnormalities, e.g. *endovascular stenting* of an abdominal aortic aneurysm.

end-tidal carbon dioxide (ETCO$_2$) partial pressure of carbon dioxide measured in the breath at the end of expiration. Used to monitor the adequacy of ventilation in mechanically ventilated patients.

enema *n* the introduction of a liquid into the bowel via the rectum, to be returned or retained. The word is usually preceded by the name of the liquid used. It can be further designated according to the function of the fluid. The evacuant enemas are usually prepared commercially in small bulk as a disposable enema: the chemicals attract water into the bowel, promoting cleansing and peristaltic contractions of the lower bowel. The enemas to be retained are usually drugs, the most common being corticosteroids. ⇒ barium enema, laxatives.

energy conservation techniques, including time management, problem solving and lifestyle planning, that enable an individual to make the best possible use of limited energy reserves. Commonly used in occupational therapy practice.

enkephalins *npl* (*syn* encephalins) neurotransmitters present in the central nervous system, pituitary gland and gastrointestinal tract. They have opioid-like analgesic effects. ⇒ endorphins.

enophthalmos *n* sunken position of an eyeball within its socket.

ensiform *adj* sword shaped; xiphoid.

ENT *abbr* ear, nose and throat.

Entamoeba *n* (*syn* Endamoeba) a genus of protozoon parasites, three species infesting humans. Two are non-pathogenic: *Entamoeba coli* in the intestinal tract and *E. gingivalis* in the mouth, whereas *E. histolytica* is pathogenic causing amoebic dysentery.

enteral *adj* within the gastrointestinal tract. *enteral diets* those which are taken by mouth or through a nasogastric tube; low residue enteral diets can be whole protein/polymeric, or amino acid/peptide. *enteral feeding* method of providing nutrition when the gastrointestinal tract is functioning. Includes via nasogastric and nasoduodenal tubes or via gastrostomy or jejunostomy tubes. Enteral feeding can be administered by bolus, gravity or pump controlled methods. ⇒ parenteral feeding, percutaneous endoscopic gastrostomy (PEG).

enteric *adj* relating to the small intestine. *enteric coating* a coating applied to a pill that prevents drug release until it reaches the small intestine. *enteric fevers* includes typhoid and paratyphoid fever.

enteritis *n* inflammation of the intestine.

enteroanastomosis *n* intestinal anastomosis.

Enterobacter *n* a genus of aerobic, nonspore-bearing, Gram-negative bacilli of the family Enterobacteriaceae. Includes two species, *Enterobacter aerogenes* and *Enterobacter cloacae*.

enterobiasis *n* infestation with *Enterobius vermicularis* (threadworms). Because of the autoinfective life cycle, treatment aims at complete elimination. Everyone in the household is given an anthelmintic, mebendazole or less commonly piperazine citrate, and hygiene measures are also necessary to prevent reinfestation during treatment.

Enterobius vermicularis (threadworm) nematode which infests the small and large intestine.

enterocele *n* prolapse of intestine. Can be into the upper third of vagina.

enteroclysis *n* the introduction of fluid into the intestine.

Enterococcus *n* a genus of Gram-positive cocci commensal in the bowel, e.g. *Enterococcus faecalis*, *E. faecium*. They cause urinary tract infection and wound infection and occasionally meningitis in neonates. It is increasingly common as a cause of hospital-acquired infection, and many strains are developing resistance to antibiotics. ⇒ vancomycin-resistant enterococci (glycopeptide-resistant enterococci).

enterocolitis *n* inflammation of the small intestine and colon. ⇒ necrotizing enterocolitis.

enterocystoplasty *n* an operation to increase the capacity of the urinary bladder by using part of the small intestine.

enterohepatic circulation the recycling of bile salts and other substances including drugs that are secreted into bile. They are absorbed from the intestine and returned to the liver via the hepatic portal vein. The returning bile salts stimulate more bile and bile acid production, but recycled drugs, such as morphine, create a pool of active drug that prolongs drug activity and can lead to toxic levels.

enterokinase *n* (*syn* enteropeptidase) a proteolytic enzyme produced by duodenal mucosa. It converts inactive trypsinogen (pancreatic enzyme) into active trypsin.

enterolithiasis *n* the presence of intestinal concretions.

enteron *n* the gut.

enteropathy *n* any disorder affecting the small intestine, such as gluten-induced enteropathy (coeliac disease).

enteropeptidase *n* ⇒ enterokinase.

enteroscope *n* an endoscope for visualization of the small intestine—**enteroscopically** *adv.*

enterostomy *n* a surgically established fistula between the small intestine and some other surface. ⇒ gastroenterostomy, ileostomy, jejunostomy—**enterostomal** *adj.*

enterotomy *n* an incision into the small intestine.

enterotoxin *n* a toxin which has its effect on the gastrointestinal tract, causing vomiting, diarrhoea and abdominal pain.

enterovesical *adj* pertaining to the bowel and the bladder.

enteroviruses *npl* a group of picornaviruses that enter the body by the gastrointestinal tract. Comprise the polioviruses, echoviruses and coxsackieviruses.

Entonox *n* proprietary name for a gaseous mixture of oxygen and nitrous oxide in equal measures that is inhaled by the patient to provide analgesia, e.g. in obstetrics and intensive care.

entropion *n* inversion of an eyelid so that the lashes are in contact with the globe of the eye.

enucleation *n* the removal of an organ or tumour in its entirety, as of an eyeball from its socket.

enuresis *n* incontinence of urine, especially bed-wetting. *nocturnal enuresis* bed wetting during sleep.

environment *n* external surroundings. Living organisms are influenced by the physical and chemical conditions of the environment external to them, and by those within the organism—**environmental** *adj.*

enzyme *n* a protein that functions as a catalyst for specific biochemical reactions involving specific substrates. Many reactions in the body would proceed too slowly without an enzyme, e.g. waste carbon dioxide would not be removed from the tissues without the enzyme carbonic anhydrase. Enzyme names often reflect their function, e.g. dehydrogenases catalyse the removal of hydrogen in oxidation reactions.

enzyme induction the ability of some chemicals, e.g. alcohol, environmental chemicals and drugs, to increase the secretion of liver enzymes. ⇒ cytochromes. The increase in enzyme production can speed up the rate at which the inducer drug and others are metabolized and excreted. There is loss of drug effectiveness, e.g. the oral contraceptive is inactivated by rifampicin (antituberculosis drug). In some situations the induction of enzyme production may increase drug effects such as the toxic metabolites formed in paracetamol overdose.

enzyme inhibitors chemicals, including many drugs that inhibit specific enzymes in the body. The inhibition may be reversible or irreversible. Some inhibitors are false substrates (very similar to the normal substrate of the enzyme) and act as competitive inhibitors, e.g. some cytotoxic drugs inhibit the enzyme needed by cancer cells for folic acid use. Others inhibit liver enzymes and increase the effects of other drugs. For example, aspirin inhibits the enzymes needed to metabolize oral anticoagulants, which causes increased anticoagulation with the risk of bleeding.

enzyme-linked immunosorbent assay (ELISA) an assay technique for measuring soluble substances based on recognition of the target antigen by specific antibodies, linked to an enzyme which causes a colour change in a substrate solution. The degree of colour change is proportional to the concentration of the substance being examined. It is used to test for the presence of antibodies to HIV. All positive tests for HIV are confirmed by the more precise Western blot test before HIV infection is confirmed.

eosin *n* a red staining agent used in histology and laboratory diagnostic procedures.

eosinophil *n* 1 cells having an affinity for eosin. 2 a type of polymorphonuclear leucocyte containing eosin-staining granules. It is associated with immune responses that involve allergies and immunoglobulin (IgE)—**eosinophilic** *adj.*

eosinophilia *n* increased number of eosinophils in the blood.

EPEC *abbr* enteropathic *Escherichia coli.*

ependymal cells a type of neuroglial cell that lines the fluid-filled cavities of the central nervous system (cerebral ventricles and the central canal of the spinal cord).

ependymoma *n* neoplasm arising in the lining of the cerebral ventricles or central canal of spinal cord. Occurs in all age groups.

ephelides *npl* freckles, an increase in pigment granules with a normal number of pigment cells. ⇒ lentigo—**ephelis** *sing*.

epicanthus *n* the congenital occurrence of a fold of skin obscuring the inner canthus of the eye—**epicanthal** *adj*.

epicardium *n* the visceral layer of the pericardium—**epicardial** *adj*.

epicondyle *n* an eminence on some bones situated above the condyles, e.g. femoral epicondyles.

epicondylitis *n* inflammation of the muscles and tendons around the elbow. Can occur if the structures are subjected to excess or repetitive stress. It may affect the structures at the lateral (outer) or medial (inner) aspect of the elbow. *lateral epicondylitis* (*syn* tennis elbow) is associated with tennis, other racquet sports and weight training. *medial epicondylitis* (*syn* golfer's elbow) is primarily an overuse injury associated with golf and poor lifting techniques. ⇒ bursitis.

epicritic *adj* describes cutaneous nerve fibres which are sensitive to fine variations of touch and vibration. Concerned with proprioception and two-point discrimination. ⇒ protopathic *opp*.

epidemic *n* a disease, such as measles, simultaneously affecting many people in an area (more than the expected number). ⇒ endemic *opp*.

epidemic myalgia ⇒ Bornholm disease.

epidemiology *n* the scientific study of the distribution of diseases. It is concerned with the incidence, distribution and control of disease—**epidemiological** *adj*, **epidemiologically** *adv*.

epidermis *n* the outer avascular layer of the skin (⇒ Figure 12); the cuticle—**epidermal** *adv*.

Epidermophyton *n* a genus of fungi affecting the skin and nails.

epidermophytosis *n* infection with fungi of the genus *Epidermophyton* such as ringworm.

epididymectomy *n* surgical removal of the epididymis.

epididymis *n* a small oblong body attached to the posterior surface of the testes (⇒ Figure 16). It consists of the seminiferous tubules which carry the spermatozoa from the testes to the deferent ducts (vas deferens).

epididymitis *n* inflammation of the epididymis.

epididymo-orchitis *n* inflammation of the epididymis and the testis.

epidural *adj* upon or external to the dura. *epidural anaesthesia* local anaesthetic injected into the space external to the dura either by single injection or intermittently via a catheter, causing loss of sensation in an area determined by the site of the injection and volume of local anaesthetic used. *epidural space* the region through which spinal nerves leave the spinal cord. It can be approached at any level of the spine, but the administering of anaesthetic is commonly done at the lumbar level or through the sacral cornua for caudal epidural block. ⇒ patient controlled analgesia.

epigastrium *n* the abdominal region lying directly over the stomach (⇒ Figure 18a)—**epigastric** *adj*.

epiglottis *n* the thin leaf-shaped flap of cartilage behind the tongue which, during the act of swallowing, covers the opening leading into the larynx (⇒ Figure 6).

epiglottitis *n* inflammation of the epiglottis.

epikeratophakia *n* surgical introduction of a biological 'lens' into the cornea to correct hypermetropia or keratoconus.

epilation *n* extraction or destruction of hair roots, e.g. by coagulation necrosis, electrolysis or forceps. ⇒ depilation—**epilate** *vt*.

epilatory *adj, n* (describes) an agent which produces epilation.

epilepsy *n* correctly called the epilepsies, a group of conditions resulting from disordered electrical activity in the brain and manifesting as epileptic seizures or 'fits'. The seizure is caused by an abnormal electrical discharge that disturbs cerebration and results in a generalized or partial seizure, depending on the area of the brain involved. (a) *Generalized seizures* may be: *tonic-clonic (grand mal)* the commonest type of epileptic seizure with loss of consciousness and generalized convulsions. *absences (petit mal)* where there is a brief alteration in consciousness. (b) *Partial seizures* occur when the electrical disturbance is limited to a particular focus of the brain and are manifested in a variety of ways, including motor problems characterized by limb twitching that may spread, known as Jacksonian epilepsy. In other types there may be paraesthesia, visual hallucinations, such as coloured patterns, and psychomotor seizures where there are changes to mood, perception and memory with more complex hallucinations and physical manifestations, such as nausea. *Secondary generalized seizures* occur when partial seizure activity spreads to involve other areas of the brain and awareness is lost. ⇒ status epilepticus.

epileptic 1 *adj* pertaining to epilepsy. **2** *n* a person with epilepsy. *epileptic aura* premonitory subjective phenomena (tingling in the hand or visual or auditory sensations) that precede an attack of major epilepsy. ⇒ aura.

epileptiform *adj* resembling epilepsy.

epileptogenic *adj* capable of causing epilepsy.

epiloia *n* ⇒ tuberous sclerosis.

epimenorrhoea *n* reduction of the length of the menstrual cycle.

epimysium outer fibrous coat surrounding an entire muscle.

epinephrine *n* ⇒ adrenaline (epinephrine).

epineurium *n* outer fibrous coat enclosing a nerve trunk.

epiphora *n* pathological overflow of tears on to the cheek.

epiphysis *n* the end of a growing bone. Separated from the shaft by the epiphyseal plate (cartilage); this is replaced with bone (ossification) when growth ceases—**epiphyses** *pl*, **epiphyseal** *adj*.

epiphysitis *n* inflammation of an epiphysis.

episclera *n* loose connective tissue between the sclera and conjunctiva—**episcleral** *adj*.

episcleritis *n* inflammation of the episclera.

episiorrhaphy *n* surgical repair of a lacerated perineum.

episiotomy *n* a perineal incision made during the birth of a child when the vaginal orifice does not stretch sufficiently.

episodic memory the part of long-term memory responsible for storing personal experiences. It is organized with respect to when and where the experience occurred, e.g. an episode from your last performance review interview.

epispadias *n* a congenital opening of the urethra on the dorsal aspect of the penis, often associated with ectopia vesicae. ⇒ hypospadias.

epistaxis *n* bleeding from the nose—**epistaxes** *pl*.

epistemology *n* theory of the grounds of knowledge. The discussion about knowledge and 'truth' and how it varies between different disciplines.

epithelialization *n* the growth of epithelium over a raw area; the final stage of healing.

epithelioma *n* a tumour arising from any epithelium.

epithelium *n* one of the four basic tissues. It lines cavities, covers the body and forms glands. It is classified according to the arrangement and shape of the cells it contains. It may be simple, single layer of squamous, cuboidal or columnar, or stratified with many layers, e.g. stratified or transitional—**epithelial** *adj*.

Epsom salts ⇒ magnesium sulphate.

Epstein–Barr virus (EBV) a herpesvirus, the causative agent of infectious mononucleosis. Also linked with the formation of some malignant tumours, including Burkitt's lymphoma and nasopharyngeal cancer.

equality of opportunity equal access to opportunities for decent housing, education, a job, health care, etc., regardless of age, gender, race or social class.

equinus *n* a condition in which the toes point down and the person walks on tiptoe. ⇒ talipes.

equity *n* fairness of distribution of resources such as health care. Access to resources is based on need and the ability to benefit. The ability of a healthcare system to provide a comparable level of health care across the entire population. Covers the following dimensions: need for health care in the population (dependent on epidemiology of disease, determinants of health); availability, accessibility of healthcare resources; distribution of healthcare resources; use (utilization) of healthcare resources; geographic variation in need and healthcare utilization.

epulis *n* a tumour growing on or from the gums.

Erb's palsy paralysis involving the shoulder and arm muscles from a lesion of the fifth and sixth cervical nerve roots. The arm hangs loosely at the side with the forearm pronated ('waiter's tip position'). Most commonly a birth injury.

ERCP *abbr* endoscopic retrograde cholangiopancreatography.

erectile *adj* upright; capable of being elevated. *erectile dysfunction* an inability to achieve or maintain penile erection. *erectile tissue* vascular tissue, which, under stimulus, becomes rigid and erect from hyperaemia.

erection *n* the state accomplished when erectile tissue is hyperaemic.

erector *n* a muscle which achieves erection of a part. *erector spinae* muscle of the back. ⇒ Figure 5.

ERG *abbr* ⇒ electroretinogram.

ergocalciferol *n* vitamin D_2 obtained from the diet. It is formed from the plant sterol ergosterol.

ergogenic *adj* a propensity to increase the output of work. *ergogenic aids* measures taken to enhance sporting performance. Some aids may be allowed within the rules of the sport but others may be prohibited. The methods include mechanical, dietary supplementation, pharmaceutical, hormonal and psychological. ⇒ blood doping, anabolic steroids.

ergometry *n* measurement of work done by muscles—**ergometric** *adj*.

ergonomics *n* the study of the work environment and efficient energy use.

ergosterol *n* a sterol provitamin found in plants and fungi, particularly yeast. It is converted to ergocalciferol (vitamin D_2) by ultraviolet radiation, which is used to fortify foodstuffs with vitamin D.

ergot *n* a fungus, *Claviceps purpurea*, which infects rye. There are two important derivatives: (a) ergometrine, used to stimulate uterine contraction thus preventing or minimizing postpartum haemorrhage, and (b) ergotamine, which may occasionally be used for migraine. It has been mostly replaced by simple analgesics or specific and more effective medications. ⇒ 5-HT$_1$ agonists.

ergotism *n* poisoning by ergot, which may cause gangrene, particularly of the fingers and toes.

ERPC *abbr* evacuation of retained products of conception.

eruption *n* the process by which a tooth emerges through the alveolar bone and gingiva.

erysipelas *n* an acute infectious disease, usually caused by haemolytic streptococci. There is a spreading inflammation of the skin and subcutaneous tissues, accompanied by systemic effects such as fever.

erysipeloid *n* a skin condition resembling erysipelas. It occurs in butchers, fishmongers or cooks. The infecting organism is the *Erysipelothrix* of swine erysipelas.

erythema *n* reddening of the skin due to vascular congestion—**erythematous** *adj*. *erythema induratum* Bazin's disease. *erythema multiforme* a form of acute toxic or allergic eruption. The lesions are in the form of target-like papules often on the hands. Severe form called Stevens–Johnson syndrome may involve mucous membranes. *erythema nodosum* an eruption of painful red nodules on the front of the legs. It may be a symptom of internal disease including tuberculosis and sarcoidosis. *erythema pernio* ⇒ chilblain.

erythroblast *n* a nucleated erythrocyte precursor found in the red bone marrow—**erythroblastic** *adj*.

erythroblastosis fetalis ⇒ haemolytic disease of the newborn.

erythrocytes *npl* non-nucleated red cells of the circulating blood. They carry oxygen and some carbon dioxide, and buffer pH changes in the blood—**erythrocytic** *adj*. *erythrocyte sedimentation rate (ESR)* citrated blood is placed in a narrow tube. The red cells fall, leaving a column of clear supernatant serum, which is measured at the end of an hour and reported in millimetres. Inflammation and tissue destruction cause an elevation in the ESR.

erythrocytopenia *n* deficiency in the number of red blood cells—**erythrocytopenic** *adj*.

erythrocytosis ⇒ polycythaemia.

erythroderma *n* excessive redness of the skin, typically involving more than 90% of the skin surface.

erythroedema polyneuropathy (*syn* acrodynia, pink disease) a condition of infancy characterized by red, swollen extremities, generalized skin rash, photophobia and irritability. May be caused by mercury poisoning.

erythropoiesis *n* the production of red blood cells by the bone marrow. ⇒ erythropoietin, haemopoiesis.

erythropoietin *n* a hormone secreted by some kidney cells in response to reduced oxygen content in the blood. It acts on the bone marrow, stimulating erythropoiesis. A recombinant human form is used therapeutically to treat anaemia associated with chronic renal failure and platinum-containing chemotherapy.

eschar *n* a slough, as results from a burn, application of caustics, diathermy, etc.

Escherichia *n* a genus of bacteria. Motile, Gram-negative bacilli that are widely distributed in nature. *Escherichia coli* is part of the normal flora in humans. Some strains are pathogens, causing gastroenteritis, peritonitis and wound infections, meningitis and urinary tract infections. The serotypes responsible for gastroenteritis are: (a) enterohaemorrhagic *E. coli* (EHEC), e.g. *E. coli* 0157, a virulent micro-organism that produces a toxin (verocytotoxin) and causes a variety of effects from mild diarrhoea to severe haemorrhagic bowel inflammation. It may cause life-threatening haemolytic uraemic syndrome; (b) enteroinvasive *E. coli* (EIEC), which causes bloodstained diarrhoea; (c) enteropathic *E. coli* (EPEC), which causes serious diarrhoea in babies, especially in developing countries; (d) enterotoxigenic *E. coli* (ETEC), responsible for outbreaks of gastroenteritis in developing countries. Leads to watery diarrhoea with fluid and electrolyte imbalance.

Esmarch's bandage a rubber roller bandage sometimes used to procure a bloodless operative field in the limbs.

esophoria *n* latent convergent strabismus.

esotropia *n* manifest convergent strabismus.

ESPs *abbr* extended scope physiotherapy practitioners.

espundia *n* ⇒ leishmaniasis.

ESR *abbr* erythrocyte sedimentation rate.

ESRD/F *abbr* end-stage renal disease/failure. ⇒ renal.

essential amino acids also known as indispensable. The amino acids that cannot be synthesized in the body and therefore have to be provided by the diet. They are isoleucine, leucine, lysine, methionine, phenylalanine, threonine, tryptophan and valine in adults. Other amino acids are considered to be conditionally essential because they become essential if the diet does not contain enough of the precursor amino acid from which they are synthesized: arginine, asparagine, cysteine, glutamine, glycine, histidine, proline, serine and tyrosine. ⇒ amino acids.

essential fatty acids (EFAs) the linoleic and α-linolenic families of fatty acids. Polyunsaturated fatty acids (PUFAs) that cannot be synthesized in the body so must be supplied by the diet. Arachidonic, eicosapentanoic and decosahexanoic acids can all be synthesized from linoleic and α-linolenic acids, and become essential if linoleic and α-linolenic acids are in short supply. They have diverse functions, which include being the precursors for many regulatory lipids, e.g. prostaglandins; they fulfil an important role in fat metabolism and are required for the integrity of cell membranes. They are present in natural vegetable seed oils.

essential oil the undiluted oil extracted from plants, usually diluted in a carrier oil prior to use during aromatherapy.

establishment *n* describes the planned staffing levels in a particular area. Usually described as the number of whole time equivalents (WTEs).

estimated average requirement (EAR) one of the UK dietary reference values. It estimates the average requirement for a group of people, usually for energy requirements. It follows that 50% of people in the group will need more and 50% will need less.

estradiol *n Am* ⇒ oestradiol.

estrogen *n Am* ⇒ oestrogen.

ESWL *abbr* extracorporeal shock-wave lithotripsy.

ETEC *abbr* enterotoxigenic *Escherichia coli*.

ETCO₂ *abbr* end-tidal carbon dioxide.

ethanol *n* ethyl alcohol. The alcohol in alcoholic drinks.

ether *n* early volatile anaesthetic agent now rarely used.

ethics *n* a code of moral principles derived from a system of values and beliefs. It is concerned with rights and obligations. *ethics committees* bodies that operate in academic institutions, Health Authorities and NHS Trusts to consider proposals for research projects. The approval of the appropriate ethics committee is usually a prerequisite for obtaining a research grant.

ethmoid *n* a spongy bone forming the lateral walls of the nose and the upper portion of the bony nasal septum.

ethmoidectomy *n* surgical removal of a part or all of the ethmoid bone.

ethnic *adj* relating to a social group who have common customs and culture.

ethnography *n* a study of individuals in their usual surroundings. Used in qualitative research by anthropologists to describe customs, culture and social life through observation, informal interviews, etc.

ethnology *n* a branch of anthropology that studies mainly the cultural differences between social groups, particularly the beliefs, attitudes and values pertaining to life events that include birth, marriage, health care, death, etc.—**ethnological** *adj*, **ethnologically** *adv*.

ethyl chloride a volatile liquid used to test the onset of regional anaesthesia by reason of the intense cold sensation produced when applied to the skin.

ethylene oxide a gas used to sterilize delicate equipment that would be damaged by high temperatures.

EUA *abbr* examination under anaesthetic.

eugenics *n* the study of genetics aimed at improving future generations—**eugenic** *adj*.

eunuch *n* a human male from whom the testes have been removed; a castrated male.

euphoria *n* in psychiatry, an exaggerated sense of well-being—**euphoric** *adj*.

eustachian tube ⇒ pharyngotympanic tube.

eustress ⇒ stress.

euthanasia *n* literally an 'easy death'. Inferring a painless death. Frequently interpreted as the act of causing a painless and planned death, such as relieving a person's extreme suffering from an incurable disease. Presently illegal in UK and opposed by many professional groups, it is practised in some European countries. ⇒ homicide.

euthyroid state denoting normal thyroid function.

eutocia *n* a natural and normal labour and childbirth without any complications.

evacuant *n* an agent which initiates an evacuation, such as of the bowel. ⇒ enema, laxatives.

evacuation *n* the act of emptying a cavity; generally refers to the discharge of faecal matter from the rectum. *manual evacuation* digital removal of faeces from the rectum. *evacuation of retained products of conception (ERPC)* emptying the uterus following an incomplete miscarriage.

evacuator *n* an instrument for procuring evacuation, e.g. the removal from the bladder of a stone, crushed by a lithotrite.

evaporate *vt, vi* to convert from the liquid to the gaseous state by the application of heat.

evaporating lotion one which, applied as a compress, absorbs heat in order to evaporate and so cools the skin.

evening primrose oil a source of γ-linoleic acid. Sometimes used to relieve the symptoms of premenstrual syndrome.

eversion *n* a turning outwards, as of the upper eyelid to expose the eyelid conjunctiva.

evidence-based medicine (EBM) practice (EBP) describes the practice of medicine or delivery of healthcare interventions that are based on systematic analysis of information available in terms of effectiveness in relation to cost-effective health outcomes. The highest level of evidence (based on the robustness of the research methodology) is that gained from meta-analysis of randomized controlled trials (RCTs). Sometimes this level of evidence is not available and at the lowest level may be based on evidence from expert committee reports or opinions and/or clinical experience of respected practitioners.

evisceration *n* removal of internal organs.

evulsion *n* forcible tearing away of a structure.

Ewing's tumour sarcoma involving a long bone, usually diagnosed in a child or young adult.

exacerbation *n* increased severity, as of symptoms.

exanthema *n* a skin eruption—**exanthemata** *pl*, **exanthematous** *adj*.

excess post-exercise oxygen consumption (EPOC) ⇒ oxygen debt.

exercise induced asthma bronchospasm caused by exercise in a cold, dry climate.

exercise physiology involves the description and explanation of functional changes in the body brought about by either a single or repeated exercise sessions.

excision *n* removal of a part by cutting—**excise** *vt*.

excitability *n* rapid response to stimuli; easily irritated such as nerve and muscle cells—**excitable** *adj*.

excitation *n* the act of stimulating an organ or tissue.

exclusion isolation ⇒ protective isolation.

excoriation *n* ⇒ abrasion.

excrement *n* faeces.

excrescence *n* an abnormal protuberance or growth of the tissues.

excreta *n* the waste material that is normally cleared from the body, particularly urine and faeces.

excretion *n* the elimination of waste material from the body, and also the eliminated material—**excretory** *adj*, **excrete** *vt*.

exenteration *n* removal of the viscera from its containing cavity, e.g. the eye from its socket, the pelvic organs from the pelvis.

exfoliation *n* **1** the scaling off of tissues in layers. **2** the shedding of the primary teeth—**exfoliative** *adj*.

exfoliative cytology ⇒ cytology.

ex gratia as a matter of favour, e.g. without admission of liability, of payment offered by a NHS Trust to a claimant.

exhibitionism *n* **1** any kind of 'showing off'; extravagant behaviour to attract attention. **2** a psychosexual disorder confined to males and consisting of repeated exposure of the genitalia to a stranger who is usually an adult female or a child. The act of exposure is sufficient and no further contact is sought with the victim—**exhibitionist** *n*.

exocrine *adj* describes glands from which the secretion passes via a duct; secreting externally. ⇒ endocrine *opp*—**exocrinal** *adj*.

exogenous *adj* of external origin. ⇒ endogenous *opp*.

exomphalos *n* (*syn* omphalocele) a condition present at birth and due to failure of the gut to return to the abdominal cavity during fetal development. The intestines protrude into the umbilical cord.

exophoria *n* latent divergent strabismus.

exophthalmos *n* protrusion of the eyeball—**exophthalmic** *adj*.

exostosis *n* an overgrowth of bone tissue forming a benign tumour.

exotoxin *n* a toxin released through the cell wall of a living bacterium, e.g. *Clostridium tetani*. They have extensive systemic effects, which include muscle spasm. ⇒ endotoxin—**exotoxic** *adj*.

exotropia *n* manifest divergent strabismus.

expected date of delivery (EDD) usually calculated as 280 days from the first day of the last normal menstrual period.

expectorant *n* a drug which may promote expectoration.

expectoration *n* **1** the elimination of secretion from the respiratory tract by coughing. **2** sputum—**expectorate** *vt*.

experimental group a research term that describes the group exposed to the independent variable (the intervention or experimental agent such as a drug). ⇒ control group, variable.

expiration *n* the process of breathing out air from the lungs—**expiratory** *adj*, **expire** *vt*, *vi*.

expression *n* **1** expulsion by force as of the placenta from the uterus; milk from the breast, etc. **2** a genetic term for the appearance of a particular trait or characteristic. **3** facial disclosure of feelings, mood, etc.

expressive motor aphasia a type of aphasia where there is difficulty in language production. Those affected have word finding difficulties and may have problems producing sentence structures. May coexist with receptive aphasia.

exsanguination *n* the process of rendering bloodless—**exsanguinate** *vt*.

extended family the wider group of family relations including grandparents, aunts, uncles, cousins, etc. ⇒ nuclear family.

extended scope physiotherapy practitioners (ESPs) specialist physiotherapists whose role has been extended to include assessment, ordering certain investigations, making referrals, etc. Currently they practise in areas that include orthopaedics, rheumatology and with neurosurgical patients.

extension *n* **1** traction upon a fractured or dislocated limb. **2** the straightening of a flexed limb or part.

extensor *n* a muscle which on contraction extends or straightens a part. ⇒ Figures 4, 5, flexor *opp*.

external cephalic version (ECV) ⇒ version.

external (lateral) rotation a limb or body movement where there is rotation away from the vertical axis of the body.

extirpation *n* complete removal or destruction of a part.

extra-articular *adj* outside a joint.

extracapsular *adj* outside a capsule. ⇒ intracapsular *opp*.

extracardiac *adj* outside the heart.

extracellular *adj* outside the cell membrane. *extracellular fluid (ECF)* that fluid outside the cells such as plasma, interstitial fluid, lymph, gastrointestinal fluid and CSF. ⇒ intracellular *opp*.

extracorporeal *adj* outside the body. *extracorporeal circulation* blood is taken from the body, directed through a machine ('heart–lung' or 'artificial kidney') and returned to the general circulation. ⇒ cardiac bypass, cardiopulmonary bypass, extracorporeal membrane oxygenation (ECMO), haemodialysis.

extracorporeal membrane oxygenation (ECMO) a cardiopulmonary bypass device which uses a membrane oxygenator (artificial lung). Venous blood from the patient circulates through the device by a roller pump. A fresh flow of oxygen into the device passes through a semipermeable membrane that allows the diffusion of oxygen whilst simultaneously removing carbon dioxide and water. Once the blood is oxygenated it is returned to the patient through an artery or a vein.

extracorporeal shock-wave lithotripsy (ESWL) ⇒ lithotriptor.

extract *n* a preparation obtained by evaporating a solution of a drug.

extraction *n* the removal of a tooth. *extraction of lens* surgical removal of the lens from the eye. It may be *extracapsular extraction*, when the capsule is ruptured

prior to delivery of the lens and preserved in part, or *intracapsular extraction*, when the lens and capsule are removed intact.

extradural *adj* external to the dura mater. *extradural haematoma* a collection of blood external to the dura mater.

extrahepatic *adj* outside the liver.

extramural *adj* outside the wall of a structure—**extramurally** *adv*.

extraperitoneal *adj* outside the peritoneum—**extraperitoneally** *adv*.

extrapleural *adj* outside the pleura, i.e. between the parietal pleura and the chest wall—**extrapleurally** *adv*.

extrapyramidal *adj* outside the pyramidal tracts. *extrapyramidal effects/disturbances* include the tremor and rigidity seen in parkinsonism and the side-effects of drugs, such as phenothiazine neuroleptics (antipsychotic drugs), that may cause a parkinsonian-like syndrome. ⇒ tardive dyskinesia. *extrapyramidal tracts* motor pathways that pass outside the internal capsule. They modify pyramidal tract motor functions and influence coarse voluntary movement and affect posture, coordination and balance.

extrarenal *adj* outside the kidney—**extrarenally** *adv*.

extrasensory *adj* outside the normally accepted senses. *extrasensory perception (ESP)* response to an external stimulus without normal contact or communication.

extrasystole *n* premature beats (ectopic beats) in the pulse rhythm: the cardiac impulse is initiated by an abnormal focus.

extrathoracic *adj* outside the thoracic cavity.

extrauterine *adj* outside the uterus. *extrauterine pregnancy* ⇒ ectopic pregnancy.

extravasation *n* an escape of fluid from its normal enclosure into the surrounding tissues.

extrinsic *adj* developing or having its origin from without; not internal. *extrinsic factor* vitamin B_{12}, essential for the maturation of erythrocytes and nerve function, cannot be synthesized in the body and must be supplied in the diet, hence it is called the extrinsic factor. Its absorption in the terminal ileum requires the presence of the intrinsic factor secreted by the stomach. *extrinsic sugars* sugars, such as lactose in milk and sucrose as table sugar, that are not contained within cell walls.

extrinsic allergic alveolitis (*syn* 'farmer's lung' or 'bird fancier's lung') an inflammatory response in the lungs to the inhalation of organic dusts. The two main causes are microbial spores present in vegetable produce such as mouldy hay and animal proteins most commonly from pigeons and budgerigars. In an acute attack flu-like symptoms and breathlessness develop several hours after exposure; the symptoms generally subside spontaneously. If exposure continues a chronic condition with pulmonary fibrosis will develop.

extrovert (extravert) *adj* Jungian description of an individual whose characteristic interests and behaviour are directed outwards to other people and the physical environment. ⇒ introvert *opp*.

extroversion *n* turning inside out. *extroversion of the bladder* ectopia vesicae. In psychology, the direction of thoughts to the external world.

extubation *n* removal of an endotracheal tube.

exudate *n* the product of exudation—**exudates** *pl*. In ophthalmology the yellow spots within the retina which accumulate secondary to fluid leakage from vessels. Previously known as hard exudates.

exudation *n* the oozing out of fluid through the capillary walls, or of sweat through the pores of the skin—**exude** *vt, vi*.

eye *n* organ of vision. There are three layers, from outside in the sclera, the uvea, which forms the pigmented choroid, ciliary body and iris, and the inner light-sensitive retina containing photoreceptors (cones and rods) and pigment cells. ⇒ Figure 15.

eye contact looking at the face of the person to whom one is talking. In many instances, it is a reciprocal activity and is such an important part of most cultures' non-verbal language that blind people are advised to turn their faces in the direction of the voice being heard. In some cultures, however, it may be perceived as bad manners or offensive to make or maintain eye contact during conversation, or when acknowledging a person.

eye teeth *n* the canine teeth in the upper jaw.

F

facet *n* a small, smooth, flat surface of a bone or a calculus.

facial *adj* pertaining to the face. *facial nerve* seventh pair of cranial nerves. They supply the facial muscles, the salivary, lacrimal and nasal glands, and part of the tongue. *facial paralysis* paralysis of muscles supplied by the facial nerve.

facies *n* the appearance or the expression of the face. *adenoid facies* open mouthed, vacant expression due to deafness from enlarged pharyngeal tonsils (adenoids). *Parkinson facies* a mask-like appearance; saliva may trickle from the corners of the mouth.

facilitated diffusion process whereby larger non-fat-soluble molecules such as glucose pass into the cell by using a protein carrier molecule. No energy is required but there must be a concentration gradient.

factitious disorder a disorder of illness behaviour in which an individual feigns symptoms repeatedly and consistently. As a result there are often repeated investigations and treatment (including surgery) in spite of repeated negative findings. ⇒ Munchausen syndrome.

factor V Leiden a genetic abnormality of factor V (one of the blood coagulation factors) which results in failure of one of the system's inbuilt antithrombotic safety mechanisms. The abnormality is found in 3–5% of populations in northern European countries, but under certain circumstances it may cause a predisposition to venous thrombosis.

facultative *adj* conditional; having the power of living under different conditions.

faecalith *n* a concretion formed in the bowel from faecal matter: it can cause obstruction and/or inflammation.

faecal-oral route describes the ingestion of micro-organisms from faeces which can be transmitted directly or indirectly. Often results in diarrhoeal disease.

faecal softeners ⇒ laxatives. ⇒ Appendix 5.

faeces *n* the waste material eliminated from the bowel, consisting mainly of indigestible cellulose, unabsorbed food, intestinal secretions, water, electrolytes and bacteria, etc.—**faecal** *adj*.

Fahrenheit *n* a thermometric scale; the freezing point of water is 32° and its boiling point 212°.

failure to thrive failure to develop and grow at the expected rate, ascertained by consistent measurement of height and weight plotted on a growth chart. It may result from an organic disorder or have non-organic causes, such as poor feeding, maternal deprivation or psychosocial problems. Careful investigation is required to establish the cause.

faint *n* syncope—**faint** *vi*.

falciform *adj* sickle-shaped.

fallopian tubes ⇒ uterine tubes.

Fallot's tetralogy a cyanotic congenital heart defect comprising a ventricular septal defect, narrowing of the right ventricular outflow tract (subvalvular pulmonary stenosis), right ventricular hypertrophy and malposition of the aorta overriding the ventricular septum. Amenable to corrective surgery.

false substrate chemicals, including some drugs, that compete with the normal substrate in a metabolic pathway. The pathway is disrupted. ⇒ enzyme inhibitors.

falx *n* a sickle-shaped structure. *falx cerebri* that portion of the dura mater separating the two cerebral hemispheres.

familial *adj* relating to the family, as of a condition such as Huntington's disease that affect several members of the same family.

familial Mediterranean fever a rare inherited disease characterized by episodes of inflammatory arthritis, pyrexia, pleurisy and peritonitis. Should not be confused with Mediterranean spotted fever caused by a rickettsial infection.

Family Health Services (FHS) community-based services provided by family doctors, dentists, opticians and pharmacists as independent contractors. They are not directly employed by the NHS, but have contractual arrangements to practise in the NHS.

family planning the methods used to space or limit the number of children born to a couple, or for enhancing conception.

Fanconi syndrome an inherited or acquired dysfunction of the proximal renal tubules. Large amounts of amino acids and glucose are excreted in the urine, and there is proximal renal tubular acidosis.

fantasy, phantasy *n* a 'day dream' in which the person's conscious or unconscious desires and impulses are fulfilled. May be accompanied by feelings of unreality. Occurs pathologically in schizophrenia.

farmer's lung ⇒ extrinsic allergic alveolitis.

FAS *abbr* fetal alcohol syndrome.

fascia *n* a connective tissue sheath consisting of fibrous tissue and fat which unites the skin to the underlying tissues. It also surrounds and separates many of the muscles, and, in some cases, holds them together—**fascial** *adj*.

fasciculation *n* visible flickering of muscle; can occur in the upper and lower eyelids.

fasciculus *n* a little bundle, as of muscle or nerve—**fascicular** *adj*, **fasciculi** *pl*.

fasciotomy *n* incision of muscle fascia. ⇒ compartment syndrome.

fat *n* **1** complex organic molecule composed of carbon, hydrogen and oxygen atoms. Fats are formed by the combination of one molecule of glycerol with three fatty acids forming a triacylglycerol or triglyceride. May be of animal or vegetable origin, and may be fats or oils. *fat embolus* ⇒ embolism. *fat-soluble vitamins* vitamins A, D, E and K are fat-soluble. ⇒ adipose, brown fat, fatty acid, glycerol, kilojoule, triacylglycerol. **2** adipose tissue, which acts as a reserve supply of energy and protects some organs—**fatty** *adj*.

Fatal Accident Enquiry ⇒ coroner.

fatigue *n* weariness. Physiological term for diminishing muscle reaction to stimulus applied. In sports medicine the failure of muscle(s) to maintain force (or power output) during sustained or repeated contractions—**fatigability** *n*. *fatigue index (FI)* the decline in power divided by the time (in seconds) interval between maximum (peak) and minimum power, recorded during an anaerobic power exercise test.

fatigue fracture ⇒ stress fracture.

fatty acid hydrocarbon component of lipids. May be unsaturated (monounsaturated or polyunsaturated) or saturated depending on the number of double chemical bonds in their structure.

fatty degeneration tissue degeneration that leads to the appearance of fatty droplets in the cytoplasm; found especially in disease of heart, liver and kidney.

fauces *n* the opening from the mouth into the pharynx, bounded above by the soft palate, below by the tongue. Pillars of the fauces, anterior and posterior, lie laterally and surround the palatine tonsil—**faucial** *adj.*

favism *n* increased breakdown of red blood cells precipitated by eating fava beans, in individuals deficient in the enzyme G6PD (glucose-6-phosphate dehydrogenase).

favus *n* a type of ringworm not common in Britain; caused by *Trichophyton schoenleini*. Yellow cup-shaped crusts (scutula) develop, especially on the scalp.

fear *n* an intense emotional state involving a feeling of unpleasant tension, and a strong urge to escape, which is a normal and natural response to a threat of danger but is abnormal when it exists without danger or is a continuous state. ⇒ anxiety, general adaptation response.

febrile *adj* feverish; accompanied by fever. *febrile convulsions* occur in children who have an increased body temperature; they do not usually result in permanent brain damage. Most common between the ages of 6 months and 5 years. ⇒ convulsions.

fecundation *n* impregnation. Fertilization.

fecundity *n* the power of reproduction; fertility.

feedback *n* a homeostatic control mechanism. It is usually *negative feedback* where a physiological process is slowed or 'turned off' by an increasing amount of product, e.g. temperature control. Much more rarely in *positive feedback* the process is speeded up by high levels of the product, e.g. normal blood clotting. *feedback treatment* ⇒ biofeedback.

Felty's syndrome enlargement of the spleen and low white blood cell count as a complication of rheumatoid arthritis.

femoral *adj* pertaining to the femur or thigh. Applied to the vein, artery, nerve and canal. ⇒ Figures 9, 10.

femoropopliteal *adj* usually, referring to the femoral and popliteal vessels.

femur *n* the thigh bone (⇒ Figures 2, 3), the longest and strongest bone in the body—**femora** *pl*, **femoral** *adj.*

fenamates *npl* a group of non-steroidal anti-inflammatory drugs. ⇒ Appendix 5.

fenestra *n* a window-like opening. *fenestra ovalis* an oval opening between the middle and internal ear. Below it lies the *fenestra rotunda*, a round opening.

fenestration *n* **1** a perforation, opening or pore. The glomerular capillaries of the nephron, which form part of the filtration membrane, are adapted for permeability and filtration by the presence of fenestrations **2** a surgical opening (or fenestra) in the inner ear to ease the deafness caused by otosclerosis.

fermentation *n* the process whereby microbial (yeasts and bacteria) enzymes break down sugars (glycolysis) and other substrates. For example in the production of bread, cheese, alcohol and vinegar.

ferric *adj* relating to trivalent iron and its salts. Ferric iron is converted to the ferrous state by gastric acid.

ferritin *n* an iron-protein complex. A storage form of iron.

ferrous *adj* pertaining to divalent iron, as of its salts and compounds. *Ferrous carbonate, ferrous fumarate, ferrous gluconate, ferrous succinate* and *ferrous sulphate* are prescribed orally in the treatment of iron deficiency anaemias.

fertilization *n* the impregnation of an oocyte by a spermatozoon.

FESS *abbr* functional endoscopic sinus surgery.

fester *vi* to become inflamed; to suppurate.

festinating gait rapid, short shuffling steps continuing until stopped by an object that gets in the way. Caused by lack of control of forward tilt of the pelvis with appearance of feet 'catching up' with centre of gravity that is too far ahead, instead of over, them; characteristic of Parkinson's disease.

festination *n* ⇒ fenestration.

fetal alcohol syndrome (FAS) stillbirth and fetal abnormality due to prenatal growth retardation caused by excessive maternal alcohol consumption during pregnancy.

fetal circulation circulation adapted for intrauterine life. Extra shunts and vessels (ductus venosus, ductus arteriosus, foramen ovale and umbilical vein) allows blood to largely bypass the liver, gastro-intestinal tract and lungs, as their functions are covered by maternal systems and the placenta.

fetishism *n* a condition in which a particular material object is regarded with irrational awe or a strong emotional attachment. Can have a psychosexual dimension in which such an object is repeatedly or exclusively used in achieving sexual excitement.

fetor *n* offensive odour, stench. *fetor oris* bad breath.

fetoscopy *n* direct visual examination of the fetus by using an appropriate fibreoptic endoscope.

fetus *n* the developmental stage from the eighth week of gestation until birth—**fetal** *adj. fetus papyraceus* a dead fetus, one of a twin which has become flattened and mummified.

FEV *abbr* forced expiratory volume. ⇒ respiratory function tests.

fever *n* (*syn* pyrexia) an elevation of body temperature above normal. Designates some infectious conditions, e.g. *paratyphoid fever, scarlet fever, typhoid fever*, etc.

fibre *n* a thread-like structure—**fibrous** *adj.* ⇒ non-starch polysaccharide.

fibreoptics *n* light is transmitted through flexible glass fibres which enable the user to 'see round corners'. The technology utilized in endoscopic equipment.

fibril *n* a component filament of a fibre; a small fibre.

fibrillation *n* uncoordinated quivering contraction of muscle; referring usually to myocardial muscle. ⇒ atrial fibrillation, cardiac arrest, ventricular fibrillation.

fibrin *n* the insoluble matrix on which a blood clot is formed. Produced from soluble fibrinogen by the action of thrombin—**fibrinous** *adj.*

fibrinogen *n* factor I of blood coagulation. A soluble plasma protein that is converted to fibrin by the action of thrombin.

fibrinolysin *n* ⇒ plasmin, plasminogen.

fibrinolysis *n* the last of four overlapping processes of haemostasis. The dissolution of the fibrin clot by the proteolytic enzyme plasmin. There is normally a balance between blood coagulation and fibrinolysis in the body. ⇒ coagulation, platelet plug, thrombolysis.

fibrinolytic drugs a group of drugs that disperse thrombi by acting as thrombolytics. ⇒ Appendix 5.

fibroadenoma *n* a benign tumour containing fibrous and glandular tissue.

fibroblast *n* (*syn* fibrocyte) a blast cell that forms connective tissues. Involved during growth and tissue repair—**fibroblastic** *adj.*

fibrocartilage *n* cartilage containing fibrous tissue—**fibrocartilaginous** *adj.*

fibrocaseous *adj* a soft, cheesy mass infiltrated by fibrous tissue, formed by fibroblasts.

fibrochondritis *n* inflammation of fibrocartilage.

fibrocyst *n* a fibroma which has undergone cystic degeneration.

fibrocystic *adj* pertaining to a fibrocyst. *fibrocystic disease of bone* cysts may be solitary or generalized. If generalized and accompanied by decalcification of bone, it is symptomatic of hyperparathyroidism. *fibrocystic disease of breast* the breast feels lumpy due to the presence of cysts, usually caused by hormone imbalance. *fibrocystic disease of pancreas* cystic fibrosis.

fibrocyte *n* ⇒ fibroblast—**fibrocytic** *adj.*

fibroid *n* a fibromuscular benign tumour usually found in the uterus. The location of fibroids can be described as *intramural* (embedded in the wall of the uterus), *subserous* (protruding from the serosal surface into the peritoneal cavity), or *submucous* (protruding into the endometrial surface).

fibroma *n* a benign tumour composed of fibrous tissue—**fibromata** *pl*, **fibromatous** *adj.*

fibromuscular *adj* pertaining to fibrous and muscle tissue.

fibromyalgia *n* a condition characterized by widespread pain and tender points. Many patients also complain of tiredness and of waking feeling unrefreshed.

fibromyoma *n* a benign tumour consisting of fibrous and muscle tissue—**fibromyomata** *pl*, **fibromyomatous** *adj.*

fibroplasia *n* the production of fibrous tissue which is a normal part of healing. *retrolental fibroplasia* older term for retinopathy of prematurity.

fibrosarcoma *n* a form of sarcoma. A malignant tumour derived from fibroblastic cells—**fibrosarcomata** *pl*, **fibrosarcomatous** *adj.*

fibrosis *n* the formation of excessive fibrous tissues in a structure. Such as pulmonary fibrosis caused by radiation, certain drugs and pneumoconiosis—**fibrotic** *adj*.

fibrositis *n* a lay term (now seldom used) that denotes non-specific soft-tissue pain. ⇒ fibromyalgia.

fibrovascular *adj* relating to fibrous tissue which is well supplied with blood vessels.

fibula *n* one of the longest and thinnest bones of the body, situated on the outer side of the leg and articulating at the upper end with the lateral condyle of the tibia and at the lower end with the lateral surface of the talus (astragalus) and tibia (⇒ Figures 2, 3)—**fibular** *adj*.

field of vision ⇒ visual field.

Filaria *n* a genus of parasitic, thread-like nematode worms found mainly in the tropics and subtropics. They include *Brugia malayi, Loa loa, Onchocerca volvulus* and *Wuchereria bancrofti*. ⇒ filariasis.

filariasis *n* infestation with *Filaria*. The adult worms may live in the lymphatics, connective tissues or mesentery, where they may cause obstruction, but the microfilariae migrate to the bloodstream and some infiltrate the eye, skin or pulmonary capillaries. The completion of the life cycle of some types is dependent upon passage through a mosquito. ⇒ elephantiasis, loiasis, onchocerciasis.

filaricide *n* an agent which destroys *Filaria*.

filiform *adj* thread-like. *filiform papillae* small projections ending in several minute processes; found on the tongue.

filter *n* a device designed to remove particles over a certain size or rays of specific wavelength while allowing others to pass through. Examples include intravenous fluid filters and optical filters.

filtrate *n* substance that passes through the filter.

filtration *n* the process of straining through a filter under gravity, pressure or vacuum. *filtration under pressure* occurs in the nephron due to high pressure blood in the afferent arteriole of the glomerulus.

filum *n* any filamentous or thread-like structure. *filum terminale* a strong, fine cord blending with the spinal cord above, and the periosteum of the sacral canal below.

fimbria *n* a fringe, e.g. of the uterine tubes (⇒ Figure 17)—**fimbriae** *pl*, **fimbrial**, **fimbriated** *adj*.

fine motor control the specific control of the muscles allowing for completion of small, delicate tasks.

fine tremor slight trembling as seen in the outstretched hands or tongue of a patient suffering from hyperthyroidism.

finger *n* a digit. *clubbed finger* swelling of terminal phalanx which occurs in many chronic respiratory and cardiac conditions.

finger spelling communication by spelling words using the fingers to make the letters of the alphabet. It may be either one-handed or two-handed finger spelling.

FiO₂ *abbr* fractional inspired oxygen concentration.

first pass metabolism (first pass effect) occurs when orally administered drugs are rapidly metabolized in the liver. This leads to a situation where the amount of the active drug reaching the circulation is insufficient to produce a therapeutic effect. Other routes of administration are used to overcome the problem, e.g. transdermal or sublingual.

fission *n* ⇒ binary fission.

fissure *n* a split or cleft. Can be moist or dry cracks in the epidermis or mucosa. They usually develop at 90° to the direction of the tension stress. Common sites include the anal mucosa and interdigitally for moist fissures, and the heel margins for dry fissures. *palpebral fissure* the opening between the eyelids.

fistula *n* an abnormal communication between two epithelial surfaces (e.g. enterovesical between bowel and bladder). May occur in conditions such as Crohn's disease, diverticulosis and cancer—**fistulae** *pl*, **fistular, fistulous** *adj*. ⇒ arteriovenous fistula.

fistulotomy *n* incision of a fistula.

fitness *n* general term used to describe a person's ability to undertake a series of different physical exercises.

fits ⇒ convulsions.

fixation *n* **1** in optics, the direct focusing of one or both eyes on an object so that the image falls on the fovea. **2** the point on the retina used to look directly at an object of interest, usually the central fovea. **3** as a psychoanalytical term, an emotional attachment, generally sexual, to a parent, causing difficulty in forming new attachments later in life.

fixed costs the costs incurred regardless of the level of activity, e.g. related to the buildings and land, equipment maintenance.

flaccid *adj* soft, flabby, not firm.

flaccidity *n* loss of muscle tone due to disturbance of the lower motor neuron, with varying degrees of paralysis depending on the extent of loss of motor supply to the muscles and associated with weakness due to lack of use.

flagellation *n* the act of whipping oneself or others to gain sexual pleasure. Can be a component of masochism and sadism.

flagellum *n* a fine, hair-like appendage capable of lashing movement. Characteristic of spermatozoa, certain bacteria and protozoa—**flagella** *pl.*

flail chest unstable thoracic cage due to fracture. ⇒ paradoxical respiration.

flap *n* a unit of skin and other subcutaneous tissues that maintains its own blood and nerve supply, used to repair defects in other parts of the body. Common in plastic surgery to treat burns and other injuries; skin flaps used to cover amputation stumps.

flat foot *n* ⇒ pes planus.

flat pelvis a pelvis in which the anteroposterior diameter of the brim is reduced.

flatulence *n* gastric and intestinal distension with gas—**flatulent** *adj.*

flatus *n* gas in the gastrointestinal tract.

flea *n* a blood-sucking wingless insect; it operates as a host and can transmit disease. Its bite provides an entry point for infection. *human flea Pulex irritans. rat flea Xenopsylla cheopis,* transmitter of plague.

flexibilitas cerea literally waxy flexibility. A condition of generalized hypertonia of muscles found in catatonic schizophrenia. When fully developed, the patient's limbs retain positions in which they are placed, remaining immobile for hours at a time. Occasionally occurs in hysteria as hysterical rigidity.

flexibility *n* the range of movement possible around a joint or series of joints. Determined by the size and shape of the bones, normal joint mechanics, mobility of soft tissues and muscle extensibility.

flexion *n* the act of bending by which the shafts of long bones forming a joint are brought towards each other.

Flexner's bacillus ⇒ *Shigella flexneri.*

flexor *n* a muscle which on contraction flexes or bends a part. ⇒ Figures 4, 5, extensor *opp.*

flexure *n* a bend, as in a tube-like structure, or a fold, as on the skin—it can be obliterated by extension or increased by flexion in the locomotor system—**flexural** *adj. left colic (splenic) flexure* is situated at the junction of the transverse and descending parts of the colon. It lies at a higher level than the *right colic* or *hepatic flexure,* the bend between the ascending and transverse colon, beneath the liver. *sigmoid flexure* the S-shaped bend at the lower end of the descending colon. It is continuous with the rectum below.

flight of ideas succession of thoughts with no rational connection. A feature of manic disorders.

floaters *npl* floating bodies in the vitreous humour (of the eye) which are visible to the person.

flocculation *n* the coalescence of colloidal particles in suspension resulting in their aggregation into larger discrete masses which are often visible to the naked eye as turbidity (cloudiness).

flooding *n* a popular term to describe excessive bleeding from the uterus.

floppy baby syndrome may be due to nervous system or muscle disorder as opposed to benign hypotonia.

flora *n* used in microbiology to describe the colonization of various areas of the body by micro-organisms, e.g. *Staphylococcus epidermidis* on the skin. They are in most instances non-pathogenic, but can become pathogenic.

flow cytometer a laboratory instrument used to measure the proportions and absolute numbers of cell populations in (e.g.) blood. Cells of interest are stained with monoclonal antibodies against particular cell surface markers. The monoclonal antibodies are conjugated to fluorescent dyes and are detected once illuminated by a laser inside the flow cytometer. CD4+ T cell counts in HIV patients are commonly measured using flow cytometry.

flowmeter *n* a measuring instrument for flowing gas or liquid.

fluctuation *n* a wave-like motion felt on digital examination of a fluid-containing tumour, e.g. abscess—**fluctuant** *adj.*

fluke *n* a trematode worm of the order Digenea. The *Chinese fluke (Clonorchis sinensis)* is usually ingested with raw fish. The adult fluke lives in the bile ducts and, while it may produce cholangitis, hepatitis and jaundice, it may be asymptomatic or be blamed for vague digestive symptoms. The *European* or *sheep fluke (Fasciola hepatica)* is usually ingested from watercress. There is fever, malaise, a large tender liver and eosinophilia. *lung fluke (Paragonimus)* usually ingested with raw crab in China and Far East. Symptoms are similar to chronic bronchitis, including bloodstained sputum. ⇒ *Schistosoma*.

fluorescein *n* orange substance which fluoresces green when exposed to blue light. Used as eye drops to detect corneal lesions. Also used in retinal angiography, by injection into a peripheral vein, to demonstrate the retinal and choroidal circulation, and chorioretinal disease. *fluorescein string test* used to detect the site of obscure upper gastrointestinal bleeding. The patient swallows a radiopaque knotted string. Fluorescein is injected intravenously and after a few minutes the string is withdrawn. If staining has occurred the site of bleeding can be determined.

fluorescent treponemal antibody absorbed test (FTA-Abs) *n* a specific serological test for syphilis.

fluoridation *n* ⇒ fluoride.

fluoride *n* an ion sometimes present in drinking water, toothpastes, tea, vegetables and sea food. It can be incorporated into the structure of bone and teeth, where it provides protection against dental caries but in gross excess it causes mottling of the teeth. As a public health preventive measure it can be added to a water supply in a strength of 1 part fluoride in a million parts of water (fluoridation).

fluorine (F) *n* halogen element.

fluoroquinolones *npl* a group of synthetic antibiotics. ⇒ Appendix 5.

fluoroscopy *n* dynamic X-ray examination of the human body, observed by means of fluorescent screen and TV system.

focal injuries those injuries that occur in a small concentrated area, usually due to a high velocity-low mass force, e.g. ice hockey puck making contact with an unguarded area of the player's body.

focus groups in research a method of obtaining data that involves interviewing people in small interacting groups.

foetor ⇒ fetor.

folate (*syn* pteroylglutamic acid) collective name for the B vitamin compounds derived from folic acid. Folates occur naturally in foods such as liver, yeasts and leafy green vegetables and are absorbed from the small intestine. They are coenzymes involved in many biochemical reactions in the body, e.g. purine and pyrimidine synthesis, and adequate amounts, along with vitamin B_{12}, are required for normal red cells and cell division generally. A deficiency results in a megaloblastic anaemia. It is recommended that supplements are taken before and during the first weeks after conception, to reduce the risk of neural tube defects (NTDs) in the fetus.

folic acid the molecule that gives rise to a large group of molecules known as folates that form part of the vitamin B complex. ⇒ folate.

folie à deux a rare psychiatric syndrome, in which one member of a close pair suffers a psychotic illness and eventually imposes his delusions on the other.

follicle *n* **1** a small secreting sac. **2** a simple tubular gland—**follicular** *adj. follicle stimulating hormone (FSH)* secreted by the anterior pituitary gland; it is trophic to the ovaries in the female, where it develops the oocyte-containing (Graafian) follicles; and to the testes in the male, where it stimulates spermatogenesis.

folliculitis *n* inflammation of follicles, such as the hair follicles. ⇒ alopecia.

fomentation *n* a hot, wet application used to produce hyperaemia when applied to the skin.

fomite *n* any article that has been in contact with infection and is capable of transmitting same.

fontanelle *n* a membranous space between the cranial bones. The diamond-shaped anterior fontanelle (bregma) is at the junction of the frontal and two parietal bones. It usually closes in the second year of life. The triangular posterior fontanelle (lambda) is at the junction of the occipital and two parietal bones. It closes within a few weeks of birth.

food allergy an abnormal immunological response to food that can be severe and life-threatening. Signs and symptoms include swelling of the mouth and throat, breathing difficulties, skin rashes and gastrointestinal disturbances. The term is often used erroneously to describe any adverse reactions to food, whether or not the underlying mechanism has been identified. ⇒ allergy.

food intolerance an abnormal reaction to a food that is not immunological in origin, e.g. lactase deficiency. Symptoms can be chronic or acute, identification of the food can be difficult and may require an exclusion diet.

food poisoning a notifiable disease characterized by vomiting, with or without diarrhoea. It results from eating food contaminated with preformed bacterial toxin (e.g. from *Escherichia coli 0157, Staphylococcus aureus* and *Clostridium perfringens*) or multiplication of live microorganisms in food (e.g. *Campylobacter jejuni, Salmonella typhimurium, Bacillus cereus* and viruses) or poisonous natural vegetation, e.g. berries, toadstools (fungi) or chemical poisons.

Food Standards Agency in the UK a body set up by the government to oversee food standards and safety.

foot *n* that portion of the lower limb below the ankle. *foot drop* inability to dorsiflex foot due normally to damage of the nerve supply to the foot. Can be a complication of bedrest.

foramen *n* a hole or opening. Generally used with reference to bones—**foramina** *pl. foramen magnum* the opening in the occipital bone through which the spinal cord passes. *foramen ovale* a fetal cardiac interatrial communication which normally closes at birth.

forced expiratory volume (FEV) volume of air exhaled during a given time (usually the first second: FEV_1).

forced vital capacity (FVC) the maximum gas volume that can be expelled from the lungs in a forced expiration. ⇒ respiratory function tests.

forceps *n* surgical instruments with two opposing blades which are used to grasp or compress tissues, swabs, needles and many other surgical appliances. The two blades are controlled by direct pressure on them (tong-like), or by handles (scissor-like). *forceps delivery* the use of various specialized obstetric forceps applied to the infant to facilitate delivery during the second stage of labour.

forensic medicine (*syn* medical jurisprudence, or 'legal medicine'). The application of medical science to questions of law.

foreskin *n* the prepuce or skin covering the glans penis.

formaldehyde *n* toxic gas used as a disinfectant. Dissolved in water (formalin), it is used mainly for disinfection and the preservation of histological specimens.

formication *n* a sensation as of ants running over the skin. Occurs in nerve lesions, particularly in the regenerative phase.

formula *n* a prescription. A series of symbols denoting the chemical composition of a substance, e.g. NaCl is the formula for sodium chloride—**formulae, formulas** *pl.*

formulary *n* a collection of formulas. The *British National Formulary* describes licensed pharmaceutical products available in the UK.

fornix *n* an arch; particularly referred to the vagina, i.e. the space between the vaginal wall and the cervix of the uterus—**fornices** *pl.*

fossa *n* a depression or furrow—**fossae** *pl.*

fostering *n* placing an 'at risk' child with a suitable family either as a short- or long-term measure. The aims are to provide a child with the security of a home environment, and to reunite the child with their natural family as soon as practical. Long-term fosterings can be 'with a view to adoption'.

Fothergill's operation ⇒ Manchester operation.

fourchette *n* a membranous fold connecting the posterior ends of the labia minora.

'four-day blues' ⇒ postnatal depression.

Fournier's gangrene a fulminating gangrene of the male external genitalia.

fovea *n* a small depression or fossa; particularly the fovea centralis retinae, the site with many cones important for distinct colour vision.

fractional inspired oxygen concentration (FiO$_2$) the concentration of oxygen in inspired gas, expressed as a fraction of 1 (e.g. FiO$_2$ 0.6 equals 60% inspired oxygen concentration).

fractionation *n* in radiotherapy, the division of the total prescribed radiation dose into smaller parts to be given over a period of time to minimize tissue damage.

fracture *n* breach in continuity of a bone as a result of injury. ⇒ Bennett's fracture, Colles' fracture. *closed fracture* there is no communication with external air. *comminuted fracture* a breach in the continuity of a bone which is broken into more than two pieces. *complicated fracture* a breach in the continuity of a bone when there is injury to surrounding organs and structures. *compression fracture* usually of lumbar or dorsal region due to hyperflexion of spine; the anterior vertebral bodies are crushed together. *depressed fracture* the broken bone presses on an underlying structure, such as brain or lung. *impacted fracture* one end of the broken bone is driven into the other. *incomplete fracture* the bone is only cracked or fissured— called *greenstick fracture* when it occurs in children. *open (compound) fracture* there is a wound permitting communication of broken bone end with air. *pathological fracture* occurring in abnormal bone as a result of force which would not break a normal bone. *spontaneous fracture* one occurring without appreciable violence; may be synonymous with pathological fracture.

fraenotomy *n* frenotomy.

fraenum *n* frenum.

fragile X syndrome X-linked disorder mainly affecting males. Individuals have relatively normal appearance, but significant learning disabilities. Males may have large testes.

fragilitas ossium ⇒ osteogenesis imperfecta.

framboesia *n* yaws.

free radical activated oxygen species, such as the superoxide ion and hydroxyl radical. They are extremely reactive chemicals produced during normal metabolism. Normally they are dealt with by complex antioxidant enzyme systems but they can cause oxidative damage to cells.

freezing *n* the sudden inability of a parkinsonian patient to take another step while walking until an external visual, auditory or cutaneous stimulus is appreciated. It is due to co-contraction of antagonistic muscle groups; a manifestation of dystonia.

Freiberg's infarction an aseptic necrosis of bone tissue which most commonly occurs in the head of the second metatarsal bone.

Frenkel's exercises special repetitive exercises to improve muscle and joint sense.

frenotomy *n* surgical severance of a frenum or frenulum, particularly for tongue-tie.

frenulum or frenum *n* a small fold of mucous membrane that checks or limits the movement of an organ, e.g. tongue, prepuce of the penis. *frenulum linguae* from the undersurface of the tongue to the floor of the mouth.

frequency distribution the number of times (frequency) each value in a variable is observed.

Freud, Sigmund (1856–1939) the originator of psychoanalysis and the psychoanalytical theory of the causation of neuroses. He first described the existence of the unconscious mind, censor, repression and the theory of infantile sexuality, and worked out in detail many mental mechanisms of the unconscious which modify normal, and account for abnormal, human behaviour.

friable *adj* easily crumbled; readily pulverized.

friction *n* rubbing. Can cause abrasion of skin, leading to a superficial pressure ulcer; the adhesive property of friction, increased in the presence of moisture, can contribute to a shearing force which can cause a more severe pressure ulcer. ⇒ frictions. *friction murmur* heard through the stethoscope when two rough or dry surfaces rub together, as in pleurisy and pericarditis.

frictions *npl* small, accurately localized, penetrating massage manipulations using the pads of the fingers and thumb. Used in a circular direction on connective tissue and muscle, or transversely across tendons, to mobilize tissues, for example to maintain and restore mobility of tissues at risk of developing adhesions following strain or injury.

Friedreich's ataxia a progressive familial disease of childhood, in which there develops a sclerosis of the sensory and motor columns in the spinal cord, with consequent muscular weakness and staggering (ataxia). The heart may also be affected.

frigidity *n* absence of normal sexual desire.

frog plaster conservative treatment of developmental dysplasia of the hip (congenital dislocation of the hip), whereby the dislocation is reduced by gentle manipulation and both hips are immobilized in plaster of Paris, both hips abducted to 80° and externally rotated.

frontal *adj* **1** pertaining to the front of a structure. *frontal plane* a vertical plane running from head to foot. It divides the body into front and back parts and is at right angles to the median plane. Also called the coronal plane. **2** the forehead bone. *frontal sinus* cavity at the inner aspect of each orbital ridge on the frontal bone (⇒ Figure 14).

frostbite *n* freezing of the skin and superficial tissues resulting from exposure to extreme cold. The lesion is similar to a burn and may become gangrenous. ⇒ trench foot.

frozen shoulder initial pain followed by stiffness, lasting several months. As pain subsides, exercises are intensified until full recovery is gained. Cause unknown.

fructose *n* (*syn* laevulose) fruit sugar, a monosaccharide found in some fruit and vegetables and in honey. Sucrose in the diet is digested to 1 molecule of fructose and 1 of glucose. Fructose can be converted to glycogen in the body, without the presence of insulin.

FSH *abbr* follicle stimulating hormone.

fugue state an apparently purposeful journey takes place with associated loss of memory. The behaviour of the person involved may appear normal or unspectacular to the casual observer. Occurs in dissociative disorder or postictally in some forms of epilepsy.

fulguration *n* destruction of tissue by diathermy.

full-term *adj* mature—when pregnancy has lasted 40 weeks.

fulminant *adj* developing quickly and with an equally rapid termination.

fumigation *n* disinfection using the fumes of a vaporized disinfectant.

function **1** the ability to adapt consistently and competently to the demands of any normal situation in any normal environment. **2** describes the specific work done by a structure or organ in its normal state.

functional *adj* **1** relating to function. **2** of a disorder, of the function but not the structure of an organ. **3** as a psychiatric term, describes a condition without primary organic disease.

functional assessment evaluation of the occupational performance components that are required in order to consistently and competently perform activities of daily living.

functional endoscopic sinus surgery minimally invasive sinus surgery using a fine nasal endoscope.

functional exercise in sports medicine the activity(ies) that mimic the stresses, demands and skills of a particular sport.

functional limitations the inability to perform functional tasks.

functional tests in sports medicine the assessment of the athlete's ability to move a body part actively, passively and against resistance. Also encompasses the normal activity of the internal and sensory organs. *functional tests (sport-specific)* the use of activities and motions that closely represent the athlete's sport and position to assess a body part's readiness to return to competition.

fundoplication *n* surgical folding of the gastric fundus to prevent reflux of gastric contents into the oesophagus.

fundoscopy *n* examination of the fundus of the eye ⇒ ophthalmoscope.

fundus *n* **1** the basal portion of a hollow structure; the part which is distal to the opening. **2** in ophthalmology the inner surface of the eye as viewed through the pupil using an ophthalmoscope—**fundi** *pl*, **fundal** *adj*.

fungi *npl* simple plants. Mycophyta, including mushrooms, yeasts, moulds and rusts, many of which cause superficial and systemic disease in humans, such as actinomycosis, aspergillosis, candidiasis and tinea—**fungus** *sing*, **fungal** *adj*.

fungicide *n* an agent that kills fungi—**fungicidal** *adj*.

fungiform *adj* resembling a mushroom, like the fungiform papillae of the tongue.

fungistatic *adj* describes an agent which inhibits the growth of fungi.

funiculus *n* a cord-like structure.

funnel chest (*syn* pectus excavatum) a congenital deformity in which the breast bone is depressed towards the spine.

furuncle *n* a boil originating in a hair follicle. ⇒ boil.

furunculosis *n* an affliction due to boils.

fusiform *adj* resembling a spindle.

FVC *abbr* forced vital capacity.

F v. West Berkshire Health Authority (1989) a professional who acts in the best interests of an incompetent person (incapable of giving consent) does not act unlawfully if he/she follows the accepted standard of care according to the Bolam test.

G

gag *n* **1** the reflex contraction of the pharyngeal muscles and elevation of the palate when the soft palate or posterior pharynx is stimulated. **2** an instrument used to keep the mouth open.

gait *n* a manner or style of walking. *ataxic gait* an incoordinate or abnormal gait. *cerebellar gait* reeling, staggering, lurching. *scissors gait* one in which the legs cross each other in progressing. *spastic gait* stiff, shuffling, the legs being held together. *tabetic gait* the foot is raised high then brought down suddenly, the whole foot striking the ground.

galactagogue *n* an agent inducing or increasing the flow of milk.

galactocele *n* a cyst containing milk, or fluid resembling milk.

galactorrhoea *n* excessive flow of milk. Usually reserved for abnormal or inappropriate secretion of milk.

galactosaemia *n* excess of galactose in the blood and other tissues. Normally lactase in the small intestine converts lactose into glucose and galactose. In the liver another enzyme system converts galactose into glucose. Galactosaemia is the result of a congenital enzyme deficiency in this system (two types) and is one cause of learning disability—**galactosaemic** *adj*.

galactose *n* a monosaccharide that is produced by the digestion of the disaccharide lactose found in milk. ⇒ galactosaemia.

gallbladder *n* a pear-shaped bag on the undersurface of the liver (⇒ Figure 18b). It concentrates and stores bile.

gallipot *n* a small vessel for lotions.

gallows traction ⇒ Bryant's 'gallows' traction.

gallstones *npl* concretions formed within the gallbladder or bile ducts; they are often multiple and faceted.

gall *n* bile.

galvanometer *n* an instrument for measuring an electrical current.

Gamblers Anonymous an organization for compulsive gamblers.

gamekeeper's thumb (*syn* skier's thumb) a colloquial expression used in sports medicine to describe force abduction of the metacarpophalangeal joint whilst the thumb is extended, leading to rupture of the ulnar collateral ligament.

gamete *n* a female or male reproductive cell with the haploid (n) chromosome number; oocyte or spermatazoon.

gamete intrafallopian tube transfer (GIFT) a technique used in assisted conception where the oocyte and sperm are placed in the uterine (fallopian) tube laparoscopically.

gametogenesis *n* production of gametes (oocytes and spermatozoa). ⇒ oogenesis, spermatogenesis.

gamma encephalography a small dose of isotope is given. It is concentrated in many cerebral tumours. The pattern of radioactivity is then measured.

gamma globulins *pl* a group of plasma proteins that have antibody activity, referred to as immunoglobulins (IgA, IgD, IgE, IgG and IgM). They are responsible for the humoral aspects of immunity.

gamma-glutamyltransferase (GGT, gamma-GT) an enzyme. Increased levels in the plasma may be indicative of liver disease, but the level may be affected by the intake of alcohol and by some drugs.

gamma rays short wavelength, penetrating rays of the electromagnetic spectrum produced by disintegration of the atomic nuclei of radioactive elements.

ganglion *n* **1** a mass of nerve cell bodies in the peripheral nervous system such as those of the autonomic nervous system and those ganglia containing the cell bodies of sensory nerves. **2** localized cyst-like swelling near a tendon, sheath or joint. Sometimes occurs on the back of the wrist due to strain such as excessive use of a word processor—**ganglia** *pl*, **ganglionic** *adj*. *Gasserian ganglion* deeply situated within the skull, on the sensory root of the fifth cranial nerve. It is involved in trigeminal neuralgia.

ganglionectomy *n* surgical excision of a ganglion.

gangliosidosis ⇒ Tay–Sachs disease.

gangrene *n* death of part of the tissues of the body. Usually the results of inadequate blood supply, but occasionally due to direct injury (traumatic gangrene) or infection (e.g. gas gangrene). Deficient blood supply may result from pressure on blood vessels (e.g. tourniquets, tight bandages and swelling of a limb); from obstruction within healthy vessels (e.g. arterial embolism, frostbite where the capillaries become blocked); from spasm of the vessel wall (e.g. ergot poisoning); or from thrombosis due to disease of the vessel wall (e.g. arteriosclerosis in arteries, phlebitis in veins)—**gangrenous** *adj*. *dry gangrene* occurs when the drainage of blood from the affected part is adequate; the tissues become shrunken and black. *moist gangrene* occurs when venous drainage is inadequate so that the tissues are swollen with fluid.

gangrenous stomatitis ⇒ cancrum oris.

Ganser's syndrome a rare dissociative disorder characterized by 'approximate answers' to questions, disorientation/changes in consciousness, amnesia and pseudohallucinations. Sometimes associated with head injury.

Gardnerella vaginalis a bacterium normally present in the vagina, but is found in increased concentrations in bacterial vaginosis.

gargle *n, vi* to wash the throat; a solution used for washing the throat.

gargoylism *n* congenital disorder of mucopolysaccharide metabolism with recessive or sex-linked inheritance. The polysaccharides chondroitin sulphate 'B' and heparitin sulphate are excreted in the urine. Characterized by skeletal abnormalities, coarse features, enlarged liver and spleen, learning disability.

gas *n* one of the three states of matter, the others being solid and liquid. A gas retains neither shape nor volume when released—**gaseous** *adj*. *gas gangrene* a serious wound infection caused by anaerobic organisms of the genus *Clostridium*, especially *Clostridium perfringens (welchii)*, a soil microbe often present in the intestine of humans and animals. ⇒ gangrene.

GAS *abbr* general adaptation syndrome.

gastralgia *n* pain in the stomach.

gas transfer factor measure of the lung's ability to exchange gases. Particularly useful in the diagnosis and surveillance of interstitial lung diseases, sarcoidosis and emphysema.

gastrectomy *n* removal of a part or the whole of the stomach. Usually for cancers but may be used for gastric ulcers that do not respond to drug therapy. *Billroth I gastrectomy* is a partial gastrectomy where the remaining portion of the stomach is anastomosed to the duodenum. *Polya partial gastrectomy* (known in the USA as *Billroth II gastrectomy*) involves removal of part of the stomach and duodenum and anastomosing the remaining part of the stomach to the jejunum. *total gastrectomy* a radical operation that may be performed for cancer in the upper part of the stomach. ⇒ Roux-en-y operation.

gastric *adj* pertaining to the stomach. *gastric juice* is acid in reaction and contains two proteolytic enzymes. *gastric suction* may be intermittent or continuous to keep the stomach empty after some abdominal operations. *gastric ulcer* an ulcer in the gastric mucosa. The majority are associated with the presence of the bacterium *Helicobacter pylori* in the stomach. Other factors include a genetic predisposition, drugs such as non-steroidal anti-inflammatory drugs (NSAIDs) and smoking. The ulcer can bleed, leading to haematemesis and/or melaena, or it can perforate, constituting an abdominal emergency. Severe scarring following chronic ulceration may produce pyloric stenosis and gastric outlet obstruction. For management ⇒ duodenal ulcer.

gastrin *n* a hormone secreted by the gastric mucosa on entry of food, which causes further gastric secretion.

gastritis *n* inflammation of the stomach.

gastrocnemius *n* the large two-headed muscle of the calf. ⇒ Figures 4, 5.

gastrocolic *adj* pertaining to the stomach and the colon. *gastrocolic reflex* sensory stimulus arising on entry of food into stomach, resulting in strong peristaltic waves in the colon.

gastroduodenal *adj* pertaining to the stomach and the duodenum.

gastroduodenostomy *n* a surgical anastomosis between the stomach and the duodenum.

gastrodynia *n* pain in the stomach.

gastroenteritis *n* food poisoning. Inflammation of mucous membranes of the stomach and the small intestine; usually due to micro-organisms, but may be caused by chemicals, poisonous fungi, etc. There is vomiting and diarrhoea due to either the multiplication of micro-organisms (invasive intestinal gastroenteritis) ingested in food or from bacterial toxins (intoxication). Microbial causes include: the bacteria *Bacillus cereus*, *Campylobacter jejuni*, *Clostridium perfringens* and *Clostridium botulinum*, *Escherichia coli*, *Salmonella enteritidis*, *Staphylococcus aureus*, or viruses such as Norwalk virus, rotavirus. Gastroenteritis is generally transmitted by the faecal-oral route, either directly or indirectly. However, droplet spread is a feature of some viruses.

gastroenterology *n* study of the digestive tract, including the liver, biliary tract and pancreas and the accompanying diseases—**gastroenterological** *adj*, **gastroenterologically** *adv*.

gastroenteropathy *n* disease of the stomach and intestine—**gastroenteropathic** *adj*.

gastroenteroscope *n* an endoscope for visualization of stomach and intestine—**gastroenteroscopic** *adj*, **gastroenteroscopically** *adv*.

gastroenterostomy *n* a surgical anastomosis between the stomach and small intestine.

gastrointestinal *adj* pertaining to the stomach and intestine.

gastrojejunostomy *n* a surgical anastomosis between the stomach and the jejunum.

gastro-oesophageal *adj* pertaining to the stomach and oesophagus. *gastro-oesophageal reflux disease* condition caused by passage of gastric contents into the oesophagus. Typically causes heartburn. Complications include ulceration, strictures and Barrett's oesophagus.

gastro-oesophagostomy *n* a surgical operation in which the oesophagus is joined to the stomach to bypass the natural junction.

gastropathy *n* any disease of the stomach.

gastropexy *n* surgical fixation of a displaced stomach.

gastrophrenic *adj* pertaining to the stomach and diaphragm.

gastroplasty *n* any reconstructive operation on the stomach.

gastroschisis *n* a congenital incomplete closure of the abdominal wall with consequent protrusion of the viscera uncovered by peritoneum.

gastroscope *n* ⇒ endoscope—**gastroscopic** *adj*, **gastroscopy** *n*.

gastrostomy *n* a surgically established fistula between the stomach and the exterior abdominal wall. A feeding tube is inserted either endoscopically, surgically or radiologically into the stomach. Allows feeding with liquid feeds. ⇒ percutaneous endoscopic gastrostomy.

gastrotomy *n* incision into the stomach during an abdominal operation for such purposes as removing a foreign body, securing a bleeding blood vessel, approaching the oesophagus from below to pull down a tube through a constricting growth.

gastrula *n* the stage following the blastocyst in embryonic development.

gastrulation *n* in early embryonic development the immense changes occurring as the blastocyst becomes the gastrula. The three primary germ layers are formed and cells move to their appointed locations in readiness for the start of structural development.

Gaucher's disease a rare inherited disorder, mainly in Jewish children, characterized by a disordered fat metabolism (lipid reticulosis) and usually accompanied by very marked enlargement of the spleen.

Diagnosis follows biopsy of the bone marrow, liver, or spleen.

gauze *n* a thin open-meshed absorbent material used in operations to dry the operative field and facilitate the procedure.

GBM *abbr* glomerular basement membrane.

GCS *abbr* Glasgow Coma Scale.

GDS *abbr* geriatric depression scale.

Geigercounter *n* a device for detecting and registering radioactivity.

gelatin(e) *n* the glue-like substance found in animal connective tissue, used in capsules, suppositories, culture medium and in food preparation. Alternative medicines may be needed for vegans and others who will not accept medicines containing gelatin—**gelatinous** *adj*.

gemellus muscles muscles arising from the ischium. ⇒ Figure 5.

gender *n* more than just biological sex. The term encompasses the socially constructed views of feminine and masculine behaviour within individual cultural groups.

gene *n* a hereditary factor consisting of DNA located at a specific locus of a specific chromosome. Genes are responsible for determining specific characteristics or traits. ⇒ dominant, recessive.

general adaptation syndrome (GAS) proposed by Hans Selye. It describes a three phase (triphasic) response of the body to a stressor. Comprising: alarm, resistance/adaptation and exhaustion.

General Medical Council (GMC) the statutory body that regulates the practice of medicine in the UK. It oversees professional quality and continuing professional development standards for professional practice, discipline and conduct. It is responsible for the establishment and maintenance of a professional register for all doctors working in the UK, and has the power to remove individuals from the register in cases of professional misconduct, or in some cases to restrict practice or order specific training.

General Medical Services the medical services provided by family doctors.

general paralysis of the insane (GPI) a manifestation of neurosyphilis in which the brain is principally affected. ⇒ neurosyphilis.

general practice in the UK the services provided by generalist doctors in first contact health care. First defined in 1948 at the inception of the National Health Service. Provides general medical services as opposed to specialist services.

general sales list (GSL) in the UK. Drugs on sale, without prescription, to the public through various retail outlets such as supermarkets.

generative *adj* pertaining to reproduction.

generic denoting a drug name not protected by brand name or manufacturer. ⇒ Recommended International Non-proprietary Name.

genetic *adj* that which relates to heredity. For example, disorders the basis of which resides in abnormalities of the genetic material, genes and chromosomes. ⇒ congenital. *genetic code* the arrangement of genetic material stored in the DNA molecule of the chromosome. It is in this coded form that the information contained in the genes is transmitted to the cells to control their activity.

genetics *n* the science of heredity and variation, namely the study of the genetic material, its transmission and its changes (mutations).

genital *adj* pertaining to the organs of generation.

genital herpes ⇒ herpes.

genital warts a very common disease caused by certain types of the human papilloma virus (HPV). Cauliflower-like lesions develop in the genital area or in the perianal region after a prepatent period that varies from several weeks to even years.

genitalia *n* the external organs of generation.

genitocrural *adj* pertaining to the genital area and the legs.

genitourinary *adj* pertaining to the reproductive and urinary organs. *genitourinary medicine (GUM)* specialty concerned with the management of sexually transmitted infections and other medical conditions of the genital tract.

genome *n* the basic set of chromosomes and the genes, equal to the sum total of gene types possessed by different organisms of a species.

genotype *n* the total genetic information encoded in the chromosomes of an individual (as opposed to the phenotype). Also, the genetic make-up of a person at a specific locus, namely the alleles present at that locus.

gentian violet ⇒ crystal violet.

genu *n* the knee.

genupectoral position the knee-chest position, i.e. the weight is taken by the knees, and by the upper chest, while the shoulder girdle and head are supported on a pillow in front.

genu valgum (bow legs) abnormal outward curving of the legs resulting in separation of the knees.

genu varum (knock knee) abnormal incurving of the legs so that there is a gap between the feet when the knees are in contact.

genus *n* a classification ranking between the family and species.

geophagia *n* the habit of eating clay or earth.

geriatric depression scale (GDS) a test of depression for use with older people.

geriatrician *n* one who specializes in geriatrics.

geriatrics *n* the branch of medical science dealing with old age and its diseases together with the medical care and nursing required by 'geriatric' patients.

germ *n* colloquial term for a micro-organism, especially a pathogen. *germ cell* ⇒ gamete.

German measles ⇒ rubella.

germicide *n* any agent capable of killing micro-organisms (germs)—**germicidal** *adj*.

gerontology *n* the scientific study of ageing—**gerontological** *adj*.

Gestalt theory a German word meaning 'organized whole'. A theory of behaviour developed early in the twentieth century. It contends that perception and learning are active, creative processes that are part of an 'organized whole'.

gestation *n* ⇒ pregnancy—**gestational** *adj*.

GFR *abbr* glomerular filtration rate.

GH *abbr* growth hormone.

Ghon focus ⇒ primary complex.

giant cell arteritis ⇒ arteritis.

giardiasis *n* (*syn* lambliasis) infection with the flagellate *Giardia intestinalis*. Often symptomless, especially in adults. Can cause diarrhoea with steatorrhoea.

GIFT *abbr* gamete intrafallopian transfer.

gigantism *n* abnormal overgrowth, especially in height, due to excess growth hormone in childhood prior to fusion of the epiphyses. Almost always due to a pituitary tumour.

gingiva *n* the keratinized oral mucosa immediately surrounding a tooth, i.e. the gum—**gingivae** *pl*, **gingival** *adj*.

gingival sulcus the invagination made by the gingiva as it joins with the tooth surface.

gingivitis *n* inflammation of the gingivae.

girdle *n* usually a bony structure of oval shape such as the shoulder and pelvic girdles.

gland *n* an organ or structure capable of making an internal or external secretion. ⇒ endocrine, exocrine—**glandular** *adj*.

glanders *n* a contagious, febrile, ulcerative disease communicable from horses, mules and asses to humans. Caused by the bacterium *Burkholderia mallei*.

glandular fever ⇒ infectious mononucleosis.

glans *n* the bulbous termination of the clitoris and penis (⇒ Figure 16).

Glasgow Coma Scale (GCS) a rating scale for neurological patients that assesses their best motor, verbal and eye opening response. Used, for example, following head injury and neurosurgery.

glaucoma *n* a group of conditions in which there is characteristic damage to the optic nerve head and visual field loss. *acute glaucoma* a painful condition of sudden onset, usually with very high intraocular pressure. *chronic glaucoma* an insidious condition causing gradual loss of vision usually over many years—**glaucomatous** *adj*.

Gleason grade system used to assess the degree of differentiation in prostate cancer.

glenohumeral *adj* pertaining to the glenoid cavity of scapula and the humerus.

glenoid *n* a cavity on the scapula into which the head of the humerus fits to form the shoulder joint.

glia *n* ⇒ neuroglia—**glial** *adj*.

glioblastoma multiforme a highly malignant brain tumour.

glioma *n* a malignant tumour that arises from neuroglial tissue, typically an astrocytoma or oligodendroglioma—**gliomata** *pl*. ⇒ astrocyte, oligodendrocyte.

gliomyoma *n* a tumour of nerve and muscle tissue—**gliomyomata** *pl.*

globin *n* the protein that joins with haem to form haemoglobin.

globulins *npl* a large group of proteins. Those in the plasma are classified as alpha and beta, which are concerned with substance transport, and gamma, which provides protection against infection. The gamma globulins comprise the immunoglobulins A, D, E, G and M.

globulinuria *n* the presence of globulin in the urine.

globus hystericus a subjective feeling of a lump in the throat. Can also include difficulty in swallowing and is due to tension of muscles of deglutition. Occurs in anxiety states, dissociative disorder and depression.

globus pallidus literally pale globe; a mass of motor grey matter situated deep within the cerebral hemispheres, lateral to the thalamus. Part of the basal nuclei.

glomerular filtration rate (GFR) the volume of plasma filtered by the kidneys in one minute. It is usually around 120 mL per min.

glomerulonephritis *n* inflammation of the glomerulus (of the nephron). The term encompasses many different disorders of varying aetiology and prognosis— **glomerulonephritides** *pl.*

glomerulosclerosis *n* fibrosis of the glomerulus (of the nephron), often as a result of glomerulonephritis—**glomerulosclerotic** *adj.*

glomerulus *n* a coil of capillaries formed from a wide-bore afferent arteriole. It lies within the invaginated blind end of the renal tubule. Together with the renal tubule it form a nephron. Part of the filtration membrane involved in the production of urine—**glomerular** *adj*, **glomeruli** *pl.*

glossa *n* the tongue—**glossal** *adj.*

glossectomy *n* excision of the tongue.

glossitis *n* inflammation of the tongue.

glossodynia *n* painful tongue without visible change.

glossopharyngeal *adj* pertaining to the tongue and pharynx. The ninth pair of cranial nerves, they innervate the tongue and pharynx.

glossoplegia *n* paralysis of the tongue.

glottis *n* the opening between the abducted vocal folds in the larynx. It allows air to enter the respiratory tract and is involved in voice production—**glottic** *adj.*

glucagon *n* hormone produced in the pancreatic islets of Langerhans. It causes the release of glucose from liver glycogen and thereby raises the blood glucose. Used by injection to reverse hypoglycaemia. ⇒ insulin.

glucagon stimulation test a test of pituitary reserve, assessing the response of growth hormone and adrenocorticotrophin (ACTH) and hence cortisol to subcutaneous or intramuscular administration of glucagon.

glucocorticoid *n* any steroid hormone which promotes gluconeogenesis and which antagonizes the action of insulin. Occurring naturally in the adrenal cortex as cortisone and cortisol, and produced synthetically as, for example, prednisolone.

glucogenesis *n* production of glucose.

gluconeogenesis *n* the formation of glucose from non-carbohydrate sources, e.g. amino acids, lactate, etc.

glucose *n* dextrose. A monosaccharide. The form in which carbohydrates are absorbed through the intestinal tract and circulated in the blood. The amount in the blood is controlled by hormones that include insulin and glucagon. It is stored as glycogen in the liver and skeletal muscle.

glucose-6-phosphate dehydrogenase (G6PD) an enzyme. Deficiencies occurring in the red blood cell may be inherited. It affects Africans, and their descendants elsewhere, people living around the Mediterranean and in the Middle East. People lacking G6PD develop anaemia when exposed to certain foods or drugs, such as antimalarial agents. ⇒ anaemia, favism.

glucose tolerance test (oral glucose tolerance test) after a period of fasting, a measured quantity (75 g) of glucose is taken orally; thereafter blood samples are tested for glucose levels at intervals. A blood glucose equal to or greater than 11.1 mmol/L 2 hours after the oral glucose meets the diagnostic criteria for diabetes mellitus. ⇒ impaired glucose tolerance.

glucuronic acid used in the liver for the conjugation of bile pigments.

glue ear an accumulation of a glue-like substance in the middle ear. A cause of conductive deafness.

glue sniffing ⇒ solvent misuse.

glutamate (glutamic acid) a non-essential (dispensable) amino acid.

glutamic oxaloacetic transaminase ⇒ aminotransferases, AST.

glutamic pyruvic transaminase ⇒ aminotransferases, ALT.

glutamine *n* a conditionally essential (indispensable) amino acid.

glutathione *n* a peptide needed for conjugation in the liver and for red cell integrity. Paracetamol overdose causes serious depletion.

gluteal *adj* pertaining to the buttocks.

gluten *n* a protein found in the cereals wheat, rye and barley and products containing these cereals, e.g. bread. A gluten-free diet is used to treat coeliac disease and dermatitis herpetiformis.

gluten-induced enteropathy ⇒ coeliac disease.

gluteus muscles muscles of the buttock. ⇒ Figure 5.

glycaemic index an index used to rank carbohydrate foods based on the effect they have on blood glucose levels. Low glycaemic index foods include pulses, high glycaemic index foods include confectionery. It is sometimes used in the planning of diets for people with diabetes mellitus.

glycerin(e) *n* a clear, syrupy liquid used as an emollient and in mouthwashes and suppositories. It has a hygroscopic action. *glycerin suppository* acts by attracting fluid to soften hardened faeces in the rectum.

glycerol *n* combines with fatty acids to form triglycerides (triacylglycerols) and phospholipids.

glycine *n* a conditionally essential (indispensable) amino acid. The amino acid with the simplest chemical structure.

glycinuria *n* excretion of glycine in the urine. Associated with learning disability.

glycogen *n* the main carbohydrate (polysaccharide) storage compound in animals. Many glucose molecules are linked together in a process called glycogenesis occurring in the liver and skeletal muscle.

The conversion of liver glycogen back to glucose is called glycogenolysis.

glycogenesis *n* glycogen formation from blood glucose.

glycogenolysis *n* the breakdown of glycogen to glucose.

glycogenosis ⇒ glycogen storage disease.

glycogen storage disease a recessively inherited metabolic disorder caused by various enzyme deficiencies. Glycogen accumulates in organs and tissues, e.g. liver. Hypoglycaemia occurs, and the body tends to use fat rather than glucose, leading to ketosis and acidosis.

glycolysis *n* a metabolic pathway where glucose is broken down to form pyruvic acid and some energy (ATP)—**glycolytic** *adj*.

glyconeogenesis ⇒ gluconeogenesis.

glycopeptide antibiotics a group of antibiotics. ⇒ Appendix 5.

glycoproteins *npl* large group of proteins conjugated with a carbohydrate, e.g. collagen, mucins.

glycosides *npl* plant substances. Many contain pharmacologically active substances, such as digitalis from foxgloves. *cardiac glycosides* such as digoxin increase myocardial contractility and cardiac output, and are defined as positive inotropes. ⇒ Appendix 5 (inotropes—positive).

glycosuria *n* the presence of sugar in the urine.

glycosylated haemoglobin (HbA₁, HbA₁c) fraction of haemoglobin that non-covalently binds glucose; assay providing a measure of average blood glucose levels and hence control of diabetes mellitus over about 8 weeks.

gnathalgia *n* jaw pain.

gnathoplasty *n* plastic surgery of the jaw or cheek.

goblet cells mucus-secreting cells, shaped like a goblet, found in the mucosa lining the gastrointestinal and respiratory tracts.

Goeckerman regimen a method of treatment for psoriasis; exposure to ultraviolet radiation alternating with the application of a tar paste.

goitre *n* thyroid gland enlargement; may be smooth (simple) or nodular, and associated with normal or abnormal thyroid function; hyperthyroid with smooth enlargement in Graves' disease, or nodular enlargement in toxic multinodular goitre; hypothyroid with glandular enlargement in Hashimoto's disease.

goitrogens *npl* agents that cause goitre. Some occur in plants, e.g. turnip, cabbage and peanuts.

gold (Au) *n* metallic element used in the management of rheumatoid arthritis. The radioactive isotope gold-198 is sometimes used in the treatment of some malignant diseases.

golfer's elbow ⇒ epicondylitis.

Golgi tendon organ specialized receptors in tendons that with skeletal muscle spindles monitor muscle stretching. Involved in proprioception.

gonad *n* the female or male primary reproductive structure, ovary, testis—**gonadal** *adj*.

gonadotrophic *adj* having an affinity for, or influencing, the gonads.

gonadotrophin *n* gonad-stimulating hormone. ⇒ follicle stimulating hormone, human chorionic gonadotrophin, luteinizing hormone.

goniometer *n* protractor used to measure a joint's position and range of movement; uses either a 180° or 360° system—**goniometric** *adj*.

gonioscopy *n* examination of the anterior chamber angle of the eye with a special lens.

goniotomy *n* operation for congenital glaucoma. Incision through the anterior chamber angle.

gonococcal *adj* resulting from infection by *Neisseria gonorrhoeae*.

Gonococcus *n* a Gram-negative diplococcus (*Neisseria gonorrhoea*), the causative organism of gonorrhoea. It is a strict parasite—**gonococci** *pl*, **gonococcal** *adj*.

gonorrhoea *n* a sexually transmitted infection in adults. Infants can become infected during delivery, resulting in gonococcal conjunctivitis. Gonococcal vulvovaginitis in girls before puberty may indicate sexual abuse. Chief manifestations of the disease in men are a purulent urethral discharge and dysuria after an average incubation period of about 6 days. The majority of women with uncomplicated infection are symptomless. Acute pelvic inflammatory disease in women, and septic arthritis with or without skin lesions, may complicate untreated gonorrhoea—**gonococcal** *adj*.

Goodpasture syndrome ⇒ anti-GBM disease.

goose flesh contraction of the tiny muscles attached to the hair follicles causing the hair to stand on end: it is a reaction to either cold or fear.

gouge *n* a chisel with a grooved blade for removing bone.

gout *n* a form of metabolic disorder in which blood levels of uric acid are raised (hyperuricaemia). Acute arthritis can result from inflammation in response to urate crystals in the joint. The big toe is characteristically involved and becomes acutely painful and swollen. Drugs that reduce uric acid levels can control the disease. If gout is untreated deposition of urate crystals can cause chronic arthritis, nodules (e.g. in the ear) and kidney damage. ⇒ pseudogout, tophus.

Graafian follicle a mature ovarian follicle. A minute vesicle in the ovarian stroma containing a single oocyte which is released when the vesicle ruptures at ovulation. After ovulation, the Graafian follicle forms the corpus luteum which, should fertilization occur, maintains the early pregnancy. In the absence of fertilization the corpus luteum only lasts for 12–14 days, after which it becomes the corpus albicans.

gracilis muscle muscle of the leg. ⇒ Figures 4, 5.

grading *n* a classification of cancers based on histopathological characteristics. The level of malignancy of the tissue is determined by comparing the amount of cellular abnormality and the rate of cell division with normal cells in the same tissue. Low grade cancer generally has slow tumour growth and spread, whereas high grade cancer is aggressive with rapid spread. The grade of the disease is more important (for some types of cancer) than the stage as an indicator of prognosis and effective treatment. ⇒ differentiation, staging.

graft *n*, *v* transplanted living tissue, e.g. skin, bone and bone marrow, cornea, kidney, heart, lungs, pancreas and liver; to transplant such tissue. Grafts may involve: tissue moved from one site to another in the same individual (autograft); between genetically identical individuals (isograft); tissue obtained from a suitably matched donor (allografts or homografts); and tissue transplanted between different species (xenografts or heterografts).

graft versus host disease (GVHD) may follow a successful transplant, especially bone marrow, where the graft 'attacks' the tissues of the immunologically compromised host. ⇒ transplant.

Gram's stain a bacteriological stain for differentiation of micro-organisms. Those retaining the blue dye are Gram-positive (+), those unaffected by it are Gram-negative (−).

grand mal ⇒ convulsions, epilepsy.

granulation *n* the outgrowth of new capillaries and connective tissue cells from the surface of an open wound. *granulation tissue* the young, soft tissue so formed—**granulate** *vi.*

granulocyte *n* a cell containing granules in its cytoplasm. Describes the polymorphonuclear leucocytes, neutrophil, eosinophil and basophil.

granulocytopenia *n* decrease of granulocytes (polymorphs) not sufficient to warrant the term agranulocytosis.

granuloma *n* a tumour formed of granulation tissue.

Graves' disease hyperthyroidism due to production of stimulating thyroid-stimulating hormone (TSH) receptor antibodies; may also cause ophthalmopathy (eye disease), often evident as prominence of the eyes, and pre-tibial myxoedema. ⇒ hyperthyroidism.

gravid *adj* pregnant; carrying fertilized eggs or a fetus.

gravitational *adj* being attracted by force of gravity. *gravitational ulcer* ⇒ venous ulcer.

gravity *n* weight. ⇒ specific gravity.

gray (Gy) *n* the derived SI unit (International System of Units) for the absorbed dose of radiation. It has replaced the rad. ⇒

green monkey disease ⇒ Marburg disease.

greenstick fracture ⇒ fracture.

gregarious *adj* showing a preference for living in a group, liking to mix and fond of company. The herd instinct is an inborn tendency of many species, including humans.

grey matter unmyelinated nerve fibres and nerve cell bodies situated in the central nervous system. ⇒ white matter.

grieving process describes the stages, denial, anger, bargaining, depression, acceptance and possibly fear, that an individual may experience in relation to bereavement and dying. Grieving is also associated with other situations of loss including: loss of employment or a pet, loss of body function, such as infertility, or of a body part, e.g. limb, breast. ⇒ bereavement.

Griffith's types subdivisions of Lancefield group A streptococci based on their antigenic structure.

gripe *n* abdominal colic.

grocer's itch contact dermatitis, especially from flour or sugar.

groin *n* the junction of the thigh with the abdomen.

grommet *n* ventilation tube inserted into the tympanic membrane. Frequently used in the treatment of glue ear in children ⇒ myringotomy.

grounded theory research study where a hypothesis is elicited from the data gathered.

group activities the simultaneous, active participation of a number of people in purposeful, productive, playful and creative tasks with a specific therapeutic goal such as encouraging social skills. Used as part of occupational therapy practice.

group C meningococcal disease serious disease caused by group C *Neisseria meningitidis*. It causes meningococcal meningitis and life-threatening septicaemia usually in children and young adults. Effective immunization is available.

group psychotherapy ⇒ psychotherapy.

growth hormone (GH) (*syn* somatotrophin). Hormone secreted by the anterior pituitary gland under the influence of two hypothalamic hormones: growth hormone releasing hormone (GHRH) and growth hormone release inhibiting hormone (GH-RIH) or somatostatin. Growth hormone has widespread effects on body tissues and influences the metabolism of proteins, fats and carbohydrates. ⇒ acromegaly, dwarfism, gigantism.

growth hormone test a test for acromegaly. Growth hormone levels are measured during an oral glucose tolerance test. In acromegaly the level of growth hormone does not show the normal suppression with glucose.

GSL *abbr* general sales list.

guar *n* a soluble form of non-starch polysaccharide (NSP) fibre derived from the locust bean. Taken orally, it absorbs water from the intestine and produces a feeling of fullness and slows the rate of carbohydrate absorption. May be used in the management of some types of diabetes mellitus to reduce postprandial blood glucose levels.

guardian ad litem an individual from a social work or childcare background who is appointed to ensure that a court is fully informed of the relevant facts that relate to a child, and that the child's wishes and feelings are clearly demonstrated.

Guedel airway a plastic oropharyngeal device used to maintain the airway. ⇒ airway.

Guillain–Barré syndrome an acquired acute demyelinating inflammatory, peripheral neuropathy that can occur after an infection such as campylobacter gastroenteritis. It may lead to pain, weakness, paralysis and in some patients respiratory problems.

guillotine *n* a surgical instrument for excision of the tonsils.

Guinea worm ⇒ *Dracunculus medinensis.*

gullet *n* the oesophagus.

GUM *abbr* genitourinary medicine. ⇒ sexually transmitted infection.

gumboil ⇒ dento-alveolar abscess.

gumma *n* a localized area of vascular granulation tissue that develops in the later stages (tertiary) of syphilis. If near the surface of the body, may form chronic ulcers—**gummata** *pl.*

gut *n* the intestines, large and small. *gut decontamination* the use of non-absorbable antibiotics to prevent endogenous infection in patients having intestinal surgery or those who are immunocompromised because of drugs or neutropenia.

Guthrie test screen test carried out within the first week of life. Drops of blood are collected on special filter paper. From these, assays are performed to screen for phenylketonuria, hypothyroidism and, in certain health regions, cystic fibrosis. Infants with a positive test must have the diagnosis confirmed.

gynaecologist *n* a surgeon who specializes in gynaecology.

gynaecology *n* the science dealing with the diseases of the female reproductive system—**gynaecological** *adj.*

gynaecomastia *n* enlargement of the male mammary gland.

gypsum *n* plaster of Paris (calcium sulphate).

gyrus *n* a convoluted portion of cerebral cortex.

Gärtner's bacillus *Salmonella enteritidis.*

H

habilitation *n* the means by which a child gradually progresses towards the maximum degree of independence of which he or she is capable. ⇒ rehabilitation.

habit *n* any learnt behaviour that has a relatively high probability of occurrence in response to a situation or stimulus. Acquisition of habits may depend on both reinforcement and associative learning.

habitual abortion ⇒ miscarriage.

habituation *n* describes a decreasing response to a stimulus when it becomes familiar through repeated presentation, for example becoming less aware of the feel of clothing on the skin. It is often used in a negative sense in relation to drug use or misuse, when repeated intake of the drug creates psychological dependence. ⇒ drug dependence.

haem *n* the iron-containing pigment portion of haemoglobin.

haemangioma *n* a malformation of blood vessels which may occur in any part of the body. When in the skin it is one form of birthmark, appearing as a red spot or a 'port wine stain'—**haemangiomata** *pl.*

haemarthrosis *n* the presence of blood in a joint cavity—**haemarthroses** *pl.*

haematemesis *n* the vomiting of blood, which may be bright red following recent bleeding. Otherwise it is of 'coffee ground' appearance due to the action of gastric juice. The bleeding is usually from the gastrointestinal tract and causes include: peptic ulcer, varices, neoplasms, drug erosions and coagulation defects, but blood swallowed from elsewhere, e.g. during epistaxis, may be vomited.

haematin *n* a ferric iron-containing derivative of haemoglobin.

haematinic *n* a substance required for the production of red blood cells.

haematocele *n* a swelling filled with blood.

haematocolpos *n* retained blood in the vagina. ⇒ cryptomenorrhoea.

haematocrit *n* ⇒ packed cell volume.

haematology *n* the science dealing with the formation, composition, functions and diseases of the blood—**haematological** *adj*, **haematologically** *adv*.

haematoma *n* a swelling composed of extravasated blood, usually traumatic in origin—**haematomata** *pl*.

haematometra *n* an accumulation of blood (or menstrual fluid) in the uterus.

haematopoiesis *n* ⇒ haemopoiesis.

haematosalpinx *n* (*syn* haemosalpinx) blood in the uterine (fallopian) tube.

haematospermia *n* the discharge of blood-stained semen.

haematozoa *npl* parasites living in the blood—**haematozoon** *sing*.

haematuria *n* blood in the urine; may be macroscopic, i.e. visible to the naked eye, microscopic when it is not—**haematuric** *adj*.

haemochromatosis *n* (*syn* bronzed diabetes) an error in iron metabolism with increased iron deposition in tissues, resulting in brown pigmentation of the skin and cirrhosis of the liver—**haemochromatotic** *adj*.

haemoconcentration *n* relative increase of volume of red blood cells to volume of plasma, usually due to loss of the latter.

haemocytometer *n* an instrument for measuring the number of blood cells.

haemodiafiltration (CVVHD) *n* similar to haemofiltration, but with the addition of dialysate. Diffusion occurs and the removal of unwanted molecules is enhanced.

haemodialysis *n* dialysis involving toxin removal directly from the bloodstream using a dialyser and dialysate both outside the body. Often requires the use of an arteriovenous fistula. A method of renal replacement therapy used in patients in end-stage renal disease/failure (irreversible) or in acute renal failure (potentially reversible).

haemofiltration (CVVH) *n* form of renal replacement therapy (artificial kidney treatment), in which the patient's blood is passed through a filter allowing separation of an ultrafiltrate containing fluid and solutes. This is discarded and replaced with an isotonic solution. Usually continuous as in continuous veno-venous haemofiltration.

haemoglobin (Hb) *n* the red, respiratory pigment in the red blood cells. A molecule comprises 4 ferrous iron-containing haem groups and 4 globin chains. It combines with oxygen and releases it to the tissues. Some carbon dioxide is carried by haemoglobin, which also acts to buffer pH changes. There is a special form of fetal haemoglobin (HbF) which has a high affinity for oxygen, and two major adult forms (HbA, HbA_2). HbF is replaced by adult forms during early childhood. ⇒ oxyhaemoglobin.

haemoglobinaemia *n* free haemoglobin in the blood plasma—**haemoglobinaemic** *adj*.

haemoglobinometer *n* an instrument for estimating the percentage of haemoglobin in the blood.

haemoglobinopathy *n* usually hereditary abnormality of the haemoglobin molecule—**haemoglobinopathic** *adj*. ⇒ sickle cell disease, thalassaemia.

haemoglobinuria *n* haemoglobin in the urine—**haemoglobinuric** *adj*.

haemolysin *n* an agent capable of causing disintegration of red blood cells.

haemolysis *n* breakdown of red blood cells, with liberation of contained haemoglobin—**haemolytic** *adj*.

haemolytic anaemia ⇒ anaemia.

haemolytic disease of the newborn (*syn* erythroblastosis fetalis) a pathological condition in the newborn child due to Rhesus incompatibility between the child's blood and that of the mother. Red blood cell destruction occurs with anaemia, often jaundice and an excess of erythroblasts or primitive red blood cells in the circulating blood. Immunization of women at risk, using anti-D immunoglobulin, can prevent haemolytic disease of the newborn. Treatment of affected infants may include; phototherapy, blood transfusion and exchange transfusion in severe cases. ⇒ hydrops fetalis, icterus gravis neonatorum, kernicterus.

haemolytic uraemic syndrome (HUS) intravascular haemolysis and acute renal failure that occurs in association with another condition, such as food poisoning due to enterohaemorrhagic *Escherichia coli* type 0157. Those affected (mainly children) may need renal replacement therapy. The majority make a full recovery, but others will have residual renal problems.

haemopericardium *n* blood in the pericardial sac. ⇒ cardiac tamponade.

haemoperitoneum *n* blood in the peritoneal cavity.

haemophilias *npl* a group of conditions with inherited blood coagulation defects. In clinical practice the most commonly encountered defects are *haemophilia A*, factor VIII procoagulant deficiency: *haemophilia B* or Christmas disease, factor IX procoagulant deficiency. Both these conditions are X-linked recessive disorders resulting in an increased tendency to bleed, the severity of which depends on the amount of residual factor VIII or IX. Bleeding typically occurs into joints and muscles. ⇒ haemophilic arthropathy, von Willebrand's disease.

haemophilic arthropathy joint disease associated with haemophilia. The extent of joint damage has been 'staged' from radiological findings: (a) synovial thickening, (b) epiphyseal overgrowth, (c) minor joint changes and cyst formation, (d) definite joint changes with loss of joint space, (e) end-stage joint destruction and secondary changes leading to deformity.

Haemophilus *n* a genus of bacteria. Small Gram-negative rods which show much variation in shape (pleomorphism). They are strict parasites. *Haemophilus aegypticus* causes acute infectious conjunctivitis. *Haemophilus ducreyi* causes chancroid. *Haemophilus influenzae* causes epiglottitis, otitis media and meningitis in young children, and respiratory infection in people with chronic lung disease. Effective immunization is available as part of routine programmes. ⇒ Hib vaccine. *Haemophilus pertussis* ⇒ *Bordetella pertussis*.

haemopneumothorax *n* the presence of blood and air in the pleural cavity.

haemopoiesis *n* (*syn* haematopoiesis) the formation of blood. ⇒ erythropoiesis—**haemopoietic** *adj*.

haemoptysis *n* the coughing up of blood—**haemoptyses** *pl*.

haemorrhage *n* loss of blood from a vessel—**haemorrhagic** *adj*. Usually refers to serious rapid blood loss. This may lead to hypovolaemic shock with tachycardia, hypotension, rapid breathing, pallor, sweating, oliguria, restlessness and changes in conscious level. Haemorrhage can be classified in several ways. (a) According to the vessel involved, arterial, venous, or capillary. (b) Timing: *primary haemorrhage* that which occurs at the time of injury or operation. *reactionary haemorrhage* that which occurs within 24 hours of injury or operation. *secondary haemorrhage* that which occurs within some days of injury or operation and usually associated with sepsis. (c) Whether it is internal (concealed) or external (revealed). *antepartum haemorrhage* ⇒ intrapartum haemorrhage, placental abruption, postpartum haemorrhage.

haemorrhagic disease of the newborn characterized by gastrointestinal, pulmonary or intracranial haemorrhage occurring from the 2nd to the 5th day of life. Caused by a physiological variation in blood clotting resulting from a transient deficiency of vitamin K which is necessary for the formation of some clotting factors. Responds to administration of vitamin K.

haemorrhagic fever ⇒ mosquito-transmitted haemorrhagic fevers, viral haemorrhagic fevers.

haemorrhoidal *adj* relating to haemorrhoids or applied to nerves and vessels in the anal region.

haemorrhoidectomy *n* surgical removal of haemorrhoids.

haemorrhoids *npl* (*syn* piles) varicosity of the veins around the anus. *external haemorrhoids* those outside the anal sphincter, covered with skin. *internal haemorrhoids* those inside the anal sphincter, covered with mucous membrane.

haemosalpinx ⇒ haematosalpinx.

haemosiderin *n* an iron-protein complex. A storage form of iron.

haemosiderosis *n* iron deposits in the tissues.

haemostasis *n* the process that controls bleeding from small vessels. Damage to the blood vessels starts a complex series of reactions between substances in the blood and others released from damaged platelets and tissue. There are four over-lapping stages: vasoconstriction, platelet plug formation, coagulation and fibrino-lysis. Also includes the measures used to stop bleeding during surgery or following injury.

haemostatic *adj* any agent which arrests bleeding. *haemostatic forceps* artery forceps.

haemothorax *n* blood in the pleural cavity.

HAI *abbr* hospital acquired infection. ⇒ infection.

hair *n* thread-like appendage present on all parts of human skin except palms, soles, lips, glans penis and that surrounding the terminal phalanges. The broken stump found at the periphery of spreading bald patches in alopecia areata is called an exclamation mark hair, from the characteristic shape caused by atrophic thinning of the hair shaft. *hair follicle* the sheath in which a hair grows. *hair root*, *hair shaft* ⇒ Figure 12.

halal *n* meat obtained from animals slaughtered according to Islamic law.

half-life (t$_{1/2}$) *n* amount of time taken for the radioactivity of a radioactive substance to decay by half the initial value. The half-life is a constant for each radioactive isotope, e.g. iodine-131 is eight days. Or the time taken for the concentration of a drug in the plasma to fall by half the initial level. *biological half-life* time taken by the body to eliminate 50% of the dose of any substance by normal biological processes. *effective half-life* time taken for a combination of radioactive decay and biological processes to reduce radioactivity by 50%.

halibut liver oil a very rich source of vitamins A and D.

halitosis *n* foul-smelling breath.

hallucination *n* a false perception occurring without any true sensory stimulus. A common psychotic symptom that can occur in schizophrenia, affective psychoses, delirium and drug intoxication.

hallucinogens *npl* (*syn* psychotomimetics) chemicals that cause hallucinations.

hallux *n* the great toe. *hallux rigidus* ankylosis of the metatarsophalangeal articulation due to osteoarthritis. *hallux valgus or hallux abducto-valgus* (*syn* bunion) a complex deformity of the medial column of the foot involving abduction and external rotation of the great toe and adduction and internal rotation of the first metatarsal (referenced to the midline of the body). Deformity exists when abduction of the hallux on the metatarsal is greater than 10 to 12°. Friction and pressure of shoes cause a bursa to develop. The prominent bone, with its bursa, is known as a bunion. *hallux varus* the great toe deviates toward the midline of the body and is commonly seen with metatarsus adductus.

halo *n* **1** a titanium ring that encircles the head. ⇒ halopelvic traction. **2** the circle of light seen by people suffering from glaucoma.

halogen *n* any one of the non-metallic elements—bromine, chlorine, fluorine, iodine.

halopelvic traction a form of external fixation whereby traction can be applied to the spine between two fixed points. The device consists of three main parts (a) a halo, (b) a pelvic loop, and (c) four extension bars.

hammer toe a permanent hyperextension of the first phalanx and flexion of second and third phalanges.

hamstring muscles flexor muscles of the posterior part of the thigh.

hand *n* that part of the upper limb below the wrist.

hand-arm vibration syndrome (HAVS) (*syn* secondary Raynaud's phenomenon) a progressive chronic condition that arises following prolonged use of hand held vibrating equipment. Early signs are 'white finger', which is caused by constriction of and damage to the digital arteries. Other symptoms include tingling and loss of sensation caused by involvement of the digital nerves leading to loss of manual dexterity.

handicapped *adj* term previously applied to a person with a defect that prevents or limits the normal activities of living and achievement.

Hand–Schüller–Christian disease a rare condition usually manifesting in early childhood with histiocytic granulomatous lesions affecting many tissues. Cause unknown and course relatively benign. ⇒ histiocytosis X.

Hansen's disease ⇒ leprosy.

haploid *adj* refers to the chromosome complement of the mature gametes (spermatozoa or oocytes) following the reduction division of meiosis. This set represents the basic complement of 23 (n) unpaired chromosomes in humans (22 autosomes and 1 sex chromosome). The normal multiple is diploid (2n) but abnormally three or more chromosome sets can be found (triploid, tetraploid, etc.). ⇒ diploid.

Harrington rod used in operations for scoliosis: it provides internal fixation whereby the curve is held by the rod and is usually accompanied by a spinal fusion.

Hartmann's solution intravenous infusion solution containing sodium lactate and chloride, potassium chloride and calcium chloride. Also called Ringer-lactate solution.

Hartnup disease an inborn error of protein metabolism, associated with diffuse psychiatric symptoms or mild learning disability.

Hashimoto's disease firm thyroid gland enlargement, often associated with hypothyroidism and rarely with hyperthyroidism, largely in middle-aged females, with high circulating levels of thyroid antibodies and due to autoimmune lymphocytic infiltration.

hashish *n* ⇒ cannabis.

haustration *n* sacculation, as of the colon—**haustrum** *sing*, **haustra** *pl*.

Hawthorne effect a positive effect occurring from the introduction of change, of which people are less aware as time passes. Researchers doing observation research make allowances for this reaction to their presence by not including data from the first few days in the final data analysis.

hay fever a form of allergic rhinitis in which attacks of inflammation of the conjunctiva, nose and throat are precipitated by exposure to pollen.

HBIG *abbr* hepatitis B immunoglobulin.

HCG *abbr* human chorionic gonadotrophin.

HDU *abbr* high dependency unit.

head injury injury resulting from a blow to the head causing haemorrhage or contusion. ⇒ extradural haematoma, Glasgow Coma Scale, papilloedema, subdural haematoma.

Heaf test skin prick test for tuberculosis. Multiple small punctures of the epidermis through a layer of filter paper soaked in tuberculin, strength 1 in 1000 or 1 in 100. An inflammatory reaction is positive for tuberculosis. Test read at 3 days; grade 0–2 negative or weakly positive, grade 3–4 strongly positive.

healing *n* **1** the natural process of cure or tissue repair. ⇒ wound healing. **2** in complementary or integrated medicine the term healing refers to a return to health; also the use of a therapy that may assist the healing process; a specific therapeutic form, such as spiritual healing and therapeutic touch—**heal** *vt, vi*.

health *n* negatively defined as a state in which no evidence of illness, disease, injury or disability is found. More positively in 1948 the World Health Organization defined health as 'a state of complete mental, physical and social well-being and not merely the absence of disease or infirmity'. The development of holistic thinking has led to the broadening of definitions of health to include social, environmental and economic influences. Health includes individuals' social and psychological resources as well as their physical capacities. A positive concept of well-being as a subjective feeling, physical fitness, normal functional capacity, resistance, resilience or hardiness. The subjective nature of what constitutes health means that individual definitions will vary from one person to another, from place to place as well as at different times.

healthcare systems national or local organizations for providing medical/health care. The structure of the system has to accommodate progress in medical interventions, consumer demand and economic efficiency. Criteria for a successful system have been formulated: (a) adequacy and equity of access to care, (b) income protection (for patients), (c) macro-economic efficiency (national expenditure measured as a proportion of gross domestic product), (d) micro-economic efficiency (balance of services provided between improving health outcomes and satisfying consumer demand), (e) consumer choice and appropriate autonomy for care providers. There are four basic types of healthcare systems: socialized (UK NHS), social insurance

(Canada, France), mandatory insurance (Germany), voluntary insurance (USA).

health centre premises from which a variety of healthcare services are provided. Includes general practice, community services such as child health, family planning and some well woman services. May be owned by local government or Primary Care Trusts, general practitioners or privately owned.

Health Development Agency a statutory body set up to improve standards in public health. It is concerned with identifying the need for evidence and for commissioning research. Other roles include: standard setting, undertaking health promotion campaigns and distributing examples of good practice.

health education providing information to the public or individuals to reduce ill health and enhance positive health by influencing people's beliefs, attitudes and behaviour. The objective is to empower individuals to make appropriate choices for healthy living.

health gain an attempt at measuring the benefit of health intervention on the population. For example, health gain from a cervical cytology screening programme may be measured as the reduction in deaths from cervical cancer; coronary heart disease prevention programme measured as a reduction in deaths from coronary heart disease in men under 65 years of age, or the number of deaths avoided over a specified period of time (e.g. 5 years).

Health Improvement Programme (HImP) a focused action plan for improving health and healthcare provision at a local level. Involves a collaborative approach between Primary Care Trust(s), health professionals, local government, voluntary organizations and patient groups, etc.

health promotion efforts to prevent ill health and promote positive health. Five key priority areas for action formulated by the World Health Organization (1986, 1998): (a) building healthy public policy, (b) creating supportive environments for health, (c) strengthening community action for health, (d) developing personal skills for health and (e) re-orientating health services (to focus on whole populations).

hearing impairment impairment resulting from hearing loss. People can experience hearing loss at any stage of life. Common causes of hearing loss include glue ear, occurring most often during childhood, and presbycusis, which is a permanent sensorineural hearing loss associated with ageing. Communication with hearing impaired people can be enhanced by some simple steps including: being in front of, fairly close to, and on the same level as the affected person, reducing background noise, speaking clearly, not shouting and maintaining speech at the normal rhythm, using sentences rather than single words, not covering your face while speaking; also, avoid talking to a hearing person accompanying the patient and always make sure that you have the hearing impaired person's attention before you start to speak. ⇒ deafness.

hearing tests ⇒ acuity.

heart *n* the hollow muscular organ which pumps the blood around the pulmonary and general circulations. It is situated behind the sternum, lying obliquely within the mediastinum (⇒ Figure 6). It weighs around 300 g and is about the size of the person's fist. *heart block* partial or complete block to the passage of impulses through the conducting system of the atria and ventricles of the heart. *heart failure* ⇒ congestive heart failure. *heart transplant* surgical transplantation of a heart from a suitable donor.

heartburn *n* retrosternal burning due to gastro-oesophageal reflux of acid.

heart-lung machine *n* a machine that bypasses both the heart and lungs and may be used in cardiac surgery to oxygenate the blood.

heat exhaustion (*syn* heat syncope) collapse, with or without loss of consciousness, occurring in conditions of heat and high humidity: mainly resulting from loss of fluid and electrolytes through sweating. If the surrounding air becomes saturated, the condition progresses to heatstroke.

heatstroke *n* (*syn* sunstroke) final stage in heat exhaustion. The body is unable to lose heat, hyperpyrexia occurs and without effective treatment the person may die.

hebephrenia *n* a type of schizophrenia characterized by affective disturbance, thought disorder and negative symptoms. Prognosis tends to be poor—**hebephrenic** *adj*.

Heberden's nodes small bony swelling at terminal (distal) interphalangeal joints occurring in osteoarthritis.

hedonism *n* excessive devotion to pleasure, so that a person's conduct is determined by an unconscious drive to seek pleasure and avoid unpleasant things.

heel bruise (*syn* stone bruise) contusion to the subcutaneous fat pad located over the inferior aspect of the calcaneus (heel bone).

heel spurs occur on the plantar surface of the calcaneus and are considered a variant of the normal point of attachment of the plantar fascia. They are insignificant when small, and may be well defined with smooth, regular cortical contours. However, when enlarged they cause pain on walking.

Hegar's sign extreme softening of the lower segment of the uterus at 8 weeks gestation detected by bimanual palpation.

Heimlich's manoeuvre abdominal thrusts. A first aid measure to dislodge a foreign body (e.g. food) obstructing the glottis, performed by holding the patient from behind and jerking the operator's clenched fists into the victim's epigastrium.

Heinz body refractile, irregularly shaped body composed of denatured haemoglobin present in red blood cells in some haemolytic anaemias.

Helicobacter pylori bacterium causing a number of gastrointestinal diseases via gastric infection. These include peptic ulceration, gastric cancer and MALToma. May be diagnosed by urea breath tests, serology or gastric biopsy. Treatment with combination therapy of antibiotics and acid suppression is usually effective.

helium *n* an inert gas. Medical uses include pulmonary function tests and to dilute other gases.

helix *n* spiral. **1** outer ridge on the auricle (pinna) of the outer ear. ⇒ Figure 13. **2** describes the structure of molecules, such as DNA.

helminthagogue *n* an anthelmintic.

helminthiasis *n* the condition resulting from infestation with worms.

helminthology *n* the study of parasitic worms.

hemianopia *n* loss of vision in the nasal or temporal half of the visual field of one or both eyes.

hemiatrophy *n* atrophy of one half or one side. *facial hemiatrophy* a congenital condition, or a manifestation of scleroderma in which the structures on one side of the face are shrunken.

hemiballismus *n* involuntary flailing movements of limbs due in some cases to contralateral damage of the subthalamic (below the thalamus) nucleus in the basal nuclei (ganglia).

hemichorea *n* choreiform movements limited to one side of the body. ⇒ chorea.

hemicolectomy *n* removal of approximately half the colon.

hemicrania *n* unilateral headache, as in migraine.

hemidiaphoresis *n* unilateral sweating of the body.

hemiglossectomy *n* removal of approximately half the tongue.

hemiparesis *n* paralysis or weakness of one side of face or body.

hemiplegia *n* paralysis of one side of the body, usually resulting from a cerebrovascular accident on the opposite side—**hemiplegic** *adj*.

Henoch–Schönlein purpura a small vessel vasculitis, mainly affecting children. Caused by hypersensitivity which may follow a streptococcal respiratory infection, or a drug allergy, but it may be idiopathic. Immune complexes are formed which damage capillaries in the skin, gut and elsewhere. It is characterized by purpuric bleeding into the skin, particularly shins and buttocks, and from the wall of the gut, resulting in abdominal colic and rectal bleeding; and bruising around joints with arthritis. The kidneys may be affected, leading to haematuria, proteinuria, acute glomerulonephritis, nephrotic syndrome or acute renal failure.

hepar *n* the liver—**hepatic** *adj*.

heparin *n* a group of naturally occurring anticoagulant substances produced by mast cells and present in liver and lung tissue. Normally it prevents inappropriate blood coagulation in the body. Used therapeutically, it inhibits blood coagulation in several ways; primarily by the prevention of fibrin formation through the inhibition of thrombin activity. Heparin is used subcutaneously or intravenously for existing thromboembolic conditions, such as deep vein thrombosis, and in prophylaxis, e.g. perioperatively. Bleeding may occur as a side-effect. Its effects can be reversed with the antidote protamine sulphate. *low molecular weight heparin* given subcutaneously has a longer action and fewer side-effects. ⇒ anticoagulant, coagulation. ⇒ Appendix 5.

hepatectomy *n* excision of the liver, or more usually part of the liver.

hepatic *adj* pertaining to the liver. *hepatic portal circulation* that of venous blood (collected from the intestine, pancreas, spleen and stomach) to the liver before return to the heart.

hepaticoenteric *adj* pertaining to the liver and intestine.

hepaticojejunostomy *n* anastomosis of the hepatic duct to the jejunum.

hepatitis *n* inflammation of the liver, commonly associated with viral infection but can be due to toxic agents, such as alcohol, drugs and chemicals, or metabolic disorders, e.g. Wilson's disease. Viral hepatitis is currently a serious public health problem. It is associated with a number of different hepatitis viruses that include: hepatitis A virus (HAV), hepatitis B virus (HBV), hepatitis C virus (HCV) and hepatitis D virus (delta virus). Other types of hepatitis identified include: hepatitis E virus, hepatitis F virus and hepatitis G virus. *hepatitis A* is caused by an RNA enterovirus. It is relatively common and may be epidemic, especially in institutions, e.g. schools. The virus is transmitted by the faeco-oral route, caused by poor hygiene or contaminated food. *hepatitis B* is caused by a DNA virus. It is usually transmitted sexually (vaginal or anal intercourse), injection of infected blood or blood products, or via contaminated equipment, such as needles. The virus is shed in vaginal discharge, semen and saliva. Individuals at high risk include, intravenous drug users, homosexual or bisexual men, prostitutes and healthcare professionals through needlestick injuries. Hepatitis B virus may

persist, causing chronic hepatitis, or a carrier state can develop. Effective vaccine exists. *hepatitis C* is caused by an RNA virus and is most common in intravenous drug users and in those who have had a transfusion of blood or blood products. The virus can remain in the blood for many years and 30 to 50% of infected people develop chronic hepatitis, cirrhosis, liver failure and possibly liver cancer. Some people become carriers of the virus. *hepatitis D (delta virus)* can only replicate in the presence of hepatitis B and is therefore found infecting simultaneously with hepatitis B, or as a superinfection in chronic carriers of hepatitis B. Delta virus may increase the severity of a hepatitis B infection, increasing the risk of chronic liver disease. *hepatitis E* is transmitted via the faeco-oral route and has been reported in travellers returning from the USA, Mexico, Asia and Africa.

hepatocellular *adj* pertaining to or affecting liver cells.

hepatoma *n* primary carcinoma of the liver—**hepatomata** *pl*.

hepatomegaly *n* enlargement of the liver. It is palpable below the costal margin.

hepatosplenic *adj* pertaining to the liver and spleen.

hepatosplenomegaly *n* enlargement of the liver and the spleen, so that each is palpable below the costal margin.

hepatotoxic *adj* having an injurious effect on liver cells such as excess alcohol—**hepatotoxicity** *n*.

herbalism *n* the therapeutic use of herbs or mineral remedies. The use of plant material by trained practitioners to promote health and recovery from illness.

hereditary *adj* inherited; capable of being inherited.

hereditary angioedema (HAE) a genetic disorder characterized by episodes of severe life-threatening angioedema and sometimes abdominal pain. It is caused by a mutation in the gene encoding C1 inhibitor, which may be absent or dysfunctional. It is treated with C1 inhibitor pooled from plasma donations.

heredity *n* transmission from parents to children of genetic characteristics by means of the genetic material; the process by which this occurs, and the study of such processes.

hermaphrodite *n* individual possessing both ovarian and testicular tissue. Although they may approximate either to male or female type, they are usually sterile from imperfect development of their gonads.

hernia *n* the abnormal protrusion of an organ, or part of an organ, through an aperture in the surrounding structures: commonly the protrusion of an abdominal organ through a gap in the abdominal wall. *diaphragmatic hernia* ⇒ hiatus hernia. *femoral hernia* protrusion through the femoral canal, alongside the femoral blood vessels as they pass into the thigh. *incisional hernia* protrusion through the site of a previous abdominal incision. *inguinal hernia* protrusion through the inguinal canal in the male. *irreducible hernia* when the contents of the sac cannot be returned to the appropriate cavity, without surgical intervention. *strangulated hernia* hernia in which the blood supply to the organ involved is impaired, usually due to constriction by surrounding structures. *umbilical hernia* (*syn* omphalocele) protrusion of a portion of intestine through the area of the umbilical scar.

hernioplasty *n* an operation for hernia in which an attempt is made to prevent recurrence by refashioning the structures to give greater strength—**hernioplastic** *adj*.

herniorrhaphy *n* an operation for hernia in which the weak area is reinforced by some of the patient's own tissues or by some other material.

herniotomy *n* an operation to cure hernia by the return of its contents to their normal position and removal of the hernial sac.

heroin *n* diamorphine.

herpangina *n* minute vesicles and ulcers at the back of the palate. Short, febrile illness in children caused by coxsackievirus group A.

herpes *n* a vesicular eruption caused by infection with the herpes simplex virus. *genital herpes* a sexually transmissible infection, caused by either herpes simplex virus type 1 or type 2 (HSV-1 or HSV-2), that is associated with painful, tender superficial ulcers of the genitalia or anal region. Without treatment first-episode lesions heal within about one month; antiviral therapy shortens the duration of the lesions. Recurrences are common, particularly with HSV-2, but the duration of lesions is shorter than during the initial episode. An individual can transmit the virus to a sexual partner even when there are no apparent genital or orolabial lesions. *herpes gestationis* a rare skin disease peculiar to pregnancy. It clears in about 30 days after delivery.

herpes simplex virus (HSV) there are two types of HSV—types 1 and 2 (HSV-1 and HSV-2). HSV-1 is associated with orolabial herpes (cold sores), but either type can cause genital herpes. Following infection, whether or not the individual develops symptoms, the virus becomes latent or hidden for the individual's lifetime in the trigeminal ganglion (in the case of orolabial herpes) or in the sacral ganglia (in the case of genital herpes). Reactivation of the virus can cause recurrent lesions, or the virus can be shed from the mucous membranes or skin without visible signs. ⇒ herpes.

herpesviruses group of DNA viruses that include: cytomegalovirus (CMV), Epstein–Barr virus (EBV), herpes simplex virus (HSV), human herpesvirus 6 (HHV6) and varicella-zoster virus (VZV).

herpes zoster (*syn* shingles) the causative organism is the varicella-zoster virus (VZV); the same virus causes chickenpox. The virus affects the sensory nerves, causing a skin eruption and pain along the course of the nerve.

herpetiform *adj* resembling herpes.

hertz (Hz) *n* a derived SI unit (International System of Units) for wave frequency.

Hess test a sphygmomanometer cuff is applied to the arm and is inflated. Petechial eruption in the surrounding area after 5 min denotes weakness of the capillary walls.

heterogenous *adj* of unlike origin; not originating within the organism; derived from a different species. ⇒ homogenous *opp*.

heterograft ⇒ xenograft.

heterologous *adj* of different origin; from a different species. ⇒ homologous *opp*.

heterophile *n* a product of one species which acts against that of another, for example human antigen against sheep's red blood cells.

heterosexual *adj, n* literally, of different sexes; often used to describe an individual who is sexually attracted to members of the opposite sex. ⇒ homosexual *opp.*

heterozygous *adj* having different genes or alleles at the same locus on both chromosomes of a pair (one of paternal origin and one maternal) ⇒ homozygous *opp.*

hexachlorophene *n* a phenolic disinfectant used in preoperative skin preparation, and as a dusting powder. It should not be used on children under two years of age, during pregnancy, or on excoriated or badly burnt skin.

HHNK *abbr* hyperglycaemic hyperosmolar non-ketotic coma.

hiatus *n* a space or opening. *hiatus hernia* migration of part of the stomach through the diaphragmatic hiatus into the chest. May be asymptomatic, cause gastro-oesophageal reflux or strangulate. ⇒ hernia—**hiatal** *adj.*

Hib vaccine *abbr Haemophilus influenzae* type B vaccine. An injectable vaccine that protects against the serious infections caused by *Haemophilus influenzae.*

hiccough *n* (*syn* hiccup) an involuntary inspiratory spasm of the diaphragm, ending in a sudden closure of the glottis with the production of a characteristic sound.

hidrosis *n* sweat secretion.

Higginson's syringe a rubber bulb with tubes leading to and from it. Compression of the rubber bulb forces fluid forward through the nozzle for irrigation of a body cavity. Rarely used and now mostly replaced by single-use items of equipment.

high-density lipoprotein (HDL) ⇒ lipoprotein.

high dependency unit (HDU) an area within a hospital with augmented levels of staff and equipment in which patients can receive levels of observation monitoring, nursing and medical care between that available on a general ward and intensive care unit. Generally excludes those needing mechanical ventilation.

hilum *n* a depression on the surface of an organ where vessels, ducts, etc. enter and leave—**hili** *pl,* **hilar** *adj. hilar adenitis* ⇒ adenitis.

hip bone (innominate bone) formed by the fusion of three separate bones—the ilium, ischium and pubis.

Hippocrates *n* Greek physician and philosopher (460–367 BC) who established a school of medicine at Cos, his birthplace. He is often termed the 'Father of Medicine'.

Hirschsprung's disease congenital intestinal aganglionosis, leading to intractable constipation or even intestinal obstruction. There is marked hypertrophy and dilation of the colon (megacolon) above the aganglionic segment. Commoner in boys and children with Down's syndrome.

hirsute *adj* hairy or shaggy.

hirsutism, hirsuties *n* any abnormal degree of coarse hairiness, (usually refers to male pattern of hair growth in a woman). ⇒ hypertrichosis.

hirudin *n* a chemical produced by the medicinal leech, which prevents the clotting of blood by acting as an anticoagulant.

hirudo *n* ⇒ leech.

histamine *n* an amine released in many tissues. It causes smooth muscle constriction, gastric secretion and vasodilation. During the inflammatory response its release from mast cells leads to capillary dilatation and increased vessel permeability. ⇒ allergy, anaphylaxis, inflammation. *histamine receptors* there are three types in the body, H_1 in the bronchial muscle, H_2 in the secreting cells in the stomach and H_3 in nerve tissue. *histamine test* test previously used to determine the maximal gastric secretion of hydrochloric acid.

histidinaemia *n* genetically determined increase in histidine in blood. Gives rise to speech defects without learning disability.

histidine *n* a conditionally essential (indispensable) amino acid which is widely distributed in the proteins present in the diet.

histiocytes *npl* macrophages or phagocytic tissue cells.

histiocytoma *n* benign tumour of histiocytes.

histiocytosis X *n* rare condition involving an overgrowth of Langerhans' cells (part of the biological barrier formed by the skin), formerly thought to be histiocytes. Variable presentation and prognosis. Hand–Schüller–Christian disease is one presentation.

histology *n* microscopic study of tissues—**histological** *adj*, **histologically** *adv*.

histolysis *n* disintegration of organic tissue—**histolytic** *adj*.

histones *npl* proteins closely associated with the chromosomal DNA of higher organisms, which coils around histone molecules.

histoplasmosis *n* an infection caused by inhaling spores of the fungus *Histoplasma capsulatum*. The primary lung lesion may be symptomless or be accompanied by fever, malaise, cough and adenopathy. Progressive histoplasmosis can be fatal.

HIV *abbr* human immunodeficiency virus. ⇒ AIDS.

hives *n* nettlerash; urticaria.

HLA *abbr* human leucocyte antigen.

HMG-CoA reductase inhibitors (3-hydroxy-3-methylglutaryl-coenzyme) known colloquially as 'statins'. A group of drugs that prevent the synthesis of cholesterol in the liver, thereby reducing its level in the blood. ⇒ Appendix 5.

Hodgkin's disease tumour of lymphoid tissue often originating in the mediastinum. Often occurs in young adults. A diagnostic feature is the presence of the large multinucleated Reed–Sternberg cells in the lymphatic system. The prognosis is related to the histological subtype and stage; cure rate is around 80%. Treatment may consist of radiotherapy and/or chemotherapy. ⇒ lymphoma.

holistic *adj* relating to the theory of holism. Describes health care that takes account of physical, psychological, emotional, social and spiritual aspects.

Homans' sign passive dorsiflexion of foot causing pain in calf muscles. Indicative of deep vein thrombosis affecting the leg.

home assessment an evaluation of the suitability of an individual's accommodation in order to identify any adaptations, resources or services needed to enable him or her to adequately perform activities of daily living in the home environment.

homeopathy *n* a method of treating disease by prescribing minute doses of drugs which, in maximum dose, would produce symptoms of the disease. First adopted by Hahnemann—**homeopathic** *adj*. ⇒ allopathy.

homeostasis *n* autoregulatory processes whereby functions such as blood pressure, blood glucose and electrolytes are maintained within set parameters.

home visit a visit (such as by an occupational therapist) made to an individual's home in order to assess the ability of an individual to function independently following discharge from hospital or other care setting.

homicide *n* killing of another person: intentional killing is murder, whereas accidental killing is manslaughter (in Scotland culpable homicide).

homocysteine *n* an intermediate which with serine forms cysteine. It is also a precursor for methionine regeneration in reactions requiring folates and cobalamins. A deficiency in folates is associated with increased amounts of homocysteine in the blood and a higher risk of CHD.

homocystinuria *n* excretion of homocystine (a sulphur-containing amino acid, homologue of cystine) in the urine. Caused by a recessively-inherited metabolic error. Gives rise to slow development or learning disability of varying degree; lens may dislocate and there is overgrowth of long bones with thrombotic episodes which are often fatal in childhood—**homocystinuric** *adj*.

homogeneous *adj* of the same type; of the same quality or consistency throughout.

homogenize *vt* to make into the same consistency throughout.

homogenous *adj* having a like nature, e.g. a bone graft from another human being. ⇒ heterogenous *opp*.

homograft *n* a tissue or organ which is transplanted from one individual to another of the same species. ⇒ allograft.

homolateral *adj* on the same side.

homologous *adj* corresponding in origin and structure. ⇒ heterologous *opp*. *homologous chromosomes* those that pair during meiosis, the process by which mature gametes are formed. Of the two homologues, one is paternal and the other maternal in origin.

homonymous *adj* consisting of corresponding halves. Pertaining to symmetrical halves of the visual fields, i.e. the nasal (inner) half of one field and the temporal (outer) half of the other. When describing a visual field defect implies loss of vision in the same side of the field in the two eyes.

homosexual *adj*, *n* literally, of the same sex; describes an individual who is sexually attracted to members of the same sex. Individuals often prefer to be described as 'gay' or 'lesbian'.

homozygous *adj* having identical genes or alleles in the same locus on both chromosomes of a pair (one is paternal in origin and the other maternal). ⇒ heterozygous *opp*.

HONK *acron* hyperosmolar non-ketotic coma.

hookworm *n* ⇒ *Ancylostoma*.

hoop traction fixed skin traction used for the treatment of fractures of the femoral shaft in children, and for the gradual abduction of the hip in children with developmental dysplasia of the hip.

hordeolum *n* ⇒ stye.

horizontal plane ⇒ transverse plane.

hormone *n* a specific chemical messenger produced by endocrine glands that is transported in the blood or lymph to regulate the functions of tissues and organs elsewhere in the body.

hormone replacement therapy a term usually applied to oestrogen therapy given to women to relieve menopausal symptoms and prevent osteoporosis. It is administered orally, by implant or transdermally with patch or gel.

Horner's syndrome loss of sympathetic innervation to the eye and upper face causing myosis (miosis) (small pupil), ptosis (drooping of the eyelid), retraction of the eyeball (enophthalmos) and anhidrosis (loss of sweating) over the forehead on that side.

Horton syndrome severe headache due to the release of histamine in the body. To be differentiated from migraine.

hospice care care provided for those with chronic or terminal illnesses and their families. The care may be at home, in a day unit and in hospice premises. Individualized symptom (especially pain) control programmes are implemented which aim to minimize the physical, emotional and spiritual distress.

hospital acquired infection (HAI) ⇒ infection.

hospital sterilization and disinfection unit (HSDU) central sterile supply units (CSSUs) that also provide disinfection of equipment.

host *n* the organic structure upon which parasites or bacteria flourish. *intermediate host* one in which the parasite passes its larval or cystic stage.

hourglass contraction a circular constriction in the middle of a hollow organ (usually the stomach or uterus), dividing it into two portions following scar formation.

housemaid's knee ⇒ bursitis.

HPV *abbr* human papilloma virus.

H_1-receptor antagonists *pl* a group of antiemetic drugs that block histamine receptors. ⇒ Appendix 5.

H_2-receptor antagonist an agent which has a selective action against the H_2 histamine receptors and thereby decreases, for example, the secretion of gastric juice. ⇒ Appendix 5.

HRmax *abbr* maximum heart rate.

HRT *abbr* hormone replacement therapy.

HSDU *abbr* ⇒ hospital sterilization and disinfection unit.

HSSU *abbr* hospital sterile supply unit. ⇒ hospital sterilization and disinfection units.

HSV *abbr* herpes simplex virus.

$5-HT_1$ agonists *npl* a group of specific antimigraine drugs. ⇒ Appendix 5.

HTLV *abbr* human T-cell lymphotropic viruses.

$5-HT_3$-receptor antagonists a group of antiemetic drugs that block 5-hydroxytryptamine$_3$ receptors. ⇒ Appendix 5.

human chorionic gonadotrophin (HCG) a hormone produced by the trophoblast cells and later the chorion. Also a tumour marker for testicular and choriocarcinoma.

human immunodeficiency virus (HIV) currently designates the AIDS virus. There are two types: HIV-1 (many strains), mainly responsible for HIV disease in Western Europe, North America and Central Africa, and HIV-2, causing similar disease mainly in West Africa.

human leucocyte antigen (HLA) the major histocompatibility complexes, so called

because they were first found on leucocytes.

human papilloma virus (HPV) there are
many types of HPV, including several that
are associated with anogenital warts
(particularly types 6 and 11), and a few
types (particularly 16 and 18) that are
associated with genital tract malignancy
such as cervical carcinoma.

human T-cell lymphotropic viruses (HTLV)
two retroviruses; HTLV-1 and HTLV-2,
both of which are linked with some forms
of leukaemia.

humerus *n* the bone of the upper arm,
between the elbow and shoulder joint (⇒
Figure 2)—**humeri** *pl*, **humeral** *adj*.

humidity *n* the amount of moisture in the
atmosphere, as measured by a hygrometer.

humoral immunity ⇒ immunity.

humour *n* any fluid of the body. ⇒
aqueous, vitreous.

Hunter syndrome one of the mucopolysaccharidoses. A sex-linked recessive condition.

Huntington's disease rare inherited incurable neurodegenerative condition of the
brain, for which the gene is known. It is
due to a dominant gene and affects both
sexes. There is slow progressive degeneration of the nerve cells of the basal
nuclei (ganglia) and cerebral cortex.
Develops in adult life (30s and 40s) or
later, causing a movement disorder
(usually chorea), mood changes and
dementia. ⇒ chorea.

Hurler syndrome one of the mucopolysaccharidoses. Inherited as an autosomal
recessive trait.

HUS *abbr* haemolytic uraemic syndrome.

Hutchinson's teeth defect of the upper
central incisors (second dentition) which
is part of the facies of congenital syphilis.
The teeth are broader at the gum than at
the cutting edge, with the latter showing
an elliptical notch.

hyaline *adj* like glass; transparent. *hyaline
degeneration* degeneration of connective
tissue especially that of blood vessels in
which tissue becomes formless in appearance. *hyaline membrane disease* ⇒ neonatal
respiratory distress syndrome.

hyaloid *adj* resembling hyaline tissue. *hyaloid membrane* ⇒ membrane.

hyaluronic acid mucopolysaccharide found
in the extracellular matrix which holds
cells together. Also present in synovial
fluid, where it contributes to viscosity.

hyaluronidase *n* enzyme that breaks down
hyaluronic acid. It is present in spermatozoa and its release by many spermatozoa allows one to penetrate and fertilize
the oocyte. Hyaluronidase may be used
therapeutically to improve the absorption
of some drugs or fluids administered
parenterally.

hydatid cyst the cyst formed by larvae of a
tapeworm, *Echinococcus granulosa*, found
in dogs and other canines. The encysted
stage normally occurs in sheep but can
occur in humans after eating with soiled
hands from contact with dogs or infected
sheep. The cysts are commonest in the
liver, but can affect the brain, lungs and
bone.

hydatidiform *adj* pertaining to or resembling a hydatid cyst. *hydatidiform mole* a
pregnancy in which the placenta shows
degenerative stoma combined with neoplastic chorionic endothelium. A *complete
hydatidiform mole* shows abnormal proliferation of the trophoblast and the presence of hydropic placental villi with no
fetal parts. An *incomplete hydatidiform mole
or partial mole* has a chromosomally
abnormal fetus (triploid chromosome
complement). Malignant transformation
to choriocarcinoma may occur, especially
in pregnancies affected by a complete
hydatidiform mole.

hydraemia *n* a greater plasma volume than
usual compared with cell volume of the
blood; normally present in late pregnancy—**hydraemic** *adj*.

hydramnios *n* an excess of amniotic fluid.

hydrarthrosis *n* a collection of synovial
fluid in a joint cavity.

hydrate *vi* combine with water—**hydration**
n.

hydroa *n hydroa aestivale* a vesicular eruption that affects exposed parts and results
from photosensitivity. *hydroa vacciniforme*
is a more severe form of this in which
scarring ensues.

hydrocele *n* a swelling due to accumulation
of serous fluid between the tunica vaginalis and tunica albuginea of the testis or
in the spermatic cord.

hydrocephalus *n* (*syn* 'water on the brain') an excess of cerebrospinal fluid inside the skull due to a disruption in normal CSF circulation, or loss of brain tissue—**hydrocephalic** *adj*. *external hydrocephalus* the excess of fluid is mainly in the subarachnoid space. *internal hydrocephalus* the excess of fluid is mainly in the ventricles of the brain. A valve (e.g. Spitz–Holter type) is used to drain excess CSF and return it to the bloodstream.

hydrochloric acid acid formed from hydrogen and chlorine; secreted by the gastric oxyntic cells and present in gastric juice.

hydrocortisone *n* ⇒ cortisol.

hydrogen (H) *n* a colourless, odourless, combustible gas. *hydrogen ion concentration (pH)* a measure of the acidity or alkalinity of a solution, ranging from pH 0 to pH 14, 7 being approximately neutral; the lower numbers denoting acidity; the higher ones denoting alkalinity. *hydrogen peroxide* H_2O_2, a powerful oxidizing and deodorizing agent, used in suitable dilution in mouthwashes.

hydrogenation *n* the addition of hydrogen to a substance. ⇒ reduction.

hydrogen (H_2) breath test a non-invasive test to detect disaccharide intolerance or bacterial overgrowth. ⇒ lactase.

hydrolysis *n* the splitting into more simple substances by adding water—**hydrolytic** *adj*, **hydrolyse** *vt*.

hydrometer *n* an instrument for determining the specific gravity of fluids—**hydrometry** *n*.

hydronephrosis *n* distension of the renal pelvis with urine, due to an obstructed outflow. If unrelieved, pressure eventually causes atrophy of kidney tissue.

hydropericarditis *n* pericarditis with effusion.

hydropericardium *n* fluid in the pericardial sac in the absence of inflammation. Can occur in heart and kidney failure.

hydroperitoneum *n* ⇒ ascites.

hydrophilic *adj* describes an affinity for water.

hydrophobia *n* fear of water. ⇒ rabies.

hydrophobic *adj* describes an aversion to water.

hydropneumopericardium *n* the presence of air and fluid in the pericardial sac surrounding the heart. It may accompany pericardiocentesis.

hydropneumoperitoneum *n* the presence of air and fluid and gas in the peritoneal cavity: it may accompany paracentesis of that cavity; it may accompany perforation of the gut; or it may be due to infection with gas-forming micro-organisms.

hydropneumothorax *n* pneumothorax further complicated by effusion of fluid into the pleural cavity.

hydrops *n* oedema—**hydropic** *adj*. *hydrops fetalis* severe haemolytic disease of the newborn.

hydrosalpinx *n* distension of a uterine tube with watery fluid.

hydrostatic pressure that exerted by a liquid on the walls of its container, such as blood on an artery.

hydrotherapy *n* the science of therapeutic bathing, or exercise for diagnosed conditions.

hydrothorax *n* the presence of fluid in the pleural cavity. Also known as a pleural effusion.

hydroureter *n* abnormal distension of the ureter with urine.

hydroxocobalamin *n* a commercially produced substance with vitamin B_{12} activity. Given by injection for those unable to absorb vitamin B_{12}. ⇒ cobalamin, cyanocobalamin, intrinsic factor.

hydroxyapatite *n* the calcium salts, carbonate, hydroxide and phosphate, that make bone extremely hard.

hydroxyl (OH⁻) *n* a monovalent ion, consisting of a hydrogen atom linked to an oxygen atom. ⇒ free radical.

5-hydroxytryptamine (5-HT) *n* also known as serotonin. A neurotransmitter. Also present in the gastrointestinal tract and platelets.

hygiene *n* the science dealing with the maintenance of health—**hygienic** *adj*. *communal hygiene* embraces all measures taken to supply the community with pure food and water, good sanitation, housing, etc. *industrial hygiene* (*syn* occupational health) includes all measures taken to preserve the individual's health whilst he or she is at work. *mental hygiene* deals with the establishment of healthy mental attitudes and emotional reactions. *personal hygiene* includes all those measures taken by the individual to preserve his own health.

hygroma *n* a cystic swelling containing watery fluid, usually situated in the neck and present at birth, sometimes interfering with birth—**hygromata** *pl*, **hygromatous** *adj*.

hygrometer *n* an instrument for measuring the amount of moisture in the air. ⇒ humidity.

hygroscopic *adj* describes substances that readily absorb water, e.g. glycerine.

hymen *n* a perforated membrane across the vaginal entrance. *imperforate hymen* a congenital condition leading to haematocolpos. ⇒ cryptomenorrhoea.

hymenectomy *n* surgical excision of the hymen.

hymenotomy *n* surgical incision of the hymen.

hyoid *n* a U-shaped bone at the root of the tongue (⇒ Figure 6).

hyperacidity *n* excessive acidity.

hyperactivity *n* excessive activity and distractibility.

hyperaemia *n* excess of blood in an area. *active hyperaemia* caused by an increased flow of blood to a part. *passive hyperaemia* occurs when there is restricted flow of blood from a part—**hyperaemic** *adj*.

hyperaesthesia *n* excessive sensitiveness of a part—**hyperaesthetic** *adj*.

hyperaldosteronism *n* excessive production of aldosterone causing hypertension, hypokalaemic alkalosis, muscle weakness and rarely tetany; *primary hyperaldosteronism, Conn's disease*: hyperplasia or adenoma of the adrenal cortex; *secondary hyperaldosteronism*, e.g. due to increased renin secretion in renal artery stenosis.

hyperalgesia *n* excessive sensibility to pain—**hyperalgesic** *adj*.

hyperbaric *adj* term applied to gas at greater pressure than normal. *hyperbaric oxygen therapy* a form of treatment in which a patient is entirely enclosed in a pressure chamber breathing 100% oxygen at greater than one atmosphere pressure. Used for patients with carbon monoxide poisoning, decompression sickness, etc.

hyperbilirubinaemia *n* excessive bilirubin in the blood—**hyperbilirubinaemic** *adj*.

hypercalcaemia *n* excessive calcium in the blood usually resulting from bone resorption as occurs in hyperparathyroidism, metastatic tumours of bone, or Paget's disease. It results in anorexia, abdominal pain, muscle pain and weakness. It is accompanied by hypercalciuria and can lead to nephrolithiasis—**hypercalcaemic** *adj*.

hypercalciuria *n* greatly increased excretion of calcium in the urine. Occurs in diseases which result in bone resorption. *idiopathic hypercalciuria* is the term used when there is no known metabolic cause. Hypercalciuria is of importance in the pathogenesis of kidney stones—**hypercalciuric** *adj*.

hypercapnia (*syn* hypercarbia) raised CO_2 tension in arterial blood usually due to hypoventilation—**hypercapnic** *adj*.

hypercarbia *n* ⇒ hypercapnia.

hypercatabolism *n* excessive breakdown of body protein. Amino acids are used as a source of energy. It occurs when energy requirements are not met by dietary sources such as in situations where nutritional requirements are increased, e.g. major trauma, sepsis, surgery and burns. ⇒ catabolism, nitrogen balance.

hyperchloraemia *n* excessive chloride in the blood. Occurs with hyperkalaemia and leads to metabolic acidosis as acid–base balance is disturbed—**hyperchloraemic** *adj*.

hyperchlorhydria *n* excessive hydrochloric acid in the gastric juice—**hyperchlorhydric** *adj*.

hypercholesterolaemia *n* excessive cholesterol in the blood. Predisposes to atheroma and gallstones. Also found in hypothyroidism (myxoedema)—**hypercholesterolaemic** *adj*.

hyperemesis *n* excessive vomiting. *hyperemesis gravidarum* severe vomiting during pregnancy that requires medical intervention.

hyperextension *n* overextension. Active or passive force which takes the joint into extension beyond its normal physiological range.

hyperflexion *n* excessive flexion.

hyperglycaemia *n* increased blood glucose, usually indicative of diabetes mellitus or impaired glucose tolerance, but sometimes due to pathological stress, e.g. myocardial infarction—**hyperglycaemic** *adj*.

hyperglycinaemia *n* excess glycine in the serum. Can cause acidosis and learning disability—**hyperglycinaemic** *adj*.

hyperhidrosis *n* excessive sweating—**hyperhidrotic** *adj.*

hyperinsulinism *n* elevated circulating levels of insulin due to pancreatic tumour, insulinoma, or factitious administration of hypoglycaemic agents; resulting in hypoglycaemia, which may lead to episodic coma, confusion or even mental health disturbance.

hyperinvolution *n* reduction to below normal size, as of the uterus after parturition.

hyperkalaemia *n* excessive potassium in the blood as occurs in renal failure. An early sign may be muscle weakness. Severe hyperkalaemia causes arrhythmias and cardiac arrest—**hyperkalaemic** *adj.*

hyperkeratosis *n* hypertrophy of the stratum corneum or the horny layer of the skin—**hyperkeratotic** *adj.*

hyperkinesis *n* excessive movement—**hyperkinetic** *adj.*

hyperkinetic syndrome usually appears between the ages of 2 and 4 years. The child is slow to develop intellectually and displays a marked degree of distractibility and a tireless unrelenting perambulation of the environment, together with aggressiveness (especially towards siblings) even if unprovoked. He or she may appear to be fearless and undeterred by threats of punishment. The parents complain of the child's cold unaffectionate character and destructive behaviour.

hyperlipaemia *n* excessive total fat in the blood—**hyperlipaemic** *adj.*

hyperlipidaemia *n* abnormally elevated plasma lipid levels. Identified as a risk factor for coronary heart disease.

hypermagnesaemia *n* excessive magnesium in the blood; found in renal failure and in people who take excessive magnesium-containing antacids—**hypermagnesaemic** *adj.*

hypermetabolism *n* production of excessive body heat. Characteristic of hyperthyroidism—**hypermetabolic** *adj.*

hypermetropia *n* longsightedness caused by low refractive power or reduced axial length of the eye, with the result that the light rays are focused beyond, instead of on, the retina—**hypermetropic** *adj.*

hypermobility *n* excessive mobility. As in a joint that has an increase in the normal range of joint movement potentially leading to instability.

hypermotility *n* increased movement, as peristalsis.

hypernatraemia *n* increased sodium concentration in the blood caused by excessive loss of water and electrolytes owing to polyuria, diarrhoea, excessive sweating or inadequate water intake—**hypernatraemic** *adj.*

hypernephroma *n* (*syn* Grawitz tumour) a malignant tumour of the kidney—**hypernephromata** *pl*, **hypernephromatous** *adj.*

hyperonychia *n* excessive growth of the nails.

hyperosmolar non-ketotic coma (HONK, HHNK) profound dehydration due to uncontrolled type 2 diabetes leading to hyperosmolar state and ultimately coma.

hyperosmolarity *n* (*syn* hypertonicity) a solution exerting a higher osmotic pressure than another is said to have a hyperosmolarity, with reference to it. In medicine, the comparison is usually made with normal plasma.

hyperostosis *n* exostosis.

hyperoxaluria *n* excessive calcium oxalate in the urine—**hyperoxaluric** *adj.*

hyperparathyroidism *n* overactivity of one or more parathyroid glands, usually due to parathyroid adenoma, and resulting in elevated serum calcium levels; rarely results in parathyroid bone disease, osteitis fibrosa cystica; may be primary, or secondary/tertiary usually in response to chronic renal failure. ⇒ hypercalcaemia, hypercalciuria, von Recklinghausen's disease.

hyperperistalsis *n* excessive peristalsis—**hyperperistaltic** *adj.*

hyperphagia *n* overeating. Can be caused by psychological disturbances and lesions of the hypothalamus. It is a symptom of Prader–Willi syndrome. ⇒ obesity.

hyperphenylalaninaemia *n* excess of phenylalanine in the blood which results in phenylketonuria.

hyperphoria ⇒ phoria.

hyperphosphataemia *n* excessive phosphates in the blood—**hyperphosphataemic** *adj.*

hyperpigmentation *n* increased or excessive pigmentation.

hyperpituitarism *n* ⇒ acromegaly, Cushing's disease, gigantism, hyperprolactinaemia.

hyperplasia *n* excessive formation of cells—**hyperplastic** *adj.*

hyperpnoea *n* rapid, deep breathing; panting; gasping—**hyperpnoeic** *adj.*

hyperprolactinaemia *n* elevation in circulating prolactin levels, sometimes due to stress; if pathological results in galactorrhoea, menstrual irregularity and subfertility; may be due to dopamine antagonists, such as metoclopramide or neuroleptic drugs, large, often non-functioning pituitary tumours, or prolactinomas.

hyperpyrexia *n* body temperature above 40–41°C—**hyperpyrexial** *adj. malignant hyperpyrexia* a rare inherited condition which presents in response to certain anaesthetic drugs and neuroleptic (antipsychotic) drugs; there is progressive increase in body temperature and, if untreated, may be fatal.

hyperreflexia *n* exaggerated reflexes.

hypersecretion *n* excessive secretion.

hypersensitivity *n* an abnormal or exaggerated immune response to an antigen, classically classified as type I, II, III or IV. Type I, or immediate-type, is caused by specific IgE against an allergen crosslinking Fc receptors on mast cells, causing the mast cell to degranulate and release inflammatory mediators including histamine. Type II hypersensitivity results from antibodies binding to antigens on cell surfaces. Type III reactions are due to the deposition of immune complexes in tissues. Type IV or delayed-type hypersensitivity reactions occur 24–72 hours later and are due to antigen-specific T cells and macrophages—**hypersensitive** *adj.*

hypersplenism *n* term used to describe depression of erythrocyte, granulocyte and platelet counts by an enlarged spleen.

hypertelorism *n* congenital defect resulting in increased interpupillary distance. May be associated with various genetic disorders.

hypertension *n* abnormally high tension, by custom abnormally high blood pressure involving systolic and/or diastolic levels. There is no universal agreement on their upper limits of normal, especially with increasing age. Many cardiologists consider a resting systolic pressure of 140 mmHg and/or a resting diastolic pressure of 90 mmHg to be abnormal at age 20 years. Hypertension is considered to be a risk factor for the development of coronary heart disease. No cause is found in the majority of patients and is termed essential hypertension. Secondary hypertension may result from coarctation of the aorta, renal artery stenosis, renal disease, phaeochromocytoma, Cushing's disease/syndrome, Conn's syndrome, various drugs, such as oral contraceptives, NSAIDs, and the pre-eclampsia of pregnancy. ⇒ portal hypertension, pulmonary hypertension—**hypertensive** *adj.*

hyperthermia *n* very high body temperature—**hyperthermic** *adj.* ⇒ hyperpyrexia.

hyperthyroidism *n* thyrotoxicosis. A condition due to excessive production of thyroid hormone (thyroxine, triiodothyronine), usually due to Graves' disease, but also multiple or solitary toxic nodules, and resulting classically in anxiety, tachycardia, sweating, increased appetite with weight loss, and a fine tremor of the outstretched hands; much commoner in women than men.

hypertonia *n* muscle tone that is too high to permit movement; increased contractility of muscle due to excessive and inappropriate excitation of the motor neuron pools of the anterior horn of the spinal cord setting the bias on the stretch reflex too low (easily triggered), causing the muscles to be more sensitive to stretch. There are two types: spasticity and rigidity—**hypertonic** *adj*, **hypertonicity** *n.* ⇒ hyperosmolarity.

hypertonic *adj* 1 pertaining to hypertonia. 2 a fluid with a higher osmotic pressure relative to another fluid. *hypertonic saline* has a greater osmotic pressure than physiological fluid.

hypertrichosis *n* excessive hairiness in a non-androgenic distribution.

hypertrophic scar an unsightly raised red scar showing continued activity and no maturation.

hypertrophy *n* increase in the size of tissues or structures, independent of natural growth. It may be congenital, compensatory, complementary or functional. ⇒ stenosis—**hypertrophic** *adj.*

hyperuricaemia *n* excessive uric acid in the blood. Characteristic of gout. ⇒ Lesch–Nyhan disease—**hyperuricaemic** *adj*.

hyperventilation *n* overbreathing. Increased respiratory rate; may occur during anxiety attacks, in salicylate poisoning or head injury, or passively as part of a technique of general anaesthesia in intensive care. Also associated with alkalosis and tetany.

hypervitaminosis *n* any condition arising from an excessive intake of a vitamin. Can develop when large quantities of vitamin supplements are taken.

hypervolaemia *n* an increase in the volume of circulating blood.

hyphaema *n* blood in the anterior chamber of the eye.

hypnogogic stage the stage between being awake and asleep. Hallucinations may occur.

hypnosis *n* a state resembling sleep, brought about by the hypnotist or the individual utilizing the mental mechanism of suggestion to produce a relaxed state and an improvement in well-being. Also used in symptom control or reduction, smoking cessation and forms of anaesthesia, as in skin suturing and pain relief such as in labour—**hypnotic** *adj*.

hypnotherapy *n* treatment that uses sleep-like state or hypnosis.

hypnotic 1 *n* a drug which produces a sleep similar to natural sleep. ⇒ narcotic. ⇒ Appendix 5. **2** *adj* pertaining to hypnotism.

hypoaesthesia *n* diminished sensitiveness of a part—**hypoaesthetic** *adj*.

hypocalcaemia *n* decreased calcium level in the blood. Causes include: disturbed kidney function, excess calcium excretion, deficiency of vitamin D, alkalosis and hypoparathyroidism. Leads to tingling in the hands and feet, and stridor and convulsions in children—**hypocalcaemic** *adj*. ⇒ carpopedal spasm, hyperventilation, tetany.

hypocapnia *n* reduced CO_2 tension in arterial blood; usually produced by hyperventilation—**hypocapnial** *adj*.

hypochloraemia *n* reduced chloride level in the blood. Leads to metabolic alkalosis as the acid–base balance is disrupted—**hypochloraemic** *adj*.

hypochlorhydria *n* decreased hydrochloric acid in the gastric juice—**hypochlorhydric** *adj*.

hypochlorite *n* salts of hypochlorous acid. They are easily decomposed to yield active chlorine, and are used as disinfectants. ⇒ chlorine.

hypochondria *n* unnecessary anxiety about one's health—**hypochondriac, hypochondriacal** *adj*, **hypochondriasis** *n*.

hypochondriacal disorder an excessive preoccupation with the possibility of having serious health problems associated with refusal to accept professional reassurance that there is no physical illness underlying the symptoms. Symptoms are often of a bodily nature or concerned with physical appearance.

hypochondrium *n* the upper lateral region (left and right) of the abdomen (⇒ Figure 18a)—**hypochondriac** *adj*.

hypochromic *adj* deficient in colouring or pigmentation. Of a red blood cell, having decreased haemoglobin.

hypodermic *adj* below the skin; subcutaneous—**hypodermically** *adv*.

hypofibrinogenaemia *n* reduced amount of fibrinogen in the blood. May be hereditary or acquired and may result in an increased tendency to bleed—**hypofibrinogenaemic** *adj*.

hypofunction *n* diminished performance.

hypogammaglobulinaemia *n* decreased gammaglobulin in the blood, occurring either congenitally or, more commonly, as a sporadic disease in adults. Lessens resistance to infection. ⇒ dysgammaglobulinaemia—**hypogammaglobulinaemic** *adj*.

hypogastrium *n* that area of the anterior abdomen which lies immediately below the umbilical region (⇒ Figure 18a)—**hypogastric** *adj*.

hypoglossal *adj* under the tongue. *hypoglossal nerve* the 12th pair of cranial nerves which innervate tongue movements.

hypoglycaemia *n* decreased blood glucose, attended by anxiety, excitement, perspiration, delirium or coma. Hypoglycaemia occurs most commonly in diabetes mellitus, when it is due either to insulin overdosage or to inadequate intake of carbohydrate—**hypoglycaemic** *adj*.

hypoglycaemic drugs oral drugs that reduce blood glucose in diabetes mellitus.

⇒ alpha (α)-glucosidases inhibitor, biguanides, sulphonylureas. ⇒ Appendix 5.

hypogonadism *n* a condition associated with failure of testicular function.

hypokalaemia *n* abnormally low potassium level of the blood. Causes include: vomiting, gastrointestinal drainage, diarrhoea, starvation, excess renal loss in Cushing's syndrome or aldosteronism and with prolonged use of diuretics and other drugs. Leads to nausea, muscle weakness, arrhythmias and cardiac arrest—**hypokalaemic** *adj.*

hypokinesia *n* poverty of movement; including: inability to maintain repetitive movements or perform rapidly alternating movements (dysdiadochokinesis), lack of trunk rotation (e.g. no arm swinging), and loss of amplitude and range of movement (e.g. writing gets smaller).

hypomagnesaemia *n* decreased magnesium level in the blood—**hypomagnesaemic** *adj.*

hypomania *n* a less intense form of mania with persistent mild elevation of mood, overactivity, increased sociability, overfamiliarity, overtalkativeness, overspending, elevated libido and decreased need for sleep. Hallucinations and delusions are usually absent—**hypomanic** *adj.*

hypometabolism *n* decreased production of body heat. Characteristic of hypothyroidism.

hypomobility *n* decrease in the normal range of joint movement.

hypomotility *n* decreased movement, as of the gastrointestinal tract.

hyponatraemia *n* decreased sodium concentration in the blood. Causes include: vomiting, diarrhoea, sweating and burns, diuretics, aldosterone deficiency, excess ADH, renal disease and diabetes mellitus, or a failure to excrete water or excess intake. Leads to cerebral oedema with convulsions and changes in conscious level. May cause hypovolaemic shock when accompanied by water loss—**hyponatraemic** *adj.*

hypo-osmolarity *n* (*syn* hypotonicity) a solution exerting a lower osmotic pressure than another is said to have a hypo-osmolarity with reference to it. In medicine the comparison is usually made with normal plasma.

hypoparathyroidism *n* underactivity of the parathyroid glands resulting in decreased serum calcium levels, producing tetany.

hypopharynx *n* that portion of the pharynx lying below and behind the larynx, correctly called the laryngopharynx.

hypophoria *n* ⇒ phoria.

hypophosphataemia *n* decreased phosphate level in the blood—**hypophosphataemic** *adj.*

hypophysectomy *n* surgical removal of the pituitary gland.

hypophysis cerebri ⇒ pituitary gland—**hypophyseal** *adj.*

hypopigmentation *n* decreased pigmentation. ⇒ albinism.

hypopituitarism *n* pituitary gland insufficiency, especially of the anterior lobe. Absence of gonadotrophins leads to failure of ovulation, uterine atrophy and amenorrhoea in women and loss of libido, pubic and axillary hair in both sexes. Lack of growth hormone in children results in short stature. Lack of adrenocorticotrophin (ACTH) and thyrotrophin (TSH) may result in lack of energy, pallor, fine dry skin, cold intolerance and sometimes hypoglycaemia. Usually due to tumour of or involving pituitary gland or hypothalamus but in other cases cause is unknown. Occasionally due to postpartum infarction of the pituitary gland.

hypoplasia *n* defective development of any tissue—**hypoplastic** *adj.*

hypoproteinaemia *n* deficient protein in blood plasma, from dietary deficiency, reduced production or excessive excretion (albuminuria)—**hypoproteinaemic** *adj.*

hypopyon *n* a collection of pus in the anterior chamber of the eye.

hyposecretion *n* deficient secretion.

hyposensitivity *n* lacking sensitivity to a stimulus.

hyposmia *n* decrease in the normal sensitivity to smell.

hypospadias *n* a congenital malformation of the male urethra. Subdivided into two types: (a) penile, when the terminal urethral orifice opens at any point along the ventral surface of the penis, and (b) perineal, when the orifice opens on the perineum and may give rise to problems of sexual differentiation. ⇒ epispadias.

hypostasis *n* **1** congestion of blood in a part due to impaired circulation. **2** a sediment—**hypostatic** *adj.*

hypotension *n* low blood pressure that is insufficient for adequate tissue perfusion and oxygenation; may be primary or secondary (e.g. reduced cardiac output, hypovolaemic shock, Addison's disease) or postural—**hypotensive** *adj.*

hypothalamus *n* literally, below the thalamus. It consists of an area of grey matter in the brain just above the pituitary gland. It has both endocrine and neural functions. The hypothalamus produces the hormones oxytocin and vasopressin (antidiuretic hormone); these are stored in the posterior pituitary prior to release. It is the major centre for the autonomic nervous system and controls physiological functions that include thirst and hunger, circadian rhythms and emotions such as anger—**hypothalamic** *adj.*

hypothenar eminence the eminence on the ulnar side of the palm below the little finger.

hypothermia *n* core body temperature below 35°C. It is ascertained by a low-reading thermometer. Occurs particularly at the extremes of age, in hypothyroidism and people exposed to cold environmental conditions such as rough sleepers. An artificially induced hypothermia can be used in the treatment of head injuries and in cardiac surgery. It reduces the oxygen consumption of the tissues and thereby allows greater and more prolonged interference of normal blood circulation. *hypothermia of the newborn* failure of the newborn child to adjust to external cold; may be associated with infection.

hypothesis *n* a declaration that can be tested by statistical (inferential) tests. It is a prediction based on the relationship between the dependent and independent variables.

hypothetico-deductive method theories are examined and hypotheses for testing are derived in a deductive manner. The particular research study tests the hypotheses by data analysis that either supports or repudiates the original theory.

hypothyroidism *n* conditions caused by low circulating levels of one or both thyroid hormones (thyroxine, triiodothyronine). Much more common in women than men and may be: (a) associated with goitre, such as autoimmune thyroiditis, lack of iodine or as a drug side-effect, e.g. with lithium; (b) due to spontaneous atrophy; or (c) after surgical treatment for hyperthyroidism. Some individuals have a subclinical form and in others it may be transient. It results in decreased metabolic rate and may be characterized by some of the following: fatigue, bradycardia, angina, hypertension, aches and pains, carpal tunnel syndrome, low temperature and cold intolerance, weight gain, constipation, hair and skin changes (dry coarse skin), puffy face, anaemia, hoarseness, slow speech, menorrhagia and depression. Treatment is with replacement thyroxine. *congenital hypothyroidism* can be detected (by routine blood testing) soon after birth and treated successfully with thyroxine. Untreated, it leads to impaired mental and physical development. It is recognized by the presence of coarse facies and protruding tongue. The term cretinism was previously used.

hypotonia *n* muscle tone that is too low to maintain posture or permit movement against gravity; loss of contractility of muscle due to disturbance of the cerebellum or links between it and other centres in the brain causing the bias on the stretch reflex to be too high and the muscles to be less sensitive to stretch. ⇒ pendular response—**hypotonic** *adj*, **hypotonicity** *n*. ⇒ hypo-osmolarity.

hypotonic *adj* **1** pertaining to hypotonia. **2** a fluid with a lower osmotic pressure relative to another fluid. *hypotonic saline* has a lower osmotic pressure than normal physiological fluid.

hypoventilation *n* diminished breathing or underventilation.

hypovitaminosis *n* any condition due to lack of vitamins.

hypovolaemia *n* reduced volume of blood in the circulation—**hypovolaemic** *adj.*

hypoxaemia *n* reduced oxygen in arterial blood, shown by decreased PaO_2 and reduced saturation—**hypoxaemic** *adj.*

hypoxia *n* reduced oxygen level in the tissues. *anaemic hypoxia* due to inadequate amounts of haemoglobin available to carry oxygen. *histotoxic hypoxia* due to inability of cells to use oxygen, e.g. due to poisoning. *hypoxic hypoxia* due to low oxygen tension in arterial blood. *stagnant hypoxia* due to insufficient blood flow to deliver oxygen.

hysterectomy *n* surgical removal of the uterus. *abdominal hysterectomy* effected via a lower abdominal incision. *subtotal hysterectomy* removal of the uterine body, leaving the cervix in the vaginal vault. *total hysterectomy* complete removal of the uterine body and cervix. *vaginal hysterectomy* carried out through the vagina. *Wertheim's hysterectomy* ⇒ Wertheim's hysterectomy.

hysteria *n* **1** a state of excitement with temporary loss of emotional control. **2** the term previously used for conversion disorder—**hysterical** *adj*.

hysterosalpingectomy *n* excision of the uterus and uterine (fallopian) tubes.

hysterosalpingography ⇒ uterosalpingography.

hysterosalpingostomy *n* anastomosis between a uterine (fallopian) tube and the uterus.

hysteroscopy *n* the passage of a small diameter telescope through the cervix to visualize the uterine cavity. Also used for treatments such as transcervical resection of endometrium.

hysterotomy *n* incision of the uterus to remove a pregnancy. The word is usually reserved for a method of abortion.

hysterotrachelorraphy *n* repair of a lacerated cervix uteri.

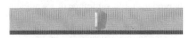

IADL *abbr* instrumental activities of daily living.

iatrogenic *adj* describes a secondary condition arising from treatment of a primary condition.

ICD *abbr* International Classification of Diseases.

ICE *acron* (ice, compress, elevation) a first aid measure used for swelling and bruising of the limbs. An ice compress is applied to the injury and the limb is elevated to assist venous return. ⇒ RICE.

ichthyoses *npl* a group of usually congenital conditions in which the skin is scaly and feels dry. Fish skin. Xeroderma.

ICP *abbr* intracranial pressure.

ICSH *abbr* interstitial cell stimulating hormone.

ICSI *abbr* intracytoplasmic sperm injection (transfer).

icterus *n* ⇒ jaundice. *icterus gravis* acute diffuse necrosis of the liver. *icterus gravis neonatorum* one of the clinical forms of haemolytic disease of the newborn. *icterus neonatorum* excess of the normal, or physiological, jaundice occurring in the first week of life as a result of excessive destruction of haemoglobin ⇒ phototherapy. *icterus index* measurement of concentration of bilirubin in the plasma. Used in diagnosis of jaundice.

ICU *abbr* intensive care unit. ⇒ intensive therapy unit.

id *n* one of the three main aspects of the personality (the others being the ego and superego); that part of the unconscious mind that comprises a system of biologically determined urges (instincts). It aspires to the immediate fulfilment of all desires and needs. According to Freud, it persists unrecognized into adult life.

IDDM *abbr* insulin dependent diabetes mellitus. ⇒ diabetes mellitus type 1.

idea *n* a concept or plan of something to be aimed at, created or discovered. *idea of reference* incorrect interpretation of casual incidents and external events as having direct reference to oneself. If of a sufficient intensity may lead to the formation of delusions.

ideation *n* the highest function of awareness, process by which ideas are imagined, conceived and formed. It includes intellect, thought and memory.

identical twins two offspring of the same sex, derived from a single fertilized ovum. ⇒ monozygotic, uniovular.

identification *n* recognition. **1** in psychology, the way in which personality is formed by modelling it on a chosen person, e.g. identification with the same sex parent— helping to form one's sex role; identification with a person of own sex such as a footballer or singer in the hero-worship of adolescence. **2** a mental defence mechanism where individuals take on the characteristics of the admired role model figure.

idiopathic *adj* of a condition, of unknown or spontaneous origin, e.g. some forms of epilepsy.

idiopathic thrombocytopenic purpura (ITP) a syndrome characterized by a low platelet count caused by the presence of autoantibodies. This results in purpura and intermittent bleeding from mucosal surfaces. In children it may appear following a virus infection. The onset in adults tends to be more insidious. Treatment in adults usually involves corticosteroids, with splenectomy in patients who fail to respond.

idiosyncrasy *n* a peculiar variation of constitution or temperament. It may relate to an unusual response to a particular protein, drug or food.

Ig *abbr* ⇒ immunoglobulin.

IHD *abbr* ischaemic heart disease.

ileal bladder ⇒ ileoureterostomy.

ileal conduit ⇒ ileoureterostomy.

ileitis *n* inflammation of the ileum.

ileocaecal *adj* pertaining to the ileum and the caecum.

ileocolic *adj* pertaining to the ileum and the colon.

ileocolitis *n* inflammation of the ileum and the colon.

ileocolostomy *n* a surgically made fistula between the ileum and the colon, usually the transverse colon. Most often used to bypass an obstruction or inflammation in the caecum or ascending colon.

ileocystoplasty *n* operation to increase the size of the urinary bladder—**ileocystoplastic** *adj*.

ileorectal *adj* pertaining to the ileum and the rectum.

ileosigmoidostomy *n* an anastomosis between the ileum and sigmoid colon.

ileostomy *n* a surgically made fistula between the ileum and the anterior abdominal wall; a type of stoma discharging liquid faecal matter. Usually permanent when the whole of the large bowel has to be removed, e.g. in severe ulcerative colitis. *ileostomy bags* special plastic bags used to collect the liquid discharge from an ileostomy.

ileoureterostomy *n* (*syn* ureteroileostomy) transplantation of the lower ends of the ureters from the urinary bladder to an isolated loop of small bowel (ileal bladder) which, in turn, is made to open on the abdominal wall (ileal conduit).

ileum *n* the lower three-fifths of the small intestine, lying between the jejunum and the caecum. Concerned with the absorption of various nutrients such as vitamin B_{12}—**ileal** *adj*.

ileus *n* intestinal obstruction. Usually restricted to paralytic as opposed to mechanical obstruction and characterized by abdominal distension, vomiting and the absence of pain. ⇒ meconium.

iliac *adj* pertaining to the ilium. *iliac arteries* carry arterial blood to the pelvis and legs. ⇒ Figure 9. *iliac crest* the highest point of the ilium. *iliac region/fossa* the abdominal region situated either side of the hypogastrium. ⇒ Figure 18a. *iliac veins* drain venous blood from the legs and pelvis. ⇒ Figure 10.

iliococcygeal *adj* pertaining to the ilium and coccyx.

iliofemoral *adj* pertaining to the ilium and the femur.

iliopectineal *adj* pertaining to the ilium and the pubis. *iliopectineal line* bony ridge on the internal surface of the ilium and pubic bones. It is the dividing line between the true and false pelvis.

iliopsoas *adj* pertaining to the ilium and the loin.

ilium *n* the upper part of the innominate (hip) bone; it is a separate bone in the fetus—**iliac** *adj*.

Ilizarov frame external fixation device used commonly in the management of fractures of the tibia.

illusion *n* a misidentification of a sensation, e.g. of sight, a bush or tree being mistaken for a person, the bush being misrepresented in consciousness as a figure.

image *n* 1 a revived experience of a percept recalled from memory. 2 the optical reproduction of an object formed on the retina as light is focused through the eye.

imagery *n* imagination. The recall of mental images of various types depending upon the specific sensory organs involved when the images were formed, e.g. smell (olfactory), sound (auditory), sight (visual), touch (tactile). *guided imagery* a technique used as part of a range of coping strategies for pain and other symptom control or anxiety in which patients are asked to imagine a particular situation, feeling or state.

imaging techniques diagnostic techniques used to investigate the condition and functioning of organs and structures. They include radiographic examination, radionuclide scans, ultrasonography, computed tomography, magnetic resonance and positron emission tomography.

imbalance *n* want of balance. Term refers commonly to the upset of acid–base relationship and the electrolytes in body fluids.

immersion foot ⇒ trench foot.

immune *adj* protected against infection by specific or non-specific mechanisms of the immune system. Altered reactivity against an antigen, caused by previous exposure to that antigen.

immune response the response of the immune system to a perceived threat, either from non-self antigens, or from self antigens during a pathological immune response. This may be against micro-organisms, malignant cells, and damaged or healthy tissues.

immunity *n* an intrinsic or acquired state of immune responsiveness to an antigen. *active immunity* is acquired, naturally during an infection or artificially by immunization. It involves the production of antibodies and specific T cells in response to exposure to an antigenic stimulus. The primary response to exposure is followed by a 2–3 week lag phase before enough antibodies are produced, but the secondary response following a subsequent exposure is more intense and has a much reduced lag phase because the memory cells are able to produce antibodies very quickly. This type of immunity tends to be of long duration. *cell mediated immunity* T-lymphocyte-dependent responses which cause graft rejection, immunity to some infectious agents and tumour rejection. *humoral immunity* from immunoglobulins produced by plasma cells derived from B lymphocytes. Immunity can be innate (from inherited qualities), or it can be acquired, actively or passively, naturally or artificially. *passive immunity* is acquired, naturally when maternal antibody passes to the fetus via the placenta or in colostrum and breast milk, or artificially by administering immunoglobulins (usually human in origin). This type of immunity tends to

be short-lived because the immune response is not stimulated to produce specific antibodies.

immunization *n* artificial means by which immunity is initiated or augmented. Achieved by using vaccines containing attenuated micro-organisms or inactive micro-organisms or bacterial products such as toxins. Antibody production (active immunity) occurs and is generally long-lasting. In certain situations, the injection of immunoglobulins obtained from immune humans, or very rarely sera from animals, can give temporary protection (passive immunization). *immunization programme* a routine programme of immunization offered during childhood and to special groups such as healthcare workers and those travelling abroad.

immunocompromised patients (*syn* immunosuppressed patients) patients with defective immune responses, which can be inherited or acquired. Often produced by treatment with drugs or irradiation. Also occurs in some patients with cancer and other diseases affecting the lymphoid system. Depending on the immune defect, different patterns of infection result. Patients with cellular defects are likely to develop infections with opportunistic organisms such as *Candida*, *Pneumocystis carinii* and *Cryptococcus neoformans*. Patients with antibody defects are more liable to infections with encapsulated bacteria such as pneumococcus.

immunocytochemistry *n* staining cells with specific antibodies for diagnostic purposes.

immunodeficiency *n* the state of having defective immune responses, leading to increased susceptibility to infectious diseases.

immunodeficiency diseases inherited or acquired disorders of the immune system.

immunogenicity *n* the ability to produce immunity.

immunoglobulins (Igs) *n* (*syn* antibodies) high molecular weight glycoproteins produced by plasma cells (derived from B lymphocytes) in response to specific antigens. The basic structure of immunoglobulins is Y-shaped, consisting of two identical heavy chains, each linked to two identical light chains. Immunoglobulins are found in the blood and other body fluids where they form part of body defences. Immunoglobulins function in a variety of ways, but all involve combining with the antigen to form an immune complex. There are five classes of immunoglobulins, IgG, IgA, IgD, IgM and IgE, each with different characteristics, functions and locations.

immunohistochemistry *n* staining tissue with specific antibodies for diagnostic purposes.

immunological response ⇒ immunity.

immunology *n* the study of the immune system of lymphocytes, inflammatory cells and associated cells and proteins, which affect an individual's response to antigens—**immunological** *adj*, **immunologically** *adv*.

immunopathology *n* the study of disease involving the immune system.

immunosuppressant drugs drugs given to suppress the immune responses. ⇒ Appendix 5.

immunosuppressed patients ⇒ immunocompromised patients.

immunosuppression *n* treatment which reduces immunological responsiveness.

immunosuppressive 1 *n* that which reduces immunological responsiveness. **2** *adj* describes an agent such as a drug that suppresses immune system function.

immunotherapy *n* can be used to mean desensitization therapy against specific allergens, e.g. insect venom, or can refer to therapeutics which use agonists or antagonists based on immune system components, e.g. treatment based on biological modifiers such as interleukin-2.

impacted *adj* firmly wedged, abnormal immobility, as of faeces in the rectum; fracture; a fetus in the pelvis; a tooth in its socket or a calculus in a duct. ⇒ fracture.

impaired fasting glucose fasting glucose levels between 6 and 7 mmol/L indicative of a pre-diabetic state.

impaired glucose tolerance glucose levels between 7.9 and 11.0 mmol/L 2 hours after a glucose load indicative of a pre-diabetic state and conferring a significantly increased risk of cardiovascular disease.

impalpable *adj* not palpable; incapable of being felt by touch (palpation).

imperforate *adj* lacking a normal opening. *imperforate anus* a congenital absence of an opening into the rectum. *imperforate hymen* a fold of mucous membrane at the vaginal entrance which has no natural outlet for the menstrual fluid. ⇒ haematocolpos.

impetigo *n* an inflammatory, pustular skin disease usually caused by *Staphylococcus*, occasionally by *Streptococcus*. *impetigo contagiosa* a highly contagious form of impetigo, commonest on the face and scalp, characterized by vesicles which become pustules and then honey-coloured crusts. ⇒ ecthyma—**impetiginous** *adj*.

implant *n* any drug, structure or substance inserted surgically into the human body, e.g. implants of progestogens for contraception, or implants used in plastic surgery. Those used to augment tissue contour may be of two types: *alloplastic* synthetic foreign body implants such as those used in breast reconstruction, or *autologous implants* tissue obtained from the same patient. *dental implant* artificial structure implanted surgically into the alveolar bone, usually made from titanium.

implantable defibrillator an implanted device to sense the heart beat. Delivers a small electric shock when ventricular tachycardia or ventricular fibrillation are detected.

implantation *n* the insertion of living cells or solid materials into the tissues, e.g. accidental implantation of tumour cells in a wound; implantation of radioactive material or solid drugs; implantation of the fertilized ovum into the endometrium.

impotence *n* inability to participate in sexual intercourse, by custom referring to the male. It can be due to erectile dysfunction or premature ejaculation.

impregnate *v* fill; saturate; render pregnant.

imprinting *n* very early learning that results in a newborn becoming attached to a model, usually a parent, but may be a carer.

impulse *n* **1** a sudden inclination, sometimes irresistible urge to act without deliberation. **2** the electrochemical process involved in neurotransmission of information and stimuli throughout the body.

IMRT *abbr* intensity modulated radiotherapy.

incarcerated *adj* describes the abnormal imprisonment of a part, as in a hernia which is irreducible or a pregnant uterus held beneath the sacral promontory.

incest *n* sexual intercourse between close blood relatives. The most common type of sexual abuse occurs between father and daughter; other types of incest such as between siblings also occur. ⇒ abuse.

incidence *n* number of new cases of a disease occurring in a population over a defined time period (usually a year).

incipient *adj* initial, beginning, in its early stages.

incised wound one which results from cutting with a sharp knife or scalpel: heals by primary intention in the absence of complications such as infection.

incision *n* the result of cutting into body tissue, using a sharp instrument—**incisional** *adj*, **incise** *vt*.

incisor tooth tooth with a cutting edge, placed first and second from the midline in both primary and secondary dentition.

inclusion bodies minute particles found in some cells of pathological and normal tissues.

incompatibility *n* usually refers to the bloods of donor and recipient in transfusion, when antigenic differences in the red cells result in reactions such as haemolysis or agglutination. When two or more medicaments are given concurrently or consecutively they can attenuate or counteract the desired effect of each.

incompetence *n* inadequacy to perform a natural function, e.g. mitral valve regurgitation—**incompetent** *adj*.

incomplete abortion ⇒ miscarriage.

incomplete fracture ⇒ fracture.

incontinence *n* inability to control the evacuation of urine or faeces. *functional incontinence* erratic and involuntary urinary incontinence in the absence of physical problems in bladder or nervous system. It may be due to immobility or cognitive defects. *neurogenic incontinence* ⇒ neurogenic bladder. *overflow incontinence* dribbling of urine from an overfull bladder. *stress incontinence* occurs when the intra-abdominal pressure is raised as in coughing, giggling and sneezing; there is usually some weakness of the urethral sphincter muscle coupled with anatomical stretching and displacement of the bladder neck. *urge incontinence* erratic bladder contraction caused by detrusor instability leads to urgency and involuntary loss of urine.

incoordination *n* inability to produce smooth, harmonious muscular movements.

incubation *n* 1 the period from entry of infection to the appearance of the first symptom. 2 the process of development, of an egg, of a bacterial culture.

incubator *n* 1 an apparatus with controlled temperature and oxygen concentration used for preterm or sick babies. 2 a low-temperature oven in which bacteria are cultured.

incus anvil-shaped bone of the middle ear. (⇒ Figure 13). ⇒ malleus, stapes.

Indian hemp ⇒ cannabis.

indicanuria *n* excess indican in the urine, associated with increased bacterial breakdown of tryptophan (an amino acid) in the bowel. ⇒ indole.

indicator *n* a substance used to make visible the completion of a chemical reaction or the achievement of a certain pH.

indigenous *adj* of a disease, etc., native to a certain locality or country.

indigestion *n* (*syn* dyspepsia) a feeling of gastric discomfort, including fullness and gaseous distension, which is not necessarily a manifestation of disease.

indirect cost a cost that cannot be attributed to any one department and its budget. It is shared between various budgets, e.g. the cost of heating a building.

indole *n* a product of the decomposition of the amino acid tryptophan in the intestines: it is excreted in urine as indican. ⇒ indicanuria.

indolent *adj* a term applied to a sluggish ulcer which is generally painless and slow to heal.

induced abortion ⇒ abortion, termination.

induction *n* the act of bringing on or causing to occur, as applied to anaesthesia and labour.

induration *n* the hardening of tissue, as in hyperaemia, infiltration by tumour, etc.—**indurated** *adj*.

industrial dermatitis ⇒ dermatitis.

industrial disease (*syn* occupational disease) a disease contracted by reason of occupational exposure to an industrial agent known to be hazardous, e.g. dust, fumes, chemicals, irradiation, etc., the notification of, safety precautions against and compensation for which are controlled by law.

industrial therapy simulation of outside industrial working conditions within a psychiatric hospital. The main purpose is preparation for patient return to the community by occupational rehabilitation.

inequalities in health differences in the distribution of health associated with social class or poverty (as opposed to physiological processes: age, sex, constitution). A considerable body of evidence shows a clear relationship between poor health and deprivation (measured by income, level of education and type of employment or unemployment). Measures of inequality include differences in standardized mortality ratios, life expectancy, infant and maternal mortality rates. Low income individuals are more likely to die prematurely, suffer acute and chronic illnesses and experience long-term disability.

inertia *n* inactivity. *uterine inertia* lack of contraction of parturient uterus.

inevitable abortion ⇒ miscarriage.

in extremis at the point of death.

infant *n* a child of less than 1 year old.

infarct *n* area of tissue affected when the end artery supplying it is occluded by atheroma, thrombosis or embolism, e.g. in myocardium or lung.

infarction *n* irreversible premature tissue death. Necrosis (death) of a section of tissue because the blood supply has been cut off. ⇒ myocardial infarction, pulmonary infarction.

infection *n* the successful invasion, establishment and growth of micro-organisms in the tissues of the host. It may be acute or chronic—**infectious** *adj*. *autoinfection* infection resulting from commensals becoming pathogenic, or when commensals or pathogens are transferred from one part of the body to another, for example by the hands. *cross infection* occurs when pathogens are transferred from one person to another. *hospital-acquired (nosocomial) infection (HAI)* one which occurs in a patient who has been in hospital for at least 72 h and did not have signs and symptoms of such infection on admission:

10–12% of hospital patients develop a HAI. Urinary tract infection is the most common type. *opportunistic infection* a serious infection with a micro-organism which normally has little or no pathogenic activity but causes disease where host resistance is reduced by a serious disease, invasive treatments or drugs.

infectious disease a disease caused by a specific, pathogenic micro-organism and capable of transmission to another individual by direct or indirect contact.

infectious mononucleosis (*syn* glandular fever) a contagious self-limiting disease caused by the Epstein–Barr virus (EBV). It mainly affects teenagers and young adults and is characterized by tiredness, headache, fever, sore throat, lymphadenopathy, splenomegaly and appearance of atypical lymphocytes resembling monocytes. Specific antibodies to EBV are present in the blood, as well as an abnormal antibody that forms the basis of the Paul–Bunnell test, which confirms a diagnosis of infectious mononucleosis.

infective *adj* infectious. Disease transmissible from one host to another. *infective endocarditis* ⇒ endocarditis. *infective hepatitis* ⇒ hepatitis.

inferential statistics also known as inductive statistics. That which uses the observations of a sample to make a prediction about other samples, i.e. makes generalizations from the sample. ⇒ descriptive statistics.

inferior *adj* lower; beneath.

infertility *n* lack of ability to reproduce. Psychological and physical causes play their part. The problem can be in either or both partners. Specialist services exist for diagnosis, treatment and counselling. ⇒ assisted conception.

infestation *n* the presence of animal parasites—**infest** *vt*.

infibulation *n* ⇒ circumcision.

infiltration *n* the entry into cells, tissues or organs of abnormal substances or cells, e.g. cancer cells, fat. Penetration of the surrounding tissues; the oozing or leaking of fluid into the tissues. *infiltration anaesthesia* analgesia produced by infiltrating the tissues with a local anaesthetic.

inflammation *n* a non-specific local defence mechanism initiated by tissue injury. The injury may be caused by trauma, micro-organisms, extremes of temperature and pH, UV radiation, or ionizing radiation. It is characterized by heat, redness, swelling, pain and loss of function. ⇒ calor, dolor, rubor, tumor.

inflammatory bowel disease (IBD) idiopathic intestinal inflammation. Mainly ulcerative colitis and Crohn's disease. Also lymphocytic and collagenous colitis.

inflammatory response a reaction of the immune system to protect the body against harmful substances or physical agents.

influenza n an acute viral infection of the nasopharynx and respiratory tract that occurs in epidemics or pandemics. Complications such as pneumonia may lead to death, especially in the very young, older adults and individuals with chronic diseases including diabetes, heart and respiratory disease—**influenzal** adj.

informal patient a patient admitted to hospital without any statutory requirements. ⇒ detained patient.

informatics n information management and technology (IM&T). Information is needed to ensure the effective running of any organization. Data are pieces of material which, when compiled effectively, form information. Information is managed in a number of different ways but increasingly it is managed using technological means (information technology, IT). Non-technological means may be more appropriate for the target group/ recipient. For example, telephone calls and notice boards are all ways in which information might be managed.

informed choice in order to make decisions about their own care and management clients/patients need information from healthcare professionals. This means the provision of accurate, appropriate information about the person's condition, and about the treatment options available. Healthcare professionals may disagree with the patient/client's decisions, but the latter takes precedence where an adult patient is deemed to be mentally competent.

informed consent in the UK consent forms must include a signed declaration by the doctor or other healthcare professional that he/she has explained the nature and purpose of the operation or treatment to the patient in non-technical terms. Any questions that the patient may have after signing the form should be referred to the doctor or other health professional who is to carry out the treatment. ⇒ consent.

infra-red rays invisible, long wavelength rays of the electromagnetic spectrum.

infundibulum n any funnel-shaped passage, e.g. the ends of the uterine tubes (⇒ Figure 17)—**infundibula** pl, **infundibular** adj.

infusion n **1** fluid flowing into the body either intravenously or subcutaneously. **2** an aqueous solution containing the active principle of a drug.

ingestion n **1** taking food or drugs into the stomach. **2** the means by which a phagocytic cell takes in material such as micro-organisms.

Ingram regimen a treatment for psoriasis using dithranol paste, tar baths and ultraviolet B radiation.

ingrowing toenail ⇒ onychocryptosis.

inguinal adj pertaining to the groin. *inguinal canal* a tubular opening through the lower part of the anterior abdominal wall, parallel to and a little above the inguinal (Poupart's) ligament. In the male it contains spermatic cord; in the female the uterine round ligaments. *inguinal hernia* ⇒ hernia.

inhalation n **1** the breathing in of air, or other vapour, etc. **2** a medicinal substance which is inhaled, such as an inhalation anaesthetic or in the aerosols used for asthma treatment.

inherent adj innate; inborn.

inhibition n the process of restraining one's impulses or behaviour as a result of both unconscious and conscious mental influences.

injected adj congested, with full vessels.

injection n **1** the act of introducing a fluid (under pressure) into the tissues, a vessel, cavity or hollow organ. (Air can be injected into a cavity. ⇒ pneumothorax.) **2** the substance injected.

inlay n in dentistry, a restoration made from cast gold or porcelain to fit a prepared cavity, into which it is then cemented.

innate adj inborn, dependent on genetic make-up.

innervation n the nerve supply to a part.

innocent adj benign; not malignant.

innominate adj unnamed. ⇒ hip bone.

inoculation *n* **1** the injection of substances, especially vaccine, into the body. **2** introduction of micro-organisms into culture medium for propagation.

inorganic *adj* neither vegetable nor animal in origin. A compound generally containing no carbon or hydrogen.

inotropes *npl* substances, such as drugs, that have an effect on myocardial contractility. Those that decrease contractility are termed negative inotropes. ⇒ beta (β)-adrenoceptor antagonists, calcium channel blockers (antagonists). Whereas those that increase contractility are positive inotropes. ⇒ beta (β)-adrenoceptor agonists, glycosides. ⇒ Appendix 5.

inotropic *adj* affecting the force of muscle contraction, applied particularly to cardiac muscle.

inquest *n* in England and Wales, a legal enquiry by a coroner into the cause of sudden or unexpected death.

insecticide *n* an agent which kills insects—**insecticidal** *adj*.

insemination *n* introduction of semen into the vagina, normally by sexual intercourse. *artificial insemination* instrumental injection of semen into the vagina ⇒ AID, AIH.

insensible *adj* without sensation or consciousness. Too tiny or gradual to be noticed.

insertion *n* **1** the act of setting or placing in. **2** the attachment of a muscle to the bone it moves.

insidious *adj* having an imperceptible commencement, as of a disease with a late manifestation of definite symptoms.

insight *n* ability to accept one's limitations while continuing to develop personally. In psychiatry means: (a) knowing that one is ill; (b) a developing knowledge of one's present attitudes and past experiences and the connection between them.

in situ in the normal position, undisturbed.

insomnia *n* sleeplessness.

inspiration *n* inhalation; breathing in—**inspiratory** *adj*, **inspire** *vt*.

inspissated *adj* thickened, as by evaporation or withdrawal of water, applied to sputum and culture media used in the laboratory.

instep *n* the arch of the foot on the dorsal surface.

instillation *n* insertion of drops into a cavity, e.g. conjunctival sac.

instinct *n* an inborn tendency to act in a certain way in a given situation, e.g. *maternal, paternal instinct* to protect children—**instinctive** *adj*, **instinctively** *adv*.

institutionalization *n* a condition of apathy resulting from lack of motivation characterizing patients and staff in institutions who have been subjected to a rigid regimen with deprivation of choice and decision-making.

instrumental activities of daily living (IADL) include activities such as child care and shopping.

insufflation *n* the blowing of air along a tube (pharyngotympanic, uterine) to establish patency. The blowing of powder into a body cavity.

insulin *n* a polypeptide hormone produced by the beta cells of the pancreas. Insulin secretion is regulated by the blood glucose level and it opposes the action of glucagon. It has an effect on the metabolism of carbohydrate, protein and fat by stimulating the transport of glucose into cells. An absolute or relative lack of insulin results in hyperglycaemia, a high blood glucose with decreased utilization of carbohydrate and increased breakdown of fat and protein; a condition known as diabetes mellitus. Three types of insulin are available commercially: bovine insulin, porcine insulin and human insulin, produced using recombinant techniques. Insulin is produced in U100 strength, i.e. 100 units per mL, a standardization replacing the previous 20, 40 and 80 unit strengths. ⇒ Appendix 5.

insulin dependent diabetes mellitus (IDDM) ⇒ diabetes mellitus type 1.

insulinoma *n* pancreatic islet beta cell adenoma.

insulin tolerance test used to assess the hypothalamic-pituitary-adrenal axis and growth hormone deficiency. Intravenous soluble insulin is administered to produce hypoglycaemia (blood glucose <2.2 mmol/L) and serial blood samples are taken to measure glucose, growth hormone and cortisol levels.

integrated medicine a term used to describe a harmonious integration of particular complementary therapies within conventional medical or other healthcare practice. Where team work and effective therapies (both allopathic and complementary) function together to promote health and well-being.

integument *n* a covering, especially the skin.

intellect *n* the ability and power of the mind for reasoning, thinking, understanding and knowing, as contrasted with the willing and feeling faculty.

intellectualization *n* a mental defence mechanism whereby people attempt to detach themselves from painful emotions or difficult situations by dealing with the issues in an abstract, intellectual manner.

intelligence *n* inborn mental ability. *intelligence quotient (IQ)* the ratio of mental age to chronological (actual) age. *intelligence tests* designed to determine the level of intelligence.

intensity modulated radiotherapy (IMRT) the use of a computer system to optimize the radiation delivery technique by evaluating millions of possible beam arrangements to create a clinically optimized treatment plan.

intensive therapy unit (ITU) an area within a hospital with augmented levels of staff and equipment in which highly specialized monitoring, resuscitation and therapeutic techniques are used to support critically ill patients with actual or impending organ failure, particularly those needing artificial ventilation. Also called intensive care unit.

intention tremor ⇒ tremor.

interaction *n* when two or more things or people have a reciprocal influence on each other. ⇒ drug interaction.

interarticular *adj* between joints.

interatrial *adj* between the two atria of the heart.

intercellular *adj* between cells.

intercostal *adj* between the ribs.

intercourse *n* **1** human communication. **2** coitus.

intercurrent *adj* describes a second disease arising in a person already suffering from one disease.

interference *n* a psychological term that describes the contest between pieces of information that may prevent learning and retrieval from long-term memory. It occurs when different pieces of information are linked to the same clue needed for retrieval.

interferons (IFNs) *npl* protein mediators that enhance cellular resistance to viruses. They are involved in the modulation of the immune response. Interferon has caused regression of some cancers and is used in the management of some types of multiple sclerosis.

interleukins (IL) *npl* large group of signalling molecules (cytokines). They are non-specific immune chemicals produced by various cells, such as macrophages. Interleukins are also involved with the regulation of haemopoiesis.

interlobar *adj* between the lobes.

interlobular *adj* between the lobules.

intermenstrual *adj* between the menstrual periods.

intermittent *adj* occurring at intervals. *intermittent claudication* ⇒ claudication. *intermittent peritoneal dialysis* ⇒ dialysis. *intermittent pneumatic compression* a stocking worn to prevent deep vein thrombosis of upper and lower limb. ⇒ phlebothrombosis. *intermittent self-catheterization* ⇒ self-catheterization.

intermittent positive pressure ventilation (IPPV) ventilation of the lungs by the intermittent application of gas under positive pressure to the airway. Used for the artificial maintenance of breathing during general anaesthesia and for critically ill patients. Synonymous with artificial, assisted, controlled and mechanical ventilation.

internal *adj* inside. *internal ear* that part of the ear which comprises the vestibule, semicircular canals and the cochlea. *internal respiration* ⇒ respiration. *internal secretions* those produced by the endocrine glands; hormones. *internal version* ⇒ version.

internal (medial) rotation a limb or body movement where there is rotation towards the vertical axis of the body.

International Classification of Diseases (ICD) list of disease categories produced by the World Health Organization.

interosseous *adj* between bones.

interphalangeal *adj* between the phalanges.

interpretive approach a research approach that incorporates the meaning and significance individuals attach to situations and behaviour. May be used in social science research.

interprofessional *adj* intense teamwork among practitioners from different health-care professions focused on a common problem-solving purpose and requiring recognition of the core expertise and core knowledge of each profession and blend-ing of common core skills to enable the team to act as an integrated whole. ⇒ multiprofessional. *interprofessional educa-tion (IPE)* shared (or common) learning of common (or generic) core skills among students and qualified practitioners of different healthcare professions that fos-ters respect for each other's core knowl-edge and expertise, capitalizes on professional differences, and cultivates integrated teamwork to solve patients' problems.

interserosal *adj* between serous membrane, as in the pleural, peritoneal and pericar-dial cavities—**interserosally** *adv.*

intersexuality *n* the possession of both male and female characteristics.

interspinous *adj* between spinous pro-cesses, especially those of the vertebrae.

interstices *npl* spaces.

interstitial *adj* situated in the interstices of a part; distributed through the connective structures.

interstitial cell stimulating hormone (ICSH) (*syn* luteinizing hormone) a hor-mone released from the anterior lobe of the pituitary gland; causes production of testosterone in the male.

interstitial fluid (tissue fluid) the extracel-lular fluid situated in the spaces around cells.

interstitial radiotherapy therapy achieved by radioactive sources inserted into the tumour.

intertrigo *n* superficial inflammation occur-ring in moist skin folds—**intertrigenous** *adj.*

intertrochanteric *adj* between trochanters such as those on the proximal femur.

interval cancer one that is discovered in the time interval between screening episodes, such as breast cancer detected between mammography examinations.

interval data measurement data with a numerical value, e.g. temperature, that has an arbitrary zero. The intervals between successive values are the same,

e.g. a one degree increase from 38 to 39 is exactly the same as one from 39 to 40. ⇒ ratio data.

interventricular *adj* between ventricles, as those of the brain or heart.

intervertebral *adj* between the vertebrae, as discs and foramina. ⇒ nucleus, prolapse.

intestinal failure failure of the intestine to absorb adequate fluid and nutrients to sustain metabolic needs due to disease or resection. ⇒ parenteral.

intestine *n* a part of the alimentary canal extending from the stomach to the anus (⇒ Figure 18b). Consists of the small and large intestine (bowel)—**intestinal** *adj.*

intima *n* the internal coat of a blood vessel—**intimal** *adj.*

intolerance *n* the manifestation of various unusual reactions to particular substances such as nutrients or medications.

intra-abdominal *adj* inside the abdomen.

intra-amniotic *adj* within or into the amnio-tic fluid.

intra-aortic *adj* within the aorta. *intra-aortic balloon pump (IABP)* device used to increase cardiac output in ventricular failure or shock.

intra-arterial *adj* within an artery—**intra-arterially** *adv.*

intra-articular *adj* within a joint.

intrabronchial *adj* within a bronchus.

intracanalicular *adj* within a canaliculus.

intracapillary *adj* within a capillary.

intracapsular *adj* within a capsule, e.g. that of the lens or a joint. ⇒ extracapsular *opp.*

intracardiac *adj* within the heart.

intracaval *adj* within the vena cava—**intra-cavally** *adv.*

intracellular *adj* within cells. *intracellular fluid (ICF)* that fluid inside the cells. ⇒ extracellular *opp.*

intracerebral *adj* within the cerebrum, such as a haemorrhage.

intracranial *adj* within the skull.

intracranial pressure (ICP) the pressure inside the cranial cavity. It is maintained at a normal level by brain tissue, intracel-lular and extracellular fluid, cerebrospinal fluid and blood. A change in any of these compartments can increase the pressure, e.g. after head injury. ⇒ raised intracra-nial pressure.

intracutaneous *adj* within the skin tis-sues— **intracutaneously** *adv.*

intracytoplasmic sperm injection (ICSI) a technique used in assisted conception where a single sperm is injected into an oocyte to achieve conception.

intradermal *adj* within the skin—**intradermally** *adv.*

intradural *adj* inside the dura mater.

intragastric *adj* within the stomach.

intragluteal *adj* within the gluteal muscle of the buttock—**intragluteally** *adv.*

intrahepatic *adj* within the liver.

intralobular *adj* within the lobule, e.g. vessels draining a hepatic lobule.

intraluminal *adj* within the lumen of a hollow tube-like structure—**intraluminally** *adv.*

intralymphatic *adj* within a lymphatic node or vessel.

intramedullary *adj* within the bone marrow.

intramural *adj* within the wall of a hollow tube or organ—**intramurally** *adv.*

intramuscular *adj* within a muscle—**intramuscularly** *adv.*

intranasal *adj* within the nasal cavity—**intranasally** *adv.*

intranatal *adj* ⇒ intrapartum—**intranatally** *adv.*

intraocular *adj* within the globe of the eye.

intraoral *adj* within the mouth, such as an intraoral appliance—**intraorally** *adv.*

intraorbital *adj* within the orbit.

intraosseous *adj* inside a bone. The intraosseous route has been developed as a way of giving fluids when rapid establishment of systemic access is vital and venous access is impossible. It provides an alternative route for the administration of drugs and fluids until venous access can be achieved.

intrapartum *adj* (*syn* intranatal) at the time of birth; during labour, as asphyxia, or infection. *intrapartum haemorrhage* that occurring during labour.

intraperitoneal *adj* within the peritoneal cavity—**intraperitoneally** *adv.*

intrapharyngeal *adj* within the pharynx—**intrapharyngeally** *adv.*

intraplacental *adj* within the placenta—**intraplacentally** *adv.*

intrapleural *adj* within the pleural cavity—**intrapleurally** *adv.*

intrapulmonary *adj* within the lungs, as intrapulmonary pressure.

intrapunitive *adj* self blaming.

intraretinal *adj* within the retina.

intraspinal *adj* within the spinal canal—**intraspinally** *adv.*

intrasplenic *adj* within the spleen.

intrasynovial *adj* within a synovial membrane or cavity—**intrasynovially** *adv.*

intrathecal *adj* within the meninges; into the subarachnoid space. A route used for the administration of certain drugs, such as antibiotic drugs for meningitis—**intrathecally** *adv.*

intrathoracic *adj* within the cavity of the thorax, such as pressures.

intratracheal *adj* within the trachea—**intratracheally** *adv.*

intrauterine *adj* within the uterus. *intrauterine contraceptive device (IUCD, IUD)* a device which is inserted in the cavity of the uterus to prevent conception. Its exact mode of action is not known. *intrauterine growth restriction (IUGR)* the impairment of fetal growth rate commonly arising due to placental insufficiency.

intravaginal *adj* within the vagina—**intravaginally** *adv.*

intravascular *adj* within the blood vessels—**intravascularly** *adv.*

intravenous (IV) *adj* within or into a vein—**intravenously** *adv. intravenous infusion (IVI)* commonly referred to as a 'drip': the closed administration of fluids from a containing vessel into a vein for such purposes as hydrating the body, correcting electrolyte imbalance or introducing nutrients. *intravenous injection* the introduction of drugs, including anaesthetics, into a vein.

intravenous immunoglobulin (IVIG) immunoglobulin, mainly IgG, produced from the pooled donations of thousands of individuals, used as replacement therapy for patients with antibody deficiencies, or in higher doses as immunomodulatory therapy for a range of inflammatory and immune-mediated disorders.

intraventricular *adj* within a ventricle, especially a cerebral ventricle.

intrinsic *adj* inherent or inside; from within; real; natural. *intrinsic factor* a protein released by gastric parietal cells, essential for the satisfactory absorption of vitamin B_{12} (the extrinsic factor). *intrinsic sugars* sugars found in the cell walls of foods originating from plants.

introitus *n* any opening in the body; an entrance to a cavity, particularly the vagina.

introjection *n* the unconscious incorporation of external ideas into one's mind.

introspection *n* study of one's own mental processes. May be associated in an exaggerated form in schizophrenia and other serious mental health disorders.

introversion *n* **1** thoughts and interests are directed inwards to the world of ideas, instead of outwards to the external world. **2** a situation where a hollow structure turns in on itself (invaginates).

introvert *n* a person whose interests and behaviour patterns are directed inwards to the self. ⇒ extrovert *opp*.

intubation *n* placing of a tube into a hollow organ. Tracheal intubation is used during anaesthesia. ⇒ endotracheal tube. *duodenal intubation* a double lumen tube is passed as far as the pyloric antrum under fluoroscopy. The inner tube is then passed along to the duodenojejunal flexure.

intussusception *n* a condition in which one part of the bowel telescopes into another, causing severe colic and intestinal obstruction. It occurs most commonly in infants around the time of weaning.

intussusceptum *n* the invaginated portion of an intussusception.

intussuscipiens *n* the receiving portion of an intussusception.

invagination *n* the act or condition of being ensheathed; a pushing inward, forming a pouch—**invaginate** *vt*.

invasion *n* the entry of bacteria into the body or the spread of cancer cells.

inversion *n* turning inside out, as inversion of the uterus. ⇒ procidentia.

in vitro in glass, as in a test tube. *in vitro fertilization (IVF)* human oocytes are fertilized by spermatozoa in test tubes in laboratories that are specialized in this technique.

in vivo in living tissue.

involucrum *n* a sheath of new bone, which forms around necrosed bone, in such conditions as osteomyelitis. ⇒ cloaca.

involuntary *adj* independent of the will, as muscle of the thoracic and abdominal organs.

involution *n* the normal shrinkage of an organ after completing its function, e.g.

uterus after labour. Or the progressive decline occurring after midlife when tissues and organs reduce in size and functional ability declines. ⇒ subinvolution—**involutional** *adj*.

iodine (I) *n* an element required for the formation of thyroid hormones (T_3, T_4). Oral iodine may be prescribed preoperatively for patients with hyperthyroidism to control the release of thyroid hormones and reduce vascularity of the gland. Radioactive isotopes of iodine, e.g. ^{131}I, are used in the diagnosis and treatment of thyroid conditions, such as cancer. Iodine is bactericidal and is used as povidone iodine for skin disinfection prior to invasive procedures. It is used within several proprietary wound dressings.

iodism *n* poisoning by iodine or iodides; presentation is similar to a common cold and the appearance of a rash.

ion *n* an atom or radical with an electrical charge—**ionic** *adj*. ⇒ anion, cation. *ion channel* water-filled channels in the cell membrane that allow certain ions to pass through as in the transmission of nerve impulses. Some drugs act at the level of the ion channels.

ion-exchange resins substances administered orally to reduce the level of specific ions (calcium and potassium) in the body such as in renal failure.

ionization *n* **1** the dissociation of a substance in solution into ions. **2** iontophoresis.

ionizing radiation form of radiation that destabilizes an atom, forming an ion. Examples include gamma rays, X-rays and particle radiation. It has the ability to cause tissue damage. ⇒ radiation.

iontophoresis *n* the introduction of ions of various soluble salts into the tissues by using an electrical current. Pilocarpine is introduced into the skin by this method in order to do a sweat test for the diagnosis of cystic fibrosis.

IOP *abbr* intraoculur pressure.

ipecacuanha *n* dried root from South America. Used in some expectorants. It is sometimes used as an emetic after poisoning but may have limited value.

IPPV *abbr* intermittent positive pressure ventilation.

ipsilateral *adj* on the same side—**ipsilaterally** *adv*.

IQ *abbr* intelligence quotient.

iridectomy *n* excision of a part of the iris.

iridium (^{192}Ir) *n* a radioactive element used in brachytherapy to treat cancers in anus, tongue, breast as implanted wires or hair pins. Can also be used as a Selectron source.

iridocyclitis *n* inflammation of the iris and ciliary body.

iridodialysis *n* a separation of the iris from its ciliary body attachment.

iridotomy *n* an incision into the iris; may be performed using a laser.

iris *n* the circular pigmented structure forming the anterior one-sixth of the middle coat of the eyeball ($\Rightarrow$ Figure 15). It is perforated in the centre by an opening, the pupil. Contraction of its muscle fibres regulates the amount of light entering the eye. *iris bombe* bulging forward of the iris due to pressure of the aqueous behind, when posterior synechiae are present around the pupil.

iritis *n* (*syn* anterior uveitis) inflammation of the iris.

iron (Fe) *n* a metallic element needed in the body as a constituent of haemoglobin and several enzymes.

irreducible *adj* unable to be brought to desired condition. *irreducible hernia* $\Rightarrow$ hernia.

irritable *adj* capable of being excited to activity; easily stimulated—**irritability** *n*. *irritable bowel syndrome (IBS)* functional intestinal symptoms not explained by organic bowel disease. Symptoms include abdominal pain, bloating and change in bowel habit (alternating constipation and diarrhoea).

irritant *adj*, *n* describes any agent which causes irritation.

ischaemia *n* deficient blood supply to any part of the body. $\Rightarrow$ angina, Volkmann's ischaemic contracture—**ischaemic** *adj*.

ischaemic heart disease (IHD) $\Rightarrow$ coronary heart disease.

ischiorectal *adj* pertaining to the ischium and the rectum, as an ischiorectal abscess which occurs between these two structures.

ischium *n* the lower part of the innominate bone of the pelvis; the bone on which the body rests when sitting—**ischial** *adj*.

islets of Langerhans collections of special cells scattered throughout the pancreas, mainly concerned with endocrine function. The pancreatic islets contain four types of hormone-secreting cells: alpha cells, which secrete glucagon; beta cells, which secrete insulin; the delta cells, which secrete several substances, including somatostatin or growth hormone inhibiting hormone (GHIH); and others that produce regulatory pancreatic polypeptide.

isoenzyme *n* one that catalyses the same reaction, but exists in several forms and at different body sites, such as lactate dehydrogenase.

isograft *n* a graft between individuals with identical genotypes, i.e. identical twins. It can also be used to describe grafts between syngeneic individuals, i.e. inbred strains of laboratory animals.

isoimmunization *n* development of anti-Rh agglutinins in the blood of an Rh-negative person who has been given an Rh-positive transfusion, or who is carrying an Rh-positive fetus.

isokinetic activity a dynamic activity in which the velocity of the movement remains the same and the resistance varies.

isokinetic dynamometer a device that quantitatively measures muscular strength through a preset speed of movement.

isolation *n* separation of a patient from others for a number of reasons. $\Rightarrow$ containment isolation, protective isolation, source isolation.

isolator *n* apparatus ranging from what is virtually a large plastic bag in which a patient can be nursed to that in which surgery can be performed. It aims to prevent pathogenic micro-organisms either gaining entry or leaving the enclosed space.

isoleucine *n* an essential (indispensable) branched chain amino acid.

isometric *adj* of equal proportions. *isometric contraction* a muscle contraction where its attachments do not move and, therefore, the muscle does not shorten and joints do not move. *isometric exercises* carried out without movement. Used to maintain muscle tone.

isotonic *adj* equal tension; applied to any solution which has the same osmotic pressure as the fluid with which it is being compared. *isotonic saline* (*syn* normal saline, physiological saline), 0.9% solution of sodium chloride in water.

isotonic exercises carried out with movement. Increases muscle strength and endurance.

isotonic muscle contraction muscle contraction that results in a change in muscle length (shortens or lengthens) and movement of its attachments.

isotopes *npl* two or more forms of the same element having identical chemical properties and the same atomic number but different mass numbers. Those isotopes with radioactive properties are used in medicine for research, diagnosis and treatment of disease.

ispaghula husk a natural dietary fibre supplement. Used as a bulk-forming laxative. ⇒ Appendix 5.

isthmus *n* a narrowed part of an organ or tissue such as that connecting the two lobes of the thyroid gland. *isthmus of the uterine tube.* ⇒ Figure 17.

itch *n* a sensation on the skin which makes one want to scratch. Often accompanies skin disease. *itch mite Sarcoptes scabiei.* ⇒ scabies.

ITU *abbr* intensive therapy unit.

IUCD *abbr* intrauterine contraceptive device.

IUD *abbr* **1** intrauterine (contraceptive) device. **2** intrauterine death (of a fetus).

IUGR *abbr* intrauterine growth restriction.

IVC *abbr* inferior vena cava.

IVF *abbr* in vitro fertilization.

IVU, IVP *abbr* intravenous urogram/pyelogram ⇒ urography.

J

Jacksonian epilepsy ⇒ epilepsy.

Jacquemier's sign darkening of the vaginal skin seen in early pregnancy.

Jakob–Creutzfeldt disease ⇒ Creutzfeldt–Jakob disease.

jargon *n* technical or specialized language that is only understood by a particular group, for example health professionals. Often used to describe the use of obscure and pretentious language, together with a roundabout way of expression.

Jarman index system for weighting general practice populations according to social conditions. A composite index of social factors that general practitioners considered important in increasing workload and pressure on services. These factors were identified through a survey of one in ten general practitioners in the UK in 1981. An underprivileged area (UPA) score was then constructed based on the level of each variable in each area, weighted by the weighting assigned from the national general practitioner survey. Eight variables were used: (a) elderly living alone, (b) children aged under five years, (c) unskilled, (d) unemployed (as % economically active), (e) lone parent families, (f) overcrowded accommodation (>1 person/room), (g) mobility (moved house within one year), (h) ethnic origin (new Commonwealth and Pakistan). Information on the variables were derived from the census.

jaundice *n* (*syn* icterus) a condition characterized by a raised bilirubin level in the blood (hyperbilirubinaemia). Minor degrees are only detectable chemically. Major degrees are visible in the yellow discoloration of skin, sclerae and mucosae. Pruritus occurs although the mechanism is not known. Jaundice without the excretion of bilirubin in the urine is termed acholuric. Jaundice may be classified as follows: (a) *haemolytic or prehepatic jaundice* where excessive breakdown of erythrocytes releases bilirubin into the blood, such as in haemolytic anaemia. ⇒ haemolysis, haemolytic disease of the newborn. (b) *hepatocellular jaundice* arises when liver cell function is impaired, such as with hepatitis or cirrhosis. (c) *obstructive or cholestatic jaundice* where the flow of bile is obstructed either within the liver (intrahepatic) or in the larger ducts of the biliary tract (extrahepatic). Causes include: cirrhosis, tumours, parasites and gallstones. ⇒ cholestasis.

jaw-bone *n* describes either the upper jaw (maxilla) or lower jaw (mandible).

jejunal biopsy ⇒ Crosby capsule.

jejunostomy *n* a surgically made fistula between the jejunum and the anterior abdominal wall; used temporarily for feeding in cases where passage of food through the stomach is impossible or undesirable.

jejunum *n* that part of the small intestine between the duodenum and the ileum— **jejunal** *adj*.

Jersey finger a colloquial term used in sports medicine to describe the rupture of the flexor digitorum longus tendon from the distal phalanx of the finger due to rapid extension of the finger while being actively flexed.

jet lag disturbance to biological processes that normally have diurnal rhythms; occurs following travel through different time zones. It is characterized by changes in sleep patterns, appetite, concentration and memory, and fatigue for some days until body rhythms return to normal. People working variable shift patterns report similar effects.

jigger *n* a sand flea, *Tunga penetrans*, found in the tropics.

joint *n* the articulation of two or more bones (arthrosis). There are three main classes: (a) fibrous (synarthroses), e.g. the sutures of the skull; (b) cartilaginous (amphiarthroses), e.g. between the manubrium and the body of the sternum; and (c) synovial or freely movable (diarthroses), e.g. shoulder or hip. ⇒ Charcot's joint.

joint reaction forces the forces that are transmitted through a joint's articular surfaces.

joule (J) *n* the SI unit for measuring energy, work and quantity of heat. The unit (J) is the energy expended when 1 kg (kilogram) is moved 1 m (metre) by a force of 1 N (newton). The kilojoule (kJ = 10^3 J) and the megajoule (MJ = 10^6 J) are used by nutritionists for measuring large amounts of energy.

jugular *adj* pertaining to the throat. *jugular veins* two veins passing down either side of the neck. ⇒ Figure 10.

Jung, Carl Swiss psychiatrist/psychoanalyst (1875–1961).

justice *n* involves the concepts of fairness and justness. May be described as acting within a set of moral laws, respecting the views and rights of others, or equity in the distribution of resources such as health care.

juvenile chronic arthritis (JCA) now more commonly termed juvenile idiopathic arthritis.

juvenile idiopathic arthritis (*syn* juvenile chronic arthritis) chronic inflammatory arthritis in children. In its systemic form (previously termed Still's disease) systemic features such as fever, rash and anaemia are prominent and may precede the arthritis.

juxtaglomerular *adj* close to the glomerulus. *juxtaglomerular apparatus (JGA)* cells in the distal tubule and the afferent arteriole of the nephron. They monitor changes in pressure and sodium levels in the blood, and initiate the release of renin. ⇒ macula densa.

juxtapose *vt* to place side by side.

K

kala-azar *n* generalized leishmaniasis occurring in the tropics. Characterized by anaemia, fever, splenomegaly and wasting. It is caused by the parasite *Leishmania donovani* and is spread by sandflies.

kaolin *n* natural aluminium silicate. Given orally it absorbs toxic substances, hence useful in diarrhoea, food poisoning and colitis. Sometimes used as a poultice.

Kaposi's disease ⇒ xeroderma pigmentosum.

Kaposi's sarcoma neoplasm characterized by new blood vessel growth producing red, purple or brown lesions, often on the skin but with metastatic potential. Originally common in Africa but now often seen in immunocompromised individuals, e.g. those with acquired immunodeficiency syndrome (AIDS).

Kaposi's varicelliform eruption widespread herpes simplex complicating atopic eczema.

karyorrhexis *n* disintegration of nuclear chromatin.

karyotype *n* an orderly array of chromosomes, usually derived from the study of cultured cells. This is usually done for diagnostic purposes, or in individuals at risk of having children with chromosomal abnormalities, or for the prenatal detection of fetal abnormality.

Kawasaki disease an inflammatory disease affecting small blood vessels (vasculitis). ⇒ mucocutaneous lymph node syndrome.

Kayser–Fleischer ring a brown/green ring in the cornea, a sign of Wilson's disease.

Kell factor a blood group factor present in about 10% of caucasians. Anti-Kell antibodies can cross the placenta.

Keller's operation for hallux valgus or rigidus. Excision of the proximal half of the proximal phalanx, plus any osteophytes and exostoses on the metatarsal head. The toe is fixed in the corrected position; after healing a pseudarthrosis results.

Kelly–Paterson syndrome ⇒ Plummer–Vinson syndrome.

keloid scar excessive scar production extending beyond the site of original injury. An elevated and progressive scar, which may produce contraction deformity. Keloid scarring occurs in some pigmented skins.

keratectomy *n* surgical excision of a portion of the cornea.

keratic precipitates (KP) clusters of cells adherent to the posterior surface of the cornea; present in inflammation of uvea.

keratin *n* a fibrous protein found in nails and the outer part of the skin and horns, etc.

keratinization *n* horn-like thickening of the skin. ⇒ keratosis.

keratitis *n* inflammation of the cornea.

keratoconjunctivitis *n* inflammation of the cornea and conjunctiva. *epidemic keratoconjunctivitis* due to an adenovirus. Present as an acute follicular conjunctivitis with preauricular and submandibular adenitis. *keratoconjunctivitis sicca* dry eye, including in Sjögren syndrome.

keratoconus *n* a cone-like protrusion of the cornea, usually due to a non-inflammatory thinning.

keratolytic *adj* having the property of breaking down keratinized epidermis.

keratoma *n* ⇒ callosity—**keratomata** *pl.*

keratomalacia *n* frequently caused by lack of vitamin A, there is keratinization of corneal and conjunctival epithelia with loss of mucin-producing cells. May lead to corneal ulceration, secondary infection and corneal perforation.

keratome *n* a special knife for incising the cornea.

keratopathy *n* any disease of the cornea.

keratoplasty *n* ⇒ corneal graft.

keratoprosthesis *n* artificial cornea.

keratosis *n* thickening of the horny layer of the skin. Also referred to as hyperkeratosis. Has the appearance of warty excrescences. *keratosis palmaris et plantaris* (*syn* tylosis) a congenital thickening of the horny layer of the palms and soles.

keratouveitis *n* inflammation of the cornea and uvea, often due to infection.

kerion *n* a boggy suppurative mass of the scalp associated with ringworm.

kernicterus *n* staining of brain cells, especially the basal nuclei with bilirubin. It is a complication of jaundice affecting preterm babies and haemolytic disease of the newborn. It can lead to a severe encephalopathy with resultant learning disabilities.

ketoacidosis *n* (*syn* ketosis) acidosis due to accumulation of ketone bodies, β-hydroxybutyric acid, acetoacetic acid and acetone, products of the metabolism of fat. Primarily a serious complication of type 1 diabetes, but also occurs in starvation and rarely in alcohol misuse. Symptoms include drowsiness, headache and deep sighing respiration (Kussmaul's). *diabetic ketoacidosis* ketone bodies are formed as fatty acids are incompletely oxidized when glucose is unavailable as an energy source. Acidosis and dehydration accompany hyperglycaemia. ⇒ Kussmaul's respiration.

ketogenic diet a high fat content producing ketosis (acidosis).

ketonaemia *n* ketone bodies in the blood—**ketonaemic** *adj.*

ketones *npl* organic compounds (e.g. ketosteroids) containing a keto group. *ketone bodies* include acetone, acetoacetate (acetoacetic acid) and β-hydroxybutyric acid produced normally during fat oxidation. Can be used as fuel but excess production leads to ketoacidosis. This may occur when blood glucose level is high, but unavailable for metabolism, as in poorly controlled diabetes mellitus.

ketonuria *n* ketone bodies in the urine—**ketonuric** *adj.*

ketosis *n* ⇒ ketoacidosis.

ketosteroids *npl* steroid hormones that contain a ketone group. The 17-ketosteroids are excreted normally in urine and are present in excess in overactivity of the adrenal glands and the gonads.

kidneys *npl* paired retroperitoneal organs situated on the upper posterior abdominal wall in the lumbar region (⇒ Figures 19, 20). Help to maintain homeostasis, by producing urine to excrete waste such as urea, control water and electrolyte balance and blood pH. They also secrete renin and renal erythropoietic factor (REF) and are involved in vitamin D metabolism. *horseshoe kidney* an anatomical variation in which the inner lower border of each kidney is joined to give a horseshoe shape. Usually symptomless, but rarely interferes with drainage of urine into ureters. *kidney failure* ⇒ renal failure. *kidney function tests* a series of tests that include: routine urine testing, urine concentration/dilution tests, serum urea and electrolytes, serum creatinine and renal clearance to estimate GFR. *kidney machine* ⇒ dialyser. *kidney transplant* surgical transplantation of a kidney from a previously tested suitable live donor or a cadaveric organ. Kidneys may also be transplanted from the renal bed to other sites in the same individual in cases of ureteric disease or trauma.

kilogram (kg) *n* one of the seven base units of the International System of Units (SI). A measurement of mass.

kilojoule (kJ) *n* a unit equal to 1000 joules. It is used to measure large amounts of energy. It replaces the kilocalorie (kcal) which is still commonly used. ⇒ calorie.

kinaesthesis *n* muscle sense; perception of movement—**kinaesthetic** *adj.*

kinanthropometry *n* the utilization of a combination of anthropometry and kinesiology.

kinase *n* **1** an enzyme activator that converts a zymogen to its active form. **2** enzymes that catalyse the transfer of a high-energy group of a donor, usually adenosine triphosphate (ATP), to some acceptor, usually named after the acceptor (e.g. fructokinase).

kineplastic surgery operative measures, whereby certain muscle groups are isolated and used to work a modified prosthesis.

kinesiology *n* the study of muscle activity that brings together the anatomy, physiology and biomechanics of parts of the body.

kinetic *adj* relating to or producing motion.

kinins *npl* biologically active peptides such as bradykinin that cause vasodilation, pain, etc.

Kirschner wire a wire drilled into a bone to apply skeletal traction. A hand or electric drill is used, a stirrup is attached and the wire is rendered taut by means of a special wire-tightener.

Klebsiella *n* a genus of anaerobic Gram-negative bacteria. They form part of the normal flora in the gut. They are opportunists and commonly cause urinary, respiratory and wound infections. Some strains are resistant to many antibiotics. *Klebsiella pneumoniae* causes serious pneumonia in critically ill patients needing respiratory support.

Klinefelter syndrome a chromosomal abnormality affecting boys, usually with 47 chromosomes including XXY sex chromosomes. Puberty is frequently delayed, with small firm testes, often with gynaecomastia. Associated with sterility, which may be the only symptom.

Klumpke's paralysis paralysis and atrophy of forearm and hand muscles, sometimes caused by birth injury. May be accompanied by Horner's syndrome with sensory and pupillary disturbances due to injury to lower roots of brachial plexus and cervical sympathetic nerves. Claw-hand results.

knee *n* the hinge joint formed by the lower end of the femur and the head of the tibia. *kneecap* the patella. *knee jerk* a reflex contraction of the relaxed quadriceps muscle elicited by a tap on the patellar tendon: usually performed with the lower femur supported behind, the knee bent and the leg limp. Persistent variation from normal usually signifies organic nervous disorder.

knuckles *npl* the dorsal aspect of any of the joints between the phalanges and the metacarpal bones, or between the phalanges.

Koebner phenomenon induction of a lesion of certain skin diseases, e.g. psoriasis, following non-specific trauma to the skin.

Köhler's disease osteochondritis of the navicular bone. Confined to children of 3–5 years.

koilonychia *n* spoon-shaped nails. The normal convex curvature of the nail is lost and it becomes slightly concave. It is more common in fingernails than toenails and is associated with iron deficiency anaemia.

Koplik's spots small white spots inside the mouth, during the first few days of the invasion (prodromal) stage of measles.

Korotkoff sounds the sounds audible when recording non-invasive arterial blood pressure with a sphygmomanometer and stethoscope. The phases are: (1) a sharp thud—systolic pressure, (2) a swishing sound, (3) a soft thud, (4) a soft blowing that becomes muffled, (5) silence. Opinion is divided as to whether phase 4 or 5 should represent diastolic pressure.

Korsakoff's (Korsakov's) syndrome chronic amnesia (defect of retrieval of recently acquired information) with denial, lack of insight and confabulation. ⇒ amnesic syndrome, Wernicke's encephalopathy.

kosher *n* food that complies with and is prepared according to the laws of Judaism.

KP *abbr* keratic precipitates.

Krabbe disease genetically determined disorder of lipid metabolism that leads to degenerative changes in the central nervous system. It is associated with learning disability.

kraurosis vulvae a degenerative condition of the vaginal introitus associated with postmenopausal lack of oestrogen.

Krebs cycle (*syn* citric acid cycle, tricarboxylic acid cycle). The final common pathway for the oxidation of fuel molecules: glucose, fatty acids, glycerol and amino acids. These enter the cycle as acetyl CoA and are oxidized to produce energy (ATP), carbon dioxide and water.

Krukenberg tumour a secondary (metastatic) malignant tumour of the ovary, usually spread from primary stomach (gastric) cancer.

Küntscher nail used for intramedullary fixation of fractured long bones, especially the femur. The nail has a 'clover-leaf' cross-section.

kuru *n* slow virus disease affecting the central nervous system. Probably transmitted by cannibalism. Rare and declining in incidence. Occurred exclusively among New Guinea highlanders.

Kussmaul's respiration deep sighing respiration typical of diabetic ketoacidosis.

Kveim test an intracutaneous test for sarcoidosis using tissue prepared from a person known to be suffering from the condition.

kwashiorkor *n* a nutritional disorder of infants and young children associated with poverty, deprivation and infection. Develops when the diet is deficient in protein; may develop at weaning when a low protein starchy porridge is fed instead of breast milk. Characteristic features are anaemia, muscle wasting, loss of appetite, pale thin hair, oedema and a fatty liver.

Kwok's syndrome ⇒ Chinese restaurant syndrome.

kymograph *n* an apparatus for recording movements, e.g. of muscles, columns of blood. Used in physiological experiments—**kymographic** *adj*, **kymographically** *adv*.

kypholordosis *n* coexistence of kyphosis and lordosis.

kyphoscoliosis *n* coexistence of kyphosis and scoliosis. May prevent proper lung expansion and respiratory problems.

kyphosis *n* as in Pott's disease, an excessive backward curvature of the dorsal spine. Commonly associated with osteoporosis—**kyphotic** *adj*.

L

labelling theory process by which socially defined labels or identities are assigned or accepted. Often linked with deviant behaviour and can make it hard for people to escape that identity.

labia *npl* lips. *labia majora* two large lip-like folds of skin extending from the mons veneris to form the vulva. *labia minora* two smaller folds lying within the labia majora—**labium** *sing*, **labial** *adj*.

labile *adj* unstable; readily changed, as many drugs when in solution; mood in some mental health problems and blood pressure.

lability *n* instability. *emotional lability* rapid change in mood.

labioglossolaryngeal *adj* relating to the lips, tongue and larynx. *labioglossolaryngeal paralysis* ⇒ bulbar palsy or paralysis.

labour *n* (*syn* parturition) the act of giving birth to a child. The first stage lasts from onset until there is full dilation of the cervical os; the second stage lasts until the baby is delivered; the third stage until the placenta is expelled.

labyrinth *n* the cavities of the internal ear including the cochlea and semicircular canals. *bony labyrinth* that part which is directly hollowed out of the temporal bone. *membranous labyrinth* the membrane lining the bony labyrinth—**labyrinthine** *adj*.

labyrinthectomy *n* surgical removal of part or the whole of the membranous labyrinth of the internal ear. Sometimes carried out for Ménière's disease.

labyrinthitis *n* inflammation of the internal ear.

laceration *n* a wound in which the tissues are torn usually by a blunt instrument or pressure; likely to become infected and to heal by second intention. ⇒ healing.

lacrimal, lachrymal, lacrymal *adj* pertaining to tears. *lacrimal bone* a tiny bone at the inner side of the orbital cavity. *lacrimal duct* connects lacrimal gland to upper conjunctival sac. *lacrimal gland* situated above the upper, outer canthus of the eye. ⇒ dacryocyst.

lacrimation *n* a flow of tears; weeping.

lacrimonasal *adj* pertaining to the lacrimal and nasal bones and ducts.

lactacid (lactic) anaerobic system a series of chemical reactions occurring within the cells whereby a very small amount of adenosine triphosphate (ATP) for energy use is produced from glucose, without oxygen. The end product being lactic acid.

lactacid oxygen debt component the amount of oxygen required to remove lactic acid from muscle tissue and blood during the process of recovery from intense exercise.

lactalbumin *n* one of the whey proteins found in milk. The proportion of protein as lactalbumin is higher in human milk than cows' milk.

lactase *n* (*syn* β-galactosidase) digestive enzyme present in the small intestine mucosa. It catalyses the hydrolysis of lactose to glucose and galactose. *lactase deficiency* an inherited or acquired deficiency of lactase. Common in African Caribbean and Asian individuals. Consumption of lactose (milk sugar) results in colic, diarrhoea, bloating and increased flatus. May be acquired in small intestinal conditions such as coeliac disease and Crohn's disease. It may occur temporarily after a gastrointestinal tract infection. The management depends on severity and may involve the exclusion or restriction of lactose-containing foods.

lactate dehydrogenase (LDH) an enzyme, of which there are five isoenzymes, that catalyses the interconversion of lactate and pyruvate in the myocardium, skeletal muscle and the liver. The level of lactate dehydrogenase in the serum increases rapidly following necrosis of metabolically active tissue, such as after myocardial infarction.

lactation *n* **1** secretion of milk. **2** the period during which an infant receives nourishment from breast milk.

lacteals *npl* the commencing lymphatic ducts in the intestinal villi; they absorb digested fats and convey them to the cisterna chyli.

lactic *adj* relating to milk. *lactic acid* an organic acid formed from the fermentation of lactose (milk sugar). It is produced when glucose is metabolized anaerobically in vigorously contracting skeletal muscle. Cramp and muscle aches may result from a build-up of lactic acid in the muscles. *lactic acidosis* results from a build-up of lactic acid in the blood and consequent reduction in pH. This type of acidosis is linked with diabetes mellitus, drugs such as biguanides, liver failure and toxins, such as alcohol, and any conditions where there is tissue hypoxia, e.g. shock.

lactiferous *adj* conveying or secreting milk.

Lactobacillus *n* a genus of non-pathogenic bacteria. A large Gram-positive rod which ferments carbohydrates, producing acid. They form part of the normal flora of the body, e.g. vagina. ⇒ Döderlein's bacillus.

lactogenic *adj* stimulating milk production. ⇒ prolactin.

lacto-ovovegetarian *adj* describes a diet consisting of milk, milk products, eggs, grain, fruit and vegetables, but no meat, poultry or fish.

lactose *n* milk sugar. A disaccharide of glucose and galactose found in all types of mammalian milks. Less soluble and less sweet than ordinary sugar. ⇒ lactase deficiency.

lactovegetarian *adj* describes a diet consisting of milk, milk products, grain, fruit and vegetables, but no meat, poultry, fish or eggs.

lactulose *n* a disaccharide that is not absorbed and reaches the colon unchanged. Used as an osmotic laxative. ⇒ Appendix 5.

lacuna *n* a space between cells; usually used in the description of bone—**lacunae** *pl*, **lacunar** *adj*.

lambliasis *n* ⇒ giardiasis.

lamella *n* **1** a thin plate-like scale or partition. **2** a gelatine-coated disc containing a drug; it is inserted under the eyelid—**lamellae** *pl*, **lamellar** *adj*.

lamina *n* a thin plate or layer, usually of bone—**laminae** *pl*.

laminectomy *n* removal of vertebral laminae—to expose the spinal cord nerve roots and meninges. Most often performed in the lumbar region, for removal of degenerated intervertebral disc.

Lancefield's groups subdivision of the genus *Streptococcus* on the basis of antigenic structure. The members of each group have a characteristic capsular polysaccharide. The most dangerous streptococci of epidemiological importance to humans belong to group A.

language *n* a system of communication based on symbols or letters and gestures. The usual interpretation involves verbal language (spoken and written) that uses an 'alphabet' of letters or symbols from which many thousands of words can be formed. Particular groups of people, such as health professionals, may construct a verbal language including jargon to explain their work and inadvertently confuse and exclude clients and patients.

lanolin *n* the fat from sheep's wool. Added to ointment bases, as such bases can form water-in-oil emulsions with aqueous constituents, and are readily absorbed by the skin. Contact sensitivity to preparations containing lanolin may develop.

lanugo *n* the soft, downy hair sometimes present on newborn infants, especially when they are premature. Usually replaced before birth by vellus hair.

laparoscopy *n* (*syn* peritoneoscopy) endoscopic examination of the internal organs by the transperitoneal route. A laparoscope is introduced through the abdominal wall after induction of a pneumoperitoneum. A variety of surgical procedures are performed in this way, including biopsy, cyst aspiration, division of adhesions, tubal ligation, assisted conception techniques, appendicectomy and cholecystectomy—**laparoscopic** *adj*, **laparoscopically** *adv*.

laparotomy *n* incision of the abdominal wall. Usually reserved for exploratory operation.

Larsen syndrome multiple joint dislocations.

larva *n* an embryo that is independent before developing the characteristic features of its parents. *larva migrans* itching tracks in the skin with formation of blisters; caused by the burrowing of larvae of some species of fly, and the normally animal-infesting *Ancylostoma*—**larvae** *pl*, **larval** *adj*.

larvicide *n* any agent which destroys larvae—**larvicidal** *adj*.

laryngeal *adj* pertaining to the larynx. *laryngeal mask airway* airway with inflatable cuff placed via the mouth into the oropharynx to maintain the airway during general anaesthesia.

laryngectomy *n* surgical removal of the larynx.

laryngitis *n* inflammation of the larynx.

laryngologist *n* a specialist in disorders of the larynx.

laryngology *n* the study of disorders affecting the larynx.

laryngoparalysis *n* paralysis of the larynx.

laryngopharyngectomy *n* excision of the larynx and part of the pharynx.

laryngopharynx *n* the lower portion of the pharynx—**laryngopharyngeal** *adj*.

laryngoscope *n* instrument for visualization of the larynx, for diagnostic or therapeutic purposes or to facilitate the insertion of an endotracheal tube into the larynx under direct vision—**laryngoscopic** *adj*.

laryngoscopy *n* direct or indirect visual examination of the interior of the larynx.

laryngospasm *n* convulsive involuntary muscular contraction of the larynx, usually accompanied by spasmodic closure of the glottis.

laryngostenosis *n* narrowing of the glottic aperture.

laryngotomy *n* surgical opening in the larynx.

laryngotracheal *adj* pertaining to the larynx and trachea.

laryngotracheitis *n* inflammation of the larynx and trachea.

laryngotracheobronchitis *n* inflammation (usually viral) of the larynx, trachea and bronchi. May be very serious when it occurs in small children. ⇒ croup.

laryngotracheoplasty *n* surgical opening of a stenosed larynx—**laryngotracheoplastic** *adj*.

larynx *n* the organ of voice situated below and in front of the pharynx and at the upper end of the trachea. (⇒ Figure 6)—**laryngeal** *adj*.

laser *acron* for Light Amplification by Stimulated Emission of Radiation. Energy is transmitted as heat which can coagulate tissue. Has many therapeutic uses that include: endometrial ablation, detached retina, skin lesions and cancer. Precautions must be taken by those using lasers as eye damage can occur.

Lassa fever one of the viral haemorrhagic fevers. Occurs as isolated cases and small outbreaks usually in West Africa. The incubation period is 3–16 days; early symptoms resemble typhoid and septicaemia. Mortality is as high as 80%. Strict isolation is required for infected people.

Lassar's paste contains zinc oxide, starch and salicylic acid in soft paraffin. Used in hyperkerototic skin conditions.

lateral *adj* at or belonging to the side; away from the median line—**laterally** *adv*.

latex allergy an allergic reaction to natural latex or one of the components used in production of latex equipment such as medical gloves and catheters. Latex allergy is becoming increasingly common in healthcare workers due to the increased use of gloves following the rise in the incidence of blood-borne viruses.

latissimus dorsi muscle of the back. ⇒ Figures 4, 5.

laughing gas ⇒ nitrous oxide.

lavage *n* irrigation of or washing out a body cavity.

laxatives *npl* (*syn* aperients) drugs used to prevent or treat constipation. Administered orally, or rectally as suppositories or by enema. They may be: bulking agents that retain water and form a large, soft stool; faecal softeners that lubricate or soften the faeces; osmotic laxatives that increase fluid in the bowel lumen; stimulants that increase peristalsis, and combined softeners and stimulants. ⇒ Appendix 5.

LDH *abbr* lactate dehydrogenase.

LE *abbr* lupus erythematosus. ⇒ systemic lupus erythematosus.

lead (Pb) *n* a soft metal with toxic salts. *lead poisoning* (*syn* plumbism) acute poisoning is unusual, but chronic poisoning due to absorption of small amounts over time does occur. For example, young children who suck objects painted with lead paint or made from lead alloys. Lead can be ingested from drinking water contaminated from lead pipes, or from cooking utensils. Abnormally high levels of lead in the environment have been linked to the use of lead in petrol. Presentation varies and may include; abdominal pain, diarrhoea and vomiting, anorexia, anaemia, and the formation of a characteristic blue line round the gums. Neurological manifestations, including convulsions, may occur in severe poisoning.

Leadbetter–Politano operation an antireflux procedure by tunnelled reimplantation of the ureter into the urinary bladder.

lead pipe rigidity increased resistance to passive stretch in any direction that is uniform throughout the whole movement, characteristic of Parkinson's disease. ⇒ cogwheel rigidity.

learning disability a general term used to describe the inability to develop intellectually. Individuals may often have problems integrating into society. Learning disability encompasses many conditions, ranging from specific learning disorders such as dyslexia, through to problems of global intellectual impairment.

lecithinase *n* enzyme that catalyses the decomposition of lecithin.

lecithins *npl* phosphatidylcholines. A group of phospholipids found in animal tissues, mainly in cell membranes. They are present in surfactant. *lecithin-sphingomyelin ratio* a test which assesses fetal lung maturity. Below 2.0 is indicative of a higher risk of neonatal respiratory distress syndrome.

leech *n Hirudo medicinalis.* An aquatic worm which can be applied to the human body to suck blood and reduce congestion. Its saliva contains hirudin, an anticoagulant.

left ventricular assist device (LVAD) mechanical pump used to increase the output of blood from the left ventricle of the heart. May be used in the short term to support critically ill patients, those waiting for a heart transplant, or to give the heart time to recover from disease.

leg *n* lower limb. *leg length discrepancy* a difference of up to 1 cm in true length is considered to be within a normal variation. The effects of discrepancy may either cause a compensatory pelvic tilt and secondary spinal scoliosis, or will force the person to walk on their toes in order to lengthen the leg. The latter will, in time, result in shortening of the Achilles tendon.

Legionella pneumophila a small Gram-negative bacillus which causes legionnaires' disease and Pontiac fever.

legionnaires' disease a severe and often fatal pneumonia caused by *Legionella pneumophila*; there is pneumonia, dry cough, and often non-pulmonary involvement such as gastrointestinal symptoms, renal impairment and confusion. A cause of both community- and hospital-acquired pneumonia, it is associated with an infected water supply in public buildings such as hospitals and hotels. There is no person-to-person spread.

legumen *n* the protein present in peas, beans and lentils.

legumes *npl* pulse vegetables—e.g. peas, beans, lentils. An essential component of a vegan diet providing protein, B vitamins and iron and soluble dietary fibre.

Leishman–Donovan bodies the rounded forms of the protozoa *Leishmania* found in certain cells, e.g. macrophages, of individuals with leishmaniasis.

Leishmania *n* genus of flagellated protozoon. *Leishmania donovani* causes leishmaniasis.

leishmaniasis *n* infestation by *Leishmania*, spread by sandflies. Generalized (visceral) manifestation is kala-azar. Old World, cutaneous forms are called an oriental sore. New World cutaneous forms may involve the nasal and oral mucosa and the lesion is called an espundia.

lens *n* **1** the small biconvex crystalline body which is supported by the suspensory ligament immediately behind the iris of the eye (⇒ Figure 15). On account of its elasticity, the lens can alter in shape, enabling light rays to focus exactly on the retina. **2** glass or plastic used to correct refractive errors (spectacles or contact lens) or in optical instruments.

lenticular *adj* pertaining to or resembling a lens.

lentigo *n* a freckle with an increased number of pigment cells. ⇒ ephelides—**lentigines** *pl*.

leontiasis *n* enlargement of the face and head giving a lion-like appearance; associated with some types of leprosy.

leprologist *n* one who specializes in the study and treatment of leprosy.

leprology *n* the study of leprosy and its treatment.

lepromata *npl* the granulomatous cutaneous eruption of leprosy—**leproma** *sing*, **lepromatous** *adj*.

leprosy (Hansen's disease) *n* a chronic and contagious disease, endemic in warmer climates and characterized by granulomatous formation in the peripheral nerves or on the skin, mucous membranes and bones with tissue destruction. Caused by *Mycobacterium leprae* (Hansen's bacillus). BCG vaccination conferred variable protection in different trials. Management includes specific care, such as that required for impaired sensation and the long-term treatment with various antimicrobial drugs, including dapsone and rifampicin—**leprous** *adj*.

Leptospira *n* a genus of bacteria. Very thin, finely coiled bacteria. Common in water as saprophytes; pathogenic species are numerous in many animals. *Leptospira interrogans* serotype *icterohaemorrhagiae* causes Weil's disease in humans: *Leptospira interrogans* serotype *canicola* infects dogs and pigs, and is transmissible to humans. ⇒ leptospirosis.

leptospiral agglutination tests serological tests used to diagnose specific leptospiral infections, e.g. Weil's disease.

leptospirosis *n* infection of humans by bacteria of the leptospira group found in rats and other rodents, cattle, dogs, pigs and foxes. Those at risk include abattoir and agricultural workers and water sports enthusiasts. Presentation varies according to which leptospira is responsible, but may include: high fever, headache, myalgia, conjunctival congestion, rash, anorexia, jaundice, severe muscular pains, rigors and vomiting. Severe infections may cause hepatitis, myocarditis, renal tubular necrosis and less frequently meningitis with an associated mortality rate of up to 20%. ⇒ Weil's disease.

lesbianism *n* sexual attraction between women.

Lesch–Nyhan disease X-linked recessive genetic disorder. Overproduction of uric acid, associated with brain damage resulting in cerebral palsy and learning disability. Victims are compelled, by a self-destructive urge, to bite away the sides of their mouth, lips and fingers.

lesion *n* pathological change in a bodily tissue.

leucine *n* an essential (indispensable) branched chain amino acid.

leucocytes *npl* generic name for white blood cells. They are nucleated, mobile and are all involved with body defences, e.g. some are phagocytic and others produce antibodies. There are two main groups: (a) polymorphonuclear cells or granulocytes (neutrophils, basophils and eosinophils)—these have a many-lobed nucleus and granules in their cytoplasm; (b) monocytes and lymphocytes—these generally have no granules, but some lymphocytes are granular.

leucocytolysis *n* destruction and disintegration of white blood cells—**leucocytolytic** *adj.*

leucocytosis *n* increased number of leucocytes in the blood. Often a response to infection—**leucocytotic** *adj.*

leucoderma *n* absent skin pigmentation, especially when it occurs in patches or bands.

leucoma *n* white opaque spot on the cornea—**leucomata** *pl.*

leuconychia *n* white areas on the nails. These may be dots, lines, or extend over the entire nail plate (totalis). They are usually indicative of minor trauma, e.g. resulting from short shoes or sporting activities.

leucopenia *n* decreased number of white blood cells in the blood—**leucopenic** *adj.*

leucopoiesis *n* formation of white blood cells from stem cells. Regulated by colony stimulating factors and cytokines—**leucopoietic** *adj.*

leucorrhoea *n* a sticky, whitish vaginal discharge—**leucorrhoeal** *adj.*

leukaemia *n* neoplastic diseases of the haematopoietic tissue with most commonly abnormal proliferation of white cells (leucocytes). Uncontrolled proliferation of the leukaemic cells causes secondary suppression of other blood components, and anaemia and thrombocytopenia result. The lack of mature white cells increases the risk of infection, thrombocytopenia increases the risk of bleeding, and anaemia is also characteristic. Causes include ionizing radiation, previous chemotherapy, retroviruses, chemicals, genetic anomalies (e.g. Down's syndrome). The classification is according to cell type—lymphocytic or myelocytic, and the course acute or chronic. The chronic leukaemias may enter a 'blast crisis' or acute phase. Therapeutic options include chemotherapy, radiotherapy, interferon alpha, monoclonal antibodies and bone marrow transplantation, either autologous or allograft. ⇒ myeloproliferative disorders.

leukoplakia *n* white, thickened patch occurring on mucous membranes. Occurs on lips, inside mouth or on genitalia. Usually patchy and often premalignant. ⇒ kraurosis vulvae.

leukotrienes *npl* regulatory lipids derived from arachidonic acid (fatty acid). They function as signalling molecules in the inflammatory response and in some allergic responses.

levator *n* **1** a muscle which acts by raising a part. *levator scapulae* ⇒ Figure 5. **2** an instrument for lifting a depressed part.

Levin tube a French plastic catheter used for gastric intubation; it has a closed weighted tip and an opening on the side.

Lewy body an inclusion body in damaged and dying nerve cells in the brain that is the pathological hallmark of Parkinson's disease and related conditions.

LGVCFT *abbr* lymphogranuloma venereum complement fixation test.

libido *n* Freud's term for the urge to obtain sensual satisfaction. Sometimes used to mean the sexual urge. Freud's meaning was satisfaction through all the senses.

lice *n* ⇒ pediculus.

lichen *n* aggregations of papular skin lesions—**lichenoid** *adj*. *lichen nitidus* characterized by minute, shiny, flat-topped, pink papules of pinhead size. *lichen planus* an eruption of unknown cause showing purple, angulated, shiny, flat-topped papules. *lichen scrofulosorum* a form of tuberculide. *lichen simplex* ⇒ neurodermatitis.

lichenification *n* thickening of the skin, usually secondary to scratching. Skin markings become more prominent and the area affected appears to be composed of small, shiny rhomboids. ⇒ neurodermatitis.

lien *n* the spleen.

lienculus *n* a small accessory spleen.

lienorenal *adj* pertaining to the spleen and kidney. ⇒ splenorenal.

life crisis describes an unforeseen unpleasant occurrence, such as becoming the victim of a violent crime, sudden and severe ill health or a life event, e.g. becoming unemployed.

life event in sociology a term describing the major occurrences occurring during the lifespan, such as starting school, getting married or ending a relationship, changing job, moving house, or suffering a bereavement.

life expectancy the average age at which death occurs. Influenced by health/illness and by social factors such as level of education; and environmental factors such as housing, sanitation and the supply of clean water.

lifestyle planning techniques used in occupational therapy practice that enable an individual to achieve a balance between occupational roles in order to reduce stress, improve quality of life, develop potentials and attain relevant personal goals. Activity analysis is used to determine the occupational performance skills required and activities are recommended that are consistent with the individual's priorities and anticipated abilities.

ligament *n* a strong band of fibrous tissue serving to bind bones or other parts together, or to support an organ—**ligamentous** *adj*.

ligand signalling chemicals that include cytokines, hormones or neurotransmitters. They can affect cell function by binding to specific cell membrane receptors. Many drugs cause their effects by being able to imitate the natural ligand.

ligate *vt* to tie off blood vessels, etc., at operation—**ligation** *n*.

ligation *n* tying off; usually reserved for *ligation of the uterine (fallopian) tubes*, a method of sterilization.

ligature *n* the material used for tying vessels or stitching the tissues. ⇒ suture.

light adaptation adjustments made by the eye in bright light. The pupils constrict, rhodopsin breakdown reduces retinal sensitivity and cone activity increases. ⇒ dark adaptation.

lightening *n* a word used to denote the relief of pressure on the diaphragm by the abdominal viscera, when the presenting part of the fetus descends into the pelvis in the last 3 weeks of a primigravida's pregnancy.

lightning pains symptomatic of tabes dorsalis. Occur as paroxysms of swift-cutting (lightning) stabs in the lower limbs.

Likert scale a scale used in questionnaire surveys. Participants are asked to specify their degree of agreement with a particular statement, i.e. strongly agree, agree, unsure, disagree and strongly disagree.

limbus *n* in ophthalmology the circumference of the cornea at which it joins the sclera.

liminal *adj* of a stimulus, of the lowest intensity that can be perceived by human sense organs. ⇒ subliminal.

linctus *n* a sweet, syrupy liquid, usually given to relieve a cough.

linea *n* a line. *linea alba* the white line visible after removal of the skin in the centre of the abdomen, stretching from the ensiform cartilage to the pubis, its position on the surface being indicated by a slight depression. *lineae albicantes* white lines which appear on the abdomen after reduction of tension as after childbirth, tapping of the abdomen, etc. ⇒ striae gravidarum. *linea nigra* pigmented line from umbilicus to pubis which appears in pregnancy.

linear accelerator a mega-voltage machine which accelerates electrons and produces high energy X-rays which are used in the treatment of various cancers.

lingua *n* the tongue—**lingual** *adj.*

liniment *n* a liquid applied to the skin using gentle friction.

linitis plastica a form of gastric cancer which infiltrates throughout the gastric wall. This leads to diffuse thickening and failure to inflate at endoscopy and barium examinations.

linoleic acid a polyunsaturated, essential fatty acid. It is found in vegetable seed oils, such as sunflower, corn and soya bean. ⇒ essential fatty acids.

linolenic acid a polyunsaturated, essential fatty acid found in vegetable oils. There are two types; α-linolenic, which is found in soya bean oil and linseed oil, and γ-linolenic found in evening primrose oil. ⇒ essential fatty acids.

lipaemia *n* increased lipoids (especially cholesterol) in the blood—**lipaemic** *adj.*

lipase *n* any fat-splitting enzyme, such as pancreatic lipase. They convert fats into fatty acids and glycerol.

lipids *npl* large group of fat-like organic molecules which include: neutral fats, such as triglycerides (triacylglycerols), phospholipids, lipoproteins, fat-soluble vitamins, steroids, prostaglandins, leukotrienes and thromboxanes. They consist of carbon, oxygen and hydrogen, and some contain phosphorus and nitrogen. They are insoluble in water, but they can be dissolved in organic solvents such as alcohol. Lipids are important in the body both structurally and functionally. Fat deposits provide an energy store, insulate and offer some protection. Other lipids are important constituents of cell membranes, are precursors for steroid hormones, act as regulatory molecules, e.g. prostaglandins, and transport fats around the body, and the fat-soluble vitamins are concerned with blood clotting, vision and antioxidant functions.

lipogenesis *n* a metabolic process where amino acids and glucose are converted to triglycerides (triacylglycerols) prior to storage in adipose tissue. It is stimulated by insulin.

lipoid *adj, n* (a substance) resembling fats or oil.

lipoidosis *n* disease due to disorder of fat metabolism—**lipoidoses** *pl.*

lipolysis *n* the chemical breakdown of fat; stored triglycerides (triacylglycerols) are released for energy. Stimulated by glucocorticoid hormones—**lipolytic** *adj.*

lipoma *n* a benign tumour of fatty tissue—**lipomata** *pl,* **lipomatous** *adj.*

lipoprotein *n* lipids combined with a protein that transport triglycerides (triacylglycerols) and cholesterol around the body in the blood. They are classified as: high-density lipoproteins (HDLs), low-density lipoproteins (LDLs) or very-low-density lipoproteins (VLDLs). A high level of LDL in the blood is associated with arterial disease whereas HDLs are considered to be protective. A high HDL:LDL is associated with a decreased risk of arterial disease. ⇒ hyperlipidaemia, lipids.

liposome *n* a spherical body comprising a phospholipid bilayer enclosing an aqueous solution.

liposome drug delivery drug administration using drugs enclosed in vesicles. Drug release occurs when the liposome is broken down in the liver by cells of the macrophage–monocyte system.

liposuction *n* in cosmetic surgery a technique of vacuum extraction of subcutaneous fat using fine cannulae.

lipotrophic substances factors which cause the removal of fat from the liver by transmethylation.

lipuria *n* (*syn* adiposuria) fat in the urine—**lipuric** *adj.*

liquor *n* a solution. *liquor amnii* fluid surrounding the fetus.

listening *n* a group of complex skills used in communicating; health professionals give their whole attention to what is being said, how it is being said, and whether or not it matches the non-verbal signals.

Listeria *n* a genus of bacteria present in animal faeces and soil. *Listeria monocytogenes* causes meningitis, septicaemia, and intrauterine or perinatal infections. ⇒ listeriosis.

listeriosis *n* infection caused by *Listeria*. Transmitted via contaminated soil, contact with infected animals and by eating unpasteurized foods, such as soft cheeses, that may be infected. It may lead to a flu-like illness but serious consequences may occur in infants, older people, debilitated or immunocompromised individuals and pregnant women. Infection during pregnancy may lead to miscarriage, stillbirth, premature labour and septicaemia and neonatal meningitis.

literature review a methodical and wide-ranging examination of the papers relevant to a topic. Research methods and results are analysed and presented critically. The literature review includes how the search was carried out, e.g. bibliographical databases such as Medline.

lithiasis *n* any condition in which there are calculi.

lithium (Li) *n* a metallic element. Lithium salts are used therapeutically in some mental health problems.

litholapaxy *n* (*syn* lithopaxy) crushing a stone within the urinary bladder and removing the fragments by irrigation.

lithopaedion *n* a dead fetus retained in the uterus, e.g. one of a pair of twins which dies and becomes mummified and sometimes impregnated with lime salts.

lithotomy *n* general term for the surgical incision of a duct or organ for the removal of calculi, especially one from the urinary tract. *lithotomy position* with the patient lying down, the buttocks are drawn to the end of the table to which a stirrup is attached on either side. Each foot is placed in a sling attached to the top of the stirrup so that the perineum is exposed for genitourinary procedures.

lithotripsy *n* destruction of calculi by crushing.

lithotriptor *n* a machine which sends shock waves through renal calculi, causing them to fragment and be passed naturally in the urine.

lithotrite *n* an instrument for crushing a stone in the urinary bladder.

litmus *n* a vegetable pigment used as an indicator of alkalinity (blue) or acidity (red). Often stored as paper strips: red litmus paper turns blue when exposed to an alkali; blue litmus paper turns red with an acid.

Little's disease diplegia of spastic type causing 'scissor leg' deformity. A congenital disease in which there is cerebral atrophy or agenesis.

liver *n* the largest gland in the body, the weight in adults is within the range 1.2–1.5 kg. The liver is situated in the right upper part of the abdominal cavity. It is vital to homeostasis and its functions include: breakdown of red blood cells with the production of bile, detoxification of drugs and hormones, nutrient metabolism, protein synthesis and storage of glycogen, vitamins and minerals. The liver is the site of considerable heat generation. *liver function tests* blood tests used to assess liver function including: alanine aminotransferase, alkaline phosphatase, aspartate aminotransferase, coagulation tests, gamma-glutamyltransferase, serum bilirubin and serum proteins. ⇒ aminotransferases. *liver transplant* liver failure may be treated by surgical transplantation of a liver from a suitable donor.

livid *adj* showing blue discoloration due to bruising, congestion or insufficient oxygenation.

living will ⇒ advance directive.

LMP *abbr* last menstrual period.

LOA *abbr* left occipitoanterior; used to describe the position of the fetus in the uterus.

Loa loa a parasitic nematode causing loiasis (filariasis).

lobe *n* a rounded section of an organ, separated from neighbouring sections by a fissure or septum, etc.—**lobar** *adj*.

lobectomy *n* removal of a lobe, for example lung, or liver.

lobule *n* a small lobe or a subdivision of a lobe—**lobular, lobulated** *adj*.

local anaesthetic ⇒ anaesthetic.

local authority in the UK, local government, e.g. regional councils, county councils, city councils, district and town councils and parish councils. All have powers to raise taxes and some have a statutory duty to provide services within a locality, such as environmental health, social services, housing, education, policing and crime prevention.

localize *vt* **1** to limit the spread. **2** to determine the site of a lesion—**localization** *n*.

local muscle endurance a person's ability to sustain a physical activity that relates to a particular muscle or group of muscles; for example, the number of press-ups possible in a given time gives an indication of upper arm and shoulder muscle endurance.

lochia *n* the vaginal discharge which occurs during the puerperium. At first pure blood, it later becomes paler, diminishes in quantity and finally ceases—**lochial** *adj*.

locked in syndrome a condition in which there is normally critical damage in the brainstem such that the patient is unable to move but can understand what is going on.

lockjaw *n* ⇒ tetanus.

locomotor *adj* can be applied to any tissue or system used in movement. Most usually refers to nerves and muscles. Sometimes includes the skeletal system. *locomotor ataxia* the disordered gait and loss of sense of position (proprioception) in the lower limbs, which occurs in tabes dorsalis. ⇒ syphilis.

loculated *adj* divided into numerous cavities.

locus of control concept in health psychology. A behaviourist theory to describe individual differences in perceived control over events in people's lives. Some people feel that events in their lives are beyond their control, a belief in an external locus of control. This would consequently determine their response to stress and health seeking (illness) behaviour with an over-reliance on medical intervention for improving health. Others may feel that they do exercise a degree of control over events, a belief in an internal locus of control. This is more likely to lead to self-help: altered behaviour to reduce the risk of ill health, adoption of healthier lifestyles, adherence to medical advice.

loiasis *n* special form of filariasis (caused by the worm *Loa loa*) which occurs in West Africa. The vector, a large horsefly, *Chrysops*, bites in the daytime. Larvae take 2–3 years to develop and may live in humans for 15 years. There is eosinophilia. The worms move about the subcutaneous tissues causing irritation and localized swellings, and sometimes a worm crosses the eye.

loin *n* that part of the back between the lower ribs and the iliac crest; the area immediately above the buttocks.

longitudinal study research study where data are collected on more than one occasion, such as the study of a cohort of people over time. ⇒ cohort study.

longsighted *adj* ⇒ hypermetropia.

long-term memory (LTM) the part of memory responsible for the retention of information for longer periods. Potentially permanent and has a much greater capacity than short-term memory.

long-term oxygen therapy (LTOT) controlled flow rate oxygen, provided for at least 15 hours per day, usually via an oxygen concentrator. Shown to prolong survival in those with severe hypoxaemia (PaO_2 <7.3 kPa with an FEV_1 < 1.5 L) secondary to obstructive lung disease with concurrent right heart failure.

loop diuretics a group of drugs that cause a diuretic effect by preventing the reabsorption of sodium, chloride and potassium in the thick part of the ascending limb of the loop of Henle. ⇒ Appendix 5.

LOP *acron* left occipitoposterior; used to describe the position of the fetus in the uterus.

lordoscoliosis *n* lordosis complicated by the presence of scoliosis.

lordosis *n* an exaggerated forward, convex curve of the lumbar spine—**lordotic** *adj*.

loupe *n* a magnifying lens often attached to spectacles.

louse *n* ⇒ *Pediculus*—**lice** *pl*.

low back pain the commonest cause seems to be posteriolateral prolapse of the intervertebral disc, putting pressure on the dura and cauda equina and causing the localized pain of lumbago. It can progress to trap the spinal nerve root, causing the nerve distribution pain of sciatica.

low birthweight term used to indicate a weight of 2.5 kg or less at birth, whether or not gestation was below 37 weeks. ⇒ small for gestational age.

low-density lipoprotein (LDL) ⇒ lipoprotein.

lower reference nutrient intake (LRNI) one of the UK dietary reference values. The amount of a nutrient that will be enough for that small group within a population (2.5%) who have a low requirement.

lower respiratory tract infection (LRTI) ⇒ pneumonia.

LP *abbr* lumbar puncture.

LRNI *abbr* lower reference nutrient intake.

LRTI *abbr* lower respiratory tract infection.

LSD *abbr* lysergic acid diethylamide.

lubb-dupp *n* words descriptive of the heart sounds as heard on auscultation.

lubricants *npl* faecal softeners that also lubricate and facilitate easy and painless defecation. ⇒ laxatives.

lucid *adj* clear; describing mental clarity. *lucid interval* a period of mental clarity which can be of variable length, occurring in people with organic mental disorder such as dementia.

Ludwig's angina ⇒ cellulitis.

lues *n* obsolete term for syphilis.

lumbago *n* incapacitating pain low down in the back.

lumbar *adj* pertaining to the loin. *lumbar nerve* ⇒ Figure 11. *lumbar vertebrae* ⇒ Figure 3.

lumbar puncture (LP) the withdrawal of cerebrospinal fluid (CSF) through a hollow needle inserted into the subarachnoid space in the lumbar region of the spine. The CSF obtained is examined for its chemical (e.g. glucose) and cellular (e.g. white blood cells) constituents and for the presence of micro-organisms; CSF pressure can be measured by the attachment of a manometer.

lumbar sympathectomy surgical removal of the sympathetic chain in the lumbar region; used to improve the blood supply to the lower limbs by allowing vasodilation.

lumbocostal *adj* pertaining to the loin and ribs.

lumbosacral *adj* pertaining to the loin or lumbar vertebrae and the sacrum.

Lumbricus *n* a genus of earthworms. ⇒ ascarides, ascariasis.

lumen *n* the space inside a tubular structure—**lumina** *pl*, **luminal** *adj*.

lumpectomy *n* the surgical excision of a tumour with removal of minimal surrounding tissue. Increasingly used, with radiotherapy and chemotherapy, for treatment of breast cancer.

Lund and Browder's charts used to calculate more accurately a burn area and illustrate the depth of area burnt, giving a calculation of burn severity.

lungs *npl* the two main organs of respiration which occupy the greater part of the thoracic cavity; they are separated from each other by the heart and other contents of the mediastinum (⇒ Figures 6, 7). They are concerned with gas exchange—the oxygenation of blood and excretion of carbon dioxide. *lung transplantation* may be single, double, heart–lung transplants, or sometimes in the case of child recipients, live-related lobar transplants.

lunula *n* the semilunar pale area at the root of the nail.

lupus *n* several destructive skin conditions, with different causes. ⇒ collagen diseases. *lupus erythematosus (LE)* ⇒ systemic lupus erythematosus (SLE). *lupus pernio* a form of sarcoidosis. *lupus vulgaris* the commonest variety of skin tuberculosis; ulceration occurs over cartilage (nose or ear) with necrosis and facial disfigurement.

luteinizing hormone (LH) a gonadotrophin secreted by the anterior pituitary gland. In females high levels in mid menstrual cycle stimulate ovulation and formation of the corpus luteum. The same hormone in males is called interstitial-cell stimulating hormone (ICSH); it stimulates the production of testosterone by the testes.

luxation *n* partial dislocation.

Lyme disease ⇒ *Borrelia*, relapsing fever.

lymph *n* the fluid contained in the lymphatic vessels. It is formed from interstitial (tissue) fluid and is similar to plasma. Unlike blood, lymph contains only one type of cell, the lymphocyte. *lymph circulation* that of lymph collected from the tissue spaces; it then passes via capillaries, vessels, nodes and ducts to be returned to the blood. *lymph nodes* accumulations of lymphatic tissue at intervals along lymphatic vessels. They mainly act as filters. They provide a site for B and T lymphocyte/cell proliferation and the production of immunoglobulins.

lymphadenectomy *n* excision of one or more lymph nodes.

lymphadenitis *n* inflammation of a lymph node.

lymphadenopathy *n* any disease of the lymph nodes—**lymphadenopathic** *adj*.

lymphangiectasis *n* dilation of the lymph vessels—**lymphangiectatic** *adj*.

lymphangiography *n* ⇒ lymphography.

lymphangioma *n* a simple tumour of lymph vessels frequently associated with similar formations of blood vessels— **lymphangiomata** *pl*, **lymphangiomatous** *adj*.

lymphangioplasty *n* any plastic surgery on lymph vessels, such as those used to improve drainage. ⇒ lymphoedema— **lymphangioplastic** *adj*.

lymphangitis *n* inflammation of a lymph vessel.

lymphatic *adj* pertaining to, conveying or containing lymph.

lymphoblast *n* an immature lymphocyte. Present in the blood and bone marrow in conditions such as acute lymphoblastic leukaemia (ALL).

lymphocyte *n* one variety of white blood cell. The lymphocytic stem cells undergo transformation to T lymphocytes/cells (in the thymus), which provide cellular immunity involved in destroying cancer cells, virus infected cells and transplanted cells (graft), or B lymphocytes/cells, which form immunoglobulins (antibodies) and provide humoral immunity. The transformation is usually complete a few months after birth—**lymphocytic** *adj*.

lymphocytosis *n* an increase in lymphocytes in the blood.

lymphoedema *n* excess fluid in the tissues from abnormality or obstruction of lymph vessels that blocks or interrupts lymph drainage. There is swelling of (usually) a limb and increased risk of cellulitis. It may occur, for example, after lymph node resection and/or radiotherapy; most common in breast cancer. Treated by compression bandaging. ⇒ elephantiasis, filariasis.

lymphoepithelioma *n* rapidly growing malignant pharyngeal tumour. May involve the tonsil. Often has metastases in cervical lymph nodes—**lymphoepitheliomata** *pl*.

lymphogranuloma venereum a sexually transmitted infection caused by *Chlamydia trachomatis*. There are ulcers on the genitalia and local lymph node enlargement. Occurs mainly in the tropics.

lymphography *n* X-ray examination of the lymphatic system after it has been rendered radiopaque. Generally replaced by CT scanning—**lymphographical** *adj*,

lymphogram *n*, **lymphograph** *n*, **lymphographically** *adv*.

lymphoid *adj* pertaining to lymph. *lymphoid tissue* tissue similar to lymph nodes, situated in a variety of locations, bone marrow, gut, liver, spleen, thymus and tonsils.

lymphokines *npl* a term applied to cytokines produced by stimulated T lymphocytes. They function during the immune response as intercellular chemical mediators.

lymphoma *n* a group of neoplastic diseases developing in lymphoid tissue. Lymphoma is characterized by lymph node enlargement, night sweats/swinging pyrexia, pain from splenic enlargement/infarction, hepatomegaly, weight loss, malaise or recurrent infection. Causes include viral infections but most are idiopathic. Classified according to histological appearances to either Hodgkin's lymphoma or non-Hodgkin's lymphoma (NHL). Staging depends on sites involved—location and number, as well as associated 'secondary' symptoms. Therapy may be radiotherapy alone for the earliest stages, and/or chemotherapy. Bone marrow transplantation may also be necessary. ⇒ Burkitt's lymphoma.

lymphorrhagia *n* an outpouring of lymph from a severed lymphatic vessel.

lymphosarcoma *n* obsolete term for some types of lymphoma.

lyophilization *n* freeze drying. Used to preserve biological substances such as plasma, tissue, etc.

lyophilized skin skin which has been subjected to lyophilization. It is reconstituted and used for temporary skin replacement.

lysergic acid diethylamide (LSD) a potent hallucinogenic agent.

lysin *n* a substance present in blood that dissolves cells. ⇒ bacteriolysin, haemolysin.

lysine *n* an essential (indispensable) amino acid necessary for growth.

lysis *n* **1** a gradual return to normal, used especially in relation to pyrexia. ⇒ crisis *opp*. **2** disintegration of the membrane of cells or bacteria.

lysozyme *n* an antibacterial enzyme present in many body fluids such as tears and saliva.

M

maceration *n* softening of the horny layer of the skin by moisture, e.g. in and below the toes (in tinea pedis), or in perianal area (in pruritus ani). Maceration reduces the protective quality of the integument and so predisposes to penetration by bacteria or fungi.

Mackenrodt's ligaments ⇒ uterine supports.

macrocephaly *n* large head, not caused by hydrocephalus—**macrocephalic** *adj*.

macrocheilia *n* excessive development of the lips.

macrocyte *n* a large red blood cell. Occurs in megaloblastic anaemia (e.g. pernicious anaemia) and in association with excess alcohol intake, liver disease and hypothyroidism—**macrocytic** *adj*.

macrocytosis an increased number of macrocytes.

macrodactyly *n* excessive development of the fingers or toes.

macroglossia *n* an abnormally large tongue.

macrolides *npl* a group of antibiotics that may be prescribed for people with penicillin hypersensitivity. ⇒ Appendix 5.

macromastia *n* an abnormally large breast.

macronutrient *n* term used to describe those nutrients required in large quantities that can be metabolized to produce energy; carbohydrate, fat and protein.

macrophages *npl* mononuclear cells, which destroy foreign bodies and cell debris by phagocytosis. Part of the monocyte-macrophage (reticuloendothelial) system, they are derived from monocytes. ⇒ histiocytes.

macroscopic *adj* visible to the unaided eye; gross. ⇒ microscopic *opp*.

macrotrauma *n* a single force resulting in trauma to body tissues.

macula *n* a spot—**macular** *adj*. *macula densa* special cells of the nephron. Forms part of the juxtaglomerular apparatus. *macula lutea* area of the retina responsible for clearest central vision. ⇒ Figure 15.

macular degeneration *n* degenerative changes of the retina in the macular region which may lead to loss of central vision. Commonly age-related. It may be atrophic or involve growth of a neovascular (new, abnormal blood vessels) membrane arising from the choroid.

macule *n* a non-palpable localized area of change in skin colour—**macular** *adj*.

maculopapular *adj* the presence of macules and raised palpable spots (papules) on the skin.

Madura foot ⇒ mycetoma.

magnesium (Mg) *n* a metallic element needed in the body for many enzyme-catalysed reactions. Magnesium is an intracellular cation and is present in bone, and its metabolism is linked to that of calcium.

magnesium salts many salts of magnesium are used therapeutically. *magnesium carbonate and trisilicate* both used as an antacid. *magnesium chloride* used intravenously for magnesium deficiency (hypomagnesaemia). *magnesium hydroxide* an antacid and osmotic laxative. *magnesium sulphate* (*syn* Epsom salts) an effective rapid-acting osmotic laxative. It is used as a paste with glycerin for the treatment of boils. Used parenterally in the treatment of eclampsia and magnesium deficiency.

magnetic resonance imaging (MRI) (*syn* nuclear magnetic resonance (NMR)) a non-invasive technique that does not use ionizing radiation. It uses radiofrequency radiation in the presence of a powerful magnetic field to produce high-quality images of the body in any plane.

magnum *adj* large or great, as foramen magnum in occipital bone.

major histocompatibility complex (MHC) both MHC class I and class II glycoproteins are members of the immunoglobulin superfamily, and present peptide antigens to the immune system to generate an immune response. The MHC genes are encoded on human chromosome 6. Class I MHC genes encode proteins that are expressed on all nucleated cells and present self antigens to CD8+ T cells. Class II MHC genes encode proteins that are present on antigen-presenting cells (dendritic cells, macrophages and B cells) that present antigens to CD4+ T cells. Class III MHC genes encode a variety of molecules including cytokines, complement components, and other molecules essential for antigen presentation.

Makaton *n* a form of sign language. It is more basic than some other languages.

mal *n* disease. *mal de mer* seasickness. *grand mal* major epilepsy. *petit mal* minor epilepsy.

malabsorption *n* defective absorption of nutrients from the digestive tract. *malabsorption syndrome* loss of weight and steatorrhoea, varying in severity. Caused by: (a) disease of the small intestine; (b) lack of digestive enzymes or bile salts; (c) surgical operations.

malacia *n* softening of a part. ⇒ keratomalacia, osteomalacia.

maladaptation an abnormal or maladaptive response to a situation or change. It may relate to personal relationships, or to a stress response that leads to poor health, e.g. headaches, body chemistry changes.

maladjustment *n* bad or poor adaptation to environment. It may have social, mental or physical components.

malaise *n* a feeling of illness and discomfort.

malalignment *n* faulty alignment—as of bones after a fracture.

malar *adj* relating to the cheek.

malaria *n* a serious infection caused by protozoa of the genus *Plasmodium* and carried by infected mosquitoes of the genus *Anopheles*. It occurs in tropical and subtropical regions and is seen in travellers returning from malarial areas. The parasite causes haemolysis during a complex life cycle. *Plasmodium falciparum* causes the most severe disease (malignant tertian malaria). *Plasmodium malariae* causes quartan malaria. *Plasmodium ovale* and *Plasmodium vivax* cause tertian malaria. The signs and symptoms depend on the type of malaria, but include: bouts of fever, rigors, headache, cough, vomiting, anaemia, jaundice, hepatosplenomegaly. Relapses are common in malaria. Various antimalarial drugs are available for both chemoprophylaxis and treatment. Elimination of the mosquito and its habitat are important in prevention—**malarial** *adj*.

malathion *n* organophosphorus compound, used in suitable dilution for the topical treatment of scabies and head lice infestation.

malformation *n* abnormal shape or structure; deformity.

malignant *adj* virulent and dangerous—**malignancy** *n*. *malignant growth or tumour*

one that demonstrates the capacity to invade adjacent tissues/organs and spread (metastasis) to distant sites; often rapidly growing and with a fatal outcome. ⇒ cancer, sarcoma. *malignant hyperpyrexia* ⇒ hyperpyrexia. *malignant pustule* ⇒ anthrax.

malingering *n* the deliberate simulation of physical or psychological illness motivated by external incentives or stressors.

malleolus *n* a part or process of a bone shaped like a hammer. *external malleolus* at the lower end of the fibula. *internal malleolus* situated at the lower end of the tibia—**malleoli** *pl*, **malleolar** *adj*.

mallet finger (*syn* hammer finger) the rupture of the extensor digitorum longus tendon from the distal phalanx. Known as baseball finger in the United States.

malleus *n* the hammer-shaped lateral bone of the middle ear (⇒ Figure 13). ⇒ incus, stapes.

malnutrition *n* the state of being poorly nourished due to the diet containing the incorrect amount of a micro- or macronutrient. Can result in disease, such as scurvy—malnutrition due to inadequate dietary intake of vitamin C, or obesity—malnutrition due to excessive energy intake.

malocclusion *n* any deviation from the normal occlusion of the teeth, often associated with an abnormal jaw relationship. ⇒ orthodontics.

malposition *n* any abnormal position of a part.

malpractice *n* improper or injurious medical or nursing treatment. Professional practice that falls below accepted standards and causes harm. It may be negligence, unethical behaviour, abuse or criminal activities.

malpresentation *n* the baby is not in the normal head-first position before or during labour.

Malta fever ⇒ brucellosis.

maltase *n* (*syn* α-glucosidase) an enzyme found in intestinal juice. It converts maltose to glucose.

MALToma *n* low grade B cell lymphoma of the mucosa-associated lymphoid tissue. It may be related to *Helicobacter pylori* infection which, when eradicated, may lead to disease regression.

maltose *n* malt sugar. A disaccharide produced by the hydrolysis of starch by amylase during digestion. Also manufactured commercially.

malunion *n* the union of a fracture in a bad position.

mamma *n* the breast—mammae *pl*, mammary *adj*.

mammaplasty *n* any plastic operation on the breast—mammaplastic *adj*. ⇒ augmentation, implant, reduction.

mammilla *n* 1 the nipple. 2 a small papilla—mammillae *pl*.

mammography *n* radiographic demonstration of the breast by use of specially low-penetration (long wavelength) X-rays. Used in the diagnosis of or screening for breast conditions including cancer—mammographic *adj*, mammographically *adv*.

Manchester operation (*syn* Fothergill's operation) anterior colporrhaphy, amputation of part of the cervix and posterior colpoperineorrhaphy, performed for genital prolapse.

manganese (Mn) *n* a metallic element needed by the body for many enzyme catalysed reactions.

mania *n* a mood disorder characterized by elation, increased energy, overactivity, pressured speech, decreased need for sleep, irritability, grandiosity, distractibility, overspending. May be accompanied by psychotic symptoms, typically grandiose/religiose/persecutory delusions and hallucinations—maniac *adj*.

manic depressive illness ⇒ bipolar affective disorder.

manipulation *n* using the hands skilfully as in reducing a fracture or hernia, or changing an abnormal fetal position to facilitate a vaginal delivery.

Mann–Whitney test a non-parametric substitute to Student's t test for independent groups.

mannitol *n* a sugar that is not metabolized in the body and acts as an osmotic diuretic. ⇒ Appendix 5.

manometer *n* an instrument for measuring the pressure exerted by liquids or gases. Used for example for measuring the pressure exerted by the cerebrospinal fluid during lumbar puncture, or for measuring central venous pressure.

Mantoux reaction a skin test for tuberculosis. 10 tuberculin units of purified protein derivative in 0.1 mL of normal saline instilled intradermally in the forearm. After 2–4 days, if induration is greater than or equal to 5 mm, the test is positive.

manual muscle testing a specific procedure used to evaluate the functional status of a muscle's innervation and contractile tissues; uses a graded strength test performed by applying manual resistance to a body segment in order to evaluate a particular muscle or group of muscles.

manubrium *n* a handle-shaped structure; the upper part of the sternum.

MAOI *abbr* monoamine oxidase inhibitor.

maple syrup urine disease genetic disorder of recessive familial type. Leucine, isoleucine and valine are excreted in excess in urine giving the smell of maple syrup. Symptoms include spasticity, poor feeding and respiratory difficulties; severe damage to the CNS may occur. A diet low in the three amino acids may be effective if started sufficiently early; otherwise the disorder is rapidly fatal. Genetic counselling may be indicated.

marasmus *n* severe protein-energy malnutrition. Wasting away of the body, especially that of a baby. ⇒ failure to thrive, kwashiorkor—marasmic *adj*.

marble bones ⇒ osteopetrosis.

Marburg disease (*syn* green monkey disease) a highly infectious viral haemorrhagic fever characterized by a sudden onset of fever, severe headache and malaise, vomiting, diarrhoea, pharyngitis and mucosal bleeding. Between days 5 and 7 a rash appears. Virus can persist in the body for 2–3 months after the initial attack. Cross infection probably occurs by the aerosol route. Incubation period believed to be 4–9 days. Treatment is symptomatic only and mortality rate in previous outbreaks has been as high as 90%.

march fracture a type of stress fracture caused by an increase in physical activity which may so stress a metatarsal (usually the second) to produce an undisplaced self-healing fracture. There is local pain, tenderness, and radiographic changes. Management usually involves moderate rest with supportive padding and strapping for a few weeks but sometimes a walking plaster is required.

Marfan's syndrome a hereditary genetic disorder of unknown cause. There is dislocation of the lens, congenital heart disease and arachnodactyly with hypotonic musculature and lax ligaments, occasionally excessive height and abnormalities of the iris.

marginal cost the cost of providing the extra resources required to carry out activity above a baseline number.

marihuana, marijuana *n* ⇒ cannabis.

marrow *n* ⇒ bone marrow.

Marshall–Marchetti–Krantz operation for stress incontinence. A form of abdominal cystourethropexy usually undertaken in patients whose loss of continence has not been controlled by a colporrhaphy.

marsupialization *n* an operation for cystic abdominal swellings, which entails stitching the margins of an opening made into the cyst to the edges of the abdominal wound, thus forming a pouch.

masochism *n* the deriving of pleasure from pain inflicted by others or occasionally by oneself. It may be a conscious or unconscious process and is frequently of a sexual nature. ⇒ sadism.

mass number the total mass of neutrons and protons within an atom.

massage *n* **1** several different soft tissue manipulations (kneading, stroking, rubbing, tapping, etc.). They are used at different depths and rates for various purposes: to improve circulation, metabolism and muscle tone, to break down adhesions, to expel gases, and to either relax or stimulate the patient. **2** a complementary therapy that involves the conscious use of gentle muscle manipulation, using stroking or light kneading, to promote relaxation.

mastalgia *n* pain in the breast.

mast cells basophils (type of leucocyte) that have migrated to the tissues. They are located around small blood vessels and bind to IgE before producing chemicals such as histamine that are involved in inflammation and anaphylaxis.

mastectomy *n* surgical removal of the breast. ⇒ lumpectomy. *simple mastectomy* removal of the breast with the overlying skin. *modified radical mastectomy* removal of the entire breast and division or excision of the pectoralis minor muscle with axillary lymph node clearance. *radical mastectomy* rarely performed operation that involves removal of the breast, pectoralis major muscle and clearance of the axillary lymph nodes.

mastication *n* chewing.

mastitis *n* inflammation of the breast. *chronic mastitis* the name formerly applied to the nodular changes in the breasts now usually called fibrocystic disease.

mastoid *adj* nipple-shaped. *mastoid air cells* extend in a backward and downward direction from the antrum. *mastoid antrum* the air space within the mastoid process, lined by mucous membrane continuous with that of the tympanum and mastoid cells. *mastoid process* the prominence of the mastoid portion of the temporal bone just behind the ear.

mastoidectomy *n* drainage of the mastoid air-cells and excision of diseased tissue. *cortical mastoidectomy* all the mastoid cells are removed making one cavity which drains through an opening (aditus) into the middle ear. The external meatus and middle ear are untouched. *radical mastoidectomy* the mastoid antrum, and middle ear are made into one continuous cavity for drainage of infection. Loss of hearing is inevitable.

mastoiditis *n* inflammation of the mastoid air-cells.

mastopexy *n* surgical fixation of a pendulous breast.

masturbation *n* non-coital sexual arousal and orgasm by stimulation of the genitalia.

materia medica the science dealing with the origin, action and dosage of drugs.

matriarchy *n* describes a situation where a female (wife, mother or daughter) inherits, dominates and controls within a social structure.

matrix *n* the foundation substance in which the tissue cells are embedded.

maturation *n* the process of attaining full development. Describes the final stage in wound healing, during which the wound is strengthened and the scar gradually fades and shrinks.

maturity onset diabetes of the young (MODY) an uncommon subtype of type 2 diabetes caused by a single gene defect.

Accounts for <5% of cases of type 2 diabetes.

maxilla *n* the jawbone; in particular the upper jaw—**maxillary** *adj*.

maxillofacial *adj* pertaining to the maxilla and face. *maxillofacial surgery* branch of surgery concerned with the surgical management of developmental disorders and diseases of the facial structure.

maximum heart rate (HRmax) a term used in sports medicine to describe an individual's maximum heart rate. HRmax is calculated by subtracting the person's age in years from 220 (HRmax = 220 − age in years).

MBC *abbr* maximal breathing capacity. ⇒ respiratory function tests.

MCA *abbr* Medicines Control Agency.

McBurney's point a point one-third of the way between the anterior superior iliac spine and the umbilicus, the site of maximum tenderness in cases of acute appendicitis.

McMurray's osteotomy division of femur between lesser and greater trochanter. Shaft displaced inwards beneath the head and abducted. This position maintained by a nail plate. Restores painless weight bearing. In developmental dysplasia of the hip, deliberate pelvic osteotomy renders the outer part of the socket (acetabulum) more horizontal.

MDA *abbr* Medical Devices Agency.

MDM *abbr* mental defence mechanism.

MDR-TB *abbr* multidrug resistant tuberculosis.

mean *n* the average. *arithmetic mean* a figure arrived at by dividing the sum of a set of values by the number of items in the set. ⇒ central tendency statistic, median, mode.

measles *n* (*syn* morbilli) an acute infectious disease caused by a virus. It is highly contagious and spreads via droplets. The incubation period is about 10 days. It starts with a cold-like illness, cough, fever, sore and watery eyes, Koplik's spots and photophobia. After 3–4 days a maculopapular rash appears. Complications include secondary bacterial infections such as pneumonia or otitis media, corneal ulceration and encephalitis. Active immunization is offered as part of routine programmes. Endemic and worldwide in distribution.

meatotomy *n* surgery to the urinary meatus for meatal stricture in men.

meatus *n* an opening or channel—**meatal** *adj*.

mechanical ventilation ⇒ intermittent positive pressure ventilation.

mechanism of labour the series of passive movements of the baby as it descends through the birth canal propelled by the uterine contractions.

Meckel's diverticulum a blind, pouch-like sac sometimes arising from the free border of the lower ileum. Occurs in 2% of the population: usually symptomless. May cause gastrointestinal bleeding or intussusception.

meconium *n* the discharge from the bowel of a neonate. It is a greenish-black, viscid substance. *meconium ileus* impaction of meconium in bowel. It is one presentation of cystic fibrosis.

media 1 *n* the middle coat of a vessel. **2** *pl* nutritive jellies used for culturing bacteria. ⇒ medium.

medial *adj* pertaining to or near the midline, or to the middle layer of a structure—**medially** *adv*.

median *adj* **1** the middle. *median line* an imaginary line passing through the centre of the body from a point between the eyes to between the closed feet. *median nerve* ⇒ Figure 11. *median plane* a vertical plane that divides the body into right and left halves. Also called the midsagittal plane. *median vein* ⇒ Figure 10. **2** a central tendency statistic; the midway or middle value in a set of scores when placed in increasing order. ⇒ mean, mode.

mediastinoscopy *n* a minor endoscopic surgical procedure for visual inspection of the mediastinum. May be combined with biopsy of the lymph nodes for histological examination, and diagnosis or staging in the case of cancer.

mediastinotomy *n* incision of the mediastinum.

mediastinum *n* the space between the lungs. Contains the heart, great vessels and the oesophagus—**mediastinal** *adj*.

Medical Devices Agency (MDA) in the UK, an agency that works with government, users and manufacturers to ensure that medical devices meet the appropriate safety, quality and efficacy standards.

medical jurisprudence ⇒ forensic medicine.

medicament *n* a medicine or remedy. ⇒ drug.

medicated *adj* impregnated with a medicine or drug.

medication *n* a therapeutic substance or drug, administered orally or by injection intra-arterially, subcutaneously, intramuscularly, intravenously, or rectally, topically, transdermally or sublingually.

medicinal *adj* pertaining to a medicine.

medicine *n* **1** science or art of healing, especially as distinguished from surgery and obstetrics. **2** a therapeutic substance. ⇒ drug.

Medicines Control Agency in the UK a government agency responsible for licensing new drugs. Decisions are made on the efficacy, quality and safety of the drug.

medicochirurgical *adj* pertaining to both medicine and surgery.

medicosocial *adj* pertaining to medicine and sociology.

mediolateral *adj* pertaining to the middle and one side.

meditation *n* an altered state achieved by rituals and exercises. It aims to produce relaxation (physical and mental). May be used as part of stress management strategies.

medium *n* a substance used in bacteriology for the growth of micro-organisms— **media** *pl*.

Medline *n* computerized database of medical science and associated literature.

medulla *n* **1** the marrow in the centre of a long bone. **2** the internal part of organs, e.g. kidneys, adrenals and lymph nodes, etc. *medulla oblongata* the lowest part of the brainstem where it passes through the foramen magnum to become the spinal cord. It contains the nerve centres controlling various vital functions, e.g. cardiac centres. ⇒ Figure 1.

medullary *adj* pertaining to the medulla.

medullated *adj* containing or surrounded by a medulla or marrow, particularly referring to myelinated nerve fibres.

medulloblastoma *n* malignant, rapidly growing tumour occurring in children; usually in the midline of the cerebellum.

megacephalic *adj* (*syn* macrocephalic, megalocephalic) large headed.

megacolon *n* dilatation of the colon. *acquired megacolon* associated with chronic constipation of any cause, or may occur in acute severe colitis of any cause (toxic megacolon). *congenital megacolon (Hirschsprung's disease)* due to absence of ganglionic cells in a distal segment of the colon with loss of relaxation resulting in dilatation of the normal proximal colon.

megakaryocyte *n* large multinucleated cells of the marrow that produce platelets (thrombocytes).

megaloblast *n* a large, nucleated, primitive red blood cell formed where there is a deficiency of vitamin B_{12} or folate— **megaloblastic** *adj*.

megaloblastic anaemia an anaemia caused by a deficiency of vitamin B_{12} or folate. It results in the formation of large red blood cells called megaloblasts.

megalocephalic *adj* ⇒ megacephalic.

megalomania *n* delusion of grandeur, characteristic of general paralysis of the insane.

meibomian cyst ⇒ chalazion.

meibomian glands sebaceous glands lying in grooves on the inner surface of the eyelids, their ducts opening on the free margins of the lids.

Meigs syndrome a benign, solid ovarian tumour associated with ascites and hydrothorax.

meiosis *n* the process which, through two successive cell divisions, results in the production of mature gametes—oocytes or spermatozoa. There is pairing of the partner chromosomes, which separate from each other at the meiotic divisions, so that the diploid (2n) chromosome number (i.e. 23 pairs) is reduced by half to 23 chromosomes, only one chromosome of each original pair: this set being the haploid (n) complement. ⇒ mitosis, gamete.

melaena *n* black, tar-like stools. Evidence of gastrointestinal bleeding.

melancholia *n* depression—from the Latin for black bile—**melancholic** *adj*.

melanin *n* a brown/black pigment found in hair, skin and the choroid of the eye.

melanocytes *npl* cells in the skin that produce melanin when stimulated by the pituitary hormone *melanocyte stimulating hormone (MSH)*.

melanoma *n* a malignant tumour arising from the pigment-producing cells (melanocytes) of the skin, or of the eye. *malignant melanoma* malignant cutaneous mole or freckle (usually), it is the most dangerous of all skin cancers. Related to overexposure to ultraviolet radiation (sunburn); most common in fair skinned, blond/red haired people. It is characterized by change in colour, shape, size of mole or with bleeding or itching in a mole. The prognosis depends on Breslow thickness; staging involves lymph node status, with sentinel node biopsy (SNB) now becoming an integral part along with computed tomography (CT) scan. Surgery is the only curative treatment with chemotherapy and radiotherapy of limited effectiveness—**melanomatous** *adj*.

melanosis *n* dark pigmentation of surfaces as in Addison's disease, etc. *melanosis coli* brown pigmentation of the colonic mucosa associated with long-term misuse of stimulant laxative drugs—**melanotic** *adj*.

melasma *n* (*syn* chloasma) hypermelanosis of the face, usually in women. Known as *melasma gravidarum* when it occurs during pregnancy.

melatonin *n* a hormone produced by the pineal body (gland) in response to the amount of light entering the eye. Influences sexual development and is involved in reproductive function. Also influences mood and various circadian rhythms, such as body temperature and sleep.

melitensis *n* ⇒ brucellosis.

membrane *n* a thin lining or covering substance—**membranous** *adj*. *basement membrane* a thin layer beneath the epithelium of mucous surfaces. *hyaloid membrane* the transparent capsule surrounding the vitreous humour of the eye. *mucous membrane* contains glands which secrete mucus. It lines the cavities and passages that communicate with the exterior of the body. *serous membrane* a lubricating membrane lining the closed cavities, and reflected over their enclosed organs. *synovial membrane* the membrane lining the intra-articular parts of bones and ligaments. It does not cover the articular surfaces. *tympanic membrane* the eardrum (⇒ Figure 13).

memory *n* the ability to retain and recall prior learning (information and events). It is a very complex process and includes different types of memory. ⇒ episodic memory, long-term memory, procedural memory, semantic memory, short-term memory.

memory lapses many adults have episodes of memory loss and some time later retrieve the appropriate information. The lapses often occur when individuals are under stress and typically increase with age. ⇒ Alzheimer's disease, dementia.

menaquinones *npl* a form of vitamin K produced by bacteria in the gastrointestinal tract.

menarche *n* when menstrual cycles commence.

Mendel's law the fundamental theory of heredity and its laws, evolved by an Austrian monk, Gregor Mendel working with peas. The laws determine the inheritance of different characters, and particularly the interaction of dominant and recessive traits in cross-breeding, the maintenance of the purity of such characters during hereditary transmission and the independent segregation of genetically different characteristics, such as the size of pea plants.

Mendelson syndrome inhalation of regurgitated stomach contents, which can cause immediate death from anoxia, or it may produce extensive lung damage or pulmonary oedema with severe bronchospasm.

Ménière's disease distension of membranous labyrinth of inner ear from excess fluid. Pressure causes failure of function of nerve of balance and hearing (vestibulocochlear); thus there is fluctuating deafness, tinnitus and repeated attacks of vertigo.

meninges *npl* the surrounding membranes of the brain and spinal cord. They are the dura mater (outer), arachnoid membrane (middle) and pia mater (inner). ⇒ meningitis—**meninx** *sing*, **meningeal** *adj*.

meningioma *n* a slowly growing fibrous tumour arising in the meninges—**meningiomata** *pl*, **meningiomatous** *adj*.

meningism *n* (*syn* meningismus) a condition describing irritation and inflammation of the meninges due normally to infection or haemorrhage and consisting of neck stiffness and photophobia.

meningitis *n* inflammation of the meninges around the brain and spinal cord that can be due to an acute bacterial (e.g. meningococcal meningitis) or viral infection, chronic infective and inflammatory conditions and occasionally malignancy.

meningocele *n* protrusion of the meninges through a bony defect. It forms a cyst filled with cerebrospinal fluid. ⇒ spina bifida.

meningococcus *n Neisseria meningitidis*—**meningococcal** *adj*.

meningoencephalitis *n* inflammation of the brain and the meninges—**meningoencephalitic** *adj*.

meningomyelocele *n* (*syn* myelomeningocele) protrusion of a portion of the spinal cord and its enclosing membranes through a bony defect in the spinal canal. It differs from a meningocele in being covered with a thin, transparent membrane which may be granular and moist.

meniscectomy *n* the removal of a semilunar cartilage of the knee joint, following injury and displacement. The medial cartilage is damaged most commonly.

meniscus *n* **1** semilunar cartilage, particularly in the knee joint. **2** the curved upper surface of a column of liquid—**menisci** *pl*.

menopause *n* the ending of menstruation. A single event occurring during the climacteric. It normally occurs between the ages of 45 and 55 years. *artificial menopause* an earlier menopause caused by surgery or radiotherapy—**menopausal** *adj*.

menorrhagia *n* an excessive regular menstrual flow.

menses *n* fluid discharged from the uterus during menstruation; menstrual flow.

menstrual *adj* relating to the menses. *menstrual or uterine cycle* the cyclical changes that occur as the endometrium responds to ovarian hormones. There are three phases: proliferative, secretory, and menstrual in which bleeding occurs for around 5 days. The cycle is repeated approximately every 28 days (21–35), except during pregnancy, from the menarche to the menopause.

menstruation *n* the flow of blood and endometrial debris from the uterus once a month in the female. It usually starts at the age of 12–13 years in developed countries, and ceases around 50 years of age.

mental *adj* pertaining to the mind. *mental aberration* a pathological deviation from normal thinking. *mental age* the age of a person with regard to his intellectual development, which can be determined by intelligence tests. *mental disorder* mental illness, arrested or incomplete development of the mind, psychopathic disorder and any other disorder or disability of the mind. As defined by Mental Health Act 1983. ⇒ mental health legislation. *Mental Health Review Tribunal* a body set up in each Regional Health Authority (in England and Wales, with a separate but similar system in Northern Ireland) to deal with patients' applications for discharge or alteration of their detention in hospital. In Scotland requests for review are made to a Mental Health Commission or by appeal to a sheriff. *Mental Health Welfare Officer* ⇒ approved social worker (ASW).

mental defence mechanism (MDM) unconscious defence mechanism by which individuals attempt to cope with stressful, difficult or threatening emotions. ⇒ compensation, conversion, denial, displacement, fantasy, identification, intellectualization, projection, rationalization, regression, repression, sublimation, suppression, withdrawal.

mental health legislation law pertaining to mental disorder. For example, in England & Wales the main body of mental health legislation is the Mental Health Act 1983, which regulates the circumstances in which the liberty of mentally disordered persons may be restricted. The Mental Health (Patients in the Community) Act 1995 amended the 1983 Act by providing for the 'supervised discharge' of those detained patients requiring a 'high degree' of supervision on discharge from hospital.

mentoanterior *adj* forward position of the fetal chin in the maternal pelvis in a face presentation.

mentoposterior *adj* backward position of the fetal chin in the maternal pelvis in a face presentation.

mercurialism *n* chronic poisoning with mercury. It may occur in individuals who are exposed to mercury at work, or it may be ingested in food, such as fish in some areas of the world, which may contain high levels. The effects of poisoning include loose teeth, stomatitis, gastrointestinal effects, renal problems, paraesthesia, ataxia, and visual and hearing problems.

mercury (Hg) *n* metallic element that is liquid at room temperature. Previously used in thermometers and sphygmomanometers. Toxicity means that local safety protocols should be followed in situations involving accidental spillage and contamination. Forms two series of salts: univalent mercurous salts and bivalent mercuric. ⇒ mercurialism.

meridians *npl* in complementary therapy the conceptual channels in which Qi energy flows. ⇒ acupuncture, shiatsu.

mesarteritis *n* inflammation of the middle coat of an artery.

mesencephalon *n* the midbrain.

messenger RNA (mRNA) ⇒ ribonucleic acid.

mesentery *n* a large sling-like fold of peritoneum passing between a portion of the intestine and the posterior abdominal wall. Contains nerves, lymphatics and blood vessels—**mesenteric** *adj*.

mesoderm *n* middle layer of the three primary germ layers of the early embryo. It gives rise to the cardiovascular system, lymphatic system, bone, muscles, blood, the dermis, pericardium, pleura, peritoneum, urogenital tract, gonads and the adrenal cortex. ⇒ ectoderm, endoderm.

mesophile *n* a bacterium that thrives within the range 25–40°C. Most human pathogens thrive best at body temperature (37°C)—**mesophilic** *adj*.

mesothelioma *n* neoplasm of the pleura (commonly), pericardium or peritoneum; usually associated with asbestos exposure at least 20 years previously. Industrially related, therefore compensation usually appropriate as few are operable and the median survival post diagnosis is around 8 months. Therapy is almost universally palliative; generally chemo- and radio-resistant.

mesovarium *n* a double fold of peritoneum that attaches the ovary to the broad ligament.

meta-analysis *n* a statistical summary of several research studies using complex quantitative analysis of the primary data.

metabolic *adj* pertaining to metabolism. *basal metabolic rate (BMR)* the expression of basal metabolism in terms of kJ per m^2 of body surface per hour—**metabolically** *adv*.

metabolism *n* the continuous series of chemical processes in the living body by which life is maintained. Nutrients and tissues are broken down (catabolism), new substances are created for growth and rebuilding (anabolism) and energy is released in catabolism and utilized in anabolism and heat production ⇒ adenosine diphosphate, adenosine triphosphate—**metabolic** *adj*. *basal metabolism* the minimum energy expended in the maintenance of essential physiological processes such as respiration.

metabolite *n* any product of or substance taking part in metabolism. An *essential metabolite* one that is necessary for normal metabolism, e.g. vitamins.

metacarpophalangeal *adj* pertaining to the metacarpus and the phalanges.

metacarpus *n* the five bones which form that part of the hand between the wrist and fingers ⇒ Figure 2—**metacarpal** *adj*.

metaplasia *n* process of substituting one type of mature epithelium for a different type of mature epithelium that is better suited to cope with the adverse environment which triggered the process.

metastasis *n* the secondary spread of malignant tumour cells from one part of the body to another. Either by the lymphatic route to the lymph nodes or to distant organs via the haematogenous (blood) route. Most solid tumours are not curable if metastasis has occurred—**metastases** *pl*, **metastatic** *adj*, **metastasize** *vi*.

metatarsalgia *n* pain under the metatarsal heads. *Morton's metatarsalgia* neuralgia caused by a neuroma on the digital nerve, most commonly that supplying the third toe cleft.

metatarsophalangeal *adj* pertaining to the metatarsus and the phalanges.

metatarsus *n* the five bones of the foot between the ankle and the toes (⇒ Figure 2). *metatarsus adductus* a deformity where the forefoot is deviated towards the midline of the body in relation to the hindfoot, as in talipes but without equinus or inversion—**metatarsal** *adj.*

methadone *n* a synthetic opioid analgesic. It is used as part of a heroin withdrawal programme.

methaemalbumin *n* abnormal compound formed in blood from combination of haem with plasma albumin, under conditions of grossly accelerated red cell breakdown (haemolysis).

methaemoglobin *n* a form of haemoglobin consisting of a combination of globin with an oxidized haem, containing ferric iron. This pigment is unable to transport oxygen. It may be formed following the administration of a wide variety of drugs, including the sulphonamides. It may also be present in the blood as a result of a congenital abnormality.

methaemoglobinaemia *n* methaemoglobin in the blood. If large quantities are present, individuals may show cyanosis, but otherwise no abnormality except, in severe cases, breathlessness on exertion, because the methaemoglobin cannot transport oxygen—**methaemoglobinaemic** *adj.*

methane *n* CH_4 a colourless, odourless, inflammable gas that results from the decomposition of organic matter.

methicillin-resistant *Staphylococcus aureus* **(MRSA)** *n* strains of *Staphylococcus aureus* that are resistant to methicillin (not used clinically) and flucloxacillin. Causes serious and sometimes fatal infections in hospitals, and patients with MRSA are increasingly encountered outside hospital. Treatment involves vancomycin or teicoplanin, or various combinations of rifampicin, sodium fusidate and ciprofloxacin. Topical mupirocin is used to eliminate nasal or skin carriage. Infection control measures that include strict adherence to hand washing, proper environmental cleaning and isolation or patient cohorting are vital in controlling MRSA. Epidemic strains (EMRSA) have developed resistance to most antibiotics except glycopeptides, i.e. vancomycin and teicoplanin.

methionine *n* one of the essential (indispensable) sulphur-containing amino acids. Occasionally used in the treatment of hepatitis, paracetamol overdose and other conditions associated with liver damage.

methylcellulose *n* a bulk-forming laxative. ⇒ Appendix 5.

metritis *n* inflammation of the uterus.

metrorrhagia *n* uterine bleeding between the menstrual periods such as after intercourse or examination.

MHC *abbr* major histocompatibility complex.

micelle tiny globules of fat and bile salts formed during fat digestion. Fatty acids and glycerol are transported into the intestinal cells (enterocytes) in this form, leaving the bile salts behind in the lumen of the bowel.

microaneurysm *n* dilatation of retinal vessel. May bleed or leak. Common in diabetic retinopathy.

microangiopathy *n* small vessel disease, with basement membrane thickening and endothelial dysfunction, usually in association with diabetes mellitus, but also seen in patients with connective tissue disease, infection and malignancy; results in retinopathy and nephropathy in patients with diabetes.

microbe *n* ⇒ micro-organism—**microbial, microbic** *adj.*

microbiology *n* the science of micro-organisms—**microbiological** *adj.*

microcephaly *n* an abnormally small head.

microcirculation *n* blood flow through the arterioles, capillaries and venules. Damage to these vessels is a cause of pressure ulcers.

Micrococcus *n* a genus of Gram-positive bacteria. Generally non-pathogenic, they are part of the skin flora.

microcyte *n* an undersized red blood cell found for example in iron deficiency anaemia.

microcytosis an increased number of microcytes—**microcytic** *adj.*

microdissection *n* dissection of tissue or cells under the microscope.

microenvironment *n* the environment at the microscopic or cellular level immediately surrounding the body.

microfilaria *n* immature filaria ⇒ filariasis.

microglial cells a type of macrophage of the central nervous system.

micrognathia *n* small jaw, especially the lower one.

microgram (μg) *n* one millionth of a gram.

micrometre (μm) *n* also still called a micron. One millionth of a metre.

micron *n* ⇒ micrometre.

micronutrients *npl* nutrients needed by the body in relatively small amounts such as vitamins. ⇒ macronutrients, trace elements.

micro-organism *n* (*syn* microbe) a microscopic cell. Often synonymous with bacterium but includes virus, protozoon, rickettsia, chlamydia and fungus.

microscopic *adj* extremely small; visible only with the aid of a microscope. ⇒ macroscopic *opp*.

Microsporum *n* a genus of fungi. Parasitic, living in keratin-containing tissues of humans and animals. *Microsporum audouini* is the commonest cause of scalp ringworm.

microsurgery *n* use of the binocular operating microscope during the performance of operations—**microsurgical** *adj*.

microtome *n* an instrument used for cutting tissue sections for microscopic study, usually in the order of 4–6 micrometres in thickness.

microtrauma *n* injury to a small number of cells due to the cumulative effect of repetitive forces.

microvascular surgery surgery carried out on blood vessels using a binocular operating microscope.

microvilli *npl* microscopic projections from the free surface of cell membranes whose purpose is to increase the exposed surface of the cell for absorption, e.g. intestinal epithelium.

micturating cystogram radiographic examination that can be used to investigate urinary incontinence. Following intravenous injection of a contrast medium or, more commonly, after contrast is introduced into the bladder via a urinary catheter until micturating begins. A series of X-rays are taken during the act of passing urine.

micturition *n* (*syn* urination) passing urine.

midbrain *n* ⇒ Figure 1.

midriff *n* the diaphragm.

midsagittal plane ⇒ median plane.

migraine *n* a type of headache that recurs and is characterized by its unilateral nature, nausea, vomiting, photophobia and phonophobia. It can be associated with neurological symptoms and signs such as visual phenomena—**migrainous** *adj*.

Mikulicz disease chronic hypertrophic enlargement of the lacrimal and salivary glands.

miliaria *n* (*syn* strophulus) prickly heat common in the tropics, and affects waistline, cubital fossae and chest. Vesicular and erythematous eruption, caused by blocking of sweat ducts and their subsequent rupture, or their infection by fungi or bacteria.

miliary *adj* resembling a millet seed. *miliary tuberculosis* ⇒ tuberculosis.

milium *n* condition in which tiny, white, cystic excrescences appear on the face, especially about the eyelids; the cysts contain keratin—**milia** *pl*.

milk *n* secretion of the mammary glands. Provided that the mother is taking an adequate diet, human milk contains all the essential nutrients in the correct proportions for the first 4–6 months of life. It contains IgA and lactoferrin which increases the newborn infant's resistance to infection. *milk sugar* lactose.

Miller–Abbott tube a double-lumen tube used for intestinal suction. The second channel leads to a balloon near the tip of the tube.

milligram (mg) *n* one thousandth part of a gram.

millilitre (mL) *n* one thousandth part of a litre. Equal to a cubic centimetre.

millimetre (mm) *n* one thousandth part of a metre.

millimole (mmol) *n* one thousandth part of a mole.

Milwaukee brace an orthotic device used in the corrective treatment of spinal curvature (scoliosis). It applies fixed traction between the occiput and the pelvis.

mineralocorticoid *n* a group of corticosteroid hormones produced by the adrenal cortex. Involved in the regulation of electrolyte and water balance. ⇒ aldosterone.

minerals *npl* inorganic elements required in the diet. They perform a vital role in body structure and functions. They are: calcium, chloride, iron, magnesium, phosphorus, potassium, sodium and zinc, and the trace elements cobalt, chromium, copper, fluoride, iodine, manganese, molybdenum and selenium.

minimally invasive surgery known colloquially as 'key hole surgery'. Surgical techniques that only require minimal access; the procedure is performed through very small incisions using endoscopic instruments. A variety of procedures are undertaken, e.g. cholecystectomy. ⇒ laparoscopy.

Mini Mental State Examination (MMSE) a test of cognitive function used to screen for dementia.

miosis (myosis) *n* constriction of the pupil of the eye.

miotic (myotic) *adj* an agent that causes miosis.

miscarriage *n* spontaneous loss of pregnancy before 24 completed weeks of gestation (previously referred to as abortion). *complete miscarriage* the entire contents of the uterus are expelled. *incomplete miscarriage* part of the fetus or placenta is retained in the uterus. ⇒ evacuation of retained products of conception. *inevitable miscarriage* loss of the pregnancy cannot be prevented. *missed miscarriage* the early signs and symptoms of pregnancy disappear and the fetus dies but is not expelled for some time. ⇒ carneous mole. *recurrent or habitual miscarriage* when miscarriage occurs in three successive pregnancies. *septic miscarriage* one associated with uterine infection. *spontaneous miscarriage* one which occurs naturally without intervention. *threatened miscarriage* characterized by slight vaginal bleeding whilst the cervix remains closed. *tubal miscarriage* an ectopic pregnancy that dies and is expelled from the fimbriated end of the uterine (fallopian) tube.

missed abortion ⇒ miscarriage.

Misuse of Drugs Act (1971, Regulations 1985) in UK. Controls the manufacture, sale, possession, supply, storage, prescribing, dispensing and administration of certain groups of habit-forming drugs that are liable to misuse and dependence. They are called controlled drugs and are available to the public by medical prescription only. Drugs subject to the Act include the opioids, synthetic narcotics,

cocaine, hallucinogens and barbiturates (with exceptions). The individual drugs include cocaine, diamorphine, methadone and pethidine.

mitochondrion *n* membrane-bound subcellular organelles situated in the cytoplasm. They are the principal sites of ATP production from the oxidation of fuel molecules. They contain nucleic acids (DNA and RNA) and ribosomes, replicate independently, and synthesize some of their own proteins. They are particularly numerous in metabolically active cells, such as skeletal muscle and liver.

mitosis *n* nuclear (and usually cell) division, in which somatic cells divide. It involves the exact replication of chromosomes, which results in two 'daughter' cells that are genetically identical to the cell of origin, i.e. they have the diploid (2n) chromosome number, 46 in humans. ⇒ meiosis—**mitoses** *pl*, **mitotic** *adj*.

mitral *adj* mitre-shaped, as the valve between the left atrium and ventricle of the heart (bicuspid valve). *mitral regurgitation (incompetence)* a defect in the closure of the mitral valve whereby blood tends to flow backwards into the left atrium from the left ventricle. *mitral stenosis* narrowing of the mitral orifice, usually due to rheumatic fever. *mitral valvulotomy (valvotomy)* an operation to correct a stenosed mitral valve.

mittelschmerz *n* abdominal pain midway between menstrual periods, at time of ovulation.

mixed venous oxygen saturation (S$\bar{v}$O$_2$) percentage of oxygenated haemoglobin in venous blood returning to the lungs, measured in blood taken from the pulmonary artery.

MLC *abbr* multi-leaf collimation.

MLNS *abbr* mucocutaneous lymph node syndrome.

MMR *abbr* measles, mumps and rubella (vaccine).

MMSE *abbr* Mini Mental State Examination.

mobilizations *npl* the manual manipulations of spinal and peripheral (limb) joints in order to free them to move more normally. Physiotherapists use several methods named for their developers, e.g. Maitland mobilizations. Whereas osteopaths and chiropractors mobilize joints with the aim of restoring function, physiotherapists also mobilize muscles, nerves and other soft tissues in order to relieve pain and restore freedom of movement.

mobilize *v* to make ready for movement. *mobilizing a patient* locomotion. *mobilize joints and soft tissues* free them to move more normally.

mode *n* the most frequent (common) value in a series of scores. ⇒ central tendency statistic, mean, median.

modelling *n* a psychological term describing the way people learn from watching and copying the behaviour of others.

MODS *abbr* multiple organ dysfunction syndrome.

MODY *abbr* maturity onset diabetes of the young.

Mohs' micrographic surgery a surgical technique for microscopically controlled excision usually of a malignant skin tumour.

moist wound healing achieved by application of an occlusive, semipermeable dressing which permits the exudate to collect under the film to carry out its bactericidal functions.

molality *n* the concentration of a solution expressed as the number of moles of solute (substance) per kilogram of solvent.

molar *adj* containing one mole of solute (substance) per litre of solution.

molarity *n* the concentration of a solution expressed as the number of moles of solute (substance) per litre of solution (mol/L).

molar tooth multi-cusped posterior grinding tooth, placed fourth and fifth from the midline in the primary dentition, and sixth, seventh and eighth in the secondary dentition.

mole *n* **1** one of the seven base units of the International System of Units (SI). The measurement of amount of substance (*abbr* mol). **2** a pigmented area on the skin, usually brown. They may be flat, some are raised and occasionally have hairs growing from them. Alterations in shape, colour, size, or bleeding may be indicative of malignant changes.

molecule *n* a combination of two or more atoms to form a specific chemical substance—**molecular** *adj. molecular weight* the sum of the atomic weights of atoms in a molecule.

mollities *n* softness. *mollities ossium* osteomalacia.

molluscum *n* a soft tumour. *molluscum contagiosum* an infectious condition common in infants caused by a virus. Tiny translucent papules with a central depression are formed. *molluscum fibrosum* the superficial tumours of von Recklinghausen's disease.

monarticular *adj* relating to one joint.

Mönckeberg's sclerosis degenerative change resulting in calcification of the median muscular layer in arteries, especially of the limbs; leads to intermittent claudication and rarely to gangrene, if atherosclerosis coexists.

Monilia *n* ⇒ *Candida*.

moniliasis *n* ⇒ candidiasis.

Monitor *n* an anglicized version of the Rush Medicus quality assurance programme for use in hospitals.

monitoring *n* sequential recording. Term usually reserved for automatic visual display of such measurements as temperature, pulse, respiration and blood pressure.

monoamine *n* organic molecules with one amine (NH_2) group. ⇒ amines.

monoamine oxidase an enzyme that breaks down monoamines, such as dopamine, 5-hydroxytryptamine (serotonin) and noradrenaline (norepinephrine) in the brain.

monoamine oxidase inhibitors (MAOIs) a group of antidepressant drugs that inhibit the action of monoamine oxidase thereby preventing the breakdown of 5-hydroxytryptamine and other monoamines. ⇒ Appendix 5.

monoarthritis *n* arthritis affecting a single joint.

monoclonal *adj* arising from a single cell and its subsequent clones, e.g. *monoclonal antibodies*. These identical specific antibodies are increasingly used in research, and for diagnosis and treatment.

monocular *adj* pertaining to one eye.

monocyte *n* a phagocytic white blood cell. It migrates to the tissues to become a macrophage—**monocytic** *adj*.

monocyte-macrophage system (*syn* reticuloendothelial system) a widely disseminated system of specialized phagocytes in the bone marrow, liver, lymph nodes, spleen, and other tissues. Functions include blood cell and haemoglobin breakdown, formation of bile pigments, removal of cell breakdown products and as part of the defences against microorganisms.

monomania *n* obsession with a single idea.

mononuclear *adj* describes a cell with a single nucleus such as a monocyte.

mononucleosis *n* an increase in the number of circulating monocytes (mononuclear cells) in the blood. ⇒ infectious mononucleosis.

monoplegia *n* paralysis of only one limb—**monoplegic** *adj*.

monosaccharide *n* a single sugar carbohydrate with the general formula CH_2O. Examples are glucose, fructose and galactose. Monosaccharide units are linked together to form disaccharides and polysaccharides.

monosomy *n* the absence of a chromosome from the normal diploid chromosome complement, resulting in 45 chromosomes rather than 46.

monovular *adj* ⇒ uniovular.

monozygotic *adj* relating to one zygote. Describes identical twins that develop from a single zygote that splits into two embryos. ⇒ dizygotic *opp*.

mons veneris the eminence formed by the pad of fat which lies over the pubic bone in the female.

mood *n* an involuntary state of mind or feeling. Mood variations are normal, but frequent swings from depression to overexcitement may be considered abnormal. ⇒ cyclothymia, depression, mania.

Mooren's ulcer peripheral ulcerative keratitis.

morbidity *n* the state of being diseased. *standardized morbidity ratio (SMBR)* the degree of self-reported limiting longterm illness indirectly standardized for variations in age and gender.

morbilli *n* ⇒ measles.

morbilliform *adj* describes a rash resembling that of measles.

moribund *adj* in a dying state.

Moro reflex on being startled a baby throws out his arms, then brings them together in an embracing movement.

morphoea *n* ⇒ scleroderma.

morphology *n* the study of the form and structure of living things—**morphological** *adj*, **morphologically** *adv*.

mortality *n* number or frequency of deaths. *mortality rate* the death rate; the ratio of the total number of deaths to the total population. There are several specialized mortality rates and ratios including: childhood mortality (children aged 1–14 years), infant mortality (first year of life), maternal mortality (deaths associated with pregnancy and childbirth), neonatal mortality (first four weeks of life), perinatal mortality (stillbirths plus deaths in the first week of life), stillbirth rate. ⇒ standardized mortality rate, standardized mortality ratio.

mortification *n* death of tissue. ⇒ gangrene.

Morton's metatarsalgia ⇒ metatarsalgia.

morula *n* a mass of cells formed from the cleavage (by mitosis) of the zygote prior to its implantation in the uterus.

mosquito-transmitted haemorrhagic fevers infections mainly occurring in tropical regions. The important ones are chikungunya, dengue, Rift Valley fever and yellow fever.

motile *adj* able to move spontaneously—**motility** *n*.

motion sickness nausea and vomiting associated with any form of motion such as car or plane.

motor *adj* pertaining to action. *motor neurone(e)* the nerve cell (or neuron) that supplies the electrical input to muscles. This can be either the lower motor neuron that directly innervates the muscles and originates in the brainstem and spinal cord or the upper motor neuron that originates from the motor cortex part of the brain and innervates the lower motor neuron. *motor neuron disease* a group of neurodegenerative disorders affecting the nerves that supply the muscles leading to weakness and eventually death. *motor skill* the ability to perform a particular task which involves significant movement of one or more joints of the body, e.g. as part of a sports skill. *motor unit* a lower motor neuron and all of the muscle fibres it innervates.

mould *n* a multicellular fungus. Often used synonymously with fungus (excluding the yeasts). It consists of filaments or hyphae, which aggregate into a mycelium. Propagates by means of spores. Occurs in infinite variety, as common saprophytes contaminating foodstuffs, and more rarely as pathogens.

moulding *n* the compression of the fetal head during its passage through the genital tract in labour.

mountain sickness symptoms of sickness, tachycardia, headache and dyspnoea caused by the reduced partial pressure of oxygen at high altitudes.

MRI *abbr* magnetic resonance imaging.

MRSA *abbr* methicillin-resistant *Staphylococcus aureus*.

MS *abbr* ⇒ multiple sclerosis.

MSP *abbr* Munchausen syndrome by proxy.

MSU *abbr* midstream specimen of urine.

mucilage *n* the solution of a gum in water—**mucilaginous** *adj*.

mucin *n* glycoprotein constituent of mucus—**mucinous** *adj*.

mucinase *n* a specific mucin-dissolving substance contained in some aerosols. Useful in cystic fibrosis.

mucinolysis *n* breakdown of mucin—**mucinolytic** *adj*.

mucocele *n* distension of a cavity with mucus.

mucocutaneous *adj* pertaining to mucous membrane and skin. *mucocutaneous lymph node syndrome (MLNS)* a disease affecting mainly babies and children. It is an inflammatory vasculitis characterized by fever, dry lips, red mouth and strawberry-like tongue. There is a rash on the trunk, and erythema with desquamation affecting the extremities. There is cervical lymphadenopathy, polymorphonuclear leucocytosis and a raised ESR. Also known as Kawasaki disease.

mucoid *adj* resembling mucus.

mucolytics *npl* drugs which reduce the viscosity of respiratory secretions. ⇒ Appendix 5.

mucopolysaccharide *n* complex polysaccharides found in connective tissue, e.g. chondroitin in cartilage.

mucopolysaccharidoses *npl* a group of inherited metabolic disorders in which the lack of specific enzymes causes the abnormal build-up of mucopolysaccharides. ⇒ gargoylism, Hunter syndrome.

mucopurulent *adj* containing mucus and pus.

mucopus *n* mucus containing pus.

mucosa *n* a mucous membrane—**mucosae** *pl*, **mucosal** *adj*.

mucositis *n* inflammation of a mucous membrane such as the mouth.

mucous *adj* pertaining to or containing mucus. *mucous membrane* ⇒ membrane. *mucous polyp* a growth (adenoma) of mucous membrane which becomes pedunculated.

mucoviscidosis *n* cystic fibrosis.

mucus *n* viscid secretion of mucous glands—**mucous, mucoid** *adj*.

mullerian ducts primitive embryonic ducts that become the internal genitalia in a genetically female embryo. ⇒ wolffian ducts.

multicellular *adj* having many cells.

multigravida *n* (*syn* multipara) a woman who has had more than one pregnancy—**multigravidae** *pl*.

multi-infarct dementia cerebrovascular dementia. A condition arising from progressive occlusion of the blood supply to regions of the brain.

multi-leaf collimation (MLC) a method of customized beam shaping in radiotherapy without the use of lead blocks.

multilobular *adj* possessing many lobes.

multilocular *adj* possessing many small cysts, loculi or pockets.

multinuclear *adj* possessing many nuclei—**multinucleate** *adj*.

multipara *n* ⇒ multigravida—**multiparae** *pl*.

multiple myeloma a form of bone marrow cancer resulting from the accumulation of malignant plasma cells—**myelomata** *pl*, **myelomatous** *adj*. ⇒ Bence Jones protein.

multiple organ dysfunction syndrome (MODS) syndrome in critically ill patients in which more than one organ system (e.g. kidneys, coagulation, gastrointestinal and respiratory) fails to function normally, may progress to multiple organ failure. It requires appropriate organ support such as mechanical ventilation and haemofiltration. ⇒ acute respiratory distress syndrome, disseminated intravascular coagulation, renal failure, systemic inflammatory response syndrome.

multiple sclerosis (MS) (*syn* disseminated sclerosis) a variably progressive inflammatory demyelinating disease of the central nervous system. It is possibly triggered by infection by one or more viruses and most commonly affects young adults in whom patchy, degenerative changes occur in nerve sheaths in the brain, spinal cord and optic nerves, followed by sclerosis. The presenting symptoms can be diverse, ranging from diplopia to weakness or unsteadiness of a limb; disturbances of micturition are common.

multiprofessional *adj* relating to teamwork among practitioners from different health-care professions working side by side. ⇒ interprofessional.

multivariate statistics analysis of three or more variables simultaneously. Used to clarify the association of two variables after allowing for other variables.

mumps *n* (*syn* infectious parotitis) an acute, specific inflammation of the parotid glands, caused by a virus. Spread is by droplets and the incubation period is around 18 days. There is fever, malaise, parotid salivary gland swelling and pain. Complications include pancreatitis, orchitis, oophoritis and meningitis. Active immunization is offered as part of routine programmes.

Munchausen syndrome ⇒ factitious disorder. *Munchausen syndrome by proxy (MSP)* the production of factitious disorders in a child by an adult, usually a parent or care giver.

mural *adj* pertaining to the wall of a structure.

murmur *n* (*syn* bruit) abnormal sound heard on auscultation of heart or great vessels. *presystolic murmur* characteristic of mitral stenosis.

Musca *n* genus of the common housefly, capable of transmitting many enteric infections.

muscarinic *adj* a type of cholinergic receptor where muscarine would, if present, bind in place of acetylcholine. ⇒ nicotinic.

muscarinic agonists (*syn* parasympathomimetic) a group of drugs that stimulate or mimic parasympathetic activity. They have structural similarities with the neurotransmitter acetylcholine. ⇒ Appendix 5.

muscarinic antagonists (antimuscarinic drugs) (*syn* parasympatholytic) a group of drugs that prevent the action of acetylcholine at the muscarinic receptors, thereby inhibiting cholinergic nerve transmission. ⇒ Appendix 5.

muscle *n* one of the four basic tissues. Composed of specialized contractile tissue formed from excitable cells. (⇒ Figures 4, 5)—**muscular** *adj*. There are three types: *cardiac muscle* makes up the middle wall of the heart; it is involuntary, striated and innervated by autonomic nerves. *skeletal muscle* is voluntary, striated and innervated by the peripheral nerves of the central nervous system. ⇒ muscle fibre, red muscle, white muscle. *smooth or involuntary muscle* is non-striated and involuntary and is innervated by the autonomic nerves.

muscle fibre a muscle cell. Skeletal muscle fibres are classified according to type of action and metabolism: *muscle fibre type I (slow twitch)* fibres are characterized by relatively slow contraction time and high aerobic capacity. They are well suited to long duration activities. *muscle fibre type IIa (fast oxidative glycolytic)* fibres that are classed as fast-twitch but have some of the aerobic characteristics of slow-twitch fibres. *muscle fibre type IIb (fast twitch glycolytic)* fibres characterized by very fast contraction time and high anaerobic capacity. They are well suited to high explosive activities. *muscle fibre type FT type C* fibres thought to function at the extreme end of the anaerobic metabolic range.

muscle relaxant drug used during general anaesthesia to produce muscle paralysis.

muscle spasm involuntary muscle contraction involving the entire muscle; may occur secondary to injury, fatigue or pain.

muscular dystrophies a group of genetically transmitted diseases; they are all characterized by progressive atrophy of different groups of muscles with loss of strength and increasing disability and deformity. Pseudohypertrophic or Duchenne type is the most severe. Presents in early childhood. ⇒ Duchenne muscular dystrophy.

muscular endurance the ability of a muscle or group of muscles to produce force over an extended period of time, i.e. to perform repeated contractions against a sub-maximal load.

muscular power the ability of a muscle(s) to produce a force at a given time.

muscular strength the amount of force a muscle or group of muscles can exert. The ability to resist or produce a force.

musculature *n* the muscular system, or any part of it.

musculocutaneous *adj* pertaining to muscle and skin.

musculoskeletal *adj* pertaining to the muscular and skeletal systems.

mutagen *n* any agent that causes a gene or chromosome mutation.

mutagenesis *n* the creation of mutations—**mutagenic**, **mutagenetic** *adj*, **mutagenetically** *adv*.

mutagenicity *n* the capacity to produce gene mutations or chromosome aberrations.

mutant *n* a cell (or organism) that has a genetic change or mutation.

mutation *n* a gene or chromosome alteration that results in genetic changes that alter the characteristics of the affected cell. The change is transmitted through succeeding generations. Mutations may be spontaneous, or induced by agents such as ionizing radiation that alter the chromosomal DNA.

mute 1 *adj* unable to speak. **2** *n* a person who is unable to speak.

mutilation *n* the condition resulting from the removal of a limb or other part of the body. It results in a change of body image, to which there has to be considerable physical, psychological and social adjustment for a successful outcome.

mutism *n* (*syn* dumbness) inability or refusal to speak. It may be due to congenital causes, the most common being deafness; it may be the result of physical disease, such as a stroke, and it can be a manifestation of mental health problems.

myalgia *n* pain in the muscles—**myalgic** *adj*. *epidemic myalgia* ⇒ Bornholm disease. *myalgic encephalomyelitis* ⇒ benign myalgic encephalomyelitis.

myasthenia *n* muscular weakness—**myasthenic** *adj*. *myasthenia gravis* an autoimmune disorder in which an antibody reduces the efficiency of transmission between the motor neuron and muscle. The antibody blocks receptor sites at the neuromuscular junctions and prevents the normal action of acetylcholine and nerve impulse transmission. In many cases there is a disorder of the thymus gland. It is characterized by marked fatigue affecting the voluntary muscles, especially following exercise. Other muscles involved include those of the eye, shoulder girdle and those required for speaking, swallowing, chewing and breathing.

myasthenic crisis a sudden deterioration with weakness of respiratory muscles due to an increase in severity of myasthenia. It is distinguished from cholinergic crisis by giving edrophonium chloride intravenously. Marked improvement confirms myasthenic crisis. ⇒ edrophonium test.

mycelium *n* a mass of branching filaments (hyphae) of moulds or fungi—**mycelial** *adj*.

mycetoma *n* (*syn* Madura foot) chronic fungal disease affecting soft tissues and bones of the limbs (usually the foot), but it may occur in other sites. It causes swelling, nodules and sinus formation.

Mycobacterium *n* a genus of Gram-positive acid-fast bacteria. *Mycobacterium avium intracellulare (MAI)* atypical mycobacterium that causes infection in humans. *Mycobacterium bovis* causes tuberculosis in cattle. It can be transmitted to humans. *Mycobacterium leprae* causes leprosy and *Mycobacterium tuberculosis* causes tuberculosis.

mycologist *n* an expert in mycology.

mycology *n* the study of fungi—**mycological** *adj*, **mycologically** *adv*.

Mycoplasma *n* a genus of very small microorganisms. They have features in common with bacteria, but lack a cell wall. Some are parasites, some are saprophytes and others are pathogens; for example *Mycoplasma pneumoniae* causes primary atypical pneumonia.

mycosis *n* disease caused by any fungus—**mycotic** *adj*.

mycosis fungoides a lymphoma that initially may present as scaly patches on the skin. In later stages, large tumours may develop. It is not fungal in origin.

mycotoxins *npl* the secondary metabolites of moulds or microfungi. Many chemical substances have been identified as mycotoxins, some of which are carcinogenic as well as causing other diseases—**mycotoxic** *adj*.

mydriasis *n* dilatation of the pupil of the eye.

mydriatics *npl* drugs which dilate the pupil (mydriasis). ⇒ Appendix 5.

myelin *n* the white, fatty substance that covers and insulates some nerve fibres. ⇒ white matter.

myelitis *n* inflammation of the spinal cord.

myeloablative *adj* describes the therapy (e.g. radiotherapy, chemotherapy) given intentionally to completely 'knock out' the bone marrow. Used in leukaemia and often precedes a bone marrow transplant.

myeloblasts *npl* the early precursor cells of the polymorphonuclear granulocytic white blood cells—**myeloblastic** *adj*.

myelocele *n* an accompaniment of spina bifida wherein development of the spinal cord itself has been arrested, and the central canal of the cord opens on the skin surface discharging cerebrospinal fluid.

myelocytes *npl* precursor cells of polymorphonuclear granulocytic white blood cells—**myelocytic** *adj*.

myelofibrosis *n* a myeloproliferative disorder characterized by the formation of fibrous tissue within the bone marrow cavity. Interferes with the formation of blood cells.

myelogenous *adj* produced in or by the bone marrow.

myelography *n* radiographic examination of the spinal canal by injection of a contrast medium into the subarachnoid space. Superseded by CT and MRI—**myelographic** *adj*, **myelogram** *n*, **myelograph** *n*, **myelographically** *adv*.

myeloid *adj* **1** pertaining to the granulocyte precursor cells in the bone marrow. ⇒ leukaemia. **2** pertaining to the bone marrow.

myeloma ⇒ multiple myeloma.

myelomatosis *n* ⇒ multiple myeloma, Bence Jones protein.

myelomeningocele *n* ⇒ meningomyelocele.

myelopathy *n* disease of the spinal cord. Can be a serious complication of cervical spondylosis—**myelopathic** *adj*.

myeloproliferative disorders condition where there is proliferation of one or more of the cellular components of the bone marrow such as myelofibrosis, primary proliferative polycythaemia and thrombocythaemia. ⇒ leukaemia, polycythaemia.

myocardial infarction death of a part of the myocardium (heart muscle) from deprivation of blood following occlusion of a coronary artery, for example from thrombosis. The patient experiences a 'heart attack' with sudden intense chest pain which may radiate to arms and lower jaw. Management includes: aspirin, thrombolytic therapy, pain relief, antiemetics, oxygen therapy, bed rest, observations including continuous ECG and later mobilization and cardiac rehabilitation. Patients should be cared for in a coronary care unit for 12–24 hours because of the risk of life-threatening arrhythmias such as ventricular fibrillation, and the need for skilled staff to monitor the effects of thrombolytic therapy. ⇒ angina pectoris; cardiac enzymes; coronary heart disease.

myocarditis *n* inflammation of the myocardium.

myocardium *n* the middle layer of the heart wall. Formed from highly specialized cardiac muscle. ⇒ muscle—**myocardial** *adj*.

myocele *n* protrusion of a muscle through its ruptured sheath.

myoclonus *n* clonic contractions of individual or groups of muscles. Normal individuals occasionally experience an isolated myoclonic jerk or two during drowsiness or light sleep. ⇒ clonus.

myoelectric *adj* relating to the electrical properties of muscle.

myofascial pain syndrome persistent pain of soft tissue, characterized by taut fibrous bands and focal areas of hypersensitivity known as trigger points.

myofibril *n* bundle of fibres contained in a muscle fibre. Formed from filaments of contractile proteins. ⇒ actin, myosin, tropomyosin, troponin.

myofibrosis *n* excessive connective tissue in muscle. Leads to inadequate functioning of part—**myofibroses** *pl*.

myogenic *adj* originating in or starting from muscle.

myoglobin *n* (*syn* myohaemoglobin) a haemprotein molecule of skeletal muscle. It is involved with the oxygen released by the red blood cells, which it stores and transports to muscle cell mitochondria where it is used to produce energy. Myoglobin escapes from damaged muscle and appears in the urine in 'crush syndrome'.

myoglobinuria *n* (*syn* myohaemoglobinuria) excretion of myoglobin in the urine as in crush syndrome.

myohaemoglobin *n* ⇒ myoglobin.

myohaemoglobinuria *n* ⇒ myoglobinuria.

myokymia *n* muscle twitching. In the lower eyelid it is benign. *facial myokymia* may result from long use of phenothiazines; has also been observed in patients with multiple sclerosis.

myoma *n* a tumour of muscle tissue—**myomata** *pl*, **myomatous** *adj*.

myomectomy *n* enucleation of uterine fibroid(s).

myometrium *n* the specialized muscular wall of the uterus.

myoneural *adj* pertaining to muscle and nerve.

myopathy *n* disease of muscle (usually applied to non-inflammatory conditions)—**myopathic** *adj*.

myope *n* a shortsighted person—**myopic** *adj*.

myopia *n* shortsightedness caused by high refractive power or increased axial length of the eye, with the result that the light rays are focused in front of, instead of on, the retina—**myopic** *adj*.

myoplasty *n* plastic surgery of muscles—**myoplastic** *adj*.

myosarcoma *n* a malignant tumour derived from muscle—**myosarcomata** *pl*, **myosarcomatous** *adj*.

myosin *n* a contractile protein, one of the filaments of a myofibril; reacts with actin in the muscle cell to cause contraction.

myosis (miosis) *n* constriction of the pupil of the eye—**myotic** *adj*.

myositis *n* inflammation of a muscle or its connective tissue. *myositis ossificans* deposition of active bone cells in muscle, resulting in hard swellings.

myotatic on-stretch reflex a reflex that involves the lengthening of a muscle followed by sudden shortening to generate power. ⇒ plyometric exercise.

myotome *n* the muscles supplied by a single spinal nerve.

myotomy *n* cutting or dissection of muscle tissue.

myotonia *n* an increase in muscle tone at rest—**myotonic** *adj*. *myotonia congenita* a genetically determined form of congenital muscular spasticity, usually presenting in infancy and due to degeneration of ante-rior horn cells in the spinal cord. Fibrillation of affected muscles is characteristic.

myringitis *n* inflammation of the eardrum (tympanic membrane).

myringoplasty *n* operation designed to close a defect in the tympanic membrane with a graft—**myringoplastic** *adj*.

myringotome *n* a delicate instrument for incising the eardrum (tympanic membrane).

myringotomy *n* incision into the eardrum (tympanic membrane). Performed for the drainage of pus or fluid from the middle ear. Middle ear ventilation is maintained by insertion of a grommet or Teflon tube.

myxoedema *n* ⇒ hypothyroidism. *myxoedema coma* rare but serious event characterized by alterations in consciousness and hypothermia, usually in an older person with hypothyroidism. There is a high mortality, and treatment involves parenteral thyroid hormone and supportive measures.

myxoma *n* a connective tissue tumour composed largely of mucoid material—**myxomata** *pl*, **myxomatous** *adj*.

myxosarcoma *n* a malignant tumour of connective tissue with a soft, mucoid consistency—**myxosarcomata** *pl*, **myxosarcomatous** *adj*.

myxoviruses *npl* RNA viruses (orthomyxoviruses and paramyxoviruses) that include the respiratory syncytial virus and those causing influenza, mumps and measles.

N

nabothian follicles cystic distension of chronically inflamed cervical glands of uterus, where the duct of the gland has become obliterated by a healing epithelial covering and the normal mucus cannot escape.

NAD *abbr* nicotinamide adenine dinucleotide.

NADP *abbr* nicotinamide adenine dinucleotide phosphate.

Näegele's obliquity tilting of the fetal head to one or other side to decrease the transverse diameter presented to the pelvic brim.

naevoid amentia ⇒ Sturge–Weber syndrome.

naevus *n* a mole; a circumscribed lesion of the skin arising from pigment-producing naevus cells or due to a developmental abnormality of blood vessels (angioma)—**naevi** *pl*, **naevoid** *adj*.

NAI *abbr* non-accidental injury.

nail *n* keratinized epithelial tissue covering the ends of the digits. *nail involution* a nail condition in which the transverse curvature increases along its longitudinal axis, reaching its maximum at the distal part. Often causes onychophosis. *pincer nail* the lateral edges of the nail practically meet. Lateral compression of the nail may cause damage to the soft tissues and reduce circulation to the nail bed. Subungual ulceration can result.

nanogram (ng) *n* one thousandth part of a microgram. 10^{-9} of a gram.

nanometre (nm) *n* one thousandth part of a micrometre. 10^{-9} of a metre.

nape *n* the nucha; back of the neck.

napkin rash erythema of the napkin area. Causes include contact with ammonia formed from the decomposition of urine, candidiasis, infantile psoriasis, allergy to detergents, excoriation from diarrhoea.

narcissism *n* self-love. In psychoanalysis the narcissistic type of personality is one where the love object is the self.

narcoanalysis *n* analysis of mental content under light anaesthesia, usually an intravenous barbiturate—**narcoanalytic** *adj*, **narcoanalytically** *adv*.

narcolepsy *n* condition occurring in 0.05% of the population. Characterized by irresistible urge to sleep, sleep paralysis and hallucinations at the onset of sleep. May also occur with cataplexy (loss of muscle tone with emotion)—**narcoleptic** *adj*.

narcosis *n* drug-induced unconsciousness. ⇒ narcotic. *carbon dioxide narcosis* full bounding pulse, muscular twitchings, confusion and eventual unconsciousness due to increased $PaCO_2$. ⇒ hypercapnia.

narcosynthesis *n* the building up of a clearer mental picture of an incident involving the patient by reviving memories of it, under light anaesthesia, so that both the patient and the therapist can examine the incident in clearer perspective.

narcotic *n, adj* (describes) a drug causing abnormally deep sleep. Strong analgesic narcotics, e.g. opioids, may cause respiratory depression which is reversible by the use of narcotic antagonists.

nares *n* (*syn* choanae) the nostrils—**naris** *sing*. *anterior nares* the pair of openings from the exterior into the nasal cavities. *posterior nares* the pair of openings from the nasal cavities into the nasopharynx.

nasal *adj* pertaining to the nose.

nasoduodenal *adj* pertaining to the nose and duodenum, as passing a *nasoduodenal tube* via this route, for feeding. ⇒ enteral.

nasogastric (NG) *adj* pertaining to the nose and stomach, as passing a *nasogastric tube* via this route, usually for aspiration, or feeding.

nasojejunal *adj* pertaining to the nose and jejunum, usually referring to a tube passed via the nose into the jejunum for feeding.

nasolacrimal *adj* pertaining to the nose and lacrimal apparatus.

naso-oesophageal *adj* pertaining to the nose and the oesophagus.

nasopharyngitis *n* inflammation of the nasopharynx.

nasopharyngoscope *n* an endoscope for viewing the nasal passages and postnasal space—**nasopharyngoscopic** *adj*.

nasopharynx *n* the portion of the pharynx above the soft palate—**nasopharyngeal** *adj*.

National Care Standards Commission (NCSC) in England a public body established in 2002 to regulate and inspect social care, private and voluntary health care, and investigate complaints, e.g. in care homes for older people, private and voluntary hospitals, etc.

National Confidential Enquiries four national enquiries that investigate clinical practice in specific areas: Maternal Deaths, Perioperative Deaths, Stillbirths and Deaths in Infancy, and Suicide and Homicide by People with Mental Illness.

National Framework for Assessing Performance a framework that includes six areas for the assessment of NHS performance: effective delivery of appropriate health care; efficiency; fair access; health improvement; health outcomes and the patient/carer experience. ⇒ Performance Indicators.

National Institute for Clinical Excellence (NICE) a Special Health Authority that generates and distributes clinical guidance based on evidence of clinical and cost effectiveness.

National Service Frameworks (NSFs) evidence-based frameworks for major care areas and particular groups of disease, e.g. diabetes, older people, that state what patients/clients can presume to receive from the NHS.

naturopathy *n* a multidisciplinary approach to health care that includes all aspects of one's lifestyle, e.g. natural foods grown without chemicals and medicines based on plants. It is founded upon the belief of the body's power to heal itself given an optimal environment for healing—**naturopathic** *adj*.

nausea *n* a feeling of impending vomiting—**nauseate** *vt*.

navel *n* ⇒ umbilicus.

navicular *adj* shaped like a canoe such as the bone in the foot.

NCSC *abbr* National Care Standards Commission.

nebula *n* a cloud-like corneal opacity.

nebulizer *n* an apparatus for converting a liquid into a fine spray. It is used to deliver medicaments for application to the respiratory tract or the skin. A very common method of drug delivery used in the management of asthma.

NEC *abbr* necrotizing enterocolitis.

Necator *n* a genus of hookworms.

necropsy *n* the examination of a dead body.

necrosectomy *n* removal of necrotic tissue, e.g. necrotic pancreas as a consequence of severe acute pancreatitis.

necrosis *n* localized death of tissue—**necrotic** *adj*.

necrotizing enterocolitis (NEC) a condition occurring primarily in preterm or low birthweight neonates. Parts of the gut wall become necrotic, leading to intestinal obstruction and peritonitis. Probably caused by a combination of ischaemia and infection.

necrotizing fasciitis rare infection caused by some strains of group A *Streptococcus pyogenes*. There is very severe inflammation of the muscle sheath and massive soft tissue destruction. The mortality rate is high.

needlestick injury an injury sustained when penetration of the skin occurs from a hypodermic needle. Risk is at its greatest when the needle is contaminated with blood from a person infected with a blood-borne virus such as hepatitis B, C and HIV.

needling *n* procedure for removal of congenital cataract, now superseded.

needs assessment estimating the need (quantifying) for services in a population. Normative, or assessed, need defined by the expert or professional in any given situation; felt need, or want, perceived by the individual; expressed need, or operationalized felt need; comparative need, using the characteristics of a population receiving a service to define those with similar characteristics as in need. Needs assessment uses broad, non-specific indicators of need obtained through repeated health surveys of the general population (e.g. General Household Survey, Health Survey for England) and more specific indicators based on surveys of particular groups (e.g. survey of disabled people, urinary incontinence). The weighted capitation formula for resource allocation uses the characteristics of populations using hospital services as indicators of need.

negativism *n* active refusal by the patient to cooperate, usually shown by the patient consistently doing the exact opposite of what is asked. Seen in catatonic schizophrenia.

negligence *n* a form of professional malpractice which includes the omission of acts that a prudent health professional would have done or the commission of acts that a prudent health professional would not do. It is a professional duty to avoid patient/client injury or suffering caused in this way. It can become the basis of litigation for damages. ⇒ Bolam test, duty of care.

Neisseria *n* a genus of Gram-negative bacteria. Some are commensals of humans and animals, e.g. *Neisseria catarrhalis*, but others are pathogens. *Neisseria gonorrhoeae* causes gonorrhoea and *Neisseria meningitidis* causes meningitis.

Nelaton's line an imaginary line joining the anterior superior iliac spine to the ischial tuberosity. The great trochanter of the femur normally lies on or below this line.

Nelson syndrome hyperpigmentation, including marked darkening of fair skin, as a result of uncontrolled adrenocorticotrophin (ACTH) secretion from a pituitary adenoma, usually after treatment of the associated Cushing's disease by bilateral adrenalectomy.

nematodes *npl* parasitic worms that can be divided into three groups: (a) those that mainly live in the intestine, e.g. *Ancylostoma duodenale* (hookworm), *Ascaris lumbricoides* (roundworm), *Enterobius vermicularis* (threadworm), *Strongyloides stercoralis* and *Trichuris trichiura* (whipworms); (b) those that are mainly in the tissues, e.g. *Dracunculus medinensis* (guinea worm) and the filarial worms that include *Loa loa*; (c) those from other species (zoonotic), e.g. *Toxocara canis*.

neoadjuvant therapy in cancer treatment the use of chemotherapy to reduce tumour size before surgery or radiotherapy.

neologism *n* the creation of a new word. A type of thought disorder seen in schizophrenia, mania and other psychotic illnesses.

neonatal *adj* relating to the first 28 days of life. *neonatal herpes* acquired during vaginal delivery from a mother actively shedding herpes simplex virus. It is a devastating illness with a 75% mortality rate and a high incidence of severe neurological sequelae among survivors. *neonatal mortality* the death rate of babies in the first month of life.

neonatal hearing screening hearing screening can be performed in small babies by otoacoustic emission testing (OAE), using a small probe linked to a computer. Where this equipment is unavailable, a less reliable distraction test using simple sounds can be performed in infants.

neonatal respiratory distress syndrome (NRDS) respiratory failure due to surfactant deficiency in the newborn. Most commonly affects premature infants.

neonatal unit (NNU/NICU/SCBU) usually reserved for preterm and small-for-dates babies between 700 and 2000 g in weight, mostly requiring the use of high technology which is available in these units.

neonate *n* a newborn baby up to 4 weeks old.

neonatology *n* the scientific study of the newborn.

neonatorum *adj* pertaining to the newborn.

neoplasia *n* literally, the formation of new tissue. Customarily refers to the pathological process in the growth of malignant tumour—**neoplastic** *adj*.

neoplasm *n* a new growth; a tumour that is either cancerous or non-cancerous.

nephrectomy *n* surgical removal of a kidney.

nephritis *n* non-specific term for inflammation within the kidney—**nephritic** *adj*.

nephroblastoma *n* the most common solid tumour of the kidney. Usually presents as an abdominal mass. Also known as Wilms tumour.

nephrocalcinosis *n* calcification within the kidney.

nephrogenic *adj* coming from or produced by the kidney.

nephrolithiasis *n* stone disease affecting the kidney.

nephrolithotomy *n* removal of a stone from the kidney by an incision through the kidney substance. *percutaneous nephrolithotomy* a minimally invasive technique where the kidney pelvis is punctured using X-ray control. A guide wire is inserted through which the stone is removed using a nephroscope (endoscope).

nephrology *n* study of diseases of the kidney.

nephron *n* the functional unit of the kidney, comprising a glomerulus and renal tubule. The tubule has a Bowman's capsule, proximal and distal convoluted tubules, loop of Henle and a collecting tubule that drains urine from many nephrons to the renal pelvis.

nephronophthisis *n* rare disorder involving the growth of many small cysts in the medulla of the kidney; often leads to renal failure.

nephropathy *n* any disease of the kidney in which inflammation is not a major component. ⇒ diabetic nephropathy—**nephropathic** *adj*.

nephropexy *n* surgical fixation of a floating kidney.

nephroptosis *n* downward displacement of the kidney. The word is sometimes used for a floating kidney.

nephroscope *n* an endoscope for viewing kidney tissue. It can be designed to create a continuous flow of irrigating fluid and provide an exit for the fluid and accompanying debris—**nephroscopic** *adj*.

nephrostomy *n* a surgically established fistula from the pelvis of the kidney to the body surface.

nephrotic syndrome disease characterized by heavy proteinuria, low serum albumin and oedema formation; there are a wide range of causes.

nephrotoxic *adj* describes any substance or process that is injurious to renal tissue or function—**nephrotoxin** *n*.

nephroureterectomy *n* removal of the kidney along with a part or the whole of the ureter.

nerve *n* an elongated bundle of fibres which serves for the transmission of impulses between the periphery and the nerve centres. *afferent nerve* one conveying impulses from the tissues to the nerve centres; also known as sensory nerves. *efferent nerve* one which conveys impulses outwards from the central nervous system to the muscles and glands; also known as; motor nerves. *nerve growth factor (NGF)* protein required for nerve growth and maintenance.

nerve stimulator apparatus used to electronically stimulate peripheral nerves to locate them and test nerve blockade.

nervous *adj* **1** relating to nerves or nerve tissue. **2** referring to a state of restlessness or timidity, *nervous system* the structures controlling the actions and functions of the body; it comprises the brain and spinal cord (central nervous system), and the peripheral nerve fibres and ganglia. ⇒ Figure 11, autonomic nervous system, peripheral nervous system, parasympathetic, sympathetic nervous system.

net oxygen cost the oxygen used during physical activity in excess of that required at rest.

nettlerash *n* ⇒ urticaria.

neural *adj* pertaining to nerves. *neural canal* the cavity within the vertebral column that houses the spinal cord; *neural tube* formed from fusion of the neural folds from which the brain and spinal cord are formed; *neural tube defect* any of a group of congenital malformations involving the neural tube including anencephaly, hydrocephalus and spina bifida. ⇒ folic acid.

neuralgia *n* pain in the distribution of a nerve—**neuralgic** *adj*.

neurapraxia *n* temporary loss of function in peripheral nerve fibres. Most commonly due to crushing or prolonged pressure. ⇒ axonotmesis.

neurasthenia *n* historically described as a form of 'nervous exhaustion'. Now regarded as an anxiety disorder characterized by persistent fatigue together with poor appetite, irritability, insomnia, headache and poor concentration—**neurasthenic** *adj*.

neurectomy *n* excision of part of a nerve.

neurilemma *n* the thin membranous covering of a nerve fibre surrounding the myelin sheath.

neuritis *n* inflammation of a nerve—**neuritic** *adj*.

neuroblast *n* a primitive nerve cell.

neuroblastoma *n* malignant tumour arising in adrenal medulla from tissue of sympathetic origin. Most cases show increased urinary catecholamine excretion—**neuroblastomata** *pl*, **neuroblastomatous** *adj*.

neurodermatitis *n* (*syn* lichen simplex) leathery, thickened patches of skin secondary to pruritus and scratching. As the skin thickens, irritation increases, scratching causes further thickening and so a vicious circle is set up.

neurofibroma *n* a tumour arising from the connective tissue of nerves—**neurofibromata** *pl*, **neurofibromatous** *adj*.

neurofibromatosis *n* a genetically determined condition in which there are many fibromata. ⇒ von Recklinghausen's disease.

neurogenic *adj* originating within or forming nervous tissue.

neurogenic bladder interference with the nerve control of the urinary bladder causing either retention of urine, which presents as incontinence, or continuous dribbling without retention. When necessary the bladder is emptied by exerting manual pressure on the anterior abdominal wall.

neuroglia *n* (*syn* glia) the supporting tissue of the central nervous system (brain and cord). ⇒ astrocytes, ependymal cells, microglial cells, oligodendrocytes—**neuroglial** *adj.*

neuroleptics (antipsychotics) *npl* drugs acting on the nervous system. Most are antagonists of dopamine receptors and other receptors. They can be divided into typical and atypical neuroleptics. ⇒ dibenzodiazepines, extrapyramidal, phenothiazines, tardive dyskinesia. ⇒ Appendix 5.

neurologist *n* a specialist in neurology. Or a medically qualified person who specializes in diagnosing and treating diseases of the nervous system.

neurology *n* **1** the science and study of nerves—their structure, function and pathology. **2** the branch of medicine dealing with diseases of the nervous system—**neurological** *adj.*

neuromuscular *adj* pertaining to nerves and muscles.

neuron(e) *n* a nerve cell. The basic unit of the nervous system comprising fibres (dendrites) which convey impulses to the nerve cell; the nerve cell itself, and the fibres (axons) which convey impulses from the cell. They are specialized excitable cells that are able to transmit an action potential ⇒ motor neuron disease—**neuronal, neural** *adj. lower motor neuron* the cell is in the anterior horn of the spinal cord and the axon passes to skeletal muscle; *upper motor neuron* the cell is in the motor cortex and the axon terminates in the anterior horn of the spinal cord.

neuropathic *adj* relating to disease of the nervous system.

neuropathy *n* loss of function of peripheral nerves which may be focal (e.g. carpal tunnel syndrome) or generalized.

neuropathology *n* a branch of medicine dealing with diseases of the nervous system—**neuropathological** *adj.*

neuropeptides *npl* neurotransmitters, including endorphins.

neuropharmacology *n* the branch of pharmacology dealing with drugs that act on the nervous system—**neuropharmacological** *adj.*

neuroplasticity *n* the ability of nerve cells to regenerate.

neuroplasty *n* surgical repair of nerves—**neuroplastic** *adj.*

neuropsychiatry *n* a subspecialty of psychiatry dealing with mental disorder and its relationship to brain/central nervous system (dys) function—**neuropsychiatric** *adj.*

neurorrhaphy *n* suturing the ends of a divided nerve.

neurosis *n* an outdated term. The traditional division between psychosis and neurosis has fallen out of favour. However, the term neurotic disorders is a grouping term for anxiety disorders, phobias and obsessive-compulsive disorder—**neurotic** *adj.*

neurosurgery *n* surgery of the nervous system—**neurosurgical** *adj.*

neurosyphilis *n* infection of brain or spinal cord, or both, by *Treponema pallidum*. The variety of clinical pictures produced is large, but the two common syndromes encountered are tabes dorsalis and general paralysis of the insane (GPI). Very often symptoms of the disease do not arise until 20 years or more after the date of primary infection—**neurosyphilitic** *adj.*

neurotomy *n* surgical cutting of a nerve.

neurotoxic *adj* poisonous or destructive to nervous tissue—**neurotoxin** *n.*

neurotropic *adj* with predilection for the nervous system. *Treponema pallidum* produces neurosyphilitic complications. Neurotropic viruses (e.g. rabies, poliomyelitis) attack nerve cells.

neutron *n* the subatomic particle that has no electrical charge.

neutropenia *n* reduction in the number of neutrophils, but not sufficient to warrant the description agranulocytosis—**neutropenic** *adj.*

neutrophil *n* the most common form of white blood cell. It is a phagocytic polymorphonuclear cell with granules.

newton (N) *n* a unit of force. Derived SI unit (International System of Units).

NGU *abbr* non-gonococcal urethritis.

NHL *abbr* non-Hodgkin's lymphoma.

NHS *abbr* National Health Service.

NHS Trusts public accountable bodies that provide NHS health care to the population, either as a hospital or community trust.

niacin *n* a generic term that includes nicotinamide and nicotinic acid.

NICE *abbr* National Institute for Clinical Excellence.

nicotinamide *n* the amide of nicotinic acid, a member of the vitamin B complex. It is part of the coenzymes *nicotinamide adenine dinucleotide (NAD)* and *nicotinamide adenine dinucleotide phosphate (NADP)*, which play essential roles in metabolism. It is obtained from the meat, pulses and wholegrain cereals in the diet, and it is formed from nicotinic acid or synthesized in the liver from the amino acid tryptophan. ⇒ niacin, pellagra.

nicotinic *adj* a type of cholinergic receptor where nicotine would, if present, bind in place of acetylcholine. ⇒ muscarinic.

nicotinic acid a member of the vitamin B complex, which has anti-pellagra properties and occurs in the diet. Has a direct vasodilatory action and is used in the management of peripheral vascular disease. ⇒ niacin, nicotinamide, pellagra.

nictitation *n* rapid and involuntary blinking of the eyelids.

NICU *abbr* neonatal intensive care unit.

nidation *n* implantation of the early embryo in the decidua.

NIDDM *abbr* non-insulin dependent diabetes mellitus. ⇒ diabetes mellitus type 2.

nidus *n* any structure resembling a nest in appearance or function. *nidus of infection* a breeding place where bacteria and other pathological agents lodge and form a focus.

Niemann–Pick disease a lipoid metabolic disturbance, chiefly in female Jewish infants. Now thought to be due to absence or inadequacy of the enzyme sphingomyelinase. There is enlargement of the liver, spleen and lymph nodes with learning disability. Now classified as a lipid reticulosis.

night blindness (*syn* nyctalopia) maladaptation of vision to darkness; may occur in vitamin A deficiency or genetic disorders of the retina.

night cry a shrill noise, made during sleep. May be of significance in hip disease when pain occurs in the relaxed joint.

night splinting the passive night time use of orthoses such as splints to maintain corrected deformities produced dynamically during walking. This may be an additional silicone digital device to maintain correction in bed, or a night splint to maintain ankle extension at 90° where there is tightening of the Achilles tendon.

Night splints for the management of hallux valgus are often used as the only corrective measure.

night sweat profuse sweating, usually during sleep; typical of tuberculosis or lymphoma.

nihilistic *adj* the belief that nothing is real. Nihilistic delusions.

Nikolsky's sign slight pressure on the skin causes 'slipping' of apparently normal skin typically adjacent to a blister. Characteristic of pemphigus.

nipple *n* the conical eminence in the centre of each breast, containing the outlets of the milk ducts.

NIPPV *abbr* non-invasive intermittent positive pressure ventilation.

nit *n* the egg of the head louse (*Pediculus capitis*). It is firmly attached to the hair.

nitrates *npl* a group of drugs that act as coronary vasodilators. There is a reduction in venous return to the heart and the work of the left ventricle. ⇒ Appendix 5.

nitric oxide (NO) an endogenous neuromodulator. It is involved with processes that include memory, learning, gastric emptying, nociception and penile erection. May be used therapeutically for patients with acute respiratory distress syndrome.

nitrogen (N) *n* **1** an almost inert gaseous element; the chief constituent of the atmosphere (78–79%), but it cannot be utilized directly by humans. However, certain organisms in the soil and roots of legumes are capable of nitrogen fixation. It is a vital constituent of many complements of living cells, e.g. proteins. **2** the essential constituent of protein foods—**nitrogenous** *adj*. *nitrogen balance* is when a person's daily intake of nitrogen from proteins equals the daily excretion of nitrogen: a negative balance occurs when excretion of nitrogen exceeds the daily intake. Nitrogen is excreted mainly as urea in the urine: ammonia, creatinine and uric acid account for a further small amount. Less than 10% total nitrogen is excreted in faeces.

nitrous oxide (N_2O) gas used widely as an adjuvant for general anaesthesia and for analgesia. Known colloquially as laughing gas.

NMR *abbr* ⇒ nuclear magnetic resonance.

NNU *abbr* neonatal unit.

nociceptors *npl* receptors that respond to harmful stimuli that cause pain, such as trauma and inflammation.

nocturia *n* passing urine at night.

nocturnal *adj* nightly; during the night.

node *n* a protuberance or swelling. A constriction. *node of Ranvier* the constriction in the neurilemma of a nerve fibre.

nodule *n* a small node—**nodular** *adj*.

no fault liability acknowledgement that compensation is payable without the requirement to prove a failure in fulfilling the duty of care.

nominal data categorical data where the classes have no particular value or order, such as road names or colours. ⇒ ordinal data.

nomogram *n* graph with several variables used to determine another related variable, such as body surface area from weight and height.

non-accidental injury (NAI) physical maltreatment, usually of children by their parents, carers, other adults, or even other children. The injuries cannot be attributed to natural disease processes or simple accident. The injuries are often multiple and typically include bruising, shaking injuries, fractures and burns, and involve the head, soft tissues, long bones and the thoracic cage. There may be evidence of neglect and usually there is associated psychological harm. ⇒ abuse.

non-compliance *n* a term used when patients who understand their drug regimen do not comply with it.

non compos mentis not mentally competent.

non-gonococcal urethritis (NGU) (*syn* non-specific urethritis—NUS) a common sexually transmitted disease in men. At least half of cases are caused by *Chlamydia trachomatis*. Uncommonly caused by *Trichomonas vaginalis* or herpes simplex virus. Aetiology in remaining cases uncertain, but the bacteria *Ureaplasma urealyticum* and *Mycoplasma genitalium* may be causes.

non-Hodgkin's lymphoma (NHL) tumour of lymphoid tissue. More common in older people. The cure rate is less good than Hodgkin's disease. ⇒ lymphoma.

non-insulin dependent diabetes mellitus (NIDDM) ⇒ diabetes mellitus type 2.

non-invasive *adj* describes any diagnostic or therapeutic technique that does not require penetration of the skin or of any cavity or organ.

non-invasive intermittent positive pressure ventilation (NIPPV) a type of respiratory support that uses a nasal or full-face mask rather than an endotracheal or tracheostomy tube.

non-maleficence *n* ethical principle of doing no harm. ⇒ beneficence.

non-milk extrinsic sugars extrinsic sugars except that found in milk (lactose).

non-parametric test statistical test that makes no presupposition about the distribution of data. ⇒ parametric tests.

non-protein nitrogen (NPN) nitrogen from nitrogenous substances other than protein, i.e. urea, uric acid, creatinine, creatine and ammonia.

non-small cell lung carcinoma (NSCLC) commonest type of lung cancer accounting for approximately 80% of tumours. The histological subtypes include squamous, adenocarcinoma and large cell. The doubling time is approximately 130 days. Clinical presentation may be with cough, haemoptysis, recurrent pneumonia, increasing breathlessness, weight loss or may be an incidental finding on chest X-ray. Therapy may include surgery (in approximately 20%), chemotherapy and/or radiotherapy.

non-specific urethritis (NSU) ⇒ non-gonococcal urethritis.

non-starch polysaccharides (NSP) polysaccharides occurring in plant material that is not digested in the human gastrointestinal tract. Can be divided into two types: non-soluble, e.g. cellulose, lignin, and soluble, e.g. pectin and mucilages. An important component of the diet to prevent constipation and colorectal cancer. Previously called dietary fibre.

non-steroidal anti-inflammatory drugs (NSAIDs) a large group of drugs with varying degrees of anti-inflammatory, antipyretic and analgesic action. They inhibit enzymes needed for the synthesis of prostaglandins and thromboxanes. ⇒ fenamates, oxicams, propionic acids, pyrazolones, salicylates. ⇒ Appendix 5.

Noonan syndrome in either males or females, with eyes set apart (hypertelorism) and other ocular and facial abnormalities; cardiac abnormalities, short stature, sometimes with neck webbing (and other Turner-like features). Generally not chromosomal; most cases sporadic; a few either dominantly or recessively inherited.

noradrenaline (norepinephrine) *n* a catecholamine neurohumoral transmitter released from adrenergic nerve endings and in small amounts from the adrenal medulla. Its physiological effects include: vasoconstriction and a rise in blood pressure. ⇒ adrenaline (epinephrine).

norm *n* a measure of a phenomenon generally accepted as an ideal against which all other measures of the phenomenon can be measured, i.e. a standard against which values are measured.

normal distribution curve in statistics. When scores are plotted they form a symmetrical bell-shaped curve that has the mean, median and mode in the centre. ⇒ skewed distribution.

normal flora ⇒ flora.

normoblast *n* a normal-sized nucleated red blood cell, the precursor of the erythrocyte—**normoblastic** *adj*.

normocyte *n* a red blood cell of normal size—**normocytic** *adj*.

normoglycaemic *adj* a normal amount of glucose in the blood—**normoglycaemia** *n*.

normotension *n* normal tension, by custom alluding to blood pressure—**normotensive** *adj*.

normothermia *n* normal body temperature, as opposed to hyperthermia and hypothermia—**normothermic** *adj*.

normotonic *adj* normal strength, tension, tone, by convention referring to muscle tissue. Spasmolytic drugs induce normotonicity in muscle, and can be used before radiography—**normotonicity** *n*.

nosocomial *adj* pertaining to a hospital. ⇒ infection.

nostalgia *n* homesickness; a longing to return to a 'place' to which, and where, one may have emotional bonds—**nostalgic** *adj*.

nostrils *npl* the anterior openings into the nose; the anterior nares; choanae.

notifiable *adj* describes incidents or occurrences and diseases that must by law be made known to the appropriate agency. For example diseases such as tuberculosis,

food poisoning and measles must be reported to the relevant department.

NPF *abbr* Nurse Prescribers' Formulary.

NRDS *abbr* neonatal respiratory distress syndrome.

NREM *abbr* non-rapid eye movement (sleep). ⇒ sleep.

NSAIDs *abbr* non-steroidal anti-inflammatory drugs.

NSCLC *abbr* non-small cell lung carcinoma.

NSP *abbr* non-starch polysaccharide.

NSU *abbr* non-specific urethritis. ⇒ non-gonococcal urethritis.

nucha *n* the nape of the neck—**nuchal** *adj*.

nuclear family in western societies the conventional family group of two married parents and their dependent children.

nuclear magnetic resonance (NMR) ⇒ magnetic resonance imaging.

nuclear medicine the use of radionuclide techniques for the diagnosis, treatment and study of disease.

nucleated *adj* possessing one or more nuclei.

nucleic acids biological macromolecules comprising many subunits called nucleotides. ⇒ deoxyribonucleic acid, ribonucleic acid.

nucleolus structures (usually two) involved in nuclear division. They are within the nuclear membrane and contain both DNA and RNA.

nucleoproteins *npl* proteins conjugated with nucleic acids found in the cell nucleus. Uric acid is an end product of nucleoprotein metabolism, which is normally excreted in the urine. ⇒ gout.

nucleotides *npl* the subunits from which nucleic acids are formed. Consist of sugars and nitrogenous bases (nucleosides) and phosphate groups.

nucleotoxic *adj* toxic to the cell nucleus, e.g. some chemicals and viruses—**nucleotoxin** *n*.

nucleus *n* 1 the membrane-bound cellular structure which contains the genetic material (chromosomes). 2 a confined accumulation of nerve cells in the central nervous system associated with a particular function—**nuclei** *pl*, **nuclear** *adj*. *nucleus pulposus* the soft core of an intervertebral disc which can prolapse into the spinal cord and cause back pain or sciatica.

null hypothesis a statement that asserts there to be no relationship between the dependent and independent variables.

nullipara *n* a woman who has not borne a child—**nulliparous** *adj*, **nulliparity** *n*.

numbers needed to treat a method of stating the benefits of a therapeutic intervention. The number of subjects who need to receive treatment before one subject has a positive outcome.

nummular *adj* coin shaped; resembling rolls of coins, as the sputum in tuberculosis.

nurse anaesthetist a nurse trained to administer general anaesthesia.

nursing home an institution where nursing care is delivered by the independent sector, charitable organizations, social services or, rarely, the NHS.

nutation *n* nodding; applied to uncontrollable head shaking.

nutrient *n, adj* a chemical substance (e.g. protein, vitamin C) found in food that can be digested and absorbed and used to promote body function. *nutrient artery* one which enters a long bone. *nutrient foramen* hole in a long bone which admits the nutrient artery.

nutrition *n* the sum total of the processes by which the living organism receives and utilizes the materials necessary for survival, growth and repair of worn-out tissues.

nutritional *adj* pertaining to nutrition. *nutritional assessment* the assessment of an individual's nutritional status used to identify those who are malnourished and those who are at risk of becoming malnourished. Factors included in the assessment are dietary intake, nutritional requirements, clinical condition, physical appearance, anthropometric and biochemical measurements. *nutritional support* intervention to improve nutrient intake. Interventions include increasing the number of meals and amounts of food provided, fortifying food with additional nutrients, sip-feeds, enteral and parenteral nutrition.

nyctalgia *n* pain occurring during the night.

nyctalopia *n* night blindness.

nyctophobia *n* abnormal fear of the night and darkness.

nymphae *npl* the labia minora.

nymphomania *n* excessive sexual desire in women—**nymphomaniac** *adj*.

nystagmus *n* jerky, involuntary and repetitive movement of the eyeball(s). It can occur under physiological situations but can also indicate diseases, especially of the cerebellum.

O

oat cell carcinoma histological subtype of small cell carcinoma most commonly of bronchogenic epithelium. It accounts for approximately 20% of all lung cancers and is characterized by rapid growth (doubling time approximately 29 days). The highest incidence is in smokers. The lung primary may present with cough, haemoptysis, recurrent pneumonia, increasing breathlessness and weight loss or may be an incidental finding on chest X-ray. Therapy generally does not include surgery, but 90% are sensitive to chemotherapy, which is usually the treatment of choice.

obesity *n* the deposition of excessive fat around the body, particularly in the subcutaneous tissue. Develops when the intake of food is in excess of the body's energy requirements, the most common nutritional disorder worldwide, the incidence is increasing. It is categorized by body mass index. ⇒ body mass index.

objective *adj* pertaining to things external to oneself. ⇒ subjective *opp. objective signs* those which the observer notes, as distinct from the symptoms of which the patient complains.

obligate *adj* distinguished by the ability to survive only in a particular set of environmental conditions.

OBS *abbr* organic brain syndrome. ⇒ dementia.

observational study research in which the researcher observes, listens and records the events of concern. Where the researcher participates and has a role it is termed a *participant observational study*. May be used in qualitative social science research.

obsessive compulsive disorder recurrent obsessional thoughts and/or compulsive acts occurring on most days for at least 2 weeks. The thoughts are usually distressing and are therefore (often unsuccessfully) resisted by the sufferer.

obstetrician *n* a qualified doctor who practises the science and art of obstetrics.

obstetrics *n* the science dealing with the care of the pregnant woman during the antenatal, parturient and puerperal stages; midwifery.

obturator *n* that which closes an aperture. *obturator foramen* the opening in the innominate bone which is closed by muscles and fascia.

occipital *adj* pertaining to the back of the head. *occipital bone* characterized by a large hole through which the spinal cord passes.

occipitoanterior *adj* describes a presentation when the fetal occiput lies in the anterior half of the maternal pelvis.

occipitofrontal *adj* pertaining to the occiput and forehead.

occipitoposterior *adj* describes a presentation when the fetal occiput is in the posterior half of the maternal pelvis.

occiput *n* the posterior region of the skull.

occlusion *n* **1** the closure of an opening, especially of ducts or blood vessels. **2** in dentistry, the contact of the upper and lower teeth in any jaw position. *centric occlusion* contact of the upper and lower teeth with maximum inter-digitation of the cusps. *traumatic occlusion* any malocclusion resulting in damage to the teeth or periodontal tissues—**occlusal** *adj*.

occult *adj* concealed. *occult blood* minute amounts of blood present in the faeces that can only be detected by chemical tests.

occupation *n* the purposeful, functional, productive, playful or creative activities of daily living performed by an individual throughout his or her life.

occupational asthma asthma caused by inhalation of specific agents in the workplace that leads to sensitization of the individual following an immune response. Symptoms do not occur on first exposure but a pattern emerges as symptoms are provoked by work exposure and relieved when away from work. Treatment is by prevention and control of exposure. Untreated the condition can become persistent and chronic.

occupational behaviour interaction with the social, temporal and physical environments in a variety of activities of daily living, throughout an individual's life. These activities should be consistent with a person's occupational role, involve achievement, and address the financial realities of life.

occupational disease ⇒ industrial disease.

occupational health the active and proactive management of health in the workplace.

occupational performance the ability to perform functional, purposeful activities of daily living in a variety of associated occupational roles and environments.

occupational role the expression of an individual's occupational behaviour through various activities of daily living that identifies his or her place in society.

occupational therapy (OT) the use of purposeful activity and meaningful occupation for people with physical and psychosocial dysfunction and disability to enable them to regain, or maintain, their health, well-being, and optimal level of functional independence in all aspects of life. Occupational therapists help people, through the analysis and application of specific, selected activities, to develop the occupational performance skills and roles required to perform consistently and competently activities of daily living in a variety of physical, temporal and social environments.

occupational therapy assessment the use of both formal and informal screening and evaluation methods, including medical records, interview, observation, standardized and non-standardized tests, to assess occupational performance areas, performance components and occupational role performance. This provides the occupational therapist with the means to develop treatment objectives and methods to remediate, or compensate for, any problems identified. Assessment can also be used to determine the effectiveness of treatment and any modifications that might be needed.

ochronosis *n* greyish discoloration of connective tissue as occurs in alkaptonuria.

ocular *adj* pertaining to the eye.

oculogyric *adj* referring to movements of the eyeball.

oculomotor *n* the third pair of cranial nerves which innervate four of the extrinsic muscles and the upper eye lid. They also alter the shape of the lens and control pupil size.

odontalgia *n* toothache.

odontoid *adj* resembling a tooth. *odontoid process* a peg-like projection of the axis (second cervical vertebra).

oedema *n* abnormal infiltration of tissues with fluid. There are many causes— including reduced blood albumin, disease of the cardiopulmonary system, the urinary system and the liver. ⇒ angiooedema, ascites—**oedematous** *adj*.

Oedipus complex an unconscious attachment of a son to his mother resulting in a feeling of jealousy towards the father and then guilt, producing emotional conflict.

oesophageal *adj* pertaining to the oesophagus. *oesophageal ulcer* ulceration of the oesophagus due to gastro-oesophageal reflux caused by hiatus hernia. *oesophageal varices* varicosity of the veins in the lower oesophagus due to portal hypertension. These varices can bleed and may cause a massive haematemesis. ⇒ Sengstaken–Blakemore tube.

oesophagectomy *n* excision of part or the whole of the oesophagus.

oesophagitis *n* inflammation of the oesophagus.

oesophagoscope *n* an endoscope for passage into the oesophagus—**oesophagoscopy** *n*, **oesophagoscopic** *adj*.

oesophagostomy *n* a surgically established fistula between the oesophagus and the skin in the root of the neck. May be used temporarily for feeding after excision of the pharynx for malignant disease.

oesophagotomy *n* an incision into the oesophagus.

oesophagus *n* the musculomembranous canal, 23 cm in length, extending from the pharynx to the stomach (⇒ Figure 18b)—**oesophageal** *adj*.

oestradiol (estradiol) *n* an endogenous oestrogen secreted by the corpus luteum.

oestriol (estriol) *n* an endogenous oestrogen. Produced by the fetus and placenta. Oestriol levels in maternal blood or urine can be used to assess fetal well-being and placental function.

oestrogens (estrogens) *npl* a generic term referring to a group of steroid hormones, oestradiol, oestriol and oestrone. Produced by the ovaries, placenta, testes and, in smaller amounts, the adrenal cortex in both sexes. Oestrogens are responsible for female secondary sexual characteristics and the development and proper functioning of the female genital organs. Used in the combined oral contraceptive and as hormone replacement—**oestrogenic** *adj*.

oestrone (estrone) *n* an endogenous oestrogen.

ointment *n* a semisolid preparation, usually greasy, for application to the skin.

olecranon process the large process at the upper end of the ulna; it forms the point of the elbow when the arm is flexed. *olecranon bursitis* ⇒ bursitis.

olfactory *adj* pertaining to the sense of smell—**olfaction** *n* the sense of smell. *olfactory nerve* the first pair of cranial nerves. They carry sensory impulses from the olfactory epithelium of the nose to the brain. *olfactory organ* the nose (⇒ Figure 14).

oligaemia *n* ⇒ hypovolaemia.

oligoclonal bands a marker of inflammation that is found in the CSF in some conditions such as multiple sclerosis.

oligodactyly *n* a developmental absence of one or more digits (fingers or toes). There is total absence of all parts of the digit, e.g. metatarsal parts and all phalanges.

oligodendrocyte *n* a neuroglial cell of the central nervous system.

oligodendroglioma *n* a tumour of glial cells (neuroglial tissue) of the brain.

oligohydramnios *n* lack of amniotic fluid.

oligomenorrhoea *n* infrequent menstruation; normal cycle is prolonged beyond 35 days.

oligospermia *n* reduction in number of spermatozoa in the semen.

oliguria *n* reduced urine output—**oliguric** *adj*.

omentum *n* a sling-like fold of peritoneum—**omental** *adj*. The functions of the omentum are support and protection, limiting infection and fat storage. *greater omentum* the fold which hangs from the lower border of the stomach and covers the front of the intestines. *lesser omentum* a smaller fold, passing between the transverse fissure of the liver and the lesser curvature of the stomach.

omphalitis *n* inflammation of the umbilicus.

omphalocele *n* ⇒ hernia.

Onchocerca *n* a genus of filarial worms such as *Onchocerca volvulus*.

onchocerciasis *n* infestation of the soft tissues, skin and eye with *Onchocerca*. Adult worms encapsulated in subcutaneous connective tissue. Larval migration to the eyes leads to 'river blindness'.

oncogene *n* a gene that may be chemically activated to induce cancer in the host cell.

oncogenic *adj* capable of tumour production.

oncology *n* the scientific study and therapy of neoplastic growths—**oncological** *adj*, **oncologically** *adv*.

onset of blood lactate accumulation (OBLA) (*syn* lactate threshold) the point during the build-up of lactic acid caused by physical activity when the blood lactate level exceeds the resting level.

onychatrophia *n* (*syn* anonychia) a nail that has reached mature size and then undergoes partial or total regression.

onychauxis *n* uniform thickening of the nail. It increases from the nail base to the free edge, and is often brownish in colour.

onychia *n* acute inflammation of the matrix and nail bed; suppuration may spread beneath the nail, causing it to become detached and fall off. Frequently originates from paronychia.

onychocryptosis *n* (*syn* ingrowing nail) occurs when a spike, shoulder or serrated edge of the nail pierces the epidermis of the sulcus and penetrates the dermal tissues, most frequently in the hallux of male adolescents. The portion of nail penetrates further into the tissues producing acute inflammation in the surrounding soft tissues, often becoming infected (paronychia) and resulting in excess granulation tissue.

onychogryphosis, oncogryposis *n* (*syn* ostler's toe, ram's horn) a ridged, thickened deformity of the nails, common in older people. There is hypertrophy, and gross deformity of the nail which develops into a curved or 'ram's horn' shape. The nail is usually dark brown or yellowish in colour, with both longitudinal and transverse ridges on its surface.

onycholysis *n* separation of the nail from the bed at the distal end and/or the lateral margins—**onycholytic** *adj*. It may be idiopathic or secondary to systemic and cutaneous diseases, or may result from local causes such as harsh manicuring. It is more common in fingernails than toenails and affects women more frequently than men.

onychomadesis *n* (*syn* onychoptosis, aplastic anonychia) the spontaneous separation of the nail, beginning at the matrix area and quickly reaching the free edge. It is often accompanied by transient arrest of nail growth, which is characterized by a Beau's line.

onychomycosis *n* (*syn* tinea unguium) a fungal infection of the nail bed and plate. The nail plate becomes thickened, brittle and becomes yellowish-brown in colour. Eventually it develops a porous appearance.

onychophosis *n* a condition where a callus and/or a corn forms in the nail sulcus. It causes pain and inflammation.

onychorrhexis *n* (*syn* reed nail) a brittle nail with a series of narrow, parallel longitudinal superficial ridges.

o'nyongnyong fever (*syn* joint-breaker fever) caused by a virus transmitted by mosquitoes in East Africa.

oocyte *n* an immature ovum.

oogenesis *n* the formation of oocytes in the ovary—**oogenetic** *adj*. ⇒ gametogenesis.

oophorectomy *n* (*syn* ovariectomy, ovariotomy) excision of an ovary.

oophoritis *n* (*syn* ovaritis) inflammation of an ovary.

oophoron *n* an ovary.

oophorosalpingectomy *n* ⇒ salpingo-oophorectomy.

opacity *n* non-transparency; cloudiness; an opaque spot, as on the cornea or lens.

open chain exercise ⇒ open kinetic chain.

open fracture ⇒ fracture.

open kinetic chain a motion during which the distal segment of an extremity moves freely in space, i.e. is non-weight-bearing. ⇒ closed kinetic chain.

operant conditioning ⇒ conditioning.

operating microscope an illuminated binocular microscope enabling surgery to be carried out on delicate tissues such as nerves and blood vessels. Some models incorporate a beam splitter and a second set of eyepieces to enable a second person to view the operation site.

operation *n* surgical procedure upon a part of the body.

operational management the management of the day-to-day activities (operations) of an organization such as a district general hospital. ⇒ strategic management.

ophthalmia *n* (*syn* ophthalmitis) inflammation of the eye. *ophthalmia neonatorum* defined as a purulent discharge from the eyes of an infant commencing within 21 days of birth. A notifiable condition. *sympathetic ophthalmia* inflammation of one eye secondary to injury or disease of the other. Also known as sympathetic ophthalmitis.

ophthalmic *adj* pertaining to the eye.

ophthalmitis *n* ⇒ ophthalmia.

ophthalmologist *n* a medically qualified specialist in ophthalmology.

ophthalmology *n* the science that deals with the structure, function, diseases and treatment of the eye—**ophthalmological** *adj*.

ophthalmoplegia *n* paralysis of one or more eye muscles leading to an inability to move the eyes normally—**ophthalmoplegic** *adj*.

ophthalmoscope *n* an instrument for examining the interior of the eye. *direct ophthalmoscope* uses a perforated illuminated mirror to visualize eye structures directly. *indirect ophthalmoscope* forms an inverted image of the fundus of the eye using an illuminating lamp, usually worn on the examiner's head, and a convex lens, usually hand-held—**ophthalmoscopic** *adj*.

opiate *n* ⇒ opioids.

opioids *npl* a large group of drugs that produce morphine-like effects and can be reversed by the specific antagonist naloxone. ⇒ Appendix 5.

opisthotonos *n* extreme extension of the body occurring in tetanic spasm. In extreme cases the patient may be resting on heels and head alone—**opisthotonic** *adj*.

opium *n* the dried juice of the opium poppy. It contains morphine and other related alkaloids.

opportunistic infection ⇒ infection.

opportunity cost when a resource is used in a particular way, the opportunity to use it for another purpose is lost. This includes money, time and the activities which cannot be undertaken. An example in health care would be the decision to use money for an expensive cancer drug leading to a lost opportunity to spend the money for another service such as cataract surgery.

opposition *n* describes the position of the thumb and fingers when objects are picked up or grasped between thumb and fingers.

opsins *npl* protein part of visual pigments found in cones and rods.

opsonic index a measurement that indicates the ability of phagocytes to ingest foreign bodies such as bacteria.

opsonin *n* complement protein or an antibody which coats an antigen. ⇒ opsonization—**opsonic** *adj*.

opsonization *n* a process where antigens are coated with opsonins thereby increasing their susceptibility to phagocytosis.

optic *adj* pertaining to sight. *optic atrophy* pathological whitening of the optic nerve head with loss of nerve axons. *optic chiasma* ⇒ chiasma. *optic disc* the point where the optic nerve enters the eyeball. ⇒ Figure 15. *optic nerves* second pair of cranial nerves. They convey impulses from the rods and cones in the retina to the brain. ⇒ Figure 15. *optic neuritis* inflammation in the optic nerve that can be first sign of multiple sclerosis. *optic neuropathy* disease of the optic nerve.

optical *adj* relating to sight. *optical aberration* any imperfection in the focus of light rays by a lens. *optical density* the light absorbed by a solution. Can be used to determine substance concentration.

optician *n* one who prescribes glasses to correct refractive errors.

optics *n* the study of the properties of light.

optimum *adj* most favourable. *optimum position* that which will be most useful and cause the least problems should a limb remain permanently paralysed such as following a stroke.

optometrist *n* practitioner of optometry. Also has a role in disease detection.

optometry *n* the study and management of human eye optics.

oral *adj* pertaining to the mouth—**orally** *adv*. *oral medicine* branch of dentistry concerned with the management of diseases of the oral mucosa and related structures, including oral manifestations of systemic diseases. *oral rehydration* solution *(ORS)* a solution for the treatment of diarrhoeal dehydration. It contains glucose and electrolytes such as sodium chloride. *oral rehydration therapy (ORT)* administration of oral rehydration solution by mouth to correct dehydration. *oral surgery* branch of dentistry concerned with minor surgery to the teeth and jaws.

oral contraceptive commonly referred to as 'the pill'. *combined oral contraceptive* contain varying amounts of the two hormones—oestrogen and progestogen. ⇒ contraceptive, progestogen-only pill.

orbicular *adj* resembling a globe; spherical or circular.

orbit *n* the bony socket containing the eyeball and its appendages—**orbital** *adj*.

orchidectomy *n* excision of a testis.

orchidopexy *n* surgical procedure of bringing an undescended testis into its correct location in the scrotum, and fixing it in this position.

orchis *n* the testis.

orchitis *n* inflammation of a testis.

ordinal data categorical data that can be ordered or ranked, e.g. general condition–good, fair or bad, or size in general terms, as in 'smaller than'. ⇒ nominal data.

orf *n* skin lesions caused by a virus normally affecting sheep and goats.

organ *n* an assembly of different tissues to form a distinct functional unit, e.g. liver, uterus, able to perform specialized functions. *organ of Corti* sited in the cochlea of the internal ear it contains the auditory receptors of the cochlear branch of the vestibulocochlear nerve.

organic *adj* pertaining to an organ. Associated with life. *organic brain syndrome* ⇒ dementia. *organic compounds* chemical compounds containing carbon and hydrogen in their structure, e.g. glucose. Include the large biological molecules, such as lipids and proteins. *organic disease* one in which there is structural change.

organism *n* a living cell or group of cells differentiated into functionally distinct parts which are interdependent.

organogenesis *n* the process whereby the body organs develop from embryonic tissue.

organophosphorus compounds several highly toxic compounds usually used as commercial insecticides.

orgasm *n* the climax of sexual excitement.

oriental sore *(syn* Delhi boil) a form of cutaneous leishmaniasis producing papular, crusted, granulomatous skin eruptions. Occurs in tropical and subtropical regions (Old World).

orientation *n* clear awareness of one's position relative to the environment. In mental conditions orientation 'in space and time' means that the patient knows where he or she is and is aware of the passage of time, i.e. can give the correct date. Disorientation means the reverse. ⇒ reality orientation.

orifice *n* a mouth or opening.

origin *n* the commencement or source of anything. *origin of a muscle* the end that remains relatively fixed during contraction of the muscle.

ornithine *n* an amino acid, obtained from arginine during the urea cycle.

ornithosis *n* human illness resulting from disease of birds. ⇒ *Chlamydia*, psittacosis.

orogenital *adj* pertaining to the mouth and the external genital area.

oropharyngeal *adj* pertaining to the mouth and pharynx.

oropharynx *n* that portion of the pharynx which is below the level of the soft palate and above the level of the hyoid bone.

ORS *abbr* oral rehydration solution.

ORT *abbr* oral rehydration therapy.

orthodontic device *n* device used to move teeth by the controlled application of force. May be removable, myofunctional (functional) or fixed.

orthodontics *n* a branch of dentistry concerned with the prevention and correction of irregularities and malocclusion of the teeth.

orthodox sleep *n* *(syn* NREM sleep) ⇒ sleep.

orthognathic surgery *n* surgery aimed at correcting abnormalities in position of the jaw to improve function and appearance.

orthopaedics *n* formerly a specialty devoted to the correction of deformities in children. It is now a branch of surgery dealing with all conditions affecting the locomotor system.

orthopnoea *n* breathlessness that occurs when the person lies flat. It occurs because this position results in the redistribution of blood, leading to an increased central and pulmonary blood volume and fluid accumulation in the lungs—**orthop-noeic** *adj*.

orthoptics *n* the study and treatment of eye movement disorders.

orthoptist *n* one who specializes in assessment and treatment of eye movement disorders.

orthosis *n* external device utilized to correct, control or counteract the effect of an actual or developing deformity. They include braces, callipers and splints. ⇒ night splint, prosthesis—**orthoses** *pl*, **orthotic** *adj*.

orthostatic *adj* caused by the upright stance. *orthostatic albuminuria* occurs in some healthy subjects only when they stand upright.

orthotics *n* the scientific study and manufacture of devices which can be applied to or around the body in the care of physical impairment or disability. ⇒ prosthesis.

orthotopic bladder substitution surgical technique of bladder reconstruction using the site of the excised native bladder with an anastomosis to the native urethra.

orthotist *n* a person who practises orthotics.

Ortolani's sign a test performed shortly after birth for the diagnosis of developmental dysplasia of the hip (congenital dislocation of the hip). It should always be undertaken by an experienced clinician. Often used in conjunction with Barlow's sign/test.

os *n* a mouth. *external os* the opening of the cervix into the vagina (⇒ Figure 17). *internal os* the opening of the cervix into the uterine cavity—**ora** *pl*.

oscillometry *n* measurement of vibration, using a special device (oscillometer).

oscilloscope *n* a device that uses a fluorescent screen to display various electrical waveforms such as that produced by the heart.

Osgood–Schlatter disease ⇒ Schlatter's disease.

Osler's nodes small painful areas in pulp of fingers or toes, or palms and soles, caused by emboli. Occurs in infective endocarditis.

osmolality *n* the number of osmoles per kilogram of solution. An expression of osmotic pressure.

osmolarity *n* the osmotic pressure exerted by a given concentration of osmotically active solute in aqueous solution, defined in terms of the number of active particles per unit volume (osmoles or milliosmoles per litre).

osmole *n* the standard unit of osmotic pressure which is equal to the gram molecular weight of a solute divided by the number of particles or ions into which it dissociates in solution.

osmosis *n* the passage of pure solvent across a semipermeable membrane under the influence of osmotic pressure. It is the movement of a dilute solution into a more concentrated solution.

osmotic diuretics inert substances such as mannitol that exert a diuretic effect. They cause an osmotic 'pull' as they are excreted by the kidney where they are filtered but not reabsorbed. ⇒ Appendix 5.

osmotic laxatives ⇒ laxatives. ⇒ Appendix 5.

osmotic pressure the pressure with which solvent molecules are drawn across a semipermeable membrane separating different concentrations of solute (such as sugars) dissolved in the same solvent, when the membrane is permeable to the solvent but impermeable to the solute.

osseous *adj* relating to or resembling bone.

ossicles *npl* small bones, particularly those contained in the middle ear; the malleus, incus and stapes. ⇒ Figure 13.

ossification *n* the conversion of cartilage, etc. into bone. Also known as osteogenesis—**ossify** *vt*, *vi*.

osteitis *n* inflammation of bone. *osteitis deformans* ⇒ Paget's disease. *osteitis fibrosa* cavities form in the interior of bone. The cysts may be solitary or the disease may be generalized. This second condition may be the result of excessive parathyroid secretion and absorption of calcium from bone.

osteoarthritis *n* sometimes termed degenerative arthritis, although the disease process is much more than simply 'wear and tear'; may be primary, or may follow injury or disease involving the articular surfaces of synovial joints. The articular cartilage becomes worn, osteophytes form at the periphery of the joint surface and loose bodies may result. ⇒ arthropathy—**osteoarthritic** *adj*.

osteoblast *n* a bone-forming cell—**osteoblastic** *adj*.

osteochondritis *n* originally an inflammation of bone cartilage. Usually applied to non-septic conditions, especially avascular necrosis involving joint surfaces, e.g. osteochondritis dissecans in which a portion of joint surface may separate to form a loose body in the joint. ⇒ Scheuermann's disease, Köhler's disease.

osteochondroma *n* a benign bony and cartilaginous tumour.

osteochondrosis *n* an idiopathic disease characterized by a disorder of the ossification of hyaline cartilage (endochondral). It encompasses a group of syndromes classified on the basis of their anatomical location. **1** primary articular epiphysis—Freiberg's disease and Köhler's disease. **2** secondary articular epiphysis—osteochondritis dissecans of the talus. **3** non-articular epiphysis (apophyseal injury)—Sever's disease. The osteochondroses occur during the years of rapid growth. Aetiology has been linked to hereditary factors, trauma, nutritional factors and ischaemia. The articular osteochondroses such as Freiberg's, Köhler's and osteochondritis dissecans are characterized by fragmentation with a centre of ossification.

osteoclasis *n* the therapeutic fracture of a bone.

osteoclast *n* cell that resorbs bone.

osteoclastoma *n* a tumour of the osteoclasts. May be benign, locally recurrent, or frankly malignant. The usual site is near the end of a long bone.

osteocyte *n* a bone cell.

osteodystrophy *n* faulty growth of bone.

osteogenesis *n* bone formation. ⇒ ossification. *osteogenesis imperfecta* a hereditary disorder usually caused by an autosomal dominant gene. It may be present at birth or develop during childhood. The congenital form is much more severe and may lead to early death. The bones are extremely fragile and may fracture following minimal trauma.

osteogenic *adj* bone-producing. *osteogenic sarcoma* malignant tumour that originates from bone-producing cells.

osteolytic *adj* destructive of bone, e.g. osteolytic malignant deposits in bone.

osteoma *n* a benign tumour of bone which may arise in the compact tissue (*ivory osteoma*) or in the cancellous tissue. May be single or multiple.

osteomalacia *n* demineralization of the mature skeleton, with softening and bone pain. It is commonly caused by insufficient dietary intake of vitamin D or lack of sunshine, or both.

osteomyelitis *n* inflammation commencing in the marrow of bone—**osteomyelitic** *adj*.

osteopath *n* one who practises osteopathy.

osteopathy *n* an established clinical discipline. It is concerned with the inter-relationship between structure and function of the body. Osteopathy may be effective for the relief or improvement of a wide variety of conditions, e.g. digestive disorders, as well as mechanical problems. Osteopathy is one of only a few complementary therapies to have achieved statutory self-regulation on a par with healthcare professions such as medicine—**osteopathic** *adj*.

osteopetrosis (*syn* Albers–Schönberg disease, marble bones) a congenital abnormality giving rise to very dense bones which fracture easily.

osteophyte *n* a bony outgrowth or spur, usually at the margins of joint surfaces, e.g. in osteoarthritis—**osteophytic** *adj*.

osteoplasty *n* reconstructive operation on bone—**osteoplastic** *adj*.

osteoporosis *n* loss of bone density caused by excessive absorption of calcium and phosphorus from the bone, due to progressive loss of the protein matrix of bone which normally carries the calcium deposits. Associated with ageing in both men and women. Common cause of fractures, particularly fractures of the wrist, crush fractures of the spine and neck of femur fractures—**osteoporotic** *adj*.

osteosarcoma *n* a malignant tumour growing from bone cells (osteoblasts)—**osteosarcomata** *pl*, **osteosarcomatous** *adj*.

osteosclerosis *n* increased density or hardness of bone—**osteosclerotic** *adj*.

osteotome *n* an instrument for cutting bone; it is similar to a chisel, but it is bevelled on both sides of its cutting edge.

osteotomy *n* division of bone followed by realignment of the ends to encourage union by healing. ⇒ McMurray's osteotomy.

ostium *n* the opening or mouth of any tubular structure—**ostia** *pl*, **ostial** *adj*.

otalgia *n* earache.

OTC *abbr* over-the-counter (medicines).

otitis *n* inflammation of the ear. *otitis externa* inflammation of the skin of the external auditory canal. *otitis media* inflammation of the middle ear cavity. The effusion can be serous, mucoid or purulent. Non-purulent effusions in children are often called glue ear. ⇒ grommet.

otoacoustic emission (OAE) a computer-linked hearing test used for screening babies soon after birth. ⇒ neonatal hearing screening.

otolaryngology *n* ⇒ otorhinolaryngology.

otoliths *npl* tiny calcareous deposits within the utricle and saccule of the internal ear.

otologist *n* a person who specializes in otology.

otology *n* the science which deals with structure, function and disorders of the ear.

otomycosis *n* a fungal (*Aspergillus, Candida*) infection of the external auditory meatus—**otomycotic** *adj*.

otoplasty *n* plastic operation to correct ear deformities.

otorhinolaryngology *n* the science that deals with the structure, function and disorders of the ear, nose and throat; each of these three may be considered a specialty. ⇒ laryngology, otology, rhinology.

otorrhoea *n* a discharge from the ear.

otosclerosis *n* abnormal bone formation affecting primarily the footplate of the stapes. A common cause of progressive conductive deafness—**otosclerotic** *adj*.

otoscope *n* an instrument for examining the ear, usually incorporating both magnification and illumination. Also called an auriscope.

ototoxic *adj* having a toxic action on the ear.

outcome measures scales developed to measure health outcome from clinical interventions: generic measures encompassing dimensions of physical, mental and social health; disease specific scales detecting the effects of treatment of specific conditions. ⇒ quality adjusted life years.

ova *npl* the female gametes (reproductive cells). More correctly known as a secondary oocyte until penetration by a spermatozoon—**ovum** *sing*.

ovarian *adj* relating to the ovaries. *ovarian cycle* the changes occurring in the ovary during the development of the follicle and oogenesis. It has two phases: follicular (days 1–14) when ovulation occurs, and luteal (days 15–28) when the corpus luteum develops. The cycle is controlled by follicle stimulating hormone and luteinizing hormone. *ovarian cyst* a tumour of the ovary, usually containing fluid—may be benign or malignant.

ovariectomy *n* ⇒ oophorectomy.

ovariotomy *n* ⇒ oophorectomy.

ovaritis *n* ⇒ oophoritis.

ovary *n* a female gonad. One of two small oval bodies situated on either side of the uterus on the posterior surface of the broad ligament (⇒ Figure 17). Controlled by pituitary hormones they produce oocytes and oestrogen and progesterones—**ovarian** *adj*. *Polycystic ovaries* ⇒ Stein–Leventhal syndrome.

overcompensation *n* a term that describes any type of behaviour which a person adopts in order to disguise a deficiency. Thus a person who is afraid may react by becoming arrogant or boastful or aggressive.

overheads *npl* the cost of services that contribute to the general upkeep and running of the organization, e.g. grounds maintenance, that cannot be linked directly to the core activity of a department.

overload principle the use of physiological overload in order to produce physiological improvements, i.e. when an individual physically demands more of the muscles than is normally required.

over-the-counter medicines describes those medicines on sale to the public without a prescription. ⇒ general sales list.

overuse injury an injury that is caused by excessive repetitive movement of a body part. Often occurs following periods of inadequate rest or recovery, over-activity, or repetitive overloading of part or structure.

overuse syndrome injury caused by accumulated microtraumatic stress placed on a structure or body area.

oviduct *n* uterine or fallopian tubes.

ovulation *n* the maturation and rupture of a Graafian follicle with the discharge of an oocyte.

oxalic acid toxic organic acid found in plants, e.g. rhubarb leaves.

oxaluria *n* excretion of oxalates (salts of oxalic acid) in the urine.

oxicams a group of non-steroidal anti-inflammatory drugs. ⇒ Appendix 5.

oxidase *n* any enzyme that encourages oxidation.

oxidation *n* the act of oxidizing or state of being oxidized. It involves the addition of oxygen, e.g. formation of oxides, or the loss of electrons or the removal of hydrogen. A part of metabolism, whereby energy is released from fuel molecules. ⇒ reduction.

oxidative phosphorylation a mitochondrial energy-producing metabolic process, whereby adenosine diphosphate (ADP) is converted to adenosine triphosphate (ATP) by the addition of a phosphate group.

oximeter ⇒ pulse oximeter.

oxygen (O) *n* a colourless, odourless, gaseous element; necessary for life and combustion. Constitutes 20% of atmospheric air. Used therapeutically as an inhalation to increase blood oxygenation. Delivered as part of a general anaesthetic to maintain life. ⇒ hyperbaric oxygen therapy. *oxygen concentrator* a device for removing nitrogen from the air to provide a high concentration of oxygen for use by patients requiring many hours of oxygen therapy each day at home.

oxygenation *n* the saturation of a substance (particularly blood) with oxygen. Arterial oxygen tension (PaO_2) indicates degree of oxgygenation (normally more than 97% saturated)—**oxygenated** *adj*. ⇒ pulse oximetry.

oxygenator *n* apparatus used to oxygenate the patient's blood during open heart surgery, or to support critically ill patients. ⇒ cardiopulmonary bypass.

oxygen consumption (VO₂) amount of oxygen consumed by the body per minute, typically 250 mL/min.

oxygen debt (*syn* excess post-exercise oxygen consumption, oxygen recovery) the total amount of oxygen needed to replace adenosine triphosphate (ATP), restore creatine phosphate (phosphocreatine) and remove lactic acid in active tissue during the recovery process following exercise. ⇒ alactacid oxygen debt

component, lactacid oxygen debt component, lactacid oxygen debt component.

oxygen delivery (DO₂) amount of oxygen delivered to the tissues per minute, product of cardiac output and arterial oxygen content, typically 1000 mL/min.

oxygen saturation percentage of oxygenated haemoglobin present in the blood. ⇒ pulse oximeter.

oxyhaemoglobin *n* oxygenated haemoglobin, an unstable compound formed from haemoglobin on contact with air in the alveoli.

oxyntic *adj* producing acid. *oxyntic cells* the cells in the gastric mucosa which produce hydrochloric acid.

oxytocic *adj, n* hastening parturition; an agent that stimulates uterine contractions. ⇒ Appendix 5.

oxytocin *n* a hormone released from the posterior pituitary. It contracts the uterine muscle and milk ducts and is involved in reflex milk ejection.

Oxyuris *n* a genus of nematodes (threadworms). Also known as *Enterobius*.

ozaena *n* atrophic rhinitis.

ozone *n* a form of oxygen. O_3. Has powerful oxidizing properties and is therefore antiseptic and disinfectant. It is both irritating and toxic to the pulmonary system.

P

^{32}**P** *abbr* radioactive phosphorus.

pacemaker *n* the region of the heart that initiates atrial contraction and thus controls heart rate. The natural pacemaker is the sinus node which is situated at the junction of the superior vena cava and the right atrium; the wave of contraction begins here, then spreads over the heart. *artificial pacemaker* ⇒ cardiac.

pachyderma *n* thick skin. ⇒ elephantiasis.

pacing *n* compensatory techniques used by occupational therapists that enable an individual to perform activities of daily living in a planned, balanced, continuous manner by strictly adhering to measurable, personal goals. It involves the use of activity analysis, timing, resting, and alternating movements in order to maximize optimal performance and minimize pain, stress and fatigue by expending effort consistently over a period of time.

packed cell volume (PCV) volume of red cells in the blood, expressed as a percentage of the total blood volume. Also called the haematocrit.

*Pa*CO$_2$ *abbr* the partial pressure or tension of carbon dioxide in arterial blood.

*P*ACO$_2$ *abbr* the partial pressure or tension of carbon dioxide in alveolar air.

PACS *abbr* picture archiving communication system.

PADL *abbr* personal activities of daily living.

paediatrician *n* a specialist in children's diseases.

paediatrics *n* the branch of medicine dealing with children and their diseases— **paediatric** *adj*.

paedophilia the sexual attraction to children.

PAFC *abbr* pulmonary artery flotation catheter.

Paget–Schroetter syndrome axillary or subclavian vein thrombosis, often associated with effort in fit young persons.

Paget's disease 1 (*syn* osteitis deformans) excess of the enzyme alkaline phosphatase causes too rapid bone formation; consequently bone is thin. There is loss of stature, crippling deformity, enlarged head and collapse of vertebrae, and neurological complications can result. Sufferers are particularly susceptible to sarcoma of bone. If the vestibulocochlear (auditory) nerve is involved, there is impairment of hearing. Calcitonin is the drug of choice. **2** erosion of the nipple caused by invasion of the dermis by intraduct carcinoma of the breast.

pain *n* unpleasant sensation experienced when nociceptors are stimulated. It is individual and subjective with a physiological and emotional component. Pain ranges from mild to agonizing, but individual responses are influenced by factors which include: information about cause, age, whether acute or chronic and pain tolerance. *pain management* involves a holistic multidisciplinary approach, and in some healthcare settings there is a designated pain team or nurse specialist. *pain threshold* the lowest intensity at which a stimulus is felt as pain. There is very little difference between people. *pain tolerance* the greatest intensity of pain

that the individual is prepared to put up with. There is substantial variation between people.

PAL *abbr* physical activity level.

palate *n* the roof of the mouth. ⇒ Figure 14—**palatal, palatine** *adj. cleft palate* ⇒ cleft palate. *hard palate* the front part of the roof of the mouth formed by the two palatal bones. *soft palate* situated at the posterior end of the palate and consisting of muscle covered by mucous membrane.

palatine *adj* pertaining to the palate. *palatine arches* the bilateral double pillars or arch-like folds formed by the descent of the soft palate as it meets the pharynx.

palatoplegia *n* paralysis of the soft palate— **palatoplegic** *adj*.

palliate *v* relieve symptoms. Often refers to option where a patient is not curable and is fit only for treatment to prevent distress from symptoms. It may involve surgery, chemotherapy, radiotherapy, nerve block, drugs (typically opioids).

palliative *adj, n* (describes) anything that serves to alleviate but cannot cure a disease. *palliative care* the specialty of symptom relief—**palliation** *n*.

pallidectomy *n* destruction of a predetermined section of globus pallidus. ⇒ chemopallidectomy, stereotactic surgery.

pallidotomy *n* surgical severance of the fibres from the cerebral cortex to the corpus striatum. Previously used for relief of tremor in Parkinson's disease.

palm *n* the anterior or flexor surface of the hand.

palmar *adj* pertaining to the palm of the hand. *palmar arches* superficial and deep, are formed by the anastomosis of the radial and ulnar arteries (⇒ Figure 9).

palpable *adj* capable of being palpated.

palpation *n* the act of manual examination—**palpate** *vt*.

palpebra *n* an eyelid—**palpebrae** *pl*, **palpebral** *adj*.

palpitation *n* rapid beating of the heart that is felt by the patient.

palsy *n* paralysis. A word that is only retained in compound forms—Bell's palsy, cerebral palsy and Erb's palsy.

panarthritis *n* inflammation of all the structures of a joint.

pancarditis *n* inflammation of all the structures of the heart.

pancreas *n* a tongue-shaped glandular organ lying below and behind the stomach (⇒ Figure 18b). Its head is encircled by the duodenum and its tail touches the spleen. It is about 18 cm long and weighs about 100 g. It secretes the hormones insulin and glucagon, and also alkaline pancreatic juice which contains digestive enzymes involved in the digestion of fats, carbohydrates and proteins in the small intestine.

pancreatectomy *n* excision of part or the whole of the pancreas.

pancreatic function tests intubation tests involve measurement of enzyme activity and bicarbonate in the duodenum after endocrine or meal stimulation. Indirect tests involve measurement of pancreatic enzyme metabolites in urine, plasma or breath.

pancreaticoduodenectomy *n* surgical excision of the duodenum and head of the pancreas, carried out in cases of cancer arising in the region of the head of the pancreas.

pancreaticojejunostomy *n* surgical procedure to establish an anastomosis between the pancreatic duct and the jejunum.

pancreatitis *n* inflammation of the pancreas which may be acute or chronic. Most commonly caused by gallstones or alcohol.

pancreozymin *n* intestinal hormone identical to cholecystokinin (CCK). Previously both names were used.

pancytopenia *n* describes peripheral blood picture when red cells, granular white cells and platelets are reduced as occurs when bone marrow function is suppressed.

pandemic *n* an infection spreading over a whole country or the world.

panniculitis *n* an inflammation of the subcutaneous fat.

pannus *n* fibrovascular membrane usually within the anterior stroma of the cornea.

panophthalmitis *n* inflammation of all the tissues of the eyeball.

panosteitis *n* inflammation of all constituents of a bone—medulla, bony tissue and periosteum.

panretinal photocoagulation (PRP) treatment of the mid-peripheral retina with laser burns to reduce proliferative retinopathy, for example in diabetes.

pantothenic acid a member of the vitamin B complex. It is part of acetyl coenzyme A (acetyl CoA). It is so widely distributed in food that dietary deficiency is very rare; if it develops it will be in association with other deficiency disorders.

PAO *abbr* peak acid output. ⇒ pentagastrin.

PaO_2 *abbr* partial pressure or tension of oxygen in arterial blood.

PAO_2 *abbr* the partial pressure or tension of oxygen in alveolar air.

PAOP *abbr* pulmonary artery occlusion pressure.

Papanicolaou test (Pap) a smear of epithelial cells taken from the cervix is stained and examined under the microscope for detection of the early stages of cancer.

papilla *n* a minute nipple-shaped eminence—papillae *pl*, papillary *adj*. *renal papilla* ⇒ Figure 20.

papillary necrosis infarction and necrosis of the renal papillae.

papillectomy *n* excision of a papilla.

papillitis *n* 1 inflammation of the optic nerve head (disc). 2 inflammation of a renal papilla.

papilloedema *n* swelling of the optic nerve head (disc), usually bilateral, caused by raised intracranial pressure. ⇒ Glasgow Coma Scale, head injury.

papilloma *n* a simple tumour arising from a non-glandular epithelial surface—papillomata *pl*, papillomatous *adj*.

papillomatosis *n* the growth of benign papillomata on the skin or a mucous membrane. Removal by laser means fewer recurrences.

papillotomy *n* incision of a papilla, e.g. duodenal papilla for endoscopic extraction of ductal calculi.

papule (*syn* pimple) a small circumscribed elevation of the skin—papular *adj*.

papulopustular *adj* pertaining to both papules and pustules.

PAR *abbr* physical activity ratio.

para-aortic *adj* near the aorta.

paracentesis *n* usually applied to the surgical puncture of the abdominal cavity for the aspiration of fluid. ⇒ aspiration—paracenteses *pl*.

paracetamol *n* a non-steroidal anti-inflammatory drug which has no anti-inflammatory action but is analgesic and antipyretic. ⇒ Appendix 5.

paradigm *n* an example, model, or set of ideas or assumptions. *paradigm shift* the changes that occur as the build-up of evidence causes a paradigm to be questioned and eventually replaced by a new set of ideas.

paradoxical respiration associated with injuries that result in the ribs on one side being fractured in two places, such as in flail chest. The injured side of the chest moves in (deflates) on inspiration and vice versa.

paradoxical sleep (*syn* REM sleep) ⇒ sleep.

paraesthesia *n* any abnormality of sensation such as tingling.

paraffin *n* medicinal paraffins are: *hard paraffin*, used in wax baths for rheumatic conditions; *liquid paraffin*, a lubricant/softener laxative; and *soft paraffin*, used as an ointment base.

paraganglioma *n* phaeochromocytoma occurring outside the adrenal medulla.

parainfluenza virus a myxovirus causing acute upper respiratory infection.

paralysis *n* complete or incomplete loss of nervous function to a part of the body. This may be sensory or motor or both. *paralysis agitans* ⇒ parkinsonism.

paralytic *adj* pertaining to paralysis. *paralytic ileus* paralysis of the intestinal muscle so that the bowel content cannot pass onwards even though there is no mechanical obstruction. ⇒ aperistalsis.

paramedian *adj* near the middle.

paramedical *adj* allied to medicine.

parametric tests statistical tests that presuppose the data are from a sample from a population that has a normal distribution curve. ⇒ non-parametric tests.

parametritis *n* ⇒ cellulitis.

parametrium *n* the connective tissues immediately surrounding the uterus—**parametrial** *adj*.

paranasal *adj* near the nasal cavities, as the various sinuses.

paraneoplastic *adj* describes symptoms or signs associated with the presence of a malignant neoplasm but not directly from the situation of the primary or the metastases.

paranoia *n* an abnormal tendency to mistrust or suspect others—**paranoid** *adj*.

paranoid behaviour acts denoting suspicion of others.

paranoid schizophrenia a form of schizophrenia characterized by (often persecutory) delusions and hallucinations.

paraoesophageal *adj* near the oesophagus.

paraparesis *n* loss of power in the legs.

paraphimosis *n* retraction of the prepuce behind the glans penis so that a tight ring of skin produces oedema of the preputial skin.

paraphrenia *n* a persistent delusional disorder with onset in later life—**paraphrenic** *adj*.

paraplegia *n* paralysis of the lower limbs, usually including the bladder and rectum—**paraplegic** *adj*. ⇒ hemiplegia, monoplegia, tetraplegia.

paraprax *n* known as a 'Freudian slip'. A verbal error caused by unconscious conflicts.

parapsychology *n* the study of extrasensory perception, telepathy and other psychic phenomena.

paraquat dichloride widely used as a herbicide. Exposure leads to local effects depending on the route, but include: oral/oesophageal damage, skin blisters, epistaxis, or severe inflammation of the conjunctiva or cornea. Systemic effects that may be delayed are usually associated with ingestion and include damage to the myocardium, lungs, liver and kidneys.

pararectal *adj* near the rectum.

parasitaemia *n* parasites in the blood—**parasitaemic** *adj*.

parasite *n* an organism that obtains nutrients or shelter from another organism, the 'host'—**parasitic** *adj*.

parasiticide *n* an agent that will kill parasites.

parasomnias *npl* a broad class of sleep-associated disturbances; it includes sleep-walking, nightmares and bruxism.

parasuicide *n* a suicidal gesture: drugs overdose or a self-mutilating act which may or may not be provoked by a real wish to die. Commonly seen in young people who are distressed but not mentally ill. May be linked to low self-esteem. ⇒ deliberate self-harm, Samaritans.

parasympathetic *adj* describes the part of the autonomic nervous system having craniosacral outflow. It is concerned with the normal at rest body processes and opposes the action of the sympathetic nervous system.

parasympatholytic *adj* usually describes a drug, that reduces or eradicates the effects of parasympathetic stimulation. ⇒ muscarinic antagonist.

parasympathomimetic *adj* describes an agent, usually a drug, that causes similar effects as or stimulates parasympathetic activity. ⇒ muscarinic agonist.

parathormone *n* parathyroid hormone. ⇒ parathyroid glands.

parathyroidectomy *n* excision of one or more parathyroid glands.

parathyroid glands four small endocrine glands lying close to or embedded in the posterior surface of the thyroid gland. They secrete *parathyroid hormone (PTH)* a protein hormone that regulates calcium and phosphate homeostasis. It is released when serum calcium level is decreased.

paratyphoid fever a variety of enteric fever, less severe and prolonged than typhoid fever. Caused by *Salmonella paratyphi A* and *B*, and more rarely *C*.

paraurethral *adj* near the urethra.

paravaginal *adj* near the vagina.

paravertebral *adj* near the spinal column. *paravertebral block anaesthesia* (more correctly, analgesia) is induced by infiltration of local anaesthetic around the spinal nerve roots as they emerge from the intervertebral foramina. *paravertebral injection* of local anaesthetic into sympathetic chain can be used as a test in ischaemic limbs to see if sympathectomy is indicated.

parenchyma *n* the parts of an organ which, in contradistinction to its interstitial tissue, are concerned with its function—**parenchymal, parenchymatous** *adj*.

parenteral *adj* not via the alimentary tract. Therapy such as fluid, drugs, or nutrition administered by a route other than the alimentary tract.

parenteral nutrition a method of providing nutrition by administering nutrients directly into the circulatory system via a venous catheter. It can be given temporarily in hospital, or permanently at home (home parenteral nutrition) in the treatment of intestinal failure. A special intravenous catheter is used to infuse various nutrient solutions into a central vein. Usually the catheter is sited centrally, through the subclavian vein into the superior vena cava. Sometimes it is possible to use peripherally inserted central catheters (PICC) which are inserted through the basilic vein (of the arm) to the superior vena cava via the right subclavian vein. Parenteral nutrition is used for patients whose gastrointestinal tract is not functioning. It should only be used if nutritional needs cannot be met via the enteral route. The term total parenteral nutrition is used in the US—**parenterally** *adv*.

paresis *n* partial or slight paralysis; weakness of a limb—**paretic** *adj*.

pareunia *n* coitus.

parietal *adj* pertaining to a wall. *parietal bones* the two bones which form the sides and vault of the skull.

parity *n* status of a woman with regard to the number of children she has borne.

parkinsonism *n* a condition resembling Parkinson's disease clinically.

Parkinson's disease an incurable neurodegenerative condition in which there is a relatively selective loss of dopamine nerve cells in the brain causing a resting tremor, bradykinesia (slowness of movement) and rigidity in the limbs. Some people differentiate between Parkinson's disease and parkinsonism, the causes of which are multiple and include repeated brain trauma (as in boxing), stroke, atherosclerosis, various toxic agents, viral encephalitis and neuroleptic drugs (typical). => neuroleptics, tardive dyskinesia.

paronychia *n* (*syn* whitlow) inflammation of the tissue around a nail plate, which may be bacterial or fungal. It frequently occurs with onychia.

parosmia *n* altered, dysfunctional sense of smell, usually of unpleasant hallucinatory nature.

parotidectomy *n* excision of a parotid (salivary) gland.

parotid gland the salivary gland situated in front of and below the ear on either side.

parotitis *n* inflammation of a parotid salivary gland. *infectious parotitis* mumps. *septic parotitis* refers to ascending infection from the mouth via the parotid duct, when a parotid abscess may result.

parous *adj* having borne a child or children.

paroxysm *n* a sudden, temporary attack.

paroxysmal *adj* coming on in attacks or paroxysms. *paroxysmal dyspnoea* occurs mostly at night in patients with cardiac disease. *paroxysmal fibrillation* occurs in the atrium of the heart and is associated with a ventricular tachycardia and total irregularity of the pulse rhythm. *paroxysmal tachycardia* may result from ectopic impulses arising in the atrium or in the ventricle itself.

parrot disease ⇒ psittacosis.

Parrot's nodes bossing of frontal bones in congenital syphilis.

partial agonist a drug that only has a partial physiological effect, having reduced efficacy compared with a full agonist.

partial pressure pressure exerted by a gas in a mixture of different gases. It is directly related to its concentration and the pressure exerted by the total mixture.

partnership working in the UK a working relationship between central government, local NHS services, local government authorities, and local communities. It enables greater coordination and cooperative multiagency/multiprofessional working that aims to improve health and well-being.

parturient *adj* pertaining to childbirth.

parturition *n* ⇒ labour.

pascal (Pa) *n* derived SI unit (International System of Units) for pressure. The kilopascal (kPa) is now frequently used for measuring blood gases. It would be used for measuring blood pressure instead of millimetres of mercury pressure (mmHg) if the change was ever made.

passive *adj* inactive. ⇒ active *opp*. *passive hyperaemia* ⇒ hyperaemia. *passive immunity* ⇒ immunity. *passive movement* performed by the physiotherapist, the patient being relaxed.

passive stretching stretching of a body part by use of a force other than tension in the antagonist muscles, e.g. by an examiner without assistance from the athlete.

Pasteurella *n* ⇒ Yersinia.

pasteurization *n* a process whereby pathogenic organisms in fluid (especially milk) are killed by heat. *flash method of pasteurization* (HT, ST—high temperature short time), the fluid is heated to 72°C, maintained at this temperature for 15 s, then rapidly cooled, *holder method of pasteurization* the fluid is heated to 63–65.5°C, maintained at this temperature for 30 min then rapidly cooled.

Patau's syndrome autosomal trisomy of chromosome 13. Closely associated with learning disability. There are accompanying physical defects.

patch test a skin test for type IV (delayed-type) hypersensitivity to allergens, which are incorporated into an adhesive patch applied to the skin. Forty-eight hours after application the skin under the patch is examined for signs of redness and swelling. Comparison is made against a negative control containing a neutral non-allergenic compound.

patella *n* a triangular, sesamoid bone; the kneecap (⇒ Figure 2)—**patellae** *pl*, **patellar** *adj*.

patellectomy *n* excision of the patella.

patent *adj* open; not closed or occluded—**patency** *n*. *patent ductus arteriosus* failure of ductus arteriosus to close soon after birth, so that an abnormal shunt between the pulmonary artery and the aorta is preserved. *patent interventricular septum* a congenital defect in the dividing wall between the right and left ventricle of the heart.

paternalism *n* over-protective or restricting, such as withholding information about potential risks of healthcare interventions, or well-meaning rules and regulations that reduce individual autonomy.

pathogen *n* a disease-producing agent, usually applied to a living agent—**pathogenic** *adj*, **pathogenicity** *n*.

pathogenesis *n* the origin and development of disease—**pathogenetic** *adj*.

pathogenicity *n* the capacity to cause disease.

pathognomonic *adj* characteristic of or peculiar to a disease.

pathological fracture ⇒ fracture.

pathology *n* the science which deals with the cause and nature of disease—**pathological** *adj*, **pathologically** *adv*.

pathophobia *n* a morbid dread of disease—**pathophobic** *adj*.

pathophysiology *n* the science that deals with abnormal functioning of the human being—**pathophysiological** *adj*, **pathophysiologically** *adv*.

patient advocacy liaison service an advocacy service to patients in NHS and

Primary Care Trusts, representing their concerns and complaints to the relevant department within the trust.

patient compliance a term used when a patient takes the prescribed drug, in the prescribed dose, at the prescribed time and by the prescribed route. ⇒ non-compliance *opp*.

patient controlled analgesia (PCA) equipment that enables patients to control the delivery of analgesic drugs, (within prescribed limits). Usually via an intravenous line, but patient controlled epidural analgesia (PCEA) may be suitable in some situations. ⇒ analgesia, epidural.

patients' forum a statutory and independent body comprising patients who will represent the views of patients about how their local NHS services are run.

patriarchy *n* a community or family where the oldest male (father) dominates, controls and is the highest authority.

patulous *adj* opened out; expanded.

Paul–Bunnell test a serological test used in the diagnosis of infectious mononucleosis.

Pawlik's grip a method of determining the engagement or otherwise of the fetal head in the maternal pelvic brim.

PBD *abbr* peak bone density.

PCA(S) *abbr* patient controlled analgesia (system).

PCEA *abbr* patient controlled epidural analgesia.

PCO_2 *abbr* the partial pressure of carbon dioxide, for example in atmospheric or expired air.

PCOS *abbr* polycystic ovary syndrome.

PCR *abbr* polymerase chain reaction.

PCT *abbr* Primary Care Trust.

PCV *abbr* packed cell volume.

peak bone density (PBD) or mass (PBM) the greatest bone density achieved by an individual, usually achieved in the 30s.

peak expiratory flow rate (PEFR) the measured amount of air in a forced expiration.

peau d'orange appearance of (usually) the breast when a cancer results in lymphatic obstruction and dimpling at the hair follicles causing the breast to look (literally) like orange skin; usually a sign of locally advanced disease.

pectoral *adj* pertaining to the breast.

pectus *n* the chest. *pectus carinatum* ⇒ pigeon chest. *pectus excavatum* ⇒ funnel chest.

pedal *adj* pertaining to the foot. *pedal pulse* the dorsalis pedis artery palpated on the dorsum of the foot.

pedicle *n* a stalk, e.g. the narrow part by which a tumour is attached to the surrounding structures.

pediculosis *n* infestation with lice (pediculi).

Pediculus *n* a genus of parasitic insects (lice) important as vectors of disease. *Pediculus capitis* the head louse. *Pediculus corporis* the body louse. *Pediculus* (more correctly, *Phthirus*) *pubis* the crab or pubic louse. In some regions of the world body lice are responsible for the transmission of typhus and other diseases.

pedopompholyx *n* ⇒ cheiropompholyx.

peduncle *n* a stalk-like structure—**peduncular, pedunculated** *adj*.

peeling *n* desquamation.

PEEP *abbr* positive end expiratory pressure.

peer support support from other members of a group to which one belongs. For example, new patients perceive established patients as providing support. Likewise, health professionals use their peer groups to gain and provide support, particularly in stressful circumstances.

PEFR *abbr* peak expiratory flow rate.

PEG *abbr* percutaneous endoscopic gastrostomy.

Pel–Ebstein fever recurring bouts of pyrexia in regular sequence found in Hodgkin's disease. A less frequent manifestation with improving treatment.

pellagra *n* a deficiency disease caused by lack of the B vitamin niacin and the amino acid tryptophan. Syndrome includes glossitis, dermatitis, peripheral neuritis and spinal cord changes (even producing ataxia), anaemia and mental confusion.

pellet *n* a small pill. ⇒ implant.

pelvic *adj* relating to the pelvis *pelvic floor* a mainly muscular partition with the pelvic cavity above and the perineum below. In the female, weakening of these muscles can contribute to urinary incontinence and uterine prolapse. *pelvic girdle* the bony pelvis comprising two innominate bones, the sacrum and coccyx.

pelvic floor repair operation performed to correct genital prolapse. ⇒ Manchester repair.

pelvic inflammatory disease (PID) acute or chronic inflammation of the ovaries, uterine (fallopian) tube and uterus. Infection may spread from adjacent pelvic structures including the bowel or appendix or through the cervix from the vagina and may be sexually transmitted. It is characterized by lower abdominal pain, and urgent antibiotic treatment is essential if tubal occlusion and infertility are to be prevented.

pelvic pain syndrome (PPS) pelvic pain which occurs in women but for which no pathological cause is evident.

pelvimeter *n* an instrument especially devised to measure the pelvic diameters for obstetric purposes.

pelvimetry *n* the measurement of the dimensions of the pelvis—**pelvimetric** *adj.*

pelvis *n* **1** a basin-shaped cavity, e.g. pelvis of the kidney (⇒ Figure 20). **2** the large bony basin-shaped cavity formed by the innominate bones and sacrum, containing and protecting the bladder, rectum and, in the female, the organs of generation—**pelvic** *adj. contracted pelvis* one in which one or more diameters are smaller than normal; this may result in difficulties in childbirth. *false pelvis* the wide expanded part of the pelvis above the brim. *true pelvis* that part of the pelvis below the brim.

pelviureteric junction (PUJ) obstruction a condition, often congenital, resulting in obstruction at the junction of the renal pelvis and proximal ureter.

PEM *abbr* protein energy malnutrition.

pemphigoid *n* a bullous eruption, usually in the latter half of life, which is of autoimmune cause. Histological examination of a blister differentiates it from pemphigus. Treated by systemic corticosteroids.

pemphigus *n* a group of rare but serious diseases called pemphigus vulgaris, pemphigus vegetans and pemphigus erythematosus. *pemphigus vulgaris* a bullous disease mostly of middle age, of autoimmune aetiology. Blister formation occurs in the epidermis, with resulting secondary infection and rupture, so that large raw areas develop. Bullae develop also on mucous membranes. The condition is treated by systemic corticosteroids and immunosuppressive drugs.

pendular response a pathological response to the stretch reflex commonly seen in cerebellar disease. When a muscle is stretched by distortion of its tendon, the stretch reflex response is sluggish and is not checked by a reciprocal response in the antagonist muscle; e.g. if the knee jerk is invoked, there will not be one sharp jerk but the leg will swing like a pendulum.

pendulous *adj* hanging down. *pendulous abdomen* a relaxed condition of the anterior wall, allowing it to hang down over the pubis.

penetrating ulcer an ulcer that is locally invasive.

penetrating wound (*syn* puncture wound) caused by a sharp, usually slim object, or a missile, which passes through the skin into the tissues beneath.

penicillinase ⇒ beta (β)-lactamase.

penicillins *npl* a large group of β-lactam antibiotics. Many are broad spectrum but they produce hypersensitivity reactions and many micro-organisms have developed resistance. Some newer penicillins are β-lactamase resistant. ⇒ Appendix 5.

Penicillium *n* a genus of moulds. The hyphae bear spores characteristically arranged like a brush. A common contaminant of food. The species *Penicillium notatum* was shown by Fleming (1928) to produce penicillin.

penis *n* the male organ of copulation (⇒ Figure 16)—**penile** *adj.*

pentagastrin *n* a synthetic hormone used in gastric function tests to produce maximal gastric acid secretion. *pentagastrin test* measures gastric acid secretion by parietal cells in the stomach.

pentose *n* a five carbon monosaccharide (sugar) such as ribose.

pepsin *n* a proteolytic enzyme secreted by the stomach, as the precursor pepsinogen, which hydrolyses proteins to polypeptides. It has an optimum pH of 1.5–2.0.

pepsinogen *n* a proenzyme secreted mainly by the chief cells in the gastric mucosa and converted to pepsin by hydrochloric acid or existing pepsin.

peptic *adj* pertaining to pepsin or to digestion generally. *peptic ulcer* a non-malignant ulcer in those parts of the digestive tract that are exposed to the gastric secretions; hence usually in the stomach or duodenum but sometimes in the lower oesophagus or with a Meckel's diverticulum.

peptidase *n* an enzyme that breaks down proteins into amino acids. ⇒ aminopeptidases, dipeptidases.

peptides *npl* organic compounds that yield two or more amino acids on hydrolysis; e.g. dipeptides and polypeptides. *peptide bond* a chemical bond formed during a dehydration reaction when two amino acids form peptides.

percept *n* the mental product of a sensation; a sensation plus memories of similar sensations and their relationships.

perception *n* the reception of a conscious impression through the sensory organs by which we differentiate objects one from another and recognize their qualities according to the different sensations they produce.

percussion *n* tapping to determine the resonance or dullness of the area examined. Normally a finger of the left hand is laid on the patient's skin and the middle finger of the right hand (plexor) is used to strike the left finger.

percutaneous *adj* through the skin. *percutaneous endoscopic gastrostomy (PEG)* gastrostomy tube inserted endoscopically through the abdominal wall. *percutaneous myocardial revascularization* a treatment for angina. A catheter with laser energy source is introduced into the heart via the femoral artery. The laser is used to produce channels through to the myocardium, thus allowing more oxygenated blood to reach the myocardium. *percutaneous nephrolithotomy* ⇒ nephrolithotomy. *percutaneous transhepatic cholangiography (PTC)* ⇒ cholangiography. *percutaneous transluminal coronary angioplasty (PTCA)* a procedure used in the treatment of angina. A balloon tipped catheter is used to dilate a stenosed coronary artery.

perforation *n* a hole in a previously intact sheet of tissue. Used in reference to perforation of the tympanic membrane, or the wall of the stomach or gut, constituting a surgical emergency.

performance components the basic skills required to perform activities of daily living, including sensorimotor, cognitive, psychosocial, psychological and spiritual skills.

performance indicators (PIs) quantitative measures of the activities and resources used in healthcare delivery. High level performance indicators, e.g. deaths from all causes (people aged 15–64), early detection of cancer, day case rate, cancelled operations, and clinical indicators, e.g. deaths in hospital after surgery, a heart attack or hip fracture, are used to assess the six areas of the National Framework for Assessing Performance.

perianal *adj* surrounding the anus.

periarterial *adj* surrounding an artery.

periarteritis *n* inflammation of the outer sheath of an artery and the periarterial tissue. *periarteritis nodosa* ⇒ polyarteritis.

periarthritis *n* inflammation of the structures surrounding a joint. Sometimes applied to frozen shoulder.

periarticular *adj* surrounding a joint.

peribulbar *adj* around the eyeball inside the orbit.

pericardectomy *n* surgical removal of the pericardium, thickened from chronic inflammation (pericarditis) and restricting the action of the heart.

pericardiocentesis *n* aspiration of the pericardial sac.

pericarditis *n* inflammation of the pericardial covering of the heart. It may or may not be accompanied by an effusion and formation of adhesions between the two layers. ⇒ pericardectomy.

pericardium *n* the double serous membranous sac which envelops the heart. The layer in contact with the heart is called visceral (or epicardium); that reflected to form the sac is called parietal. Between the two is the pericardial cavity, which normally contains a small amount of serous fluid—**pericardial** *adj*.

perichondrium *n* the membranous covering of cartilage—**perichondrial** *adj*.

pericolic *adj* around the colon.

pericranium *n* the periosteal covering of the cranium—**pericranial** *adj*.

perifollicular *adj* around a follicle.

perilymph *n* the fluid contained in the internal ear, between the membranous and bony labyrinth.

perimetrium *n* the peritoneal covering of the uterus—**perimetrial** *adj*.

perimetry *n* measurement of the field of vision.

perinatal *adj* pertaining to the period around birth. The weeks before a birth, the birth and the week following. ⇒ mortality.

perineometer *n* a pressure gauge inserted into the vagina to register the strength of contraction in the pelvic floor muscles.

perineorrhaphy *n* an operation for the repair of a torn perineum.

perineotomy *n* episiotomy.

perinephric *adj* surrounding the kidney.

perineum *n* the wedge-shaped structure situated between the rectum and the external genitalia—**perineal** *adj*.

perineurium *n* connective tissue enclosing a bundle of nerve fibres.

periodic breathing a period of apnoea in a newborn baby of 5–10 seconds followed by a period of hyperventilation at a rate of 50–60 breaths a minute, for a period of 10–15 seconds. The overall respiratory rate remains between 30 and 40 breaths per minute.

periodontal disease ⇒ periodontitis.

periodontics *n* branch of dentistry concerned with prevention and treatment of diseases of the supporting tissues of the teeth.

periodontitis *n* inflammatory disease of the periodontium, resulting in destruction of the periodontal ligament.

periodontium *n* collective name given to the tissues supporting a tooth and comprising the gingiva, periodontal ligament, cementum and surrounding alveolar bone.

perioperative *adj* refers to the period during which a surgical operation is carried out, as well as to the pre- and postoperative periods.

perioral *adj* around the mouth.

periosteum *n* the membrane which covers a bone. In long bones only the shaft as far as the epiphysis is covered. It protects and allows regeneration—**periosteal** *adj*.

periostitis *n* inflammation of the periosteum. *diffuse periostitis* that involving the periosteum of long bones. *haemorrhagic periostitis* that accompanied by bleeding between the periosteum and the bone.

peripartum *n* at the time of delivery. A precise word for what is more commonly called perinatal.

peripheral *adj* relating to the outer parts of any structure. *peripheral nervous system (PNS)* describes that part of the nervous system outside the brain or spinal cord. Usually applied to those nerves which supply the musculoskeletal system and surrounding tissues to differentiate from the autonomic nervous system. *peripheral resistance (PR)* the force exerted by the arteriolar walls which is an important factor in the control of normal blood pressure. *peripheral vascular disease (PVD)* any abnormal condition arising in the blood vessels outside the heart, the main one being atherosclerosis, which can lead to thrombosis and occlusion of the vessel, resulting in gangrene. *peripheral vision* that surrounding the central field of vision.

periportal *adj* surrounding the hepatic portal vein.

perirenal *adj* around the kidney.

perisplenitis *n* inflammation of the peritoneal coat of the spleen and of the adjacent structures.

peristalsis *n* a rhythmic wave-like contraction and dilatation occurring in a hollow structure, e.g. ureter, gastrointestinal tract. In the intestine it is the movement by which the contents (food and waste) are propelled along the lumen. It consists of a wave of contraction preceded by a wave of relaxation—**peristaltic** *adj*.

peritomy *n* incision of the conjunctiva around the corneal limbus.

peritoneal dialysis a form of dialysis in which the peritoneum is the porous membrane, and synthetic fluid is inserted into, and removed from the peritoneal cavity via a catheter. Different techniques exist, such as automated peritoneal dialysis and continuous ambulatory peritoneal dialysis.

peritoneoscopy ⇒ laparoscopy.

peritoneum *n* the delicate serous membrane which lines the abdominal and pelvic cavities (parietal layer) and also covers some of the organs (visceral layer) contained in them—**peritoneal** *adj*.

peritonitis *n* inflammation of the peritoneum, usually secondary to disease of one of the abdominal organs.

peritonsillar abscess (quinsy) abscess formation in the loose tissue around the palatine tonsil.

peritrichous *adj* applied to a bacterium that has flagella on all sides of the cell. ⇒ *Bacillus*.

periumbilical *adj* surrounding the umbilicus.

periurethral *adj* surrounding the urethra, as a periurethral abscess.

perivascular *adj* around a blood vessel.

perlèche *n* lip licking. An intertrigo at the angles of the mouth with maceration, fissuring, or crust formation. May result from use of poorly fitting dentures, bacterial and fungal infection, vitamin deficiency, drooling or thumb sucking.

permeability *n* in physiology, the extent to which substances dissolved in the body fluids are able to move through cell membranes or layers of cells (e.g. the walls of capillaries or absorptive tissues).

pernicious anaemia ⇒ anaemia.

perniosis *n* chronic chilblains.

peromelia *n* a teratogenic malformation of a limb.

peroneal nerve ⇒ Figure 11.

peroneus muscles ⇒ Figures 4, 5.

peroral *adj* through the mouth.

perseveration *n* constant repetition of words or phrases. Seen in organic brain disease (OBS). ⇒ delirium, dementia.

personal activities of daily living (PADL) include activities such as washing and dressing.

personality *n* the various mental attitudes, traits and characteristics which distinguish a person. The sum total of the mental make-up. ⇒ psychopathic personality.

personality disorder a disturbance of personality together with deeply ingrained maladaptive behavioural patterns established by late adolescence/early adulthood resulting in personal and social difficulties.

perspiration *n* the excretion from the sweat glands through the skin pores. *insensible perspiration* the water lost by evaporation through the skin surface other than by sweating. It is significantly increased in inflamed skin. *sensible perspiration* the term used when there are visible drops of sweat on the skin.

Perthes' disease (*syn* pseudocoxalgia) avascular degeneration of the upper femoral epiphysis occurs in children; revascularization occurs, but residual deformity of the femoral head may subsequently lead to arthritic changes.

pertussis *n* (*syn* whooping cough) a serious infectious respiratory disease caused by the bacterium *Bordetella pertussis*. It is spread by droplets and has an incubation period of 7–14 days. It is characterized by conjunctivitis, rhinitis, dry cough and later bouts of paroxysmal coughing with a 'whoop' and vomiting. Complications may include pneumonia, bronchiectasis and convulsions. Active immunization is available as part of the routine programme in infancy.

pes *n* a foot or foot-like structure. *pes cavus (high arched foot)* (*syn* claw-foot) a pathological elevation of the longitudinal arch caused by plantar flexion of the forefoot relative to the rearfoot. The medial longitudinal arch is most affected but the lateral longitudinal arch can also be elevated. There is dorsal humping of the midfoot and associated forefoot and rearfoot deformities. These may include clawing or retraction of the lesser toes, a trigger first toe, and a depressed first metatarsal with either heel varus or equinus. It may be acquired or congenital. *pes planus (syn flat-foot)* a generic term for a foot with an abnormally low arch. The medial longitudinal arch is depressed or absent, and the foot has an increased contact area with the ground. During weightbearing the foot appears to have no longitudinal arch. It may be congenital or acquired. When young children first stand the feet appear to be flat, as adipose tissue under the medial longitudinal arch is pressed close to the ground. Older children very frequently have flattening of the medial longitudinal arch on standing but the arch reappears on standing on tiptoe (a mobile flat foot). *flexible pes planus* is generally asymptomatic in children but may become a semi-rigid condition in adulthood. It has been linked with excess laxity of the joint capsule and the ligaments supporting the arch, which allows it to collapse when weight is applied. *rigid pes planus* in adults may be a progression from flexible to semi-rigid to rigid as part of the ageing process. Structural changes due to the existing abnormal position become fixed, as soft and osseous tissues adapt. Rigidity is increased where there are significant osteoarthritic changes or inflammatory arthritic destruction.

pessary *n* **1** a device inserted into the vagina to correct uterine displacements. A *ring* or *shelf pessary* is used to support a prolapse. A *Hodge pessary* is used to correct a retroverted uterus. **2** a suppository containing a medication inserted into the vagina.

PET *abbr* positron emission tomography.

petechia *n* a small, haemorrhagic spot—**petechiae** *pl*, **petechial** *adj*.

petit mal minor epilepsy. ⇒ epilepsy.

pétrissage *n* rhythmical massage manipulations of muscle and other soft tissues where pressure is used to help venous and lymphatic drainage and to mobilize skin and connective tissue. It may be slow and deep to produce relaxation and reduce spasm, or brisk to invigorate. The manipulation may be performed with one hand alone, or with both hands working alternately.

petrous *adj* resembling stone.

Peyer's patches aggregates of lymphatic tissue situated in the ileum. Function to prevent micro-organisms entering the blood. Site of infection in typhoid fever.

Peyronie's disease deformity and painful erection of penis due to fibrous tissue formation from unknown cause. Can be associated with Dupuytren's contracture.

PGD *abbr* preimplantation genetic diagnosis.

PGDRS *abbr* psychogeriatric dependency rating scale.

pH *abbr* hydrogen ion concentration, expressed as a negative logarithm. A neutral solution has a pH 7.0. With increasing acidity the pH falls with increasing alkalinity it rises.

phacoemulsification *n* (*syn* pakoemulsification) ultrasonic vibration is used to liquefy nuclear lens fibres. The liquid lens matter is then sucked out in an action similar to that of a vacuum cleaner.

phaeochromocytoma *n* (*syn* paraganglioma) a condition in which there is a tumour of the adrenal medulla, or of the structurally similar tissues associated with the sympathetic chain. It secretes adrenaline (epinephrine) and allied hormones and the symptoms are due to the excess of these substances. Results in hypertensive crises, with associated headache, flushing and tachycardia.

phage typing identifying bacterial strains by their bacteriophages.

phagocyte *n* a cell capable of engulfing bacteria and other particulate material—**phagocytic** *adj*.

phagocytosis *n* the process by which phagocytes engulf particles such as bacteria.

phalanges *n* the small bones of the fingers and toes (⇒ Figures 2, 3)—**phalanx** *sing*, **phalangeal** *adj*.

phallus *n* the penis—**phallic** *adj*.

phantasy *n* ⇒ fantasy.

phantom limb the sensation that a limb is still attached to the body after it has been amputated. Pain may seem to come from the amputated limb.

phantom pregnancy (*syn* pseudocyesis) signs and symptoms simulating those of early pregnancy; it may occur in a childless person who has an overwhelming desire to have a child.

pharmaceutical *adj* relating to drugs.

pharmacist *n* a person who is qualified and registered to dispense drugs. They also provide advice and information for other health professionals and the public.

pharmacodynamics *n* the study of how a drug acts in a living system and how it alters cell metabolism to have an effect.

pharmacokinetics *n* the study of the way the body deals with a drug over time. It considers drug absorption, distribution, metabolism and excretion.

pharmacology *n* the science dealing with drugs—**pharmacological** *adj*, **pharmacologically** *adv*.

pharmacopoeia *n* an authorized book detailing drugs available for prescribing in a specific country, such as the British pharmacopoeia (BP) or United States pharmacopoeia.

pharmacy *n* **1** the place where drugs are prepared and dispensed. **2** the science of preparing drugs. *pharmacy only medicine (P)* medicines that may be bought by the public from a pharmacy but only when a pharmacist is in attendance.

pharyngeal pouch pathological dilatation of the lower part of the pharynx.

pharyngectomy *n* surgical removal of the pharynx (partial or total).

pharyngismus *n* spasm of the pharynx.

pharyngitis *n* inflammation of the pharynx.

pharyngolaryngeal *adj* pertaining to the pharynx and larynx.

pharyngolaryngectomy *n* surgical removal of the pharynx and larynx.

pharyngoplasty *n* any plastic operation to the pharynx.

pharyngotomy *n* a surgical opening into the pharnynx.

pharyngotympanic tube (*syn* eustachian tube) a canal, partly bony, partly cartilaginous, connecting the pharynx with the tympanic cavity ($\Rightarrow$ Figure 13). It allows air to pass into the middle ear, so that the air pressure is kept even on both sides of the eardrum.

pharynx *n* the cavity at the back of the mouth ($\Rightarrow$ Figures 6, 14). It is cone shaped and is lined with mucous membrane; at the lower end it opens into the oesophagus. The pharyngotympanic (eustachian) tubes pierce its lateral walls and the posterior nares pierce its anterior wall. The larynx lies immediately below it and in front of the oesophagus—**pharyngeal** *adj*.

PHC *abbr* primary health care.

phenol *n* (*syn* carbolic acid) a powerful disinfectant. Phenolic disinfectants are used in suitable dilution for environmental use. They are toxic and corrosive.

phenothiazines *npl* a group of typical neuroleptics. $\Rightarrow$ tardive dyskinesia. $\Rightarrow$ Appendix 5.

phenotype *n* the physical characteristics of an organism that result from genotype and environment.

phenylalanine *n* an essential (indispensable) amino acid. Those unable to metabolize it develop phenylketonuria.

phenylketonuria (PKU) *n* metabolites of phenylalanine (e.g. phenylketones) in urine. Occurs in hyperphenylalaninaemia, owing to the lack of or inactivity of the liver enzyme that normally converts dietary phenylalanine into tyrosine. Autosomal recessive disease, resulting in learning disability unless discovered by screening and treated with an appropriate diet from birth—**phenylketonuric** *adj*.

pheromones *npl* chemicals with a specific odour. They are present in the sweat produced by the apocrine sweat glands. They may influence sexual behaviour.

Philadelphia chromosome (Ph) an anomaly of chromosome number 22. It is found in the blood cells of most people with chronic myeloid leukaemia.

phimosis *n* tightness of the prepuce so that it cannot be retracted over the glans penis.

phlebectomy *n* excision of a vein. *multiple cosmetic phlebectomy (MCP)* removal of varicose veins through little stab incisions which heal without scarring.

phlebitis *n* inflammation of a vein—**phlebitic** *adj*.

phlebography $\Rightarrow$ venography.

phlebolith *n* a concretion that forms in a vein.

phlebothrombosis *n* thrombosis in a vein. $\Rightarrow$ deep vein thrombosis, embolism, pulmonary embolus.

phlebotomist *n* a technician who is trained to take blood samples from patients.

phlebotomy *n* $\Rightarrow$ venesection, venotomy.

phlegm *n* sputum. Mucus expectorated (coughed up) from the bronchi.

phlegmatic *adj* describes a person who is emotionally stable.

phlyctenule *n* a small inflammatory nodule which occurs on conjunctiva or cornea close to the corneal limbus.

phlyctenulosis *n* eye disease characterized by phlyctenules.

phobia *n* a morbid fear—**phobic** *adj*.

phocomelia *n* teratogenic malformation. Arms and feet attached directly to trunk giving a seal-like appearance. Many cases in the 1960s were associated with the use of thalidomide during pregnancy.

phonation *n* voice production by vibration of the vocal cords.

phonocardiography *n* the graphic recording of heart sounds and murmurs by electric reproduction. The fetal heart rate and its relation to uterine contraction can be measured continuously. $\Rightarrow$ cardiotocography—**phonocardiographic** *adj*, **phonocardiogram** *n*, **phonocardiograph** *n*, **phonocardiographically** *adv*.

phonophobia *n* a dislike of noise such as with migraine.

phoria *n* latent strabismus. May be used as a suffix.

phosphatases *npl* enzymes needed in the reactions concerning phosphate esters, e.g. phospholipids. ⇒ acid phosphatase, alkaline phosphatase.

phosphates *npl* salts of phosphoric acid.

phosphaturia *n* excess phosphates in the urine—**phosphaturic** *adj*.

phosphocreatine ⇒ creatine.

phospholipids *npl* organic molecules comprising a lipid plus nitrogen and phosphate groups, vital in the formation of the cell (plasma) membrane.

phosphorus (P) *n* a poisonous element. Forms an important constituent (as phosphates) of nucleic acids, bone and all cells. *radioactive phosphorus* (^{32}P) is used in the treatment of thrombocythaemia.

phosphorylases *npl* a group of enzymes needed for the addition of phosphate groups to other molecules, e.g. phosphofructokinase concerned with glucose metabolism.

phosphorylation *n* the metabolic process of introducing a phosphate group into an organic molecule.

photochemical *adj* chemically reactive in the presence of light.

photochemotherapy *n* drug effects improved by exposing the individual to ultraviolet light.

photocoagulation *n* burning of the tissues with a powerful, focused light source.

photoendoscope *n* an endoscope incorporating a camera, thus allowing a permanent record of clinical findings to be made—**photoendoscopic** *adj*, **photoendoscopy** *n*, **photoendoscopically** *adv*.

photophobia *n* dislike of bright light, usually associated with eye pain, such as in migraine and meningism—**photophobic** *adj*.

photosensitive *adj* reactive to light.

photosensitivity *n* an exaggerated inflammatory reaction of the skin in response to light.

phototherapy *n* exposure to artificial blue light. Used most commonly for treatment of jaundice in neonates. Effectiveness most likely due to its ability to convert bilirubin to water soluble forms that are easily excreted.

phren *n* the diaphragm—**phrenic** *adj*.

phrenicotomy *n* division of the phrenic nerve to paralyse one-half of the diaphragm.

phrenoplegia *n* paralysis of the diaphragm—**phrenoplegic** *adj*.

phthiriasis *n* infestation with the pubic louse, *Phthirus pubis*. Most commonly transmitted by sexual contact, but non-sexual acquisition of the insect is also possible.

phylloquinone *n* a member of the vitamin K family of compounds found in green vegetables.

physical abuse ⇒ abuse, non-accidental injury.

physical activity level (PAL) the ratio of daily physical energy expenditure to BMR. This factor reflects the average activity both at work and at leisure and is used to estimate average energy requirement. Average energy requirement = PAL × BMR. Examples of PALs for population groups are estimated to be: 1.4 for inactive men and women, 1.6 for moderately active women, and 1.7 for moderately active men.

physical activity ratio (PAR) the ratio of the energy cost of a specific activity to the BMR. Factors range from 1 for complete rest to 9 for very vigorous sporting activities, and are used to estimate the energy requirement of a specific activity.

physician *n* a registered doctor who practises medicine rather than surgery.

physicochemical *adj* relating to physics and chemistry.

physiological *adj* often used to describe a normal process or structure, to distinguish it from an abnormal or pathological feature (e.g. the physiological level of glucose in the blood). *physiological advantage* a muscle's ability to shorten. Its greatest physiological advantage is when a muscle is at rest. *physiological saline* ⇒ isotonic. *physiological solution* a fluid isotonic with the body fluids and containing similar salts.

physiology *n* the science dealing with normal functioning of the body—**physiological** *adj*, **physiologically** *adv*.

physiotherapy *n* traditionally describes treatment to improve, restore and sometimes cure, using manipulation, electrotherapy, and exercise therapy and rehabilitation following injury or disease, e.g. stroke. Contemporarily, it also includes assessment and diagnosis, health promotion and education, and prevention of disability. ⇒ extended scope physiotherapy practitioners.

phytates, phytic acid chemicals present in wholegrain cereals. They can decrease intestinal absorption of some minerals, e.g. calcium, zinc and iron.

phyto-oestrogens chemicals with oestrogen-like effects (oestrogenic) that originate in plants that include soya beans.

pia mater the innermost of the meninges; the vascular membrane which lies in close contact with the brain and spinal cord.

pica *n* a desire for extraordinary types of food. Seen in pregnancy.

Pick's disease 1 syndrome of ascites, hepatomegaly, oedema and pleural effusion that occurs with constrictive pericarditis. **2** a type of cerebral atrophy producing dementia during midlife.

picornavirus *n* derived from pico (very small) and RNA (ribonucleic acid). Small RNA viruses. Includes the enteroviruses (polio, coxsackie, hepatitis A and echovirus) and the rhinoviruses. ⇒ virus.

picture archiving communications system (PACS) in radiography. A networked system of viewing monitors connected to a central image database that allows integration of image and demographic information.

PID *abbr* **1** pelvic inflammatory disease. **2** prolapse of an intervertebral disc. ⇒ prolapse.

pigeon chest (*syn* pectus carinatum) a narrow chest, bulging anteriorly in the breast bone region.

pigment *n* any colouring matter of the body.

pigmentation *n* the deposit of pigment, especially when abnormal or excessive.

piles *npl* ⇒ haemorrhoids.

pili *npl* hair-like appendages of many bacteria, and used for the transfer of genetic material—**pilus** *sing*.

pilomotor nerves tiny nerves that innervate the hair follicle, causing the hair to become erect and give the appearance of 'goose flesh'.

pilonidal *adj* hair-containing. *pilonidal sinus* a sinus containing hairs which is usually found in hirsute people in the cleft between the buttocks. In this situation it is liable to infection.

pilosebaceous *adj* pertaining to the hair follicle and the sebaceous gland opening into it.

pilot study an early smaller-scale study carried out before the main research project to evaluate viability and to identify problems with the research methodology.

pimple *n* ⇒ papule.

pineal body (gland) a small reddish-grey conical structure on the dorsal surface of the midbrain. It secretes various substances which include 5-hydroxytryptamine and melatonin. The release of melatonin is connected to the amount of light entering the eye. Melatonin levels fluctuate during the 24 hours and appear to influence gonadotrophin secretion, diurnal rhythms such as sleep, and mood. ⇒ depression, seasonal affective disorder.

pinguecula *n* a yellowish, slightly elevated thickening of the bulbar conjunctiva between the eyelids. Associated with the ageing eye.

pin index system designed to prevent the wrong connection of a gas cylinder to an anaesthetic machine.

pink disease ⇒ erythroedema polyneuropathy.

pinna *n* the auricle. That part of the ear which is external to the head. (⇒ Figure 13).

pinta *n* a mild contagious disease, caused by *Treponema pallidum* (ssp. *carateum*) similar to yaws but confined to the Central and South Americas. Only the skin is affected. ⇒ bejel, yaws.

pitting *n* making an indentation, e.g. in the nails as in psoriasis, or in oedematous tissues.

pituitary gland (*syn* hypophysis cerebri) a small oval endocrine gland lying in the pituitary fossa of the sphenoid bone. The anterior lobe (adenohypophysis) produces and secretes several hormones; growth hormone, adrenocorticotrophic hormone, thyroid-stimulating hormone, luteinizing hormone, follicle stimulating hormone, prolactin and melanocyte stimulating hormone. The posterior lobe (neurohypophysis) stores and secretes oxytocin and vasopressin (antidiuretic hormone). These hormones are made by nerve fibres in the hypothalamus.

pityriasis *n* scaly (branny) eruption of the skin. *pityriasis alba* a common eruption in children characterized by scaly hypopigmented macules on the cheeks and upper arms. *pityriasis capitis* dandruff. *pityriasis rosea* a slightly scaly eruption of ovoid erythematous lesions which are widespread over the trunk and proximal parts of the limbs. It is a self-limiting condition. *pityriasis rubra pilaris* a chronic skin disease characterized by coalescing red papules of perifollicular distribution. *pityriasis versicolor* called also 'tinea versicolor', is a yeast infection which causes the appearance of buff-coloured patches on the trunk.

Pityrosporum *n* genus of yeasts. *P. orbiculare (Malassezia furfur)* is associated with pityriasis versicolor.

PKU *abbr* phenylketonuria.

placebo *n* a harmless substance given as medicine. In a randomized placebo-controlled trial, an inert substance, identical in appearance with the material being tested. When neither the researcher nor the subject knows which is which, the trial is said to be double blind. *placebo effect* a therapeutic effect is observed after the administration of a placebo.

placenta *n* the afterbirth, a hormone-secreting vascular structure developed and functioning about the third month of pregnancy and attached to the inner wall of the uterus. Through it the fetus is supplied with nourishment and oxygen and through it the fetus gets rid of its waste products. In normal labour it is expelled, with the fetal membranes, during the third stage of labour. When this does not occur it is termed a *retained placenta* and may be an *adherent placenta*. The placenta is usually attached to the upper segment of the uterus; where it lies in the lower uterine segment it is called a *placenta praevia* and usually causes placental abruption with painless antepartum bleeding—**placental** *adj*.

placental abruption premature placental separation from the uterine wall prior to the delivery of the fetus resulting in haemorrhage.

placental insufficiency inefficiency of the placenta. Can occur due to maternal disease or postmaturity of fetus giving rise to a 'small for dates' baby.

placentography *n* X-ray examination of the placenta now superseded by ultrasound.

plague *n* very contagious epidemic disease caused by the bacterium *Yersinia pestis*, and spread by infected rats. Transfer of infection from rat to human is through bites from rat fleas, but droplet spread may occur between humans. The main clinical types are bubonic, pneumonic or septicaemic.

plantar *adj* pertaining to the sole of the foot. *plantar arch* the union of the plantar and dorsalis pedis arteries in the sole of the foot. *plantar flexion* downward movement of the big toe.

plaque *n* an elevated area of skin. ⇒ dental plaque.

plasma *n* the fluid part of blood. *plasma cell* an immune cell that produces antibodies. It is derived from B lymphocytes/cells.

plasmapheresis *n* taking blood from a donor, removing some desired fraction, then returning the red cells and repeating the whole process. It can be used in the treatment of some diseases which are caused by antibodies or immune complexes circulating in the patient's plasma. Removing the plasma and replacing it with human plasma protein fraction (PPF) or a plasma substitute can improve the prognosis of the disease and prevent or delay the onset of renal failure.

plasmid *n* DNA present in some bacteria. The transfer of this genetic material between bacteria during sexual reproduction allows the exchange of genes for antibiotic resistance.

plasmin *n* proteolytic enzyme produced when plasminogen is activated. It breaks down fibrin clots when healing is complete. Also called fibrinolysin. ⇒ fibrinolysis.

plasminogen *n* precursor of plasmin. Release of activators, e.g. tissue plasminogen activator (t-PA), from damaged tissue promotes the conversion of plasminogen into plasmin.

Plasmodium *n* a genus of protozoa. Parasites in the blood of warm-blooded animals which complete their sexual cycle in blood-sucking arthropods such as mosquitoes. Malaria is caused by four species of *Plasmodium*—**plasmodial** *adj*.

plaster of Paris ⇒ gypsum.

plastic *adj* capable of taking a form or mould. *plastic surgery* transfer of healthy tissue to repair damaged area and to restore form and function.

platelet *n* ⇒ thrombocyte. Cellular fragments concerned with blood coagulation. *platelet plug* one of the four overlapping stages of haemostasis. Platelets aggregate and adhere to form a temporary plug at the site of blood vessel damage.

platyhelminth *n* flat worm; cestodes (tapeworms) and trematodes (flukes). ⇒ *Echinococcus*, schistosomiasis, *Taenia*.

play therapist a person who uses play constructively to help children to come to terms with having to be in hospital.

pleomorphism *n* denotes a wide range in shape and size of individuals in a bacterial population—**pleomorphic** *adj*.

plethora *n* fullness; overloading—**plethoric** *adj*.

plethysmograph *n* an instrument which accurately measures blood flow. Used to measure and record changes in the volume and size of organs or an extremity—**plethysmographic** *adj*.

pleura *n* the serous membrane covering the surface of the lung (visceral pleura), the diaphragm, the mediastinum and the chest wall (parietal pleura)—**pleural** *adj*, **pleurae** *pl*.

pleurectomy *n* surgical stripping of the pleura to achieve a surgical pleurodesis.

pleurisy, pleuritis *n* inflammation of the pleura. May be fibrinous (dry), be associated with an effusion (wet), or be complicated by empyema—**pleuritic** *adj*.

pleurodesis *n* adherence of the visceral to the parietal pleura. Used therapeutically to prevent recurrence of metastatic pleural effusions, or recurrent pneumothoraces. Achieved by the use of sclerosing agents such as talc. ⇒ pleurectomy.

pleurodynia *n* intercostal myalgia or muscular rheumatism (fibrositis). ⇒ Bornholm disease.

pleurolysis *n* surgical separation of the pleura from its attachments.

pleuropulmonary *adj* relating to the pleura and lung.

pleurotomy *n* incision of the pleura.

plexus *n* a network of vessels or nerves (⇒ Figure 11).

plication *n* a surgical procedure of making tucks or folds to decrease the size of an organ—**plica** *sing*, **plicae** *pl*, **plicate** *adj*, *vt*.

plombage *n* extra-pleural compression of a tuberculous lung cavity to deprive tubercle of oxygen. Widely used surgical technique before the introduction of antibiotic therapy for tuberculosis. Now sometimes used in multidrug resistant tuberculosis.

plumbism *n* ⇒ lead poisoning.

Plummer–Vinson syndrome (*syn* Paterson–Brown–Kelly syndrome) a combination of glossitis with postcricoid web and iron deficiency anaemia.

pluriglandular *adj* pertaining to several glands, as cystic fibrosis.

plyometric exercise explosive exercise that maximizes the myotatic on-stretch reflex, i.e. a lengthening of a muscle followed by a sudden shortening in order to produce power.

PMS *abbr* premenstrual syndrome.

pneumaturia *n* the passage of flatus with urine, usually as a result of a vesicocolic (bladder–bowel) fistula.

pneumococcus *n* *Streptococcus pneumoniae*. A Gram-positive diplococcus. Causes lobar pneumonia and other infections, e.g. meningitis—**pneumococcal** *adj*.

pneumoconiosis *n* (*syn* dust disease) fibrosis of the lung caused by long continued inhalation of dust in industrial occupations. The most important complication is the occasional superinfection with tuberculosis—**pneumoconioses** *pl*. *rheumatoid pneumoconiosis* fibrosing alveolitis occurring in patients suffering from rheumatoid arthritis. ⇒ anthracosis, asbestosis, byssinosis, siderosis, silicosis.

Pneumocystis carinii an opportunistic micro-organism that causes pneumonia in immunocompromised individuals, such as infants, debilitated and immunosuppressed patients and those with AIDS: mortality is high.

pneumocytes *npl* cells lining the alveolar walls in the lungs. Type I are flat, Type II are cuboidal and secrete surfactant.

pneumoencephalography *n* radiographic examination of cerebral ventricles after injection of air by means of a lumbar or cisternal puncture—**pneumoencephalogram** *n*.

pneumolysis *n* separation of the two pleural layers, or the outer pleural layer from the chest wall, to collapse the lung.

pneumomycosis *n* fungal infection affecting the lung, e.g. actinomycosis, aspergillosis, candidiasis—**pneumomycotic** *adj*.

pneumonectomy *n* excision of a lung.

pneumonia *n* acute infection of the lung by an invading organism associated with new pulmonary shadowing on a radiograph. Can be subdivided into community-acquired, hospital-acquired, and pneumonia associated with profound immunosuppression.

pneumonitis *n* inflammation of lung tissue.

pneumoperitoneum *n* air or gas in the peritoneal cavity. Can be introduced for diagnostic or therapeutic purposes.

pneumothorax *n* air or gas in the pleural cavity separating the visceral from the parietal pleura so that lung tissue is compressed. Occurs spontaneously when an over-dilated pulmonary air sac ruptures, permitting communication of respiratory passages with the pleural cavity. Associated with many lung diseases, including asthma, bronchial cancer, COPD, congenital cysts, tuberculosis, trauma, and positive pressure ventilation. *tension pneumothorax* a valve-like wound or tear in the lung allows air to enter the pleural cavity with each inspiration, but not to escape on expiration, thus progressively increasing intrathoracic pressure and constituting an acute medical emergency. Signs are of hyperinflation, midline shift and increasing respiratory distress.

PNF *abbr* proprioceptive neuromuscular facilitation.

PNI *abbr* psychoneuroimmunology.

PO₂ *abbr* the partial pressure of oxygen, for example in atmospheric or expired air.

podalic version ⇒ version.

podiatrist *n* a primary healthcare professional responsible for the assessment, diagnosis and management of conditions affecting the foot and lower limb without referral from medical practitioners. Podiatrists adopt holistic approaches to the assessment and treatment of individuals and utilize a wide range of treatment modalities many of which are performed under local anaesthesia.

podiatry *n* a term that is generally used in Western Europe and the rest of the English speaking countries to describe chiropody. The practice of podiatry involves maintaining the feet in a healthy condition. It recognizes the interdependence of the health of the foot with the rest of the body.

podopompholyx *n* pompholyx on the feet.

polarized *adj* describes the resting state of the plasma membrane of an excitable cell where there is no impulse transmission. The inside of the membrane is electrically negative relative to the outside. ⇒ depolarization.

poliomyelitis *n* (*syn* infantile paralysis) an epidemic virus infection which attacks the motor neurons of the anterior horns in a healthy brainstem (*bulbar poliomyelitis*) and spinal cord. An attack may or may not lead to paralysis of the lower motor neuron type with loss of muscular power and flaccidity. Immunization, using oral vaccine, is available as part of routine programmes. Poliomyelitis has followed immunization, and handwashing is strongly advised after defaecation or contact with recently vaccinated babies, especially after handling napkins. ⇒ Sabin vaccine, Salk vaccine.

polioviruses *npl* three enteroviruses that cause poliomyelitis. ⇒ virus.

pollenosis *n* an allergic condition arising from sensitization to pollen.

pollicization *n* a surgical procedure whereby the index finger is rotated and shortened to produce apposition as a thumb.

polyarteritis *n* inflammation of many arteries. In *polyarteritis nodosa* (*syn* periarteritis nodosa) aneurysmal swellings and thrombosis occur in the affected vessels. Further damage may lead to haemorrhage and the clinical picture presented depends upon the site affected. ⇒ collagen.

polyarthralgia *n* pain in several joints.

polyarthritis *n* inflammation of several joints.

polycystic *adj* composed of many cysts.

polycystic kidney diseases a number of conditions which have variable effects on kidney function. Many lead to end-stage renal failure and the need for dialysis. Often associated with cystic disease of other organs, especially the liver and meninges.

polycystic ovary syndrome (PCOS) a syndrome of oligomenorrhoea, infertility, hirsutism and occasionally obesity.

polycythaemia *n* increase in the number of circulating red blood cells. This may result from dehydration or be a compensatory phenomenon to increase the oxygen carrying capacity, as in congenital heart disease. *primary proliferative polycythaemia (polycythaemia vera)* is an idiopathic condition in which the red cell count is very high. The patient may complain of headache and lassitude, and there is danger of thrombosis and haemorrhage.

polydactyly, polydactylism *n* having more than the normal number of fingers or toes. On the foot the extra digits may develop from one metatarsal or there may be duplication of metatarsal segments. Sometimes selective amputation at an early age is indicated. This ensures optimum foot function, thus facilitating shoe fitting in childhood and adult life.

polydipsia *n* excessive thirst.

polygene inheritance describes physical characteristics, such as hair colour that are determined by the combined effects of several paired genes at different locations.

polygraph *n* instrument which records several variables simultaneously.

polyhydramnios *n* an excessive amount of amniotic fluid.

polymer *n* a molecule made up of many smaller molecules or subunits, such as glycogen; a polymer of glucose molecules.

polymerase chain reaction (PCR) an in vitro method for the enzymic synthesis of specific DNA sequences and hence the capacity to amplify these segments of DNA. A modification of the method also allows the rapid detection and analysis of RNA.

polymorphonuclear *adj* having a many-shaped or lobulated nucleus, usually applied to the phagocytic leucocytes (granulocytes), neutrophils, basophils and eosinophils.

polymyalgia rheumatica a syndrome occurring in older people comprising a sometimes crippling ache in the shoulders, pelvic girdle muscles and spine, with pronounced morning stiffness and a raised ESR. There is an association with temporal arteritis. Clinically different from rheumatoid arthritis. ⇒ arthritis.

polymyositis *n* manifests as muscle weakness, most commonly in middle age. Microscopic examination of muscle reveals inflammatory changes that respond to corticosteroids. ⇒ dermatomyositis.

polyneuritis *n* multiple neuritis—**polyneuritic** *adj*.

polyopia *n* seeing many images of a single object.

polyp, polypus *n* a pedunculated tumour arising from any epithelial surface, e.g. cervical, uterine, nasal, intestinal. Usually benign but may be malignant. Adenomatous polyps are premalignant. ⇒ polyposis. Tissue overgrowth underlying the epithelium may also be the cause of polyp formation—**polypous** *adj*.

polypectomy *n* surgical removal of a polyp such as from the bowel or nose.

polypeptides *npl* molecules comprising several amino acids joined by peptide bonds. They are between peptides and proteins in size.

polypharmacy *n* describes a situation when many drugs are prescribed for the same patient. It increases the risk of adverse effects and non-compliance.

polypoid *adj* resembling a polyp.

polyploidy *n* a multiple of the normal haploid (n) chromosome number of 23, other than the normal diploid (46) number, e.g. 69. Not compatible with life. ⇒ triploid.

polyposis *n* a condition in which there are numerous intestinal polyps. *familial adenomatous polyposis* a dominantly inherited condition in which multiple polyps occur throughout the large bowel and which invariably leads to colon cancer. Polyps also occur in the stomach and duodenum.

polysaccharide *n* complex carbohydrates ($C_6H_{10}O_5$) containing a large number of monosaccharide units. Starch, inulin, glycogen, dextrin and cellulose are examples. ⇒ non-starch polysaccharides.

polyserositis *n* inflammation of several serous membranes. A genetic type is called familial Mediterranean fever. ⇒ amyloidosis.

polyunsaturated fatty acid (PUFA) a fatty acid with two or more double bonds in its structure. ⇒ essential fatty acids.

polyuria *n* excretion of an excessive volume of urine—**polyuric** *adj*.

POM *abbr* prescription only medicine.

pompholyx *n* vesicular skin eruption on the skin associated with itching or burning. ⇒ cheiropompholyx, podopompholyx.

POMR *abbr* problem-orientated medical record.

pons *n* a bridge; a process of tissue joining two sections of an organ. *pons varolii* part of the brainstem which serves to connect the various lobes of the brain (⇒ Figure 1)—**pontine** *adj*.

Pontiac fever a flu-like illness with little or no pulmonary involvement and no mortality caused by *Legionella pneumophila*. ⇒ legionnaires' disease.

POP *abbr* **1** progestogen only pill. **2** plaster of Paris.

popliteal *adj* pertaining to the popliteus. *popliteal space* the diamond-shaped depression behind the knee, bounded by muscles and containing the popliteal nerve and vessels (artery and vein) ⇒ Figures 9, 10.

popliteus *n* a muscle in the popliteal space which flexes the leg and aids rotation.

pore *n* a minute surface opening. One of the mouths of the ducts (leading from the sweat glands) on the skin surface; they are controlled by fine papillary muscles, closing in the cold and opening in the presence of heat.

porphyria *n* inborn error in porphyrin metabolism, usually hereditary, causing pathological changes in nervous and muscular tissue in some varieties and photosensitivity in others, depending on the level of the metabolic block involved. Excess porphyrins or precursors are found in the urine or stools or both. In some cases attacks are precipitated by certain drugs.

porphyrins *npl* group of organic compounds that form the basis of respiratory pigments, including haemoglobin. Naturally occurring porphyrins are uroporphyrin and coproporphyrin. ⇒ porphyria.

porphyrinuria *n* excretion of porphyrins in the urine. Such pigments are produced as a result of an inborn error of metabolism.

porta *n* the depression (hilum) of an organ at which the vessels enter and leave—**portal** *adj*. *porta hepatis* the transverse fissure through which the hepatic portal vein, hepatic artery and bile ducts pass on the under surface of the liver.

portacaval, portocaval *adj* relating to the hepatic portal vein and inferior vena cava. *portacaval anastomosis* the hepatic portal vein is joined to the inferior vena cava with the object of reducing the pressure within the hepatic portal vein in cases of hepatic portal hypertension.

portal circulation ⇒ hepatic portal circulation.

portal hypertension more properly called hepatic portal hypertension. Increased pressure in the hepatic portal vein. Usually caused by cirrhosis of the liver; results in splenomegaly, with hypersplenism and alimentary bleeding. ⇒ oesophageal varices.

portal vein more properly called hepatic portal vein. That conveying blood into the liver; it is about 75 mm long and is formed by the union of the superior mesenteric and splenic veins.

positive end expiratory pressure (PEEP) the maintenance of positive pressure in the airway of a ventilated patient at the end of expiration. Analogous to continuous positive airway pressure in a spontaneously breathing patient.

positive pressure ventilation (PPV) positive pressure inflation of lungs to produce inspiration. ⇒ mechanical ventilation.

positron emission tomography (PET) uses cyclotron produced isotopes of extremely short half-life that emit positrons. PET scanning is used to evaluate physiological function of organs, e.g. the brain.

positrons *npl* positively charged particles that combine with electrons (negative charge), causing gamma rays to be emitted.

posseting *n* regurgitation of small amounts of curdled milk in infants.

postabsorptive state the metabolic state existing between meals, such as late afternoon and at night. Fuel molecules for immediate energy use are in short supply and the body uses catabolic processes (e.g. glycogenolysis) to break down complex substances to provide energy. ⇒ absorptive state.

postanaesthetic *adj* after anaesthesia.

postanal *adj* behind the anus.

postcoital *adj* after sexual intercourse. The word describes the 'morning after' contraceptive.

postconcussional syndrome 1 the association of headaches, giddiness and a feeling of faintness, which may persist for a considerable time after a head injury. **2** a term used in sports medicine to describe a progressive deterioration of cognitive function following repeated brain trauma such as that caused during boxing.

postdiphtheritic *adj* following an attack of diphtheria. Refers especially to the paralysis of limbs and palate.

postepileptic *adj* following on an epileptic seizure. *postepileptic automatism* is a fugue state, following on a fit, when the patient may undertake a course of action, even involving violence, without having any memory of this (amnesia).

posterior *adj* situated at the back. ⇒ anterior *opp. posterior chamber of the eye* situated between the anterior surface of the lens and the posterior surface of the iris. ⇒ aqueous—**posteriorly** *adv.*

postganglionic *adj* situated distal to a collection of nerve cells (ganglion), as a postganglionic nerve fibre.

postgastrectomy syndrome covers two sets of symptoms, those of hypoglycaemia when the patient is hungry, and those of a vasovagal attack immediately after a meal.

posthepatic *adj* behind the liver.

postherpetic *adj* after herpes infection such as *postherpetic neuralgia* following shingles.

posthitis *adj* inflammation of the prepuce.

posthumous *adj* occurring after death. *posthumous birth* **1** delivery of a baby by caesarean section after the mother's death, or birth occurring after the father's death.

postmature *adj* past the expected date of delivery. A baby is postmature when labour is delayed beyond the usual 40 weeks—**postmaturity** *n.*

postmenopausal *adj* occurring after the menopause has been established. *postmenopausal bleeding (PMB)* vaginal bleeding occurring after the menopause.

postmortem *adj* after death, usually implying dissection of the body. ⇒ antemortem *opp*, autopsy.

postmyocardial infarction syndrome Dressler's syndrome. A late complication presenting as pericarditis developing from 2 weeks to a few months after myocardial infarction. Due to an autoimmune response to products released from dead muscle.

postnasal *adj* behind the nose and in the nasopharynx—**postnasally** *adv.*

postnatal *adj* after delivery. ⇒ antenatal *opp. postnatal depression* describes a low mood experienced by some mothers for a few days following the birth of a baby; sometimes called 'four day blues'. Less severe than puerperal psychosis. *postnatal examination* routine examination 6 weeks after delivery—**postnatally** *adv.*

postoperative *adj* after operation—**postoperatively** *adv.*

postpartum *adj* after a birth (parturition). *postpartum haemorrhage* excessive bleeding after delivery of the child. It may be due to incomplete placental separation during the third stage of labour. Secondary postpartum haemorrhage is excessive uterine bleeding occurring more than 24 h after delivery. It is usually caused by infection associated with the retention of placental tissue.

postprandial *adj* following a meal.

post-traumatic stress disorder (PTSD) a mixed emotional disorder arising in response to an exceptional trauma. Symptoms include autonomic arousal, intrusive images ('flashbacks' or nightmares), emotional numbness, anhedonia and avoidance of reminders of the trauma.

postural *adj* relating to posture. *postural albuminuria* ⇒ orthostatic albuminuria. *postural drainage* techniques that use gravity and position to drain respiratory secretions. The airways of infected lung lobes or segments are positioned as vertically as possible. Also known as tipping because the lower lobes need to be raised higher than the mouth for secretions to drain into the trachea to stimulate the cough reflex. Apical segments of the upper lobe drain in sitting. The chest is percussed with clapping and vibrated and sputum coughed into a suitable disposable container or removed by suctioning. Children with cystic fibrosis must have this treatment at home and family members learn the techniques required. Small children are usually tipped across an adult's thighs but bigger children and adults can be tipped by raising the foot end of the bed, or over a roll or special frame. ⇒ tapotement. *postural hypotension* orthostatic hypotension. A reduction in blood pressure when a person stands up from lying or sitting. It may occur as a side-effect of some drugs such as alpha-adrenoceptor antagonists (alpha blockers). ⇒ Appendix 5. *postural reflex* describes any of the reflexes concerned with establishing or maintaining an individual's posture, particularly against the pull of gravity.

posture *n* the manner in which the body is held in lying, sitting, standing and walking; a particular position or attitude of the body. *hemiplegic posture* the position of the head, neck, trunk and limbs after a stroke. *opisthotonic posture* characterized by the arched position of complete extension of the head, spine and limbs typically in severe meningeal irritation and other serious neurological conditions. ⇒ opisthotonos.

potassium (K) *n* a metallic element. A major intracellular cation essential for proper neuromuscular conduction. ⇒ hyperkalaemia, hypokalaemia. *potassium chlorate* a mild antiseptic used in mouthwashes and gargles. *potassium chloride* used in potassium deficiency, and as a supplement with some diuretic drugs. *potassium citrate* alkalinizes urine; still used in cystitis to minimize discomfort. *potassium permanganate* used in solution for wounds and some skin conditions for its cleansing and deodorizing properties.

potassium deficiency ⇒ hypokalaemia.

potassium sparing diuretics a group of diuretic drugs that act to retain potassium and increase loss of sodium and water, or by reducing potassium loss and sodium reabsorption. ⇒ Appendix 5.

Pott's disease spondylitis; spinal caries; spinal tuberculosis. The resultant necrosis of the vertebrae causes kyphosis.

Pott's fracture a fracture-dislocation of the ankle joint. A fracture of the lower end of the tibia and fibula, 75 mm above the ankle joint, and a fracture of the medial malleolus of the tibia.

potter's rot one of many lay terms for silicosis arising in workers in the pottery industry.

pouch *n* a pocket or recess. *pouch of Douglas* the rectouterine pouch.

poverty *n* may be *absolute poverty* where people have insufficient resources to maintain physical health, such as not having food, shelter or the means to keep warm, or *relative poverty* when an individual's living standards are less than those that generally exist in a particular population. Definitions of what constitutes relative poverty show considerable variation between different communities and the same community over time.

povidone iodine ⇒ iodine.

power calculation a measure of statistical power. The likelihood of the research study to generate statistically significant results.

powerlessness *n* a feeling of being trapped and unable to control or influence the situation. People may feel powerless in their dealings with healthcare professionals and healthcare systems.

pox *n* a slang name for syphilis.

PPLO *abbr* pleuropneumonia-like organism. ⇒ *Mycoplasma*.

PPS *abbr* pelvic pain syndrome.

PQRST complex the letters used to denote the five parts of the ECG waveform.

PR *abbr* per rectum: describes the route used for examination of the rectum, or introduction of drugs or fluids into the body.

Prader–Willi syndrome an inherited condition that arises from mutations in the paternal chromosome 15 during the formation of the gamete. There is learning disability, hypotonia, short stature, hyperphagia and obesity. ⇒ Angleman syndrome.

praecordial *adj* ⇒ precordial.

preanaesthetic *adj* before an anaesthetic.

precancerous outdated term. ⇒ carcinoma in situ.

precipitin *n* an antibody that is capable of forming an immune complex with an antigen and becoming an insoluble precipitate, which can be detected in laboratory assays. This reaction forms the basis of many delicate diagnostic serological tests for the identification of antigens in serum and other fluids ⇒ immunoglobulins.

preconceptual *adj* before conception. Pre-conception care refers to the physical and mental preparation for childbearing of both parents before pregnancy. Health promoting activity focuses on measures aimed at reducing the risk of fetal problems and maternal complications during pregnancy and labour. The measures include the importance of an adequate diet, such as the provision of sufficient folic acid in the diet of women of childbearing age, and the avoidance of alcohol, drugs (prescribed, over the counter and illegal) and smoking in the months before a couple decide to have a baby.

preconscious *adj* information in the subconscious mind that can be evaluated and allowed to enter the conscious mind if we so wish.

precordial, praecordial *adj* relating to the area of the chest immediately over the heart.

precursor *n* forerunner.

prediabetes *n* ⇒ impaired fasting glucose, impaired glucose tolerance.

predisposition *n* a natural tendency to develop or contract certain diseases.

prejudice *n* a preconceived opinion or bias which can be negative or positive. It can be for or against members of particular groups and may lead to discrimination, racism, sexism or intolerance.

pre-eclampsia *n* a condition characterized by proteinuria, hypertension and oedema, arising usually in the latter part of pregnancy. ⇒ eclampsia.

prefrontal *adj* situated in the anterior portion of the frontal lobe of the cerebrum.

preganglionic *adj* proximal to a collection of nerve cells (ganglion), as a preganglionic nerve fibre.

pregnancy *n* being with child, i.e. gestation from last menstrual period to parturition, normally 40 weeks or 280 days. ⇒ ectopic pregnancy, phantom pregnancy.

preimplantation genetic diagnosis (PGD) a technique used in assisted conception to determine the genetic constitution of an embryo prior to implantation in the uterus.

preload *n* the degree of stretch present in the myocardial muscle fibres at the end of diastole. ⇒ afterload, stroke volume.

premature *adj* occurring before the proper time. *premature beat* ⇒ extrasystole. *premature birth* in English law, the birth of a baby after 24 weeks but before 37 weeks gestation.

premedication *n* drugs given before the administration of another drug, e.g. those given before a general anaesthesia to reduce anxiety.

premenstrual *adj* preceding menstruation. *premenstrual (cyclical) syndrome (PMS)* a group of physical and mental changes occurring any time between 2 and 14 days before menstruation. They are relieved almost immediately when menstruation starts.

premolar tooth permanent tooth with two cusps (bicuspid), placed fourth and fifth from the midline. They succeed the primary molars.

prenatal *adj* pertaining to the period between the last menstrual period and birth of the child, normally 40 weeks or 280 days—**prenatally** *adv*.

preoperative *adj* before operation—**preoperatively** *adv*.

preparalytic *adj* before the onset of paralysis, usually referring to the early stage of poliomyelitis.

prepatellar *adj* in front of the patella, as applied to a large bursa. ⇒ bursitis.

prepubertal *adj* before puberty.

prepuce *n* the foreskin of the penis (⇒ Figure 16).

prerenal *adj* literally, before or in front of the kidney, but usually refers to perfusion of the kidneys.

presbycusis *n* idiopathic sensorineural hearing loss caused by or associated with ageing.

presbyopia *n* failure of accommodation in those of 45 years and onwards—**presbyopic** *adj*, **presbyope** *n*.

Prescribing Analysis and Costs the information supplied to family doctors about their prescribing.

prescription *n* a written formula, signed by the authorized prescriber, instructing the pharmacist to supply the required drugs. *prescription only medicine* a drug that requires a written prescription, except in an emergency when the pharmacist may dispense the drug if certain criteria are met.

presenile dementia ⇒ dementia.

presenility *n* a condition occurring before senility is established. ⇒ dementia—**presenile** *adj*.

presentation *n* the part of the fetus which first enters the pelvic brim and will be felt by the examining finger through the cervix in labour. May be vertex, face, brow, shoulder or breech.

pressor *n* a substance which raises the blood pressure.

pressure areas any body area subjected to pressure sufficient to compress the capillaries and disrupt the microcirculation. Usually occurs where tissues are compressed between a bone and a hard surface, e.g. theatre table, trolley, bed, chair, splint, or where two skin surfaces are in contact such as under the breasts. Pressure areas include: head, spine, sacrum, shoulders, elbows, hips, buttocks, heels, ankles. ⇒ pressure ulcer.

pressure garment a skin-coloured, Lycra material garment used to exert firm, even pressure to a specific part of the body. Often used in the treatment of varicose veins; and burns and scalds to prevent keloid scarring.

pressure groups organizations formed to exert pressure on government (central and local) in order to further the interests of certain groups, such as older people.

pressure point a place at which an artery passes over a bone, against which it can be compressed, to stop bleeding.

pressure sore ⇒ pressure ulcer.

pressure support mode of positive pressure ventilation, which augments the size of a patient's spontaneous breaths.

pressure transducer device that converts pressure into calibrated electrical signals which can be displayed on a monitor.

pressure ulcer (*syn* decubitus ulcer, pressure sore) previously called a bedsore. Defined as an area of localized damage to the skin and underlying tissue caused by pressure, shear, friction, or a combination of these factors. Pressure ulcers develop when any area of the body is subjected to unrelieved pressure that leads to local hypoxia, ischaemia and necrosis with inflammation and ulcer formation. Shearing forces also disrupt the microcirculation when they cause the skin layers to move against one another. Shearing damages the deeper tissues and can lead to an extensive pressure ulcer. Friction from continual rubbing leads to blisters, abrasions and superficial pressure ulcers, and is made worse by moisture such as urine or sweat. Factors that increase the risk of pressure ulcer formation include: poor oxygenation, incontinence, age over 65–70, immobility, altered consciousness, dehydration and malnutrition.

presystole *n* the period preceding the systole or contraction of the heart muscle—**presystolic** *adj*.

pretibial laceration injury on the front of the shin especially common in older adults.

pretibial myxoedema purple/pink indurated areas of skin, usually on anterior aspect of the leg and dorsum of the foot. It is a feature of Graves' disease. The skin may be itchy and coarse hair is present.

prevalence *n* total number of cases of a disease existing in a population at a single point in time. *prevalence ratio* the prevalence of a disease, expressed as a ratio of population size.

priapism *n* prolonged penile erection in the absence of sexual stimulation.

prickly heat ⇒ miliaria.

prima facie 'at first sight', or sufficient evidence brought by one party to require the other party to provide a defence.

primary *adj* first in order. *primary tumour* the neoplasm at the site of origin.

Primary Care Trust (PCT) in England a body that works with Social Services and other local government departments and other relevant bodies, e.g. voluntary sector, to assess local health needs, plan, develop and provide community and primary healthcare services, and commission secondary services for the local population, in order to improve health, and reduce inequalities in health and improve access. They employ staff, run community hospitals, own property, and are responsible for public health. ⇒ Strategic Health Authority.

primary complex (*syn* Ghon focus) the initial tuberculous infection in a person, usually in the lung, manifesting as a small focus of infection in the lung tissue and enlarged caseous, hilar lymph nodes. It usually heals spontaneously.

primary health care 1 the first level contact with the healthcare system. For example general practitioner or practice nurse. 2 defined by WHO-UNICEF declaration (Alma-Ata 1978) as 'Essential health care based on practical, scientifically sound and socially acceptable methods and technology, made universally available to individuals and families in the community through their full participation and at a cost that the community and the country can afford, to maintain every stage of their development in the spirit of self-reliance and self-determination.' In its original and narrowest sense, primary health care refers to first contact care where patients contact healthcare workers directly. Principles on which effective primary health care is based are education about diseases, healthcare problems and their control; safe water and sanitation; maternal and child health, including family planning; immunization against major infectious diseases; appropriate treatment of common diseases and injuries; providing essential drugs.

primary healthcare team in the UK an interdependent multiprofessional group of individuals with a common purpose and responsibility, each member clearly understanding his or her own role, and those of other team members, in offering an equitable, efficient and effective primary healthcare service. The health professionals involved may include: community nurses, counsellors, general practitioners, health visitors, midwives, occupational therapists, physiotherapists, podiatrists, practice nurses, speech and language therapists.

primary prevention ⇒ disease prevention.

primigravida *n* a woman who is pregnant for the first time—**primigravidae** *pl*.

primipara *n* a woman who has given birth to a child for the first time—**primiparous** *adj*.

primordial *adj* primitive, original; applied to the ovarian follicles present at birth.

prion *n* an infectious agent consisting of protein, similar to viruses but containing no nucleic acids.

prion disease a range of disorders in which there is an abnormal deposition of prion protein in the brain of which the most common example is Creutzfeldt–Jakob disease.

Private Finance Initiative (PFI) a joint venture between private and public sector to build a facility, e.g. a hospital, using private finance. The NHS then leases the building. Some non-clinical services may also be provided under the lease agreement.

proband *n* in the genetically inherited diseases, the first family member to present for investigation.

problem-orientated medical record a multiprofessional system of keeping patient records. Entries are made using the SOAP formula: S = subjective, O = objective, A = analysis of the subjective and objective data, P = plan.

procedural memory that part of memory that stores information needed to do things, e.g. take a venous blood sample or record a television programme.

process *n* a prominence or outgrowth of any part.

procidentia *n* complete prolapse of the uterus, so that it lies within the vaginal sac but outside the contour of the body.

proctalgia *n* pain in the rectal region.

proctitis *n* inflammation of the rectum.

proctoclysis *n* introduction of fluid into the rectum for absorption. ⇒ enteroclysis.

proctocolectomy *n* surgical excision of the rectum and colon.

proctocolitis *n* inflammation of the rectum and colon.

proctoscope *n* a speculum or rigid tubular instrument for examining the anal canal and rectum. ⇒ endoscope—**proctoscopic** *adj*.

proctoscopy *n* inspection of the anal canal and rectum using a rigid instrument.

proctosigmoiditis *n* inflammation of the rectum and sigmoid colon.

prodromal *adj* preceding, as the transitory rash before the true rash of an infectious disease.

prodrug *n* a drug administered as an inactive form that may be activated in a numbers of ways, e.g. by bowel bacteria, in the brain or by liver enzymes. Used for a variety of reasons such as avoiding gastrointestinal side-effects, or crossing the blood–brain barrier.

proenzyme *n* the inactive (or precursor) form of a proteolytic enzyme, such as pepsinogen. Also called a zymogen.

professional self-regulation the professional quality and continuing professional development standards set by various professional regulatory bodies for health professionals, e.g. GMC, for professional practice, discipline and conduct.

profiling (community) process of producing a profile of a specific community. It includes demographic information such as the age profile, social and economic make-up, existing facilities, networks and services. The profile may be produced by people living in the community with varying degrees of support from the local authority, development agencies or health services.

progestational *adj* before pregnancy. Favouring pregnancy—**progestation** *n*.

progesterone *n* a steroid hormone secreted by the corpus luteum, placenta and, in limited amounts, by the adrenal glands. Progesterone acts on the endometrium, myometrium, cervical mucus and breasts. It is important in the preparation for and maintenance of pregnancy.

progestogen *n* any natural or synthetic progestational hormone including progesterone. *progestogen-only pill* an oral contraceptive that is taken continuously and at regular time intervals to provide effective contraception.

proglottis a sexually mature segment of tapeworm—**proglottides** *pl*.

prognosis *n* a forecast of the probable course and termination of a disease—**prognostic** *adj*.

projection *n* a mental mechanism occurring in normal people unconsciously, and in exaggerated form in some mental health problems, whereby the person fails to recognize certain motives and feelings in him or herself but attributes them to other people.

projective techniques the therapeutic use of creative media such as art and music to encourage individuals to express themselves and to explore and interpret their thoughts and feelings.

prolactin (PRL) *n* a hormone secreted by the anterior pituitary, concerned with lactation and reproduction.

prolactinoma *n* prolactin secreting pituitary adenoma. ⇒ hyperprolactinaemia.

prolapse *n* descent; the falling of a structure. *prolapse of an intervertebral disc (PID)*

protrusion of the disc nucleus into the spinal canal. Most common in the lumbar region where it causes low back pain and/or sciatica. *prolapse of the iris* iridocele. *prolapse of the rectum* the lower portion of the intestinal tract descends outside the external anal sphincter. *prolapse of the uterus* the uterus descends into the vagina and may be visible at the vaginal orifice. ⇒ procidentia.

proliferate *vi* increase by cell division—**proliferation** *n*, **proliferative** *adj*.

prolific *adj* fruitful, multiplying abundantly.

proline *n* a conditionally essential (indispensable) amino acid.

promontory *n* a projection; a prominent part.

pronate *vt* to place ventral surface downward, e.g. on the face; to turn (the palm of the hand) downwards. ⇒ supinate *opp*—**pronation** *n*.

pronator *n* that which pronates, usually applied to a muscle. ⇒ supinator *opp*. *pronator teres* ⇒ Figure 4.

prone *adj*. **1** lying on the anterior surface of the body with the face turned to the side. **2** of the hand, with the palm downwards. ⇒ supine *opp*.

prophylaxis *n* (attempted) prevention, e.g. immunization—**prophylactic** *adj*, **prophylactically** *adv*.

propionic acids a group of non-steroidal anti-inflammatory drugs. ⇒ Appendix 5.

proprietary name (*syn* brand name) the name given to e.g. a drug by the pharmaceutical company which developed it. It should always be spelt with a capital letter to distinguish it from the approved (generic) name which can be used by other companies.

proprioception *n* appreciation of balance and the position of the body and individual body parts in relation to each other, especially as they change during movement.

proprioceptive neuromuscular facilitation (PNF) exercises that stimulate proprioceptors in muscles, tendons and joints in order to improve strength and flexibility.

proprioceptor *n* a sensory receptor located in a muscle, tendon, ligament or vestibular apparatus of the ears whose reflex function is locomotor or postural.

proptosis *n* forward protrusion, especially of the eyeball.

prosody *n* describes the phonological features of speech that include rate, rhythm, stress, loudness and pitch.

prospective study research that deals with future data, moving forward in time. ⇒ retrospective study.

prostacyclin *n* a substance formed by endothelial cells lining blood vessels. It inhibits platelet aggregation and is concerned with preventing intravascular clotting.

prostaglandins *npl* a large group of regulatory lipids. Found in most body tissues where they regulate physiological functions including: smooth muscle contraction, inflammation, gastric secretion and blood clotting. Used pharmaceutically to terminate pregnancy, induce labour and for asthma and gastric hyperacidity. ⇒ Appendix 5.

prostate *n* a small conical gland at the base of the male bladder and surrounding the first part of the urethra. Adds alkaline fluid containing enzymes into the semen (⇒ Figure 16)—**prostatic** *adj*.

prostatectomy *n* surgical removal of the prostate gland. *retropubic prostatectomy* the prostate is reached through a lower abdominal (suprapubic) incision, the bladder being retracted upwards to expose the prostate behind the pubis. *transurethral prostatectomy (TUR/TURP)* the operation whereby chippings of prostatic tissue are cut from within the urethra using an electric cautery. ⇒ resectoscope. *transvesical prostatectomy* the operation in which the prostate is approached through the bladder, using a lower abdominal (suprapubic) incision.

prostate specific antigen (PSA) protein secreted by prostatic tissue. Acts as a tumour marker for prostate cancer, and its detection in the blood forms the basis for a screening test. Conditions other than prostate cancer can cause an increase in PSA level.

prostatic *adj* relating to the prostate. *benign prostatic hyperplasia (BPH)* benign enlargement of the prostate gland occurring mainly in older men. Leads to urinary problems such as poor stream and retention. *prostatic acid phosphatase* ⇒ acid phosphatase.

prostatism *n* term used to describe the symptom complex associated with bladder outflow obstruction.

prostatitis *n* inflammation of the prostate gland.

prosthesis *n* an artificial substitute for a missing part—**prostheses** *pl*, **prosthetic** *adj*.

prosthetics *n* the branch of surgery which deals with prostheses.

protease *n* an enzyme which digests protein (proteolytic).

protective isolation reverse barrier nursing. Involves separating patients who are immunocompromised and susceptible to infection, either by disease or treatment. The type of patients needing protection from infection include those with leukaemia, those having immunosuppressant treatment for organ transplantation, chemotherapy or radiation or neutropenic patients. ⇒ containment isolation, source isolation.

protein-energy malnutrition (PEM) previously known as protein calorie malnutrition (PCM). Describes a condition in which individuals have depleted body fat and protein resulting from a diet that is deficient in both protein and energy. It develops during famine, during illness and childhood due to inappropriate weaning. ⇒ kwashiorkor, marasmus.

proteins *npl* highly complex nitrogenous compounds found in all animal and vegetable tissues. They are built up of amino acids and are essential for growth and repair of the body. Those from animal sources are of high biological value since they contain the essential amino acids. Those from vegetable sources contain not all, but some of the essential amino acids. Proteins are hydrolysed in the body to produce amino acids, which are then used to build up new body proteins.

proteinuria *n* excretion of abnormally high levels of protein in the urine. ⇒ albuminuria.

proteolysis *n* the hydrolysis of the peptide bonds of proteins with the formation of smaller polypeptides—**proteolytic** *adj*.

proteolytic enzymes enzymes that promote proteolysis; they are used in the management of leg ulcers to remove slough.

Proteus *n* a bacterial genus of Gram-negative motile rods. Found in damp surroundings. A commensal of the intestinal tract but causes urinary tract and wound infection.

prothrombin *n* inactive precursor of the enzyme thrombin produced in the liver. Factor II in blood coagulation. *prothrombin time* assesses the activity of the extrinsic coagulation pathway. It is the time taken for plasma to clot in vitro following the introduction of thromboplastin in the presence of calcium. It is inversely proportional to the amount of prothrombin present, a normal person's plasma being used as a standard of comparison. The prothrombin time is extended in people taking anticoagulant drugs and in some haemorrhagic conditions.

proton *n* subatomic particle having a positive charge.

proton pump inhibitors a group of drugs that decrease gastric acid secretion by irreversibly blocking the proton pump (H^+/K^+-ATPase). ⇒ Appendix 5.

proto-oncogene *n* a gene with the potential to become a cancer-causing oncogene if stimulated by mutagenic carcinogens. ⇒ oncogene.

protopathic *adj* the term applied to the somatic sensations of fast localized pain; slow, poorly localized pain; and temperature. ⇒ epicritic *opp.*

protoplasm *n* ⇒ cytoplasm.

protozoa *npl* unicellular microscopic animals. Some are pathogenic. Includes the genera *Plasmodium*, *Leishmania* and *Entamoeba*—**protozoon** *sing*, **protozoal** *adj.* ⇒ amoebiasis, giardiasis, leishmaniasis, malaria, toxoplasmosis, trichomoniasis.

protraction *n* a forward movement such as thrusting out the jaw. ⇒ retraction *opp.*

proud flesh excessive granulation tissue.

provitamin *n* a vitamin precursor, e.g. β-carotene is converted into vitamin A.

proximal *adj* nearest to the head or source. ⇒ distal *opp*—**proximally** *adv.*

prune belly syndrome a condition found in male infants with obstructive uropathy and atrophy of the abdominal musculature. The term is descriptive.

prurigo *n* a chronic, itching disease often associated with skin lichenification.

pruritus *n* itching. *pruritus ani* and *pruritus vulvae* may be due to a number of causes, e.g. vaginitis. Generalized pruritus may be a symptom of systemic disease, as in renal failure, Hodgkin's disease, cancer or jaundice—**pruritic** *adj.*

PSA *abbr* prostate specific antigen.

pseudoangina *n* false angina. Sometimes referred to as 'left mammary pain', it occurs in anxious individuals. Usually there is no cardiac disease present. May be part of effort syndrome.

pseudoarthrosis *n* a false joint, e.g. due to ununited fracture; also congenital, e.g. in tibia.

pseudobulbar paralysis there is disturbance in the higher control of the tongue and pharynx typically with cognitive and limb abnormalities, and found most often in the context of amyotrophic lateral sclerosis (ALS) or a succession of 'strokes'.

pseudocoxalgia *n* ⇒ Perthes' disease.

pseudocrisis *n* a rapid reduction of body temperature resembling a crisis, followed by further fever.

pseudocyesis *n* ⇒ phantom pregnancy.

pseudogout *n* an arthritis (usually monoarthritis) caused by crystals of calcium pyrophosphate dihydrate within the joint.

pseudohermaphrodite *n* a person in whom the gonads of one sex are present, whilst the external genitalia comprise those of the opposite sex.

pseudologia fantastica a tendency to tell, and defend, fantastic lies plausibly.

pseudomembranous colitis inflammation of the colon coated in pale plaques (pseudomembranes). Usually caused by superinfection with *Clostridium difficile*. Recent antibiotic usage predisposes.

Pseudomonas *n* a bacterial genus. Gram-negative motile rods. Found in water and decomposing vegetable matter. Some are pathogenic to plants and animals and *Pseudomonas aeruginosa* is a cause of urinary, wound and respiratory infection in humans. It can cause superinfection where the normal commensals have been eliminated by antibiotic usage. Produces blue-green exudate or pus with a characteristic musty odour.

pseudomucin *n* a gelatinous substance (not mucin) found in some ovarian cysts.

pseudophakia *n* presence of an artificial lens. Describes an eye after cataract surgery with intraocular lens implantation.

pseudopolyposis *n* widely scattered polypi, usually the result of previous inflammation—sometimes ulcerative colitis.

pseudoseizures *npl* attacks that can look like epileptic seizures but which have no electrical basis and are normally related to psychiatric problems.

psittacosis *n* disease of parrots, pigeons and budgerigars which is occasionally responsible for atypical pneumonia in humans. Caused by *Chlamydia psittaci*.

psoas *n* muscles of the loin. *psoas abscess* a cold abscess in the psoas muscle, resulting from tuberculosis of the vertebrae. The abscess appears as a firm smooth swelling which does not show signs of inflammation—hence the adjective 'cold'.

psoralen *n* a naturally occurring photosensitive compound, used in PUVA treatment.

psoriasis *n* a genetically determined chronic skin disease in which erythematous scaly plaques characteristically occur on the elbows, knees and scalp—**psoriatic** *adj*.

psoriatic arthritis arthritis occurring in association with psoriasis.

psyche *n* Greek term for 'life force', used to describe that which makes up the mind and all its processes, and sometimes used to describe 'self'.

psychiatry *n* the branch of medicine that addresses the diagnosis and treatment of mental illness—**psychiatric** *adj*.

psychic *adj* of the mind.

psychoactive *adj* substances and drugs that may alter mental processes.

psychoanalysis *n* a specialized branch founded by Freud. It is a method of diagnosis and treatment of neuroses. Briefly the method is to revive past forgotten experiences and effect a cure of the neurosis by helping the patient readjust his attitudes to those experiences—**psychoanalytic** *adj*.

psychodrama *n* a psychotherapy technique whereby patients act out their personal problems by adopting roles in spontaneous dramatic performances. Group discussion aims at giving the patients a greater awareness of the problems presented and possible strategies for dealing with them.

psychodynamics *n* the science of the mental processes, especially of the factors causing mental activity.

psychogenesis *n* the development of the mind.

psychogenic *adj* arising from the mind. *psychogenic symptom* originates in the mind.

psychogeriatric *adj* outdated term, relating to the application of psychology to geriatrics. The phrase elderly mentally ill (EMI) has also been used. *psychogeriatric dependency rating scales* construction of these scales was based on three basic dimensions—psychological deterioration, physical infirmity and psychological agitation.

psychology *n* the study of the behaviour and mental processes.

psychometry *n* the science involved with mental testing.

psychomotor *adj* pertaining to the motor effects of mental activity.

psychoneuroimmunology (PNI) *n* study of the integration of neural and immune response in relation to psychological state. Psychological distress/stress is associated with the impairment of immune system function.

psychoneurosis *n* ⇒ neurosis.

psychopath *n* one who is morally irresponsible and intent on instant gratification—**psychopathic** *adj*.

psychopathic personality a persistent disorder of the mind (whether or not including learning disability) which results in abnormally aggressive or seriously irresponsible behaviour that requires, or is susceptible to, medical treatment. ⇒ Mental Health Act.

psychopathology *n* the pathology of abnormal mental states—**psychopathological** *adj*, **psychopathologically** *adv*.

psychopharmacology *n* the study and use of drugs which influence the affective and emotional state—**psychopharmacological** *adj*, **psychopharmacologically** *adv*.

psychophysics *n* a branch of experimental psychology concerned with stimuli and sensations—**psychophysical** *adj*.

psychoprophylactic *adj* that which aims at preventing mental health problems.

psychosexual *adj* pertaining to the mental aspects of sexuality. *psychosexual development* according to Freud's theory, development occurs through five stages (oral, anal, phallic, latent and genital). Each stage is characterized by a different area of pleasurable stimulation. *psychosexual counselling* usually sought by one or both members of a partnership because one or both is unable to obtain emotional and sexual satisfaction within the relationship. Psychosexual counselling of otherwise 'healthy' people is provided by specialists and is rarely provided by the NHS in the UK. Healthcare professionals need to be aware that any health disturbance may create actual or potential psychosexual problems.

psychosis *n* ⇒ neurosis. The term psychotic is used as a grouping term for disorders where a lack of contact with reality occurs, e.g. by hallucinations or delusions—**psychoses** *pl*, **psychotic** *adj*.

psychosomatic *adj* pertaining to the mind and body *psychosomatic disorder* a physical condition where psychological factors such as stress may be involved in the cause, such as some types of peptic ulcer.

psychotherapy *n* treatment of emotional and psychological problems by individual or group interaction. Usually by talking but many other approaches exist—**psychotherapeutic** *adj*. *group psychotherapy or group therapy* a therapist enables and encourages people to understand and analyse their own problems and those of other group members.

psychotropic *adj* that which exerts its specific effect upon the brain cells.

pteroylglutamic acid ⇒ folic acid.

pterygium *n* **1** a wing-shaped degenerative condition of the conjunctiva which encroaches on the cornea. **2** adhesion of the eponychium (cuticle) to the nail bed. It follows destruction of the matrix due to diminished circulation or some systemic diseases. The entire nail plate is eventually shed.

ptosis *n* a drooping, particularly that of the upper eyelid. Common in old age—**ptotic** *adj*.

ptyalin *n* ⇒ amylase.

puberty *n* the period during which the reproductive organs become functionally active and the secondary sexual characteristics develop—**pubertal** *adj*.

pubes *n* the hair-covered area over the pubic bone.

pubiotomy *n* rarely performed surgery that involves cutting the pubic bone to facilitate delivery of a child.

pubis *n* the pubic bone or os pubis. The two bones that meet at the symphysis pubis—**pubic** *adj*.

public health broadly defined as health activity for populations in small areas, regions, nations and worldwide. In the UK public health involves the following functions: Health surveillance, monitoring and analysis. Investigation of disease outbreaks, epidemics and risks to health. Establishing, designing and managing health promotion and disease prevention programmes. Enabling and empowering communities and citizens to promote health and reduce inequalities. Creating and sustaining cross-governmental and inter-sectoral partnerships to improve health and reduce inequalities. Ensuring compliance with regulations and laws to protect and promote health. Developing and maintaining a well-educated and trained, multidisciplinary public health workforce. Ensuring the effective performance of the NHS services to meet goals in improving health, preventing disease and reducing inequalities. Research, development, evaluation and innovation. Quality assuring the public health function.

pudendal block the rendering insensitive of the pudendum by the injection of local anaesthetic. Used mainly for episiotomy and forceps delivery. ⇒ transvaginal.

pudendum *n* the external reproductive organs, especially of the female—**pudenda** *pl*, **pudendal** *adj*.

puerperal *adj* pertaining to childbirth. *puerperal psychosis* a mental illness (psychosis) occurring in the puerperium. ⇒ postnatal depression. *puerperal sepsis* infection of the genital tract occurring within 21 days of abortion or childbirth.

puerperium *n* the period immediately following childbirth to the time when involution is completed, usually 6–8 weeks—**puerperia** *pl*.

PUFA *abbr* polyunsaturated fatty acid.

pulmonary *adj* pertaining to the lungs. *pulmonary artery* ⇒ Figures 7, 8, 9. *pulmonary circulation* deoxygenated blood leaves the right ventricle, flows through the lungs where it loses carbon dioxide, becomes oxygenated and returns to the left atrium of the heart. ⇒ circulation. *pulmonary emphysema* overdistension and subsequent destruction of alveoli and reduced gas exchange in the lungs. Associated with tobacco smoking, it is a form of chronic obstructive pulmonary disease (COPD). ⇒ bronchitis. *pulmonary hypertension* raised blood pressure within the pulmonary circulation, due to increased resistance to blood flow within the pulmonary vessels. It may be primary (genetic), or secondary due to chronic lung disease or chronic pulmonary embolism. *pulmonary infarction* necrosis of lung tissue resulting from an embolus. *pulmonary oedema* fluid within the alveoli. The lungs are 'waterlogged' and gas exchange is reduced, such as in left ventricular failure, mitral stenosis, or fluid excess in renal failure. *pulmonary stenosis* narrowing of the pulmonary valve. *pulmonary tuberculosis* ⇒ tuberculosis. *pulmonary valve* semilunar valve situated between the pulmonary artery and right cardiac ventricle. *pulmonary veins* ⇒ Figures 7, 8. *pulmonary ventilation* or minute volume. The amount of air moved in and out of the lungs in one minute.

pulmonary artery flotation catheter (PAFC) specialized balloon tipped catheter which is 'floated' from the central veins, through the heart and into the pulmonary artery. Allows measurement of pulmonary artery pressure, pulmonary artery occlusion pressure and cardiac output.

pulmonary artery occlusion pressure (PAOP) pressure in the left atrium measured by inflating a balloon on the tip of a pulmonary artery catheter thereby temporarily occluding the pulmonary artery; also known as wedge pressure.

pulmonary artery pressure blood pressure in the pulmonary artery usually measured using a pulmonary artery catheter.

pulmonary embolus (PE) an embolism which occurs in the pulmonary arterial system; most commonly as a result of deep vein thrombosis in the leg or pelvic veins. Prophylaxis includes deep breathing and foot exercises, early mobilization, antithromboembolic stockings with the administration of heparin in at-risk groups.

pulmonary rehabilitation combination of graded physical exertion, educational, psychological and behavioural interventions

designed to improve symptoms in those with chronic lung disease.

pulp *n* the soft, interior part of some organs and structures. *digital pulp* the tissue pad of the finger tip. ⇒ dental pulp.

pulsatile *adj* beating, throbbing.

pulsation *n* beating or throbbing, as of the arteries or heart.

pulse *n* the impulse transmitted to arteries by contraction of the left ventricle, and customarily palpated in the radial artery at the wrist. The *pulse rate* is the number of beats or impulses per minute and is about 130 in the newborn infant, 70–80 in the adult and 60–70 in old age. The *pulse rhythm* is its regularity—and can be regular or irregular; the *pulse volume* is the amplitude of expansion of the arterial wall during the passage of the wave; the *pulse force* or tension is its strength, estimated by the force needed to obliterate it by pressure of the finger. *pulse deficit* the difference in rate of the heart (counted by stethoscope) and the pulse (counted at the wrist), as seen in atrial fibrillation. *pulse pressure* is the difference between the systolic and diastolic pressures. ⇒ beat.

pulseless disease progressive obliterative arteritis of the vessels arising from the aortic arch resulting in diminished or absent pulse in the neck and arms. Thromboendarterectomy or a bypass procedure may prevent blindness by improving the carotid blood flow at its commencement in the aortic arch.

pulseless ventricular tachycardia a form of cardiac arrest. ⇒ ventricular tachycardia.

pulse oximeter an instrument attached to the finger, ear or nose to 'sense' the oxygen saturation of arterial blood. An accurate non-invasive technique.

pulsus alternans a regular pulse with alternate beats of weak and strong amplitude; associated with left ventricular heart failure.

pulsus bigeminus double pulse wave produced by interpolation of extrasystoles. A coupled beat.

pulsus paradoxus arterial pulsus paradoxus is alteration of the volume of the arterial pulse sometimes found in pericarditis. The volume becomes greater with expiration. Venous pulsus paradoxus (Kusman's sign) is an increase in the height of the venous pressure with inspiration, the reverse of normal. Sometimes found in pericardial or right ventricular disease.

pulvis *n* a powder.

punctate *adj* dotted or spotted, e.g. punctate basophilia describes red cells in which there are droplets of blue-staining material in the cytoplasm.

punctum *n* entrance to lacrimal drainage system on eyelid margin—**puncta** *pl*.

puncture *n* a stab; a wound made with a sharp pointed hollow instrument for withdrawal or injection of fluid or other substance. ⇒ cisternal puncture, lumbar puncture, penetrating wound.

PUO *abbr* pyrexia of unknown origin.

pupil *n* the opening in the iris of the eye, which allows the passage of light—**pupillary** *adj*.

pupillary *adj* relating to the pupil. *pupillary reflex* the reflex dilatation and constriction of the pupil in response to the amount of light entering the eye. Controlled by the oculomotor nerves (third cranial).

purgative *n* a drug that causes the evacuation of fluid faeces.

purines *npl* nitrogenous bases needed as constituents of nucleoproteins. Uric acid is produced when purines are broken down. Increased uric acid in the blood is associated with disorders of metabolism and excretion of uric acid, and leads to the development of gout.

purpura *n* superficial haemorrhage, less than 1 cm, into the skin. A disorder characterized by extravasation of blood from the capillaries into the skin, or into or from the mucous membranes. May be either small red spots (petechiae) or large bruises (ecchymoses) or by oozing from minor wounds confined to the mucous membranes. It may be due to impaired integrity of the capillary walls, or to defective quality or quantity of platelets. Purpura can be caused by many different conditions, e.g. infective, toxic, allergic, etc. ⇒ Henoch-Schönlein purpura.

purulent *adj* pertaining to or resembling pus.

pus *n* a liquid, usually yellowish in colour, formed in certain infections and composed of tissue fluid containing bacteria and leucocytes. Various types of bacteria are associated with pus having distinctive features, e.g. the faecal smell of pus due to

Escherichia coli; the green colour of pus due to *Pseudomonas aeruginosa*.

pustule *n* a visible collection of free pus in a blister usually indicates an infection (e.g. furuncle) but not always (e.g. pustular psoriasis)—**pustular** *adj. malignant pustule* ⇒ anthrax.

putrefaction *n* rotting; bacterial destruction of organic material.

PUVA *abbr* psoralen with ultra violet radiation of a long wavelength used for the treatment of skin diseases, particularly psoriasis.

PV *abbr* per vaginam: describes the route used for examination of the vagina, or the administration of drugs.

P value in research, the symbol used to denote the probability of the results of a test occurring by chance. A P value is given in all inferential statistics. This is the probability that the results found have occurred by chance alone. The P value is measured on a scale of 0–1, so for example a P value of $P=0.05$ means 5% or a one in twenty chance. A lower case p is used for proportions.

PVD *abbr* peripheral vascular disease.

pyaemia *n* the presence in the circulation of septic emboli. They can lodge in organs, such as the liver, brain, kidneys and lungs, to form multiple abscesses—**pyaemic** *adj*.

pyarthrosis *n* pus in a joint cavity.

pyelitis *n* obsolete term. ⇒ pyelonephritis.

pyelography *n* ⇒ urography.

pyelolithotomy *n* the operation for removal of a stone from the renal pelvis.

pyelonephritis *n* infection within the substance of the kidney, often derived either from the urine or from the blood—**pyelonephritic** *adj*.

pyeloplasty *n* a reconstructive operation on the kidney pelvis. ⇒ hydronephrosis.

pyelostomy *n* surgical formation of an opening into the kidney pelvis.

pyloroduodenal *adj* pertaining to the pylorus and the duodenum.

pyloromyotomy *n* (*syn* Ramstedt's operation) incision of the pyloric sphincter muscle as in pyloroplasty.

pyloroplasty *n* a plastic operation on the pylorus designed to widen the passage.

pylorospasm *n* spasm of the pylorus; usually due to the presence of a duodenal ulcer.

pylorus *n* region containing the opening of the stomach into the duodenum, controlled by a sphincter muscle—**pyloric** *adj*.

pyocolpos *n* pus in the vagina.

pyodermia, pyoderma *n* any purulent condition of the skin—**pyodermic** *adj*.

pyogenic *adj* relating to pus formation.

pyknosis darkening and condensation of nuclear chromatin.

pyometra *n* pus retained in the uterus and unable to escape through the cervix—**pyometric** *adj*.

pyonephrosis *n* distension of the renal pelvis with pus—**pyonephrotic** *adj*.

pyopericarditis *n* pericarditis with purulent effusion.

pyopneumothorax *n* pus and gas or air within the pleural sac.

pyorrhoea *n* a flow of pus.

pyosalpinx *n* a uterine (fallopian) tube containing pus.

pyothorax *n* pus in the pleural cavity.

pyramidal *adj* applied to some conical eminences in the body. *pyramidal cells (Betz cells)* nerve cells in the precentral motor area of the cerebral cortex, from which originate impulses to voluntary muscles. *pyramidal tracts* main motor tracts in the brain and spinal cord, which transmit impulses arising from the pyramidal cells. Most decussate (cross over) in the medulla.

pyrazolones *npl* a group of non-steroidal anti-inflammatory drugs. ⇒ Appendix 5.

pyrexia *n* body temperature above normal, usually between 37°C and 40/41°C. *pyrexia of unknown origin* where the reason for the raised body temperature is not known. ⇒ fever, hyperpyrexia—**pyrexial** *adj*.

pyridoxine *n* vitamin B_6; may be connected with the utilization of unsaturated fatty acids or the synthesis of fat from proteins. Deficiency may lead to dermatitis and neuritic pains. Used in nausea of pregnancy and radiation sickness, muscular dystrophy, pellagra, the premenstrual syndrome, etc.

pyrimidines *npl* nitrogenous bases needed as constituents of nucleic acids.

pyrogen *n* a substance producing fever—**pyrogenic** *adj*.

pyrosis *n* (*syn* heartburn, waterbrash) eructation of acid gastric contents into the mouth, accompanied by a burning sensation felt behind the sternum.

pyrotherapy *n* production of fever by artificial means. ⇒ hyperthermia.

pyruvic acid an important metabolic molecule. Converted to acetyl CoA which is used in the Krebs cycle, or forms lactic acid during anaerobic glucose metabolism.

pyuria *n* pus in the urine (more than three leucocytes per high-power field)—**pyuric** *adj*.

Q

QALYs *abbr* quality adjusted life years.

Q fever a febrile disease caused by *Coxiella burnetii*. It is transmitted to humans from sheep and cattle or in unpasteurized milk. Pasteurization of milk kills *Coxiella burnetii*.

Qi energy also known as chi, yin/yang. In complementary medicine, the person's inborn energy focused on maintaining health and well-being. The concept of Qi energy is fundamental to therapies such as acupuncture where the energy is believed to flow through meridians.

quadrantanopia *n* loss of vision in one quadrant of the visual field.

quadriceps *n* large four-part extensor muscle of the thigh, comprises the rectus femoris, vastus medialis, vastus lateralis and vastus intermedius. ⇒ Figure 4.

quadriparesis *n* weakness of all four limbs.

quadriplegia *n* ⇒ tetraplegia—**quadriplegic** *adj*.

qualitative *adj* relating to quality. *qualitative research* research study based on observation and/or interviews to ascertain people's opinions, feelings or beliefs. Non-statistical methods often used in analysis. ⇒ quantitative research.

quality adjusted life years (QALYs) measure of years of life gained through a health intervention adjusted for the quality of life. For example, if an intervention prolongs life by 5 years, but at only half the quality of normal life, this produces 2.5 QALYs. Quality of life (QoL) is a patient-centred subjective outcome measure to complement clinical outcomes. Usually measures the presence or absence of symptoms (e.g. pain), side-effects of treatment (e.g. tiredness, loss of hair), feelings of well-being, impact on income, family, work and social life.

quality assurance systematic monitoring and evaluation of agreed levels of service provision which are followed by modifications in the light of the evaluation and or audit. ⇒ benchmarking, clinical audit, performance indicators.

quality circles an initiative to improve the quality of care in a specific area. The health professionals in a clinical area investigate a healthcare intervention systematically and relate it to good standards of practice.

quantitative *adj* relating to quantity. *quantitative research* research study based on the measurement and analysis of observations using statistical methods. ⇒ qualitative research.

quarantine *n* a period of isolation of infected or suspected people with the objective of preventing spread to others. For contacts it is usually the same period as the longest incubation period for the specific disease.

quartan *adj* recurring every 72 hours (fourth day), such as the fever of quartan malaria.

Queckenstedt's test during lumbar puncture compression on the internal jugular vein normally produces a rise in cerebrospinal fluid (CSF) pressure if there is no obstruction to circulation of fluid.

quellung reaction swelling of the capsule of a bacterium when exposed to specific antisera. It allows the identification of bacteria causing a disease.

quickening *n* the first perceptible fetal movements felt by the mother, usually at 16–18 weeks gestation.

quiescent *adj* becoming quiet or inactive.

quinine *n* an alkaloid of cinchona, previously standard treatment for malaria. Use is increasing in regions where resistance to newer antimalarials is a problem.

quininism *n* toxic effects such as headache, tinnitus and partial deafness, disturbed vision and nausea arising from an overdose or long-term use of quinine.

quinsy *n* ⇒ peritonsillar abscess.

quotient *n* a number obtained by division. ⇒ respiratory quotient. *intelligence quotient* ⇒ intelligence.

R

rabid *adj* infected with rabies.

rabies *n* (*syn* hydrophobia) fatal infection of the central nervous system caused by a virus; infection follows the bite of a rabid animal, e.g. dog, cat, fox, vampire bat. It is distributed worldwide; human and animal vaccines are available—**rabid** *adj*.

race *n* often mistakenly linked to ethnicity. However, race only applies to biological characteristics such as facial features, skin colour or hair type that distinguish a specific group. ⇒ ethnic.

racemose *adj* resembling a bunch of grapes.

racism *n* an opinion of particular groups that is founded on race alone. It results in negative stereotyping, prejudice and discrimination. Racism may be overt, where individuals are subjected to oppressive acts, or covert, where a climate of institutional racism permits one section of society to oppress and subordinate other groups.

radial *adj* pertaining to the radius. Applied to the nerve, artery and vein. ⇒ Figures 9, 10.

radiation *n* emanation of radiant energy in the form of electromagnetic waves including: gamma rays, infrared, ultraviolet rays, X-rays and visible light rays. Subatomic particles, such as neutrons or electrons, may also be radiated. Radiation may be non-ionizing or ionizing and has many diagnostic and therapeutic uses. ⇒ ionizing radiation. *radiation sickness* tissue damage from exposure to ionizing radiation leads to diarrhoea, vomiting, anorexia and bone marrow failure.

radiation oncologist medical specialist in the treatment of disease by X-rays and other forms of radiation.

radical *adj* pertaining to the root of a thing. *radical surgery* usually extensive and aims to be curative, not palliative.

radiculography *n* X-ray of the spinal nerve roots after rendering them radiopaque to locate the site and size of a prolapsed intervertebral disc. Superseded by CT and MRI—**radiculogram** *n*.

radiculopathy *n* entrapment of the nerve as it passes out from the spinal cord to the arm or leg, and usually occurs as a result of intervertebral disc prolapse and degenerative disease in the facet joints of the spine.

radioactive *adj* exhibiting radioactivity. Describes an unstable atomic nucleus which emits charged particles as it disintegrates. ⇒ radioisotope. *radioactive decay* the spontaneous disintegration of radioactive atoms within a radioactive substance. ⇒ half-life. *radioactive fallout* release of radioactive particles into the atmosphere. Results from industrial processes or accidents, and the testing or use of nuclear weapons.

radioallergosorbent test an obsolete test for IgE antibodies against specific allergens. Now largely replaced by non-radioactive enzyme-based assays.

radiobiology *n* the study of the effects of radiation on living tissue—**radiobiological** *adj*, **radiobiologically** *adv*.

radiocarbon *n* a radioactive form of the element carbon, such as carbon-14 (^{14}C), used for investigations, e.g. absorption tests and research.

radiograph *n* a photographic image formed by exposure to X-rays; the correct term for an 'X-ray'—**radiographic** *adj*.

radiographer *n* there are two distinct professional disciplines within radiography, diagnostic and therapeutic; they are health professionals qualified in the use of ionizing radiation and other techniques, either in diagnostic imaging or radiotherapy.

radiography *n* the use of X-radiation (a) to create images of the body from which medical diagnosis can be made (diagnostic radiography); or (b) to treat a person suffering from a (malignant) disease, according to a medically prescribed regimen (therapeutic radiography). ⇒ radiotherapy.

radioimmunoassay *n* the use of radioactive substances to measure substances such as hormones and drugs in the blood.

radioiodinated human serum albumin (RIHSA) used for detection and localization of brain lesions, determination of blood and plasma volumes, circulation time and cardiac output.

radioisotope *n* (*syn* radionuclide) forms of an element which have the same atomic number but different mass numbers,

exhibiting the property of spontaneous nuclear disintegration. When taken orally or by injection, can be traced by a Geigercounter. *radioisotope scan* pictorial representation of the amount and distribution of radioactive isotope present in a particular organ.

radiologist *n* a medical specialist in diagnosis by using X-rays and other allied imaging techniques.

radiology *n* the study of the diagnosis of disease by using X-rays and other allied imaging techniques—**radiological** *adj*, **radiologically** *adv*.

radiomimetic *adj* exerting effects similar to those of ionizing radiation.

radionuclide *n* ⇒ radioisotope.

radiopaque *adj* having the property of significantly absorbing X-rays, thus becoming visible on a radiograph. Barium and iodine compounds are used, as contrast media, to produce artificial radiopacity—**radiopacity** *n*.

radiosensitive *adj* applied to tissue sensitive to the killing effects of ionizing radiation.

radiosurgery *n* (*syn* stereotactic radiotherapy) a radiotherapy treatment based on a 3D coordinate system designed to achieve a high concentration of absorbed dose to an intracranial target.

radiotherapist *n* ⇒ radiation oncologist.

radiotherapy *n* the treatment of proliferative disease, especially cancer, by X-rays and other forms of radiation.

radium (Ra) *n* a radioactive element occurring in nature, historically a mainstay of radiotherapy.

radius *n* bone of the forearm. ⇒ Figures 2, 3.

radon seeds capsules containing radon—a radioactive gas produced by the disintegration of radium atoms. Historically used in radiotherapy.

raised intracranial pressure (RIP) an elevation in intracranial pressure is a serious situation. Causes include: tumours, intracranial haemorrhage, trauma causing oedema or haematoma and obstruction to the flow of cerebrospinal fluid. The features depend on the cause, but there may be headache, vomiting, papilloedema, fits, bradycardia, arterial hypertension and changes in the level of consciousness. ⇒ benign intracranial hypertension.

RA latex test used in rheumatoid arthritis. A blood test used to detect the presence of the rheumatoid factor. ⇒ SCAT.

râle *n* abnormal sound heard on auscultation of lungs when fluid is present in bronchi.

Ramsay Hunt syndrome herpes zoster causing vesicles on the ear lobe with pain, facial paralysis and loss of taste.

Ramstedt's operation ⇒ pyloromyotomy.

randomized controlled trial (RCT) research study using two or more randomly selected groups: experimental and control. It produces high level evidence for practice.

random sampling in research. The selection process whereby every person in the population has an equal chance of being selected.

range *n* describes the span of values (lowest–highest) observed in a sample.

range of motion (ROM) the movements possible at a joint.

ranula *n* a cystic swelling beneath the tongue due to blockage of a duct—**ranular** *adj*.

rape *n* unlawful sexual intercourse without consent which is achieved by force or deception. Full penetration of the vagina (or other orifice) by the penis and ejaculation of semen is not necessary to constitute rape. Most rapes include force and violence, but acquiescence because of verbal threats should not be interpreted as consent. Where women are admitted to hospital, a police surgeon will perform an examination to obtain the necessary specimens in the presence of specially trained female police officers who then support the victim throughout the interviews and subsequent investigation. Male rape, the rape of a man by another man, is increasingly recognized.

raphe *n* a seam, suture, ridge or crease.

rapid plasma reagin test (RPR) a non-specific serological test for syphilis.

rarefaction *n* becoming less dense, as applied to diseased bone—**rarefied** *adj*.

rash *n* skin eruption. *nettle rash* ⇒ urticaria.

RAST *abbr* radioallergosorbent test.

rat-bite fever *n* a relapsing fever caused by *Spirillum minus* or by *Streptobacillus moniliformis*. Usually transmitted by rat bites. There is also local inflammation, rash, splenomegaly and lymphadenitis.

ratio data measurement data with a numerical score, e.g. height, that has a true zero of 0. It is interval data with an absolute zero. ⇒ interval data.

rationalization *n* a mental process whereby a person justifies his or her actions following the event, so it looks more rational or socially acceptable.

Raynaud's disease paroxysmal spasm of the digital arteries producing pallor or cyanosis of fingers or toes, and occasionally resulting in gangrene. Disease of young women.

Raynaud's phenomenon episodic discoloration of the fingers and sometimes the toes (classically the fingers turn white, then blue, then red) usually in response to temperature change or stress. ⇒ hand-arm vibration syndrome, CREST syndrome.

RBC *abbr* red blood cell. ⇒ blood.

RCT *abbr* randomized controlled trial.

RDA *abbr* recommended daily allowance.

RDS *abbr* respiratory distress syndrome.

reaction *n* **1** response to a stimulus. **2** a chemical change. *allergic reaction* ⇒ allergy.

reactive arthritis (*syn* Reiter's syndrome) arthritis that develops in response to infection, usually urogenital, gastrointestinal or throat infection. ⇒ sexually acquired reactive arthritis.

reagent *n* a substance that participates in a chemical reaction, in order to detect, measure, or produce other substances.

reality orientation (RO) *n* a form of therapy useful for withdrawn, confused and depressed patients: they are frequently reminded of their name, the time, place, date and so on. Reinforcement is provided by clocks, calendars and signs prominently displayed in the environment.

reasonable doubt to secure a conviction in criminal proceedings, the prosecution must establish beyond reasonable doubt the guilt of the accused.

rebore *n* ⇒ disobliteration.

recalcitrant *adj* refractory. Describes medical conditions that are resistant to treatment.

recall *n* part of the process of memory. Memory consists of memorizing, retention and recall.

recannulation *n* re-establishment of the patency of a vessel.

receptaculum *n* receptacle, often forms a reservoir.

receptive aphasia a type of aphasia where there are problems of varying severity with language comprehension. Those affected may also have expressive aphasia.

receptor *n* **1** sensory afferent nerve ending capable of receiving and transmitting stimuli. **2** a protein situated on or inside a cell membrane. Reacts with various molecules, drugs, hormones or cell mediators.

recessive *adj* receding; having a tendency to disappear. *recessive trait* a genetic character or trait that is expressed when the determining allele is present at both paired chromosomal loci (i.e. homozygous or 'in double dose'). When the specific allele is present in single dose the characteristic is not expressed as it is overpowered by the dominant allele at the other locus. However, recessive X-linked genes in males will be expressed in a single dose. ⇒ dominant.

recipient *n* the individual who receives something from a donor such as blood, an organ such as a kidney or bone marrow. ⇒ blood groups.

reciprocal inhibition a technique in which an active contraction of the agonist muscle is used to produce a reflex relaxation of the antagonist, thereby allowing the antagonist muscle to be stretched.

Recklinghausen's disease ⇒ von Recklinghausen's disease.

recombinant DNA DNA produced by recombining chemically the DNA of two different organisms. Used for the study of both normal and abnormal genes and so, for example, of genetic disorders. The practical applications include diagnosis (including prenatal diagnosis) and in the manufacture of therapeutic products, e.g. human insulin.

recommended daily allowance (RDA) (*syn* recommended daily intake—RDI) refers to national and international standards that recommend the intake level of a particular nutrient for specific groups of people. The term RDA is still used in some countries but in the UK it has been replaced by dietary reference values (DRVs).

Recommended International Non-proprietary Name (rINN) the system of non-proprietary drug names in use internationally.

reconstituted family a family with step-parents resulting from divorce or remarriage.

recovery *n* a return to a normal state or health. It may be total or only partial. *recovery position* a first aid measure where a person with altered level of consciousness is positioned so as to maintain the airway and prevent aspiration of secretions or vomit.

recrudescence *n* the return of symptoms.

rectal varices haemorrhoids.

rectocele *n* prolapse of the rectum, so that it lies outside the anus. Usually reserved for herniation of anterior rectal wall into posterior vaginal wall caused by injury to the levator muscles during childbirth. Repaired by a posterior colporrhaphy. ⇒ cystocele, procidentia.

rectosigmoid *adj* pertaining to the rectum and sigmoid colon.

rectouterine *adj* pertaining to the rectum and uterus, as the rectouterine pouch.

rectovaginal *adj* pertaining to the rectum and vagina.

rectovesical *adj* pertaining to the rectum and bladder.

rectum *n* the lower part of the large intestine between the sigmoid flexure and anal canal (⇒ Figure 18b)—**rectal** *adj*, **rectally** *adv*.

rectus abdominis abdominal muscle. ⇒ Figure 4.

recumbent *adj* lying or reclining—**recumbency** *n*. *recumbent position* lying on the back with the head supported on a pillow: the knees can be flexed and parted to facilitate inspection of the perineum.

recurrent (habitual) abortion ⇒ miscarriage.

recurring costs regular and ongoing costs, such as planned maintenance and staff salaries.

red muscle describes muscle consisting mainly of slow-twitch fibres. The red colour is derived from the plentiful blood supply and myoglobin.

reduction *n* **1** the process of reducing or state of being reduced. It is the removal of oxygen or the addition of hydrogen or electrons to a substance. ⇒ oxidation. **2** making smaller. Commonly applied to plastic surgical procedures used to decrease the size of structures, for example the nose or breast. **3** returning to the normal position, e.g. a hernia or after dislocation or fracture.

Reed–Sternberg cell a large, abnormal multinucleated cell found in the lymphatic system in Hodgkin's disease.

reference nutrient intake (RNI) one of the UK dietary reference values. The amount of a nutrient required to make sure that the needs of most people in a group (97.5%) are met. Commonly used as an estimate of the micronutrient, e.g. specific vitamins, requirement of a population.

referred pain pain occurring at a distance from its source, e.g. pain felt in the upper limbs from angina pectoris; that from the gallbladder felt in the scapular region.

reflex 1 *adj* literally, reflected or thrown back; involuntary, not controlled by will. *reflex action* an involuntary motor or secretory response by tissue to a sensory stimulus, e.g. tendon stretch, sneezing, blinking, coughing. Reflexes may be postural or protective. Testing reflexes provides valuable information in the localization and diagnosis of neurological diseases. **2** *n* a reflex action. *accommodation reflex* constriction of the pupils and convergence of the eyes for near vision. *conditioned reflex* a reaction acquired by practice or repetition. *corneal reflex* a reaction of blinking when the cornea is touched.

reflexology *n* a complementary therapy based upon the assertion that the internal body structures are 'mapped out' on the soles and palms. It is thought that gentle pressure upon the areas corresponding to specific structures can lead to a therapeutic response. ⇒ zones.

reflex sympathetic dystrophy rare pain syndrome in which there are autonomic changes in the area of the body (usually limb) from which the pain derives. It is now more correctly termed complex regional pain syndrome as the pathophysiology is more complex and varied than first thought.

reflux *n* backward flow. ⇒ vesicoureteric reflux.

refraction *n* the bending of light rays as they pass through media of different densities. In normal vision, this occurs so that the image is focused on the retina—**refractive** *adj*.

refractory *adj* resistant to treatment or unmanageable.

regeneration *n* renewal of tissue.

regional ileitis ⇒ Crohn's disease.

regression *n* in psychiatry, reversion to an earlier stage of development, becoming more childish. Occurs in dementia, especially senile dementia, and more normally, in a young child following the birth of a sibling.

regression techniques various analytical methods used in multivariate statistics. Used to predict dependent variable(s) from independent variable(s).

regurgitation *n* backward flow, e.g. of stomach contents into, or through, the mouth, or blood through an incompetent (regurgitant) heart valve.

rehabilitation *n* a planned programme in which convalescent or disabled people progress towards, or maintain, the maximum degree of physical and psychological independence of which they are capable.

rehabilitation clinician in sports medicine a medical professional who is responsible for the design, progression, supervision and administration of a rehabilitation programme for an injured athlete or sports participant.

rehearsal in memory memory processing depends on two forms of rehearsal of facts: *maintenance rehearsal* where information re-enters short-term memory (STM) by repetition (such as repeating the names of a new group); each time the information enters short-term memory (STM) appears to enhance its chance of storage in long-term memory (LTM); and *elaborative rehearsal* processing information in STM so that it can be coded for storage in LTM. It may use sensory factors, such as sound, or focus on the meaning of the information.

reinforcement *n* a psychological term that describes the methods employed during conditioning to increase the probability and strength of a response.

Reiter's syndrome ⇒ reactive arthritis, sexually acquired reactive arthritis.

rejection *n* **1** the act of excluding or denying affection to another person. **2** the process which leads to the destruction of grafted tissues.

relapsing fever louse-borne or tick-borne infection caused by spirochaetes of the genus *Borrelia*. Characterized by a febrile period of a week or so, with apparent recovery, followed by a further bout of fever.

relaxant *n* a drug or technique that reduces tension. ⇒ muscle.

relaxation *n* a state of consciousness where individuals feel calm and peaceful. Muscle tension, anxiety and stress are all released. *relaxation techniques* often used in health care and health promotion activities such as stress management. They include meditation, progressive muscle relaxation, visual guided imagery and yoga. ⇒ biofeedback, hypnosis.

relaxin *n* polypeptide hormone secreted by the placenta and ovaries to soften the cervix and loosen the ligaments in preparation for birth.

releaser/releasing mechanism a stimulus that launches a cycle of instinctive behaviour.

reliability *n* in research a term meaning consistency of results. The likelihood of achieving the same findings using the same research conditions over a period of time or with different researchers.

reminiscence therapy a technique, also known as nostalgia therapy, that provides older persons with the opportunity to reflect on, and validate, their memories of the past through the use of old pictures, music and objects. These are used to prompt shared discussion of personal experiences.

remission *n* the period of abatement of a fever or other disease.

remittent *adj* increasing and decreasing at periodic intervals.

REM sleep *abbr* rapid eye movement sleep. Also known as paradoxical sleep. ⇒ sleep.

renal *adj* relating to the kidney. *renal artery* ⇒ Figures 9, 19, 20. *renal calculus* stone in the kidney. *renal capsule* ⇒ Figure 20. *renal colic* ⇒ colic. *renal erythropoietic factor (REF)* a substance released by the kidneys in response to renal (and therefore systemic) hypoxia. Once secreted into the blood, it reacts with a plasma protein to produce erythropoietin. *renal failure* can be described as acute or chronic. Acute renal failure (ARF) occurs when previously healthy kidneys suddenly fail because of a variety of problems affecting the kidney and its perfusion with blood. This condition is potentially reversible. ARF is treated by haemofiltration or haemodiafiltration until kidney function improves. Chronic renal failure (CRF) occurs when irreversible and progressive pathological destruction of the kidney leads to end-stage renal disease (ESRD). This process usually takes several years but once ESRD is reached, death will follow unless the patient is treated with some type of renal replacement therapy such as dialysis, or renal transplant. ⇒ crush syndrome, acute tubular necrosis, uraemia. *renal function tests* ⇒ kidney function tests. *renal glycosuria* occurs in patients with a normal blood sugar and a lowered renal threshold for glucose. *renal rickets* ⇒ rickets. *renal transplant* kidney transplant. *renal vein* ⇒ Figures 19, 20.

renin *n* an enzyme released by the kidney (juxtaglomerular apparatus) in response to low serum sodium or low blood pressure. Renin starts the angiotensin-aldosterone response. A plasma protein (angiotensinogen) is activated to produce angiotensin I, which in turn is converted into angiotensin II.

rennin *n* milk curdling enzyme found in the gastric juice of human infants and ruminants. It converts caseinogen into casein.

renogram *n* radioisotope study of the kidney.

reovirus *n* a group of RNA viruses that includes the rotavirus, which causes gastroenteritis.

repetitive strain injury (RSI) a misleading term used to describe diffuse pain and inflammation randomly occurring in the hand and forearm arising from repetitive activities in the workplace, aggravated by static posture. ⇒ work-related upper limb disorder.

repolarization *n* the process whereby the membrane potential returns from the depolarized state to its polarized resting (negative) state.

repression *n* a mental defence mechanism whereby painful events, unacceptable thoughts and impulses are impelled into, and remain in, the unconscious mind.

reproductive system the structures necessary for reproduction. In the male it includes the testes, deferent ducts (vas deferens), prostate gland, seminal vesicles, urethra and penis (⇒ Figure 16). In the female it includes the ovaries, uterine tubes, uterus, vagina and vulva (⇒ Figure 17).

RES *abbr* reticuloendethelial system. ⇒ monocyte-macrophage system.

research *n* systematic investigation of data, reports and observations to establish facts or principles, in order to produce organized scientific knowledge. *research design* how a research study is to be undertaken such as data collection method, statistical analysis, etc.

resection *n* surgical excision. *submucous resection (of nasal septum)* incision of nasal mucosa, removal of deflected nasal septum, replacement of mucosa.

resectoscope *n* an instrument passed along the urethra; it permits resection of tissue from the base of the bladder and prostate under direct vision. ⇒ prostatectomy.

reservoirs of infection the skin, respiratory tract and bowel are colonized by bacteria and fungi which form the normal flora in humans. The normal flora may become pathogenic under certain circumstances.

residential home the premises where residential care is delivered by the independent sector, social services or voluntary organizations.

residual *adj* remaining. *residual air* the air remaining in the lung after forced expiration. *residual urine* the volume of urine remaining in the bladder after micturition.

resistance *n* power of resisting. In psychology, describes the force which prevents repressed thoughts from re-entering the conscious mind from the unconscious. *resistance to infection* the capacity to withstand infection. ⇒ immunity. *peripheral resistance* ⇒ peripheral.

resisted range of movement (ROM) a range of movement that occurs with resistance being applied.

resolution *n* the subsidence of inflammation; describes the earliest indications of a return to normal, as when, in lobar pneumonia, the consolidation begins to liquefy.

resonance *n* the musical quality elicited on percussing a cavity which contains air. *vocal resonance* is the reverberating note

heard through the stethoscope when the patient is asked to say 'one, one, one' or '99'.

resorption *n* the act of absorbing again, e.g. absorption of (a) callus following bone fracture, (b) roots of the deciduous teeth, (c) blood from a haematoma.

respiration *n* the gaseous exchange between a cell and its environment— **respiratory** *adj. external respiration* is the exchange of gases between alveolar air and pulmonary capillary blood. Oxygen in the alveolar air moves into the blood, and carbon dioxide moves from the blood into the air in the lungs for excretion. *internal* or *tissue respiration* is the reverse process involving gaseous exchange between the cells and blood. Oxygen moves from the blood, via the tissue fluid, to the cells, and waste cellular carbon dioxide moves into the blood for onward transport to the lungs. ⇒ abdominal breathing, Cheyne–Stokes respiration, Kussmaul respiration, paradoxical respiration.

respirator *n* an apparatus worn over the nose and mouth and designed to purify the air breathed through it.

respiratory failure failure of the lungs to adequately oxygenate the blood. May be *type 1 respiratory failure* characterized by hypoxaemia alone (PaO_2 <8 kPa, $PaCO_2$ <6.6 kPa), or *type 2 respiratory failure*, when decreased respiratory drive supervenes and hypercapnia is seen in association with hypoxia (PaO_2 <8 kPa, $PaCO_2$ >6.6 kPa).

respiratory function tests tests available for assessing respiratory function and aiding in diagnosis of respiratory disease. Include spirometry to measure FEV_1 (forced expiratory volume in one second), and FVC (forced vital capacity) and in more specialized laboratories measurements of total lung volume and gas transfer factor.

respiratory quotient the ratio between inspired oxygen and expired carbon dioxide during a specified time.

respiratory syncytial virus (RSV) a myxovirus that causes bronchiolitis and pneumonia in infants and small children. Infants under six months may be severely affected.

respiratory system deals with gaseous exchange. Comprises the nose, nasopharynx, larynx, trachea, bronchi and lungs (⇒ Figures 6, 7).

respite care short-term or temporary care provided within a health or social care facility to allow relief for family and other home carers. May be residential or on a daily basis.

restless leg syndrome restless legs characterized by paraesthesiae like creeping, crawling, itching and prickling.

rest re-injury cycle a pattern of injury that occurs when an athlete returns to activity after an injury and subsequently aggravates that injury due to inadequate recovery.

resuscitation n restoration to life of one who is collapsed or apparently dead—**resuscitative** adj. ⇒ cardiopulmonary resuscitation.

retardation n **1** the slowing of a process which has already been carried out at a quicker rate or higher level. **2** arrested growth or function from any cause.

retching n straining at vomiting.

retention n **1** retaining of facts in the memory. **2** accumulation of that which is normally excreted. *retention cyst* a cyst caused by the blocking of a duct. ⇒ ranula. *retention of urine* accumulation of urine within the bladder due to interference of nerve supply, obstruction or psychological factors.

reticular adj resembling a net.

reticular activating system (RAS) part of the brainstem involved in level of consciousness, state of cortical arousal and the prevention of sensory overload.

reticulocyte n an immature circulating red blood cell which still contains traces of the nucleus. Accounts for up to 2% of circulating red cells.

reticulocytosis n an increase in the number of reticulocytes in the blood indicating active red blood cell formation in the marrow. ⇒ reticulocyte.

reticuloendothelial system (RES) ⇒ monocyte-macrophage system.

retina n layer of tissue in the eye that converts light into electrical signals. Consists of a multiple-layer complex of neurosensory retina containing nerve cells including photoreceptors (rods and cones), and a layer of pigmented cells beyond the neurosensory retina.(⇒ Figure 15)—**retinal** adj.

retinitis n inflammation of the retina. *retinitis pigmentosa* a non-inflammatory degenerative condition of the retina due to genetic disorder.

retinoblastoma n a malignant tumour of the neuroglial element of the retina; occurs exclusively in children.

retinochoroiditis ⇒ chorioretinitis.

retinoids npl a group of vitamin A derivatives. ⇒ Appendix 5.

retinol n also known as retinene. A light-absorbing molecule formed from vitamin A. It combines with a protein (opsin) to form rhodopsin (visual pigment).

retinopathy n disease of the retina. *retinopathy of prematurity* circulatory disorder occurring in preterm babies.

retinoscope n instrument for detection of refractive errors by illumination of retina using a mirror.

retinotoxic adj toxic to the retina.

retractile adj capable of being drawn back, i.e. retracted.

retraction n a backward movement. ⇒ protraction opp.

retractor n a surgical instrument for holding apart the edges of a wound to reveal underlying structures.

retrobulbar adj pertaining to the back of the eyeball. *retrobulbar neuritis* inflammation of the optic nerve behind the eyeball.

retrocaecal adj behind the caecum.

retroflexion n the state of being bent backwards. ⇒ anteflexion opp.

retrograde adj going backward. *retrograde urography/pyelography* ⇒ urography.

retroperitoneal adj behind the peritoneum.

retropharyngeal adj behind the pharynx.

retroplacental adj behind the placenta.

retropubic adj behind the pubis.

retrospection n morbid dwelling on the past.

retrospective study research that deals with past data, moving backwards in time. ⇒ prospective study.

retrosternal adj behind the sternum.

retrotracheal adj behind the trachea.

retroversion n turning backward. ⇒ anteversion opp. *retroversion of the uterus* tilting of the whole of the uterus backward with the cervix pointing forward—**retroverted** adj.

retroviruses *npl* family of RNA viruses that include the human immunodeficiency viruses (HIV 1 and 2) and the human T-cell lymphotropic viruses (HTLV 1 and 2).

Rett's syndrome a neurodegenerative disorder occurring in girls. X-linked dominant inheritance. There is progressive neurological and developmental regression from early childhood. Death occurs by second or third decade.

revascularization *n* the regrowth of blood vessels into a tissue or organ after deprivation of its normal blood supply.

revenue budget the budget allocation for day to day running costs, e.g. salaries, telephone, electricity and drugs, etc. ⇒ capital budget.

reverse barrier nursing ⇒ protective isolation.

reverse transcriptase inhibitors (nucleoside/non-nucleoside) a group of drugs that act by inhibiting the enzyme reverse transcriptase, required for viral replication. ⇒ Appendix 5.

Reye syndrome 'wet brain and fatty liver' as described in 1963. There is cerebral oedema without cellular infiltration, and diffuse fatty infiltration of liver and other organs, including the kidney. The age range of recorded cases is 2 months–15 years. Presents with vomiting, hypoglycaemia and disturbed consciousness, jaundice being conspicuous. There is an association with salicylate administration and chicken pox.

Rh *abbr* Rhesus factor. ⇒ blood groups.

rhabdomyolysis *n* disease of skeletal muscle where muscle injury leads to myoglobinuria. It may also be due to crush injury or compression, which can result in acute renal failure.

rhagades *npl* superficial elongated scars radiating from the nostrils or angles of the mouth and which are found in congenital syphilis. One of the stigmata of the disease.

Rhesus factor (Rh) ⇒ blood groups.

Rhesus incompatibility, isoimmunization this problem arises when a Rhesus negative mother carries a Rhesus positive fetus. During or before the birth there is mixing of fetal and maternal bloods. The mother's body then develops antibodies against the Rhesus positive blood. If a subsequent fetus is also Rhesus positive, then maternal antibodies will attack the fetal blood causing severe haemolysis.

rheumatic *adj* pertaining to rheumatism, a non-specific term. *rheumatic diseases* a diverse group of diseases affecting connective tissue, joints and bones. They include: inflammatory joint disease, e.g. rheumatoid arthritis, septic arthritis and gout; connective tissue disease, e.g. systemic lupus erythematosus; osteoarthritis; non-articular/soft tissue rheumatism, e.g. fibromyalgia. *rheumatic heart disease (RHD)* chronic cardiac disease with valve damage resulting from rheumatic fever.

rheumatic fever (*syn* acute rheumatism) a disorder, tending to recur but initially commonest in childhood, classically presenting as fleeting polyarthritis of the larger joints with swelling and pain, tachycardia, pyrexia, rash and pancarditis (involving all layers) of varying severity within 3 weeks following a streptococcal throat infection. Atypically, but not infrequently, the symptoms are trivial and ignored, but carditis may be severe and result in permanent cardiac damage, particularly of heart valves. It may also lead to neurological problems. ⇒ chorea.

rheumatism *n* a non-specific term embracing a diverse group of diseases and syndromes which have in common disorder or diseases of connective tissue and hence usually present with pain, or stiffness, or swelling of muscles and joints. Used colloquially to describe ill-defined aches and pains. ⇒ rheumatic diseases.

rheumatoid arthritis a disease of unknown aetiology, characterized by polyarthritis usually affecting firstly the smaller peripheral joints, before extending to involve larger joints accompanied by general ill health and resulting eventually in varying degrees of joint destruction and deformity with associated muscle wasting. It is not just a disease of joints; and most body systems can be affected, e.g. lung, peripheral nerves. Many rheumatologists therefore prefer the term 'rheumatoid disease'. There is some question of it being an autoimmune process. *rheumatoid factors* autoantibodies found in most people with rheumatoid arthritis. It is not yet known whether they are the cause of, or the result of, arthritis.

rheumatology *n* the science or the study of the rheumatic diseases.

rhinitis *n* inflammation of the nasal mucous membrane.

rhinology *n* the study of disorders of the nose—**rhinologist** *n*.

rhinomanometry *n* a test used for assessment of the nasal airway and to measure the nasal airflow and pressure during respiration.

rhinophyma *n* nodular enlargement of the skin of the nose.

rhinoplasty *n* plastic surgery of the nasal framework.

rhinorrhoea *n* nasal discharge.

rhinoscopy *n* inspection of the nose using a nasal speculum or other instrument—**rhinoscopic** *adj*.

rhinosinusitis *n* inflammation of the nose and paranasal sinuses.

rhinosporidiosis *n* a fungal condition affecting the mucosa of the nose, eyes, ears, larynx and occasionally the genitalia.

Rhinosporidium *n* a genus of fungi parasitic to humans.

rhinovirus *n* group of picornaviruses responsible for the common cold (coryza).

rhizotomy *n* surgical division of a root; usually the posterior root of a spinal nerve. *chemical rhizotomy* accomplished by injection of a chemical, often phenol.

rhodopsin *n* the visual purple (pigment) found in the rods. Required for vision in low intensity light. Its colour is maintained in darkness; bleached by daylight. Vitamin A is needed for its formation.

rhomboid *adj* diamond shaped.

rhonchus *n* an adventitious sound heard on auscultation of the lung. Passage of air through bronchi obstructed by oedema or exudate produces a musical note.

riboflavin(e) *n* a constituent of the vitamin B group. Given in Ménière's disease, angular stomatitis and a variety of other conditions.

ribonuclease *n* an enzyme that breaks down ribonucleic acid.

ribonucleic acid (RNA) nucleic acids present in all living cells. Composed of a single chain of nucleotides formed from ribose (a 5-carbon sugar), phosphates and the nitrogenous bases: adenine (A), guanine (G), cytosine (C) and uracil (U). There are three forms: messenger (mRNA), ribosomal (rRNA) and transfer (tRNA), which have specific functions during protein synthesis. ⇒ deoxyribonucleic acid, transcription, translation.

ribosomal RNA (rRNA) ⇒ ribonucleic acid.

ribosomes *npl* submicroscopic protein-making structures inside all cells.

ribs *npl* the twelve pairs of bones which articulate with the twelve dorsal vertebrae posteriorly and form the walls of the thorax (⇒ Figures 2, 3, 6). The upper seven pairs are *true ribs* and are attached to the sternum anteriorly by costal cartilage. The remaining five pairs are the *false ribs*; the first three pairs of these do not have an attachment to the sternum but are bound to each other by costal cartilage. The lower two pairs are the *floating ribs* which have no anterior articulation. *cervical ribs* are an extension of the transverse process of the seventh cervical vertebra in the form of bone or fibrous tissue; this causes an upward displacement of the subclavian artery.

RICE *acron* for rest, ice, compression and elevation. Used in the management of acute injuries to minimize inflammatory processes and to accelerate the recovery process by eliminating swelling.

rice-water stool the stool of cholera. The 'rice grains' are desquamated intestinal epithelium.

rickets *n* bone disease caused by vitamin D deficiency during infancy and childhood (prior to ossification of the epiphyses) which results from poor dietary intake or insufficient exposure to sunlight. There is abnormal metabolism of calcium and phosphate with poor ossification and bone growth. There is muscle weakness, anaemia, respiratory infections, bone tenderness and pain and hypocalcaemia. Delays occur in motor development such as walking, eruption of teeth and closure of the fontanelles. Later there may be bony deformities, e.g. bow legs. Rickets may be secondary to vitamin D malabsorption, or impaired metabolism, such as with chronic renal failure. The same condition in adults is known as osteomalacia.

Rickettsia *n* small pleomorphic parasitic Gram-negative micro-organisms that have similarities with both viruses and bacteria. Like viruses, they are obligate intracellular parasites. Rickettsia are intestinal parasites of arthropods such as fleas, lice, mites and ticks; transmission to humans is by bites from these arthropods. They cause various types of typhus group and Rocky mountain spotted fever. ⇒ rickettsial fevers, spotted fever.

rickettsial fevers a group of rickettsial diseases that include epidemic typhus caused by *Rickettsia prowazekii*, endemic typhus caused by *R. mooseri*, scrub typhus caused by *R. tsutsugamushi* and Rocky Mountain spotted fever caused by *R. rickettsii*. They are transmitted by ticks, fleas, lice and mites and are associated with overcrowding and poor hygiene (e.g. after natural disasters, or in refugee camps).

rickety rosary a series of protuberances (bossing) at junction of ribs and costal cartilages in children suffering from rickets.

rider's bone a bony mass in the origin of the adductor muscles of the thigh, from repeated minor trauma in horse riding.

Riedel's thyroiditis a chronic fibrosis of the thyroid gland; ligneous goitre.

Rift Valley fever one of the mosquito-transmitted haemorrhagic fevers.

rights *npl* the recognition in law that certain inalienable rights, such as the right to life, should be respected, e.g. Human Rights Act 1998.

rigidity *n* (*syn* lead pipe rigidity, parkinsonian rigidity) increased tension or tone of muscle (hypertonia) with increased resistance to passive stretch in any direction that is uniform throughout the whole movement. ⇒ cogwheel rigidity.

rigor *n* a sudden chill, accompanied by severe shivering. The body temperature rises rapidly and remains high until perspiration ensues and causes a gradual fall in temperature. *rigor mortis* the stiffening of the body after death.

Ringer's solution an intravenous infusion solution containing sodium chloride with potassium chloride and calcium chloride. *lactated Ringer's solution (Ringer-lactate or Hartmann's solution)* one that also contains sodium lactate.

ringworm *n* (*syn* tinea) generic term used to describe contagious fungal infection of the skin, because of the common circular (circinate) scaly patches. ⇒ dermatophytes.

rINN *abbr* Recommended International Non-proprietary Name.

Rinne's test a test to distinguish between conductive and sensorineural deafness.

RIP *abbr* raised intracranial pressure.

risk *n* a potential hazard. *attributable risk* the disease rate in people exposed to the risk factor minus the occurrence in unexposed people. *relative risk* the ratio of disease rate in people exposed to the risk factor to those not exposed. It is related to the odds ratio, which is the odds (as in betting) of disease occurring in an exposed person divided by the odds of the disease occurring in an unexposed person.

risk assessment a structured and methodical assessment of risk carried out for a particular area or activity. For example moving and handling patients in the operating theatre.

risk factors factors associated with an increase in the likelihood of ill health, disease, handicap or disability. Demonstration of the association has to fulfil Sir Austin Bradford Hill's eight criteria (e.g. smoking and lung cancer): (a) biological plausibility—tobacco tar contains known carcinogens, the stages of tumour development following exposure are clearly demonstrated, (b) reversibility—smoking cessation reduces subsequent increase in risk of lung cancer by half in the first year, to nil after ten years, (c) animal demonstration—model of beagles in laboratory experiments, (d) dose response—risk of lung cancer in smokers shown to increase progressively with the number of cigarettes smoked per day, (e) follows exposure—temporal relationship demonstrated, lung cancer always follows exposure to cigarettes with a time lag of 20 to 30 years, (f) over time and overseas—relationship consistent between different case series and different places (in the world), (g) experimental design—must be reliable. Randomized controlled trials most convincing, but may be unethical. Observational studies (case control, cohort) useful if correctly carried out. (h) strength of the effect—the larger the increase in risk, the more likely the causal relationship.

risk management managing risk in health-care settings involves: identification of the risk, analysis of the risk and controlling the risk.

risus sardonicus the spastic grin of tetanus.

river blindness ⇒ onchocerciasis.

RNA *abbr* ribonucleic acid.

RNA viruses viruses that contain RNA as their nucleic acid such as picornavirus, retrovirus.

RNI *abbr* reference nutrient intake.

RO *abbr* reality orientation.

ROA *abbr* right occipitoanterior; used to describe the position of the fetus in the uterus.

Rocky Mountain spotted fever a tick-borne rickettsial infection. Characterized by fever, myalgia, headache and petechial rash. Occurs in the USA. ⇒ rickettsial fevers.

rodent ulcer a basal cell carcinoma often seen on the face which, although locally invasive, does not give rise to metastases.

rods *npl* photoreceptors in the retina for appreciation of coarse detail vision in low light conditions. They contain the visual pigment rhodopsin.

role *n* the characteristic social behaviour of a person in relation to others in the group, for example that of a physiotherapist vis-à-vis that of the doctor. *role model* an individual who acts as a model for another individual's behaviour in a particular role. Important for development during childhood, and also as part of professional education and development. *role playing* may be used during professional education when a student assumes the role of a patient/client so that other students may practise a particular skill, such as communication. Also used in therapeutic situations, e.g. patients with mental health problems.

ROM *abbr* **1** range of motion. **2** resisted range of movement.

Romberg's sign a sign of impaired balance. Inability to stand erect (without swaying) when the eyes are closed and the feet together. Also called 'Rombergism'.

rooting reflex a primitive reflex present in newborns. The infant will turn his or her head to that side when the cheek is touched.

ROP *abbr* right occipitoposterior; used to describe the position of the fetus in the uterus.

rosacea *n* a skin disease which shows on flush areas of the face. In areas affected there is chronic dilation of superficial capillaries and hypertrophy of sebaceous follicles, often complicated by a papulo-pustular eruption.

rose bengal a staining agent used to detect diseased corneal and conjunctival epithelium.

rotation *n* a limb movement around the axis down the centre of a long bone.

rotator *n* a muscle that acts to turn a part. *rotator cuff* four muscles; subscapularis, supraspinatus, infraspinatus and teres minor. Their insertional tendons converge to form a cuff over the shoulder joint. Controls and produces rotation of the shoulder.

rotaviruses *npl* viruses mainly associated with gastroenteritis in children and infants.

Roth spots round white spots in the retina in some cases of infective endocarditis; thought to be of embolic origin.

roughage *n* an outdated term. ⇒ non-starch polysaccharides.

rouleaux *n* a stack of red blood cells, resembling a roll of coins.

round ligaments uterine supports that run from the uterus, through the inguinal canal, to the labia majora. ⇒ Figure 17.

roundworm *n* (*Ascaris lumbricoides*) intestinal nematodes with worldwide distribution. Parasitic to humans. Eggs passed in stools; ingested; hatch in bowel; migrate through tissues, lungs and bronchi before returning to the bowel as mature worms. During migration worms can be coughed up. Heavy infections can produce pneumonia. They cause abdominal discomfort and may be vomited or passed per rectum. A tangled mass can cause intestinal obstruction or appendicitis. Adult worms can obstruct pancreatic and bile ducts. ⇒ *Toxocara*.

Roux-en-Y operation originally the distal end of divided jejunum was anastomosed to the stomach, and the proximal jejunum containing the duodenal and pancreatic digestive juices was anastomosed to the jejunum about 75 mm below the first anastomosis. The term is now used to include joining of the distal jejunum to a divided bile duct, oesophagus or pancreas, in major surgery of these structures.

Rovsing's sign pressure in the left iliac fossa (see Figure 18a) causes pain in the right iliac fossa in appendicitis.

RSI *abbr* repetitive strain injury.

RSV *abbr* respiratory syncytial virus.

rubefacients *npl* substances which, when applied to the skin, cause redness (hyperaemia).

rubella *n* (*syn* German measles) an acute, infectious, eruptive fever (exanthema) caused by a virus and spread by droplet infection. There is mild fever, a scaly, pink, macular rash and enlarged occipital and posterior cervical lymph nodes. Complications are rare, except when contracted in the first trimester of pregnancy, when it may produce fetal deformities, such as heart abnormalities, cataracts, deafness and brain damage. Immunization is available as part of routine programmes during childhood and to non-pregnant woman of childbearing age with insufficient immunity.

Rubinstein–Taybi syndrome includes mental and motor retardation, broad thumbs and toes, growth retardation, susceptibility to infection in the early years and characteristic facial features.

rubeosis *n* neovascularization (growth of new, abnormal blood vessels) of the iris.

rubor *n* redness; usually used in the context of being one of the five classical signs and symptoms of inflammation—the others being calor, dolor, loss of function and tumor.

runner's nipples a colloquial expression used in sports medicine to describe the irritation of the nipples due to friction caused by the runner's shirt rubbing over their nipples.

S

Sabin vaccine live attenuated poliomyelitis vaccine, given orally.

sacculation *n* appearance of several saccules.

saccule *n* a minute sac. A fluid-filled sac in the internal ear. Part of the vestibular apparatus concerned with static equilibrium; contains hair cells and otoliths—**saccular, sacculated** *adj.* ⇒ utricle.

sacral *adj* pertaining to the sacrum. *sacral nerve* ⇒ Figure 11.

sacroanterior *adj* describes the position of the breech in the pelvis when the fetal sacrum is in the anterior part of the maternal pelvis—**sacroanteriorly** *adv.*

sacrococcygeal *adj* pertaining to the sacrum and the coccyx.

sacroiliac *adj* pertaining to the sacrum and the ilium.

sacroiliitis *n* inflammation of a sacroiliac joint. Involvement of both joints characterizes such conditions as ankylosing spondylitis, Reiter's syndrome and psoriatic arthritis.

sacrolumbar *adj* pertaining to the sacrum and the loins.

sacroposterior *adj* describes the position of the breech in the pelvis when the fetal sacrum is in the posterior part of the maternal pelvis—**sacroposteriorly** *adv.*

sacrum *n* the triangular bone lying between the fifth lumbar vertebra and the coccyx ⇒ Figure 3. It consists of five vertebrae fused together, and it articulates on each side with the innominate bones of the pelvis, forming the sacroiliac joints—**sacral** *adj.*

SAD *acron* seasonal affective disorder.

saddle nose one with a flattened bridge; may be a sign of congenital syphilis.

sadism *n* the obtaining of pleasure from inflicting pain, violence or degradation on another person. ⇒ masochism.

sagittal *adj* resembling an arrow. *sagittal plane* the anteroposterior plane of the body. *sagittal sinuses* venous channels (sinuses) that drain blood from the brain. *sagittal suture* the immovable joint between the two parietal bones.

SAID *acron* specific adaptation to imposed demands.

salicylates *npl* a group of non-steroidal anti-inflammatory drugs. ⇒ Appendix 5.

salicylic acid used topically, it is keratolytic and has fungicidal and bacteriostatic properties. Used in a variety of hyperkeratotic skin conditions such as corns and psoriasis.

saline *n* a solution of sodium chloride and water. Normal or physiological saline is a 0.9% solution with the same osmotic pressure as that of blood. ⇒ hypertonic, hypotonic, isotonic.

saliva *n* fluid secreted by the salivary glands. It contains water, mucus and salivary amylase—**salivary** *adj*.

salivary *adj* pertaining to saliva. *salivary calculus* a stone formed in the salivary ducts. *salivary glands* the glands which secrete saliva, i.e. the parotid, submandibular (submaxillary) and sublingual glands.

salivation *n* an increased secretion of saliva.

Salk vaccine a preparation of killed poliomyelitis virus used as an antigen to produce active artificial immunity to poliomyelitis. It is given by injection.

Salmonella *n* a genus of bacteria. Gram-negative rods. Parasitic in many animals and humans in whom they are often pathogenic. Some species, such as *Salmonella typhi*, are host-specific, infecting only humans, in whom they cause typhoid fever. Others, such as *Salmonella typhimurium*, may infect a wide range of host species, usually through contaminated foods. *Salmonella enteritidis* a motile Gram-negative rod, widely distributed in domestic animals, particularly poultry, and in rodents, and sporadic in humans as a cause of food poisoning.

salpingectomy *n* excision of a uterine (fallopian) tube.

salpingitis *n* acute or chronic inflammation of the uterine (fallopian) tubes. ⇒ hydrosalpinx, pyosalpinx.

salpingogram *n* radiological examination of tubal patency by retrograde introduction of opaque medium into the uterus and along the uterine tubes. Being superseded by ultrasound examination—**salpingographic** *adj*, **salpingography** *n*, **salpingographically** *adv*.

salpingo-oophorectomy *n* excision of a uterine (fallopian) tube and ovary.

salpingostomy *n* the operation performed to restore tubal patency.

salpinx *n* a tube, especially the uterine (fallopian) tube or the eustachian tube.

salt *n* a substance produced by the combination of an acid and an alkali (base), e.g. potassium chloride.

Samaritans *npl* a voluntary befriending service available 24 hours/day to support suicidal and despairing people who make contact.

sample *n* the particular subset chosen from a population.

sandfly *n* an insect (*Phlebotomus*) responsible for transmitting viral sandfly fever and the protozoa that causes leishmaniasis.

sanguineous *adj* pertaining to or containing blood.

SaO₂ *abbr* arterial oxygen saturation. ⇒ pulse oximeter.

saphenous *adj* apparent; manifest. The name given to two superficial veins in the leg, the great (long) and the small (short) (⇒ Figure 10), and to the nerves (⇒ Figure 11) accompanying them.

saprophyte *n* free-living micro-organisms obtaining nutrients from dead and decaying animal or plant tissue—**saprophytic** *adj*.

SARA *abbr* sexually acquired reactive arthritis.

sarcoid *adj* a term applied to a group of lesions in skin, lungs or other organs, which resemble tuberculous foci in structure, but the true nature of which is still uncertain.

sarcoidosis *n* a granulomatous disease of unknown aetiology in which histological appearances resemble tuberculosis. May affect any organ of the body, but most commonly presents as a condition of the skin, lymph nodes or the bones of the hand.

sarcoma *n* malignant tumour of connective tissue, muscle, nerve, bone (osteosarcoma). Treatment options include surgery, radiotherapy and chemotherapy usually in combination. ⇒ Ewing's tumour—**sarcomata** *pl*, **sarcomatous** *adj*.

sarcomatosis *n* a condition in which sarcomata are widely spread throughout the body.

Sarcoptes scabiei *n* a species of itch mite responsible for scabies.

sartorius *n* the 'tailor's muscle' of the thigh, since it flexes one leg over the other (⇒ Figures 4, 5).

saturated fatty acids those having no double bonds in their structure. Most originate from animal sources. High dietary intake is associated with arterial disease.

scab *n* a dried crust forming over an open wound.

scabies *n* a parasitic skin disease caused by the itch mite. Highly contagious.

scald *n* an injury caused by moist heat.

scalenus syndrome pain in arm and fingers, often with wasting, because of compression of the lower trunk of the brachial plexus behind scalenus anterior muscle at the thoracic outlet.

scalp *n* the hair-bearing skin which covers the cranium. *scalp cooling* technique used to minimize or prevent alopecia associated with the administration of cytotoxic drugs such as doxorubicin.

scalpel *n* a surgeon's knife, which may or may not have detachable blades.

scan *n* an image built up by movement along or across the object scanned, either of the detector or of the imaging agent, to achieve complete coverage, e.g. ultrasound scan.

scaphoid *n* boat-shaped, as a bone of the tarsus and carpus. *scaphoid fracture* commonly occurs as a result of compression of the scaphoid, when there is a fall onto the outstretched hand in hyperextension. Commonly, if the fracture involves the proximal third of the scaphoid, there is a high risk of non-union and threat of avascular necrosis, due to the poor blood supply.

scapula *n* the shoulder-blade—a large, flat triangular bone (⇒ Figure 3)—**scapular** *adj.*

scar *n* (*syn* cicatrix) the dense, avascular white fibrous tissue, formed as the end result of healing, especially in the skin. ⇒ hypertrophic scar, keloid.

scarification *n* the making of a series of small, superficial incisions or punctures in the skin for the purpose of introducing a vaccine.

scarlet fever *n* (*syn* scarlatina) infection by β-haemolytic streptococcus (Lancefield Group A). Occurs mainly in children. Starts commonly with a throat infection, leading to fever, and a punctate erythematous rash on the skin of the trunk that is followed by desquamation. Characteristically the area around the mouth escapes (circumoral pallor).

SCAT *abbr* sheep cell agglutination test. Rheumatoid factor in the blood is detected by the sheep cell agglutination titre.

SCBU *abbr* special care baby unit. ⇒ neonatal unit.

SCC *abbr* 1 spinal cord compression. 2 squamous cell carcinoma.

Scheuermann's disease osteochondritis of the spine affecting the ring epiphyses of the vertebral bodies. Occurs in adolescents.

Schick test a skin test used to determine susceptibility or immunity to diphtheria. It consists of the intradermal injection of diphtheria toxin. A positive reaction (susceptibility to diphtheria) is indicated by the appearance of a round red area within 24–48 hours. Whereas the absence of any skin reaction to the toxin indicates immunity to the disease.

Schilder's disease a genetically determined degenerative disease associated with learning disability. ⇒ adrenoleucodystrophy.

Schilling test estimation of absorption of radioactive vitamin B_{12} for investigation of the cause of vitamin B_{12} deficiency.

Schistosoma *n* (*syn Bilharzia*) a genus of blood flukes which require freshwater snails as an intermediate host before infesting humans. Includes: *Schistosoma haematobium* in Africa and the Middle East, *Schistosoma japonicum* in Japan, the Philippines and Eastern Asia and *Schistosoma mansoni* in the Middle East, Africa, South America and the Caribbean.

schistosomiasis *n* (*syn* bilharziasis) infestation by *Schistosoma* that enter via the skin or mucosae. A single fluke can live in one part of the body, depositing eggs over many years. Prevention is by water chlorination, safe disposal of human waste and eradication of freshwater snails. There may be irritation at the entry site and after 3–5 weeks signs of larval migration, e.g. fever, eosinophilia, pneumonitis and hepatitis. Later, effects depend on where the eggs are deposited and the type, e.g. hepatitis, colitis, skin lesions, cystitis and haematuria. Many years later there may be organ damage due to fibrosis such as hepatic fibrosis and portal hypertension, urinary tract damage and pulmonary hypertension.

schistosomicide *n* any agent lethal to *Schistosoma*—**schistosomicidal** *adj.*

schizophrenia *n* a group of psychotic disorders characterized by disturbances of thinking, perceiving and affect. The course can be at times chronic, at times marked by acute episodes—**schizophrenic** *adj.*

Schlatter's disease (*syn* Osgood–Schlatter disease) osteochondritis of the tibial tubercle.

Schlemm's canal a channel in the inner part of the sclera, close to its junction with the cornea. It drains excess aqueous humour and maintains normal intraocular pressure. ⇒ glaucoma.

Schönlein's disease ⇒ Henoch–Schönlein purpura.

Schultz–Charlton test a blanching produced in the skin of a patient showing scarlet fever rash, around an injection of serum from a convalescent case, indicating neutralization of toxin by antitoxin.

Schwann cells neuroglial cells of the peripheral nervous system. They are concerned with the production of the myelin sheath that surrounds some nerve fibres.

sciatica *n* entrapment of the sciatic nerve during its course from the lower back to the leg causing pain which runs down the back of the leg to the heel and which can lead on to weakness such as foot drop and sensory loss in the lower leg.

SCID *abbr* severe combined immunodeficiency.

scintillography *n* (*syn* scintiscanning) visual recording of radioactivity over selected areas after administration of suitable radioisotope.

scissor leg deformity the legs are crossed in walking—following double hip-joint disease, or as a manifestation of Little's disease (spastic cerebral diplegia).

scissors gait ⇒ gait.

sclera *n* the 'white' of the eye (⇒ Figure 15); the opaque bluish-white fibrous outer coat of the eyeball covering the posterior five-sixths; it merges into the cornea at the front—**sclerae** *pl*, **scleral** *adj*.

sclerema *n* a rare disease in which hardening of the skin results from the deposition of mucinous material.

scleritis *n* inflammation of the sclera.

sclerocorneal *adj* pertaining to the sclera and the cornea, as the circular junction of these two structures.

sclerodactyly *n* deformity affecting the fingers. There is fixed, partial flexion of the fingers with subcutaneous calcification. Ulceration of the finger tips may occur. Associated with scleroderma. ⇒ CREST syndrome.

scleroderma *n* a disease in which localized oedema of the skin is followed by hardening, atrophy, deformity and ulceration. Occasionally it becomes generalized, producing immobility of the face, contraction of the fingers; can involve internal organs with diffuse fibrosis of the myocardium, kidneys, digestive tract and lungs (systemic sclerosis). When confined to the skin it is termed morphoea. ⇒ collagen, CREST syndrome, dermatomyositis.

sclerosis *n* a word used in pathology to describe abnormal hardening or fibrosis of a tissue. ⇒ multiple sclerosis, tuberous sclerosis—**sclerotic** *adj*.

sclerotherapy *n* injection of a sclerosing agent for the treatment of varicose veins. When, after the injection, rubber pads are bandaged over the site to increase localized compression, the term *compression sclerotherapy* is used. Sclerotherapy for oesophageal varices involves the use of an endoscope—**sclerotherapeutic** *adj*, **sclerotherapeutically** *adv*.

sclerotomy *n* incision of sclera of the eye.

scolex *n* the head of the tapeworm which it uses to attach itself to the intestine, and from which the segments (proglottides) develop.

scoliosis *n* lateral curvature of the spine, which can be congenital or acquired and is due to abnormality of the vertebrae, muscles and nerves. *idiopathic scoliosis* is characterized by a lateral curvature together with rotation and associated rib hump or flank recession. The treatment is by spinal brace or traction or internal fixation with accompanying spinal fusion. ⇒ halopelvic traction, Harrington rod, Milwaukee brace—**scoliotic** *adj*.

scotoma *n* a blind spot in the field of vision. May be normal or abnormal. *arcuate scotoma* a visual field defect in the area extending from the normal blind spot in an arc either above or below the central field. *central scotoma* a defect affecting the central field of vision. *centrocaecal scotoma* a defect extending from the normal blind spot to the central field of vision—**scotomata**.

scotopic vision dark-adapted vision.

scrapie *n* a prion disease of sheep and goats.

screening *n* a preventive measure to identify potential or incipient disease at an early stage when it may be more easily treated. It is carried out in a variety of settings, including primary care, hospitals, and clinics for antenatal care, and well babies, well men and well women clinics. Screening checks include: mammography, cervical cytology, blood pressure checks, checks for diabetes mellitus, faecal occult blood, prostatic specific antigen test for prostate cancer, ultrasound and triple blood test during pregnancy. The screening process may cause anxiety even when no abnormality is found (negative result).

scrotum *n* the pouch of pigmented skin in the male which contains the testes (⇒ Figure 16)—**scrotal** *adj*.

scurf *n* a lay term for dandruff.

scurvy a deficiency disease caused by lack of vitamin C (ascorbic acid). Clinical features include fatigue and haemorrhage. Latter may take the form of oozing at the gums or large ecchymoses. Tiny bleeding spots on the skin around hair follicles are characteristic. In children painful subperiosteal haemorrhage (rather than other types of bleeding) is pathognomonic.

scybala *n* rounded, hard, faecal lumps—**scybalum** *sing*.

SD *abbr* standard deviation.

SE *abbr* standard error.

seasonal affective disorder (SAD) a form of mood disorder (usually depression) with a strong association to winter. Thought to be related to a lack of exposure to light. Can be successfully treated with exposure to light with 'light boxes'.

sebaceous *adj* literally, pertaining to fat; usually refers to sebum. *sebaceous cyst* (*syn* wen) a cyst that actually contains keratin. Such cysts are most commonly found on the scalp, scrotum and vulva. *sebaceous glands* the cutaneous glands which secrete an oily substance called sebum. The ducts of these glands are short and straight and open into the hair follicles. (⇒ Figure 12).

seborrhoea *n* greasy condition of the scalp, face, sternal region and elsewhere due to overactivity of sebaceous glands.

sebum *n* the secretion of the sebaceous glands; it contains fatty acids, cholesterol and dead cells.

secondary *adj* second in order. *secondary care* health care indirectly accessed via primary care. Usually refers to specialist medical and surgical services provided in hospitals. *secondary prevention* ⇒ disease prevention. *secondary tumour* refers to a primary cancer that has spread to other distant sites in the body, such as colorectal cancer spreading to the liver. ⇒ metastasis.

secretin *n* a hormone produced in the duodenal mucosa, which causes secretion of pancreatic juice, and with other regulatory peptides inhibits gastric secretion and motility.

secretion *n* a fluid or substance, formed or concentrated in a gland and passed into the gastrointestinal tract, the blood or to the exterior.

secretory *adj* involved in the process of secretion: describes a gland which secretes.

secular *adj* describes the civil, state or non-religious influences on society. *secular beliefs* those not overtly or specifically religious. The strong non-religious convictions/values that guide concepts of morality that affect everyday life. ⇒ spiritual beliefs.

sedation *n* the production of a state of lessened functional activity.

sedative *n* an agent which reduces functional activity by its action on the nervous system. ⇒ anxiolytic.

segregation *n* a genetic term. The separation of the two alleles, each carried on one of a pair of chromosomes; this happens during meiosis when the haploid (n) gametes (spermatozoa, oocytes) are made. ⇒ Mendel's law.

Seldinger catheter a special catheter and guide wire for insertion into an artery, along which it is passed to, for example, the heart.

selective (o)estrogen receptor modulators (SERMs) a group of tissue specific drugs that modulate oestrogen receptors in some tissues but not others. They may cause oestrogen-agonist or oestrogen-antagonist effects. ⇒ Appendix 5.

selective serotonin reuptake inhibitors (SSRIs) a group of antidepressant drugs that act by preventing the reuptake of the neurotransmitter serotonin (5-hydroxytryptamine). ⇒ Appendix 5.

Selectron *n* a proprietary device which stores sealed radioactive sources of caesium or iridium in a shielded container in readiness for intracavitary treatment in the uterus, cervix or vagina. In recent years extended to other body sites such as bronchus and oesophagus.

selenium (Se) *n* an antioxidant. A trace element needed in the diet to facilitate reactions that protect cells from oxidative damage.

self-catheterization *n* both male and female patients can be taught to pass a catheter into the urinary bladder to evacuate urine intermittently.

self-concept *n* the view that the individual has of their total characteristics, ideas, feelings, qualities and negative features.

self-esteem *n* the value or worth an individual places on themselves.

self-fulfilling prophecy a situation whereby our expectations of another person cause us to behave in such a way as to cause the exact response that we anticipated.

self-infection the unwitting transfer of micro-organisms from one part of the body to another, in which it produces infection.

self-inflating bag a bag used for ventilation of a patient during anaesthesia or resuscitation.

self-monitoring of blood glucose (SMBG) use of capillary blood, usually obtained by a finger prick, for glucose estimation by a hand-held meter allowing patient monitoring and management of their diabetes.

sella turcica pituitary fossa located on sphenoid bone.

semantic memory that part of memory that stores general information about the world, e.g. where lions and tigers are found.

semen *n* seminal fluid. Fluid ejaculated during coitus. It comprises spermatozoa from the testes and the secretions from the prostate gland, seminal vesicles and bulbourethral glands.

semicircular canals three fluid-filled canals contained within the bony labyrinth of the internal ear (⇒ Figure 13). Orientated in the three planes of space they are part of the vestibular apparatus concerned with dynamic equilibrium and balance.

semicomatose *adj* describes a condition bordering on the unconscious. ⇒ Glasgow Coma Scale (GCS).

semilunar *adj* shaped like a crescent or half moon. *semilunar cartilages* the crescentic interarticular cartilages of the knee joint (menisci).

seminal *adj* pertaining to semen. *seminal vesicle* two tubular accessory glands behind the male bladder. They produce a thick alkaline fluid, which forms some 60% of semen volume. ⇒ Figure 16.

seminiferous *adj* carrying or producing semen such as the *seminiferous tubules*, the site of spermatogenesis.

seminoma *n* a neoplasm of the testis; subtype of germ cell tumour—**seminomata** *pl*, **seminomatous** *adj*.

semipermeable *adj* describes a membrane which is permeable to some substances in solutions, but not to others.

senescence *n* normal physical and mental changes in increasing age—**senescent** *adj*.

Sengstaken–Blakemore tube incorporates gastric and oesophageal balloons which when inflated apply pressure to bleeding oesophageal varices.

senile *adj* suffering from senescence complicated by morbid processes commonly called degeneration—**senility** *n*.

senna *n* leaves and pods of a purgative plant. Used as a stimulant laxative. ⇒ Appendix 5.

sensation *n* consciousness of a feeling that results from nerve impulses from the sensory organs reaching the brain.

sensible *adj* **1** endowed with the sense of feeling. **2** detectable by the senses.

sensitivity *n* the ability of a test to accurately identify affected individuals, such as mammography screening for breast cancer.

sensitivity training group individuals learn about what occurs during their interactions with other people within a supportive environment. They can test and refine different behavioural responses in the light of feedback, and are encouraged to try the positively modified behaviours in situations outside the group.

sensitization *n* rendering sensitive. Persons may become sensitive to a variety of substances, which may be food (e.g. shellfish), bacteria, plants, chemical substances, drugs, sera, etc. Liability is much greater in some persons than others. ⇒ allergy, anaphylaxis.

sensorineural *adj* pertaining to sensory neurons. *sensorineural deafness* a discriminating term for nerve deafness.

sensory *adj* pertaining to sensation. *sensory nerves* those which transmit impulses from peripheral receptors to the brain and spinal cord.

sentinel node biopsy (SNB) procedure used in staging (mainly) breast cancer and melanoma where (blue) dye is injected at the primary tumour site and traced to the nearest nodal basin where the first node involved with tumour will accumulate the dye; resection of that node may improve the cure rate.

sepsis *n* the state of being infected with pyogenic (pus-forming) micro-organisms—**septic** *adj*.

septic abortion ⇒ miscarriage.

septicaemia *n* the multiplication of living bacteria in the bloodstream causing infection—**septicaemic** *adj*.

septic arthritis arthritis caused by infection in the joint.

septoplasty *n* conservative operation to straighten the nasal septum, usually undertaken for deviations and dislocations of the quadrilateral cartilage. The nasal septum is repositioned in the midline with minimal removal of nasal cartilage.

septum *n* a partition between two cavities, e.g. between the nasal cavities—**septa** *pl*, **septal, septate** *adj*.

sequela *n* pathological consequence of a disease—**sequelae** *pl*.

sequestrectomy *n* excision of a sequestrum.

sequestrum *n* a piece of dead bone which separates from the healthy bone but remains within the tissues—**sequestra** *pl*.

serine *n* a conditionally essential (indispensable) amino acid.

SERMs *abbr* selective (o)estrogen receptor modulators.

seropurulent *adj* containing serum and pus.

serosa *n* a serous membrane, e.g. the peritoneal covering of the abdominal viscera—**serosal** *adj*.

serositis *n* inflammation of a serous membrane.

serotonin *n* a monoamine formed from tryptophan (amino acid). Liberated by blood platelets after injury and found in high concentrations in the CNS and gastrointestinal tract. It is a vasoconstrictor, inhibits gastric secretion, stimulates smooth muscle and acts as a central neurotransmitter. It is also involved in pain transmission and perception, and sleep–wake cycles. Also called 5-hydroxytryptamine (5-HT).

serotyping *n* classification of micro-organisms based on specific antigenic features.

serous *adj* pertaining to serum. *serous membrane* ⇒ membrane.

serpiginous *adj* snakelike, coiled, irregular; used to describe the margins of skin lesions, especially ulcers and ringworm.

Serratia *n* a genus of Gram-negative bacilli capable of causing infection in humans. *Serratia marcescens* is an endemic hospital resident and causes nosocomial urinary tract infection and pneumonia.

serration *n* a saw-like notch—**serrated** *adj*.

serum *n* the clear fluid remaining after blood has clotted—**sera** *pl*. *serum sickness* the allergic illness occurring 7–10 days following the injection of foreign serum for treatment or prophylaxis of infection. Rarely seen now that serum from other species has been replaced by the use of human immunoglobulins. ⇒ anaphylaxis.

sesamoid bone a small area of bone formation in muscle tendons such as the patella.

severe acute asthma (*syn* status asthmaticus) severe life-threatening asthma attack. Typically there is respiratory distress, cyanosis (central), tachycardia, sweating, an unproductive cough, exhaustion and severe hypoxia. It is a medical emergency requiring immediate treatment with high concentration oxygen, intravenous access, systemic corticosteroids and inhaled β_2-adrenoceptor agonists. ⇒ Appendix 5. Some patients may need respiratory support.

severe combined immunodeficiency (SCID) a group of immunodeficiency disorders presenting in infancy, characterized by failure of cellular and humoral immunity due to a genetic defect in a critical immune system component. SCID is generally fatal unless treated by bone marrow transplantation or gene therapy. Examples include adenosine deaminase (an enzyme) deficiency (ADA-SCID) and X-linked SCID caused by a defective cytokine.

Sever's disease calcaneal epiphysitis. Occurs in children and is caused by damage to the bone-cartilage layer in the heel resulting in pain.

sex chromatin in females the chromatin in one of the sex chromosomes (pair of X chromosomes) is inactive and appears in a somatic cell nucleus as a densely staining mass called a Barr body.

sex chromosomes the two chromosomes that determine genetic sex; XX in females and XY in males.

sexism *n* a view that members of one sex are superior to the other. Leads to discrimination and may be a limiting influence in education, professional development, etc.

sex-linked *adj* refers to genes located on the sex chromosomes or, more especially, on the X chromosome. By convention it is usual to refer to the latter genes (and the characters that they determine) as X-linked.

sexual abuse performing a sexual act with a child or with an adult against the person's wishes. The commonest type is that occurring between a father (or father figure) and daughter. ⇒ abuse, incest.

sexual dysfunction a lack of desire or the ability to achieve coitus in one or both partners. ⇒ dyspareunia, erectile dysfunction, frigidity, impotence, libido, vaginismus.

sexual intercourse coitus.

sexuality *n* the sum of the structural, functional and psychological characteristics as they are expressed by a person's gender-identity and sexual behaviour.

sexual orientation describes an individual's sexual attraction: towards people of the same sex (homosexuality), the opposite sex (heterosexuality) or both sexes (bisexuality). The particular preference may be transitory or life-long.

sexually acquired reactive arthritis (SARA) *n* (*syn* Reiter's disease) often caused by infection with *Chlamydia trachomatis*, but intestinal infections can also be the triggering event. Arthritis occurs together with conjunctivitis or uveitis, urethritis (or cervicitis in women), and sometimes psoriasis. ⇒ reactive arthritis.

sexually transmitted disease (STD) previously called venereal disease. ⇒ sexually transmitted infection.

sexually transmitted infection (STI) the infections, including those defined legally as venereal, which are usually transmitted through sexual contact, but not exclusively so. They include: gonorrhoea, syphilis, HIV, candidiasis, chlamydial infection, genital herpes, genital warts, and trichomoniasis.

SGOT *abbr* serum glutamic oxaloacetic transaminase. ⇒ aminotransferase.

SGPT *abbr* serum glutamic pyruvic transaminase. ⇒ aminotransferase.

shearing force when any part of the supported body is on a gradient, the tissues nearest the bone 'slide' towards the lower gradient while the skin stays in contact with the supporting surface because of friction which is increased in the presence of moisture. The deep blood vessels are stretched and bent and the deeper tissues become ischaemic with consequent necrosis. ⇒ pressure ulcers.

shelf operation an operation to deepen the acetabulum in developmental dysplasia of the hip, involving the use of a bone graft. Performed at 7–8 years, after failure of conservative treatment.

shiatsu *n* a form of Japanese health care similar in principle to acupuncture. Specific points along the body surface are pressed using the thumbs, fingers or palms to stimulate energy flow and to start self-healing processes. The belief is that an imbalance in a person's energy may result in physical symptoms. The aims of shiatsu are to rebalance self-healing energy and so promote health and well-being.

Shigella *n* a genus of Gram-negative bacilli. Several species cause dysentery. *Shigella boydii*, *S. dysenteriae* and *S. flexneri* in tropical and subtropical areas. *S. sonnei* causes dysentery in temperate regions and is the most common type in the UK. Commonly affects young children and is spread by the faecal-oral route. ⇒ dysentery.

shin bone ⇒ tibia.

shingles *n* a condition arising when the infecting agent (herpes zoster virus) attacks sensory nerves causing severe pain and the appearance of vesicles along the nerve's distribution (usually unilateral). ⇒ herpes zoster virus.

Shirodkar's operation placing of a purse-string suture around an incompetent cervix during pregnancy. It is removed when labour starts.

shock *n* condition in which there is inadequate flow of oxygenated blood to the tissues. There is cell hypoxia and inadequate tissue perfusion. Causes include haemorrhage and dehydration (hypovolaemic shock), heart failure (cardiogenic shock), infection (septic shock) and allergic reaction (anaphylactic shock).

Short Portable Mental State Questionnaire a test of cognitive function used to screen for dementia.

shortsightedness ⇒ myopia.

short-term memory (STM) working memory. The portion of memory that is responsible for the retention of information for a few seconds only. It can only be retained if it is rehearsed or moved to long-term memory (LTM). ⇒ chunking, rehearsal in memory.

shoulder girdle formed by the clavicle and scapula on either side.

'show' *n* a popular term for the blood-stained vaginal discharge at the commencement of labour.

shunt *n* a term applied to the passage of fluid through other than the usual channel. This may refer to shunting of blood (e.g. arteriovenous shunt) or cerebrospinal fluid (e.g. ventriculoperitoneal shunt).

SI *abbr* Système International d'Unités.

SIADH *abbr* syndrome of inappropriate ADH secretion.

sialagogue *n* an agent which increases saliva production.

sialogram *n* radiographic image of the salivary glands and ducts, after injection of an opaque contrast medium—**sialography** *n*, **sialographic** *adj*, **sialographically** *adv*.

sialolith *n* a stone in a salivary gland or duct.

sickle cell disease an inherited haemoglobinopathy. It is due to an abnormal haemoglobin (HbS) and affects people from areas where falciparum malaria is endemic (equatorial Africa, part of India and part of the eastern Mediterranean) and their descendants in Europe, West Indies and the USA. The red blood cells

become sickle-shaped, if the person becomes dehydrated, hypoxic or has an infection. The change in red cell shape leads to reduced oxygen-carrying capacity, blood vessel blockage with pain and infarction and chronic haemolytic anaemia as the abnormal red cells are destroyed in the spleen. When a sickle-cell crisis occurs, the person requires urgent rehydration and pain relief. At-risk populations should be screened for the abnormal HbS. ⇒ malaria, thalassaemia.

side-effect *n* any physiological change other than the wanted one from a drug, e.g. oral iron causes the side-effect of black faeces. Also covers undesirable drug reactions. Some are predictable, being the result of a known metabolic action of the drug, e.g. hair loss with cytotoxic drugs. Unpredictable reactions can be: (a) immediate: anaphylaxis, angiooedema, (b) erythematous: all forms of erythema, including nodosum and multiforme and purpuric rashes, (c) cellular eczematous rashes and contact dermatitis, (d) specific, e.g. light-sensitive eruptions with griseofulvin (antifungal).

siderosis *n* excess of iron in the blood or tissues. Inhalation of iron oxide into the lungs can cause one form of pneumoconiosis.

SIDS *abbr* sudden infant death syndrome.

sievert (Sv) the SI unit (International System of Units) for radiation dose equivalent. It has replaced the rem.

sigmoid *adj* shaped like the letter S. *sigmoid colon* ⇒ Figure 18b. *sigmoid flexure* ⇒ flexure.

sigmoidoscope *n* an instrument for visualizing the rectum and sigmoid colon. ⇒ endoscope—**sigmoidoscopic** *adj*.

sigmoidoscopy *n* endoscopic examination of the rectum and distal colon (sigmoid colon). ⇒ colonoscopy.

sigmoidostomy *n* the formation of a colostomy in the sigmoid colon.

sign *n* any objective evidence of disease.

sign language a form of non-verbal language using the hands and upper body to make signs, whereby hearing impaired people can communicate with each other and with family and friends. ⇒ British sign language, finger spelling, Makaton.

silicone *n* a water-repellent compound. Used in dressings, as sheets, foams and gels, where it fits exactly the contours of the granulating wound to provide an ideal environment for wound healing. Also used as implants in breast reconstruction.

silicosis *n* a form of pneumoconiosis or industrial dust disease found in metal grinders, stone-workers, etc.

Silverman score a method of rating respiratory distress by assessing movement of accessory muscles and degree of expiratory grunt.

silver nitrate used as a caustic for warts.

SIMA *abbr* system for identifying motivated abilities.

simple fracture ⇒ fracture.

Sims' position an exaggerated left lateral position with the right knee well flexed and the left arm drawn back over the edge of the bed.

Sims' speculum a type of vaginal speculum.

SIMV *abbr* synchronized intermittent mandatory ventilation.

sinoatrial node ⇒ sinus node.

sinus *n* **1** a hollow or cavity, especially the nasal air sinuses (⇒ Figure 14). **2** a channel containing blood, especially venous blood, e.g. the sinuses of the brain. ⇒ cavernous. **3** a recess or cavity within a bone. **4** any abnormal blind tract or channel opening onto the skin or a mucous surface. ⇒ pilonidal.

sinus arrhythmia an increase of heart rate on inspiration, decrease on expiration.

sinusitis *n* inflammation of a sinus, used exclusively for the paranasal sinuses.

sinus node (sinoatrial) the pacemaker of the heart. Part of the specialized tissue that forms the conducting system of the heart. It is situated at the junction of the superior vena cava and the right atrium. It initiates the wave of cardiac contraction. ⇒ pacemaker.

sinusoid *n* a dilated channel into which arterioles or veins open in some organs, e.g. liver, and which act in place of the usual capillaries.

sinus rhythm normal rhythm of the heart. ⇒ PQRST complex.

SIRS *abbr* systemic inflammatory response syndrome.

sitz-bath *n* a hip bath.

Sjögren–Larsson syndrome genetically determined congenital ectodermosis. Associated with learning disability.

Sjögren syndrome deficient secretion from lacrimal, salivary and other glands, mostly in postmenopausal women. There is keratoconjunctivitis, dry tongue and hoarse voice. Thought to be due to an autoimmune process. Also called keratoconjunctivitis sicca.

skeleton *n* the bony framework of the body, supporting and protecting the soft tissues and organs and acting as attachments for muscles. (⇒ Figures 2, 3)—**skeletal** *adj*. *appendicular skeleton* the bones forming the pectoral girdle, upper limbs, pelvic girdle and lower limbs. *axial skeleton* the bones forming the head and trunk.

Skene's glands two small glands at the entrance to the female urethra; the lesser vestibular or paraurethral glands.

skewed distribution a statistical term that describes any distribution of scores where there are a greater number of values on one side of the mean than the other, i.e. not symmetrical. ⇒ normal distribution curve.

skill *n* the ability to competently and consistently perform a specific task with minimum effort and maximum effect.

skill mix the level, range and variety of skills of the staff in a department, unit or team which is needed to meet the organizational outcomes.

skin *n* the tissue which forms the outer covering of the body; it consists of two layers, the outer epidermis (cuticle), dermis (true skin) and the appendages; nails, glands and hair. ⇒ Figure 12. *skin fold thickness* an anthropometric measurement used as part of nutritional assessment. *skin shedding* skin is continually shedding its outer keratinized cells as scales. As the skin has a natural bacterial flora, the scales are a potential source of infection for susceptible patients. ⇒ psoriasis.

skin expansion a technique utilizing an inflatable prosthesis to distend and expand the skin and subcutaneous tissue.

skin flap ⇒ flap.

skin graft sheet of skin containing dermis and epidermis separated from its blood supply and applied to a raw surface. *full thickness (Wolfe) graft* full thickness skin graft that requires closure of the donor site. *split thickness (Thiersch) graft* partial thickness skin graft where the donor site heals spontaneously.

skull *n* the bony framework of the head, the face and cranium (⇒ Figure 2).

SLE *abbr* systemic lupus erythematosus.

sleep *n* a naturally altered state of consciousness occurring in humans in a 24 h biological rhythm. A *sleep cycle* consists of alternating cycles of non-rapid eye movement sleep (NREM) or orthodox sleep, which has four stages, and rapid eye movement sleep (REM) or paradoxical sleep. *sleep deprivation* a cumulative condition arising when there is interference with a person's established rhythm of paradoxical sleep. It can result in slurred rambling speech, irritability, disorientation, slowed reaction time, malaise, progressing to illusions, delusions, paranoia and hyperactivity. *sleep study* usually monitoring oxygen and heart rate overnight. Used to diagnose nocturnal hypoxaemia and apnoeic episodes.

sleep apnoea recurrent periods of apnoea while sleeping due to repeated upper airway obstruction. Associated with transient hypoxaemia, severe headaches and daytime somnolence. More often seen in obese individuals, or those with soft palate abnormalities. ⇒ continuous positive airway pressure.

sleeping sickness a disease endemic in Africa; there is increasing somnolence caused by infection of the brain by trypanosomes. ⇒ trypanosomiasis.

sleep walking ⇒ somnambulism.

slipped disc *n* prolapsed intervertebral disc. ⇒ prolapse.

slipped epiphysis displacement of an epiphysis, especially the upper femoral one. ⇒ epiphysis.

slough *n* septic tissue which becomes necrosed and separates from the healthy tissue.

slow release drugs drug formulations which do not dissolve until they reach the small intestine, where the drug is slowly released and absorbed. Many slow release preparations are now incorporated into transdermal patches.

slow virus an infective agent (prion) that only causes infection after a long latent period. Many cases may never develop overt symptoms but may still be a link in the chain of infectivity. ⇒ Creutzfeldt–Jakob disease.

small for dates small for gestational age.

small for gestational age (SGA) babies who weigh less than expected for a given gestational age. They are either constitutionally small or suffer from growth restriction. ⇒ low birthweight.

smallpox *n* (*syn* variola) caused by a virus: eradicated following WHO worldwide campaign. Vaccination may be required for laboratory staff working with pox viruses and others at risk of exposure. ⇒ vaccinia.

SMBG *abbr* self-monitoring of blood glucose.

smear *n* a film of material spread out on a glass slide for microscopic examination. *cervical smear* microscopic examination of cells obtained from the surface of the cervix. ⇒ carcinoma, cervical intraepithelial neoplasia (CIN), colposcope, cytology.

smegma *n* the sebaceous secretion which accumulates beneath the prepuce and clitoris.

Smith-Petersen nail a trifin, cannulated metal nail used to provide internal fixation for intracapsular fractures of the femoral neck.

smoking (passive) passive smoking is described as the involuntary inhalation of smoke from burning tobacco generated by another person over a period of time. It is associated with an increased risk of smoking-related illnesses such as coronary heart disease, hypertension, bronchial cancer and chronic obstructive pulmonary disease, and can also trigger an asthma attack. Passive smoking is an occupational hazard, for example for those working in bars and clubs, and efforts to reduce the risk may include encouraging employers to support smoking cessation programmes and the introduction of no smoking policies. Babies and children are especially vulnerable and have little choice about exposure to tobacco smoke. ⇒ sudden infant death syndrome.

SMR *abbr* **1** standardized mortality ratio. **2** submucous resection.

snapping hip syndrome a snapping sensation either heard or felt in the hip during movement of the joint. The nature of the signs and symptoms will indicate whether the structure at fault is more likely to be the iliotibial band or the iliopsoas tendon.

snare *n* a surgical instrument with a wire loop at the end; used for removal of polypi.

SNB *abbr* sentinel node biopsy.

Snellen test type chart a chart for testing visual acuity.

snuffles *n* a snorting inspiration due to congestion of nasal mucous membrane. It is a sign of early congenital (prenatal) syphilis when the nasal discharge may be purulent or blood-stained.

social class the classification of people into social groups. Various classifications are used, and one such is a five category socioeconomic classification based on the householder's occupation. I, professional, e.g. lawyer; II, intermediate, e.g. nurse; III, skilled (non-manual), e.g. secretary and (manual), e.g. carpenter; IV, semi-skilled, e.g. agricultural worker; V, unskilled, e.g. cleaner.

social deprivation measurement composite index of deprivation (poverty) in a defined population based on census-derived social and economic variables. Geographically defined populations include residents within a strategic health authority (population up to several million) or district (population half to one million), administrative (electoral) wards (several thousands) or enumerator districts (25 households). Deprivation indices may also be attributed to general practice populations based on the wards or enumerator districts from which the practice draws its registered patients.

social exclusion the lack of social connections, social support or access to social networks for particular groups in the population (community). Groups affected include rough sleepers, teenage mothers, refugees and many young people. Research has reported higher levels of ill health (illness, psychological ill health, disease, disability, mortality) in people with low levels of social support and integration, independent of physical health, socio-economic status and lifestyle. Two main theories: social support affects health directly; social support protects against life stresses. Conversely, social exclusion increases the risk of physical and psychological ill health. ⇒ underclass.

social isolation a term that can be applied to an individual, a family or a group of individuals. Interaction with other people does not conform to the usual pattern, for reasons that may include immobility, poverty, etc.

socialization *n* the means by which individuals learn the social norms and the value of abiding by them. It may occur informally in the family, and more formally at school and at work.

social norms describes socially acceptable behaviour. Norms may prescribe some forms of behaviour and prohibit others. ⇒ anomie.

social stratification the means of dividing populations into unequal strata using different characteristics, for example: age, gender, income, ethnicity, etc.

sociocultural *adj* pertaining to culture in its sociological context.

sociology *n* the scientific study of interpersonal and intergroup social relationships—**sociological** *adj*. *sociology of sport* area of study concerned with the social structure, social patterns and social organization of groups and subcultures in sport.

sociomedical *adj* relating to sociology and medicine. For example how social influences may predispose to diseases, e.g. sleeping rough may increase the risk for hypothermia, etc.

sodium (Na) *n* metallic element. A major extracellular cation concerned with the composition of fluid compartments and neuromuscular function. *sodium bicarbonate (hydrogen carbonate)* acts as a buffer in the blood. Administered intravenously to correct metabolic acidosis. *sodium chloride* often used in intravenous fluids to replace fluids and correct electrolyte levels. *sodium citrate* used as an in vitro anticoagulant, e.g. for stored blood. *sodium hypochlorite* a powerful disinfectant used, in suitable dilutions, in many situations, such as dealing with environmental contamination with blood and other body fluids. *sodium pump* an active transport mechanism (needing ATP) that pumps sodium ions through semipermeable cell membranes.

soft sore chancroid.

soft tissue mobilization physiotherapists and sports therapists use pétrissage or kneading techniques using the whole hand or the finger pads to stretch retracted muscles and tendons, relieve spasm and help to remove metabolic waste products from muscles. Kneading with the finger pads is also used during some natural childbirth methods. Physiotherapists use percussive manipulations, collectively called tapotement, to move thick secretions from the respiratory tract and assist expectoration.

solar plexus a large network of sympathetic (autonomic) nerve ganglia and fibres in the upper abdomen. It supplies the abdominal organs. *solar plexus punch* a blow to the abdomen that results in an immediate inability to breathe freely.

solute *n* substance dissolved in a solvent.

solution *n* a fluid that contains a dissolved substance or substances. *saturated solution* one in which the maximum amount of a particular substance is dissolved.

solvent *n* an agent that is capable of dissolving other substances (solutes). The component of a solution that is present in excess. *solvent misuse* the practice of inhaling volatile substances, such as those in some adhesives, solvents and fuels, to produce euphoria and intoxication. Characterized by odour on clothes and hair, redness and blistering around the nose and mouth, and behaviour changes. Dependence, local damage to the nasal mucosa and organ damage, e.g. the brain, may result. Death may be caused by asphyxia or toxicity. ⇒ drug misuse.

somatic *adj* relating to the body such as somatic cells (body cells), as distinct from the gametes. *somatic nerves* nerves controlling the function of voluntary, skeletal muscle.

somatostatin *n* growth hormone release-inhibiting hormone (GH-RIH).

somatotrophin *n* ⇒ growth hormone.

somnambulism *n* (*syn* sleepwalking) dissociated consciousness in which sleeping and waking states are combined. Considered normal in children but abnormal in adults.

sonograph *n* graphic record of sound waves.

sonography *n* the means by which a sonograph is recorded and interpreted.

soporific *adj*, *n* (describes) an agent which induces deep sleep.

souffle *n* puffing or blowing sound. *funic souffle* auscultatory murmur of pregnancy. Synchronizes with the fetal heart beat and is caused by pressure on the umbilical cord. *uterine souffle* soft, blowing murmur which can be auscultated over the uterus after the fourth month of pregnancy.

sound *n* an instrument introduced into a hollow organ or duct to detect a stone or to dilate a stricture.

source isolation is used for patients who are sources of micro-organisms that may be transmitted from them to infect others. *strict source isolation* is for highly transmissible and dangerous diseases. *standard source isolation* is for other communicable diseases/infections.

soya protein a protein that is extracted from soya bean, a legume used in Asiatic countries in place of meat. It is useful in dietetic preparations for those people who are allergic to cows' milk. Soya protein is a constituent of soya milk used as a substitute for cows' milk by vegans.

spansule *n* a drug preparation designed to produce controlled release when given orally.

spasm *n* **1** a sudden, involuntary contraction of a muscle. **2** sustained contraction of a muscle or group of muscles due to pain. **3** a seizure or convulsion of the whole body.

spasmodic dysmenorrhoea ⇒ dysmenorrhoea.

spasmolytic *adj*, *n* ⇒ antispasmodic.

spasticity *n* increased tension or tone of muscle (hypertonia) with increased resistance to passive movement out of the tonic posture proportional to the rate of stretch and characterized by the clasp-knife phenomenon, exaggerated deep tendon reflexes, Babinki's sign and clonus. Spasticity of one side of the body following stroke (cerebrovascular accident) is accompanied by loss of voluntary movement and postural reactions of one side of the body (spastic hemiplegia)—**spastic** *adj*.

spatula *n* a flat flexible instrument with blunt edges for spreading creams, ointment, etc. *tongue spatula* a rigid, blade-shaped instrument for depressing the tongue.

species *n* a systematic category, subdivision of genus. Individuals within a species group have common characteristics and differ, fairly obviously, from a related species.

specific *adj* special; characteristic; peculiar to. *specific disease* one that is always caused by a specified organism.

specific adaptation to imposed demands (SAID) principle in sports medicine the principle of specificity of training. ⇒ training.

specific dynamic action (SDA) the increase in body temperature and metabolism that occurs when energy is used in the assimilation of ingested food. Protein foods in particular cause a sustained increase in basal metabolic rate that lasts for some hours.

specific gravity the weight of a substance, as compared with that of an equal volume of pure water, the latter being represented by 1000.

specificity *n* the ability of a test to accurately identify non-affected individuals, such as a screening test.

spectrophotometer *n* a spectroscope combined with a photometer for quantitatively measuring the relative intensity of different parts of a light spectrum—**spectrophotometric** *adj*.

spectroscope *n* an instrument for observing spectra of light.

speculum *n* an instrument used to hold the walls of a cavity apart, so that the interior of the cavity can be examined or treated—**specula** *pl*. *nasal speculum* used for examination of the nose and for treatments, such as nasal cautery and packing to stop bleeding. *vaginal speculum* used to examine the vagina and cervix, for taking high vaginal swabs and cervical smears and for some treatments. Types include Cuscoe's bivalve and Sims' speculum.

speech and language therapist the professional responsible for the assessment, diagnosis and treatment of speech and language disorders in children and adults. In the USA and Australia they are known as speech pathologists.

speech and language therapy (SLT) one of the professions allied to medicine. Describes the therapy provided by a speech and language therapist to people with impaired communication, e.g. aphasia.

Speech and language therapy is provided for people who are dysfluent (stammer), have impaired hearing, have language difficulties (grammar and vocabulary and the social use of language), have problems producing the correct sounds for speech so that they are difficult to understand, or have difficulties with their voice. Speech and language therapy referrals are also made for people who have dysphagia (difficulty in swallowing). Speech and language therapy includes assessment and treatment of these difficulties. In the UK therapy with adults is usually carried out within an NHS setting, including hospitals and nursing homes. Children may be seen in health centres but increasingly speech and language therapy services are being offered in educational settings, including mainstream schools. Speech and language therapy aims to achieve the best level of communication possible for the person concerned. As well as being provided for individuals, speech and language therapy may be provided for small groups. Programmes may also be set up for other staff such as nurses to carry out. Speech and language therapists are a valuable resource for other members of the multidisciplinary team and can provide advice on how to achieve optimum communication with people with difficulties in communicating.

speech mechanism normal speech involves several processes, breathing, phonation, articulation, resonance and prosody. It is disturbed in various combinations and degrees in dysarthria and dysphasia.

sperm *n* an abbreviated form of the word spermatozoon or spermatozoa. *sperm count* an infertility test where semen is examined for volume, sperm numbers, morphology, motility and chemical composition.

spermatic *adj* pertaining to or conveying semen. *spermatic cord* suspends the testis in the scrotum and contains the testicular artery and vein and the deferent duct (vas deferens) (⇒ Figure 16).

spermatogenesis *n* the formation and development of spermatozoa—**spermatogenetic** *adj*.

spermatorrhoea *n* involuntary discharge of semen without orgasm.

spermatozoon *n* a mature, male gamete (germ cell)—**spermatozoa** *pl*.

spermicide, spermatocide *n* an agent that kills spermatozoa—**spermicidal** *adj*.

sphenoid *n* a wedge-shaped bone at the base of the skull containing the sphenoidal sinus—**sphenoidal** *adj*.

spherocyte *n* round red blood cell, as opposed to biconcave—**spherocytic** *adj*.

spherocytosis *n* a hereditary disorder transmitted as a dominant gene. It is present at birth, but symptoms may vary from non-existent to severe; thus it is sometimes discovered by 'accidental' examination of the blood, which reveals that the red cells are predominantly spherocytic. ⇒ jaundice.

sphincter *n* a circular muscle, contraction of which serves to close an orifice (⇒ Figure 19).

sphincterotomy *n* surgical incision of a sphincter.

sphincteroplasty *n* plastic surgical reconstruction of a sphincter.

sphingolipid *n* sphingosine combined with a lipid. A constituent of biological membranes, especially in the brain.

sphingomyelin *n* a phospholipid formed from sphingosine found as part of biological membranes.

sphingomyelinase *n* an enzyme concerned with the metabolism and storage of lipids.

sphingosine *n* a constituent of sphingolipids and sphingomyelin.

sphygmomanometer *n* an instrument used for non-invasive measurement of arterial blood pressure. Some utilize a column of mercury, but are generally being replaced with aneroid (not containing a liquid) devices that contain no mercury.

spica *n* a bandage applied in a figure-of-eight pattern.

spicule *n* a small, spike-like fragment, especially of bone.

spigot *n* plastic peg used to close a tube.

spina bifida a congenital defect in which there is incomplete closure of the neural canal, usually in the lumbosacral region. *spina bifida occulta* the defect does not affect the spinal cord or meninges. It is often marked externally by pigmentation, a haemangioma, a tuft of hair or a lipoma which may extend into the spinal canal. *spina bifida cystica* an externally protruding spinal lesion. It may vary in severity

from meningocele to myelomeningocele. The condition can be detected during pregnancy by an increased concentration of alphafetoprotein in the amniotic fluid or by ultrasonography.

spinal *n* pertaining to the spine. *spinal anaesthetic* a local anaesthetic solution injected into the subarachnoid space, so that it renders the area supplied by the selected spinal nerves insensitive. *spinal canal* ⇒ vertebral canal. *spinal column* ⇒ vertebral column. *spinal cord* the continuation of nervous tissue of the brain down the spinal canal to the level of the first or second lumbar vertebra (⇒ Figures 1, 11). *spinal nerves* 31 pairs leave the spinal cord and pass out of the spinal canal to supply the periphery.

spinal accessory nerve the eleventh pair of cranial nerves. They supply the muscles of the larynx and pharynx, and the muscles of the neck and shoulder to control movement of the head and shoulders.

spinal cord compression (SCC) pressure on the spinal cord. Often caused by tumour (which is commonly metastatic tumour from lung, breast or gastrointestinal cancers). Early diagnosis is vital to prevent permanent effects such as paralysis. Treatment usually involves corticosteroids and radiotherapy.

spine *n* **1** a popular term for the bony spinal or vertebral column. **2** a sharp process of bone—**spinous, spinal** *adj*.

spinhaler *n* a nebulizer (atomizer) which delivers a preset drug dose.

Spirillum n a genus of small spiral bacteria. *Spirillum minus* is found in rodents and causes one type of rat-bite fever—**spirilla** *pl*, **spirillary** *adj*.

spiritual beliefs may be a belief system ascribed by a particular religion; a modified version of these, reached following questioning, thinking and reasoning. Other people form a strong non-religious belief system to guide their concept of morality, and to find meaning in life. ⇒ secular beliefs.

spiritual distress may occur when a person's spiritual beliefs are derived from a particular religion, which requires the person to observe certain practices in everyday living activities, e.g. the preparation of food, types of food eaten, fasting, attending public worship, prayer, personal hygiene and type of clothing. Distress is likely if they are unable to conform to the teachings of their religious faith such as might occur during illness and hospitalization.

spirochaetaemia *n* spirochaetes in the bloodstream such as occurs in the secondary stage of syphilis—**spirochaetaemic** *adj*.

spirochaete *n* an order of tiny spiral bacteria that includes the genera *Borrelia*, *Leptospira* and *Treponema* such as *Treponema pallidum*, the cause of syphilis—**spirochaetal** *adj*.

spirograph *n* an apparatus which records the movement of the lungs—**spirographic** *adj*, **spirography** *n*, **spirographically** *adv*.

spirometer *n* an instrument for measuring the volume of inhaled and exhaled air—**spirometric** *adj*, **spirometry** *n* ⇒ respiratory function tests.

Spitz–Holter valve a special valve used to drain hydrocephalus.

splanchnic *adj* pertaining to or supplying the viscera.

splanchnicectomy *n* surgical removal of the splanchnic nerves, whereby the viscera are deprived of sympathetic impulses; occasionally performed in the treatment of hypertension or for the relief of certain kinds of visceral pain.

splanchnology *n* the study of the structure and function of the viscera.

spleen *n* a lymphoid, vascular organ immediately below the diaphragm, at the tail of the pancreas, behind the stomach. It is part of the monocyte-macrophage (reticuloendothelial) system. Functions include the destruction of worn out blood cells, filtering the blood of debris and providing a site for lymphocyte proliferation and antibody production.

splenectomy *n* surgical removal of the spleen.

splenitis *n* inflammation of the spleen.

splenocaval *adj* pertaining to the spleen and inferior vena cava, usually referring to anastomosis of the splenic vein to the latter.

splenomegaly *n* enlargement of the spleen.

splenoportal *adj* pertaining to the spleen and hepatic portal vein.

splenoportogram *n* radiographic demonstration of the spleen and hepatic portal vein after injection of radiopaque contrast medium. Superseded by ultrasound examination.

splenorenal *adj* pertaining to the spleen and kidney, as anastomosis of the splenic vein to the renal vein; a procedure carried out in some cases of portal hypertension.

splint ⇒ orthosis.

SPMSQ *abbr* Short Portable Mental State Questionnaire.

SPOD *abbr* sexual problems of the disabled. Part of the Royal Association of Disability and Rehabilitation offering specific advice and support to people with disabilities.

spondyl(e) *n* a vertebra.

spondylitis *n* inflammation of the spine—**spondylitic** *adj*. ankylosing spondylitis an inflammatory condition affecting the spine and sacroiliac joints and characterized (in its later stages) by ossification of the spinal ligaments and ankylosis of sacroiliac joints. It occurs most commonly in young men.

spondylography *n* a method of measuring and studying the degree of kyphosis by directly tracing the line of the back.

spondylolisthesis *n* forward displacement of lumbar vertebra(e)—**spondylolisthetic** *adj*.

spondylosis *n* degenerative disease of the whole spine, with osteophyte formation on either side of the intervertebral disc. Often associated with osteoarthritis of the apophyseal (facet) joints.

spontaneous abortion ⇒ miscarriage.

spontaneous fracture ⇒ fracture.

sporadic *adj* scattered; occurring in isolated cases; not epidemic—**sporadically** *adv*.

spore *n* **1** a phase in the life cycle of a limited number of bacterial genera (*Clostridium* and *Bacillus*) where the cell is encapsulated and metabolism almost ceases. Spores are highly resistant to environmental conditions such as heat and desiccation. The spores are ubiquitous so that sterilization procedures must ensure their removal or death. ⇒ endospore. **2** reproductive body produced by some plants, particularly fungi, and by protozoa.

sporicidal *adj* lethal to spores—**sporicide** *n*.

sporotrichosis *n* chronic infection of a wound by the fungus *Sporotrichum schenkii*. A sore, ulcer or abscess forms with lymphangitis and subcutaneous painless granulomata. Occurs amongst agricultural workers.

sport biomechanics the study of determining optimal techniques for sport performance, the design of sports equipment and investigation of the stresses placed upon the athlete's body during performance. ⇒ biomechanics.

sport psychology the study of human behaviour and mind in sport. Includes the areas of motor learning, sport skill acquisition and psychological skills training.

sports medicine branch of medicine concerned with the diagnosis, treatment, rehabilitation and prevention of traumatic and non-traumatic injuries and disease affecting the athlete. May also be used to describe both medical and scientific aspects of sport and exercise. ⇒ sports science.

sports science a broad discipline that is mainly concerned with the processes that explain behaviour in sport and how athletic performance can be improved. Includes kinesiology, kinanthropometry, sport biomechanics, exercise physiology, sport psychology and sociology of sport.

spotted fever ⇒ Rocky Mountain spotted fever.

sprain *n* injury to the soft tissues surrounding a joint, resulting in discoloration, swelling and pain. There is stretching or tearing of a ligament or capsular structure of a joint.

Sprengel's shoulder deformity congenital high scapula, a permanent elevation of the shoulder, often associated with other congenital deformities, e.g. the presence of a cervical rib or the absence of vertebrae.

sprue *n* a chronic malabsorption disorder. ⇒ coeliac, tropical sprue.

spurious *adj* not genuine or what it appears to be. *spurious diarrhoea* the leakage of fluid faeces past a solid impacted mass of faeces. More common in children and older people.

sputum *n* the mucus and other matter expectorated (coughed up) from the lower respiratory tract.

squamous *adj* scaly. *squamous cell carcinoma* carcinoma arising in squamous epithelium; epithelioma. *squamous epithelium* the

non-glandular epithelial covering of the external body surfaces.

squint *n* ⇒ strabismus.

SSRIs *abbr* selective serotonin reuptake inhibitors.

SSPE *abbr* subacute sclerosing panencephalitis.

staging *n* process of measuring how advanced a tumour is and to which sites it has spread; may be locally advanced or metastatic. Usually involves imaging with computed tomography, bone scan and often surgery. It includes tumour (T) size, nodal (N) status and metastatic (M) sites present/absent.

stagnant loop syndrome ⇒ blind loop syndrome.

standard *n* a level or measure against which the performance of an activity can be monitored.

standard deviation (SD) in statistics, a measure of dispersion of scores around the mean value. It is the square root of variance.

standard error (SE) in statistics, a measure of variability of many mean values of different samples from a population. Used to calculate the chance of a sample mean being smaller or bigger than that for the population.

standardized mortality rate the number of deaths per specific population standardized for age.

standardized mortality ratio (SMR) allows comparisons to be made between the death rates in populations with different demographic structures. It involves the application of national age-specific mortality rates to local populations so that a ratio of expected deaths to actual deaths can be calculated. The comparative national figure is, by convention, 100 and, for example, a local figure of 106 means that there is an increased risk of 6%, whereas a local figure of 94 indicates a risk 6% lower.

St Anthony's fire historical term for the mental abnormalities and painful vasoconstriction leading to gangrene of the extremities caused by ergot poisoning. Occurred through eating rye infested with a fungus containing alkaloids of ergot.

stapedectomy *n* surgical removal of stapes for otosclerosis. After stapedectomy, stapes can be replaced by a prosthesis.

Normal hearing is restored in 90% of patients.

stapedial mobilization, stapediolysis release of a stapes rendered immobile by otosclerosis.

stapes *n* the stirrup-shaped medial bone of the middle ear. (⇒ Figure 13). ⇒ incus, malleus.

Staphylococcus *n* a genus of Gram-positive bacteria occurring in clusters. Some types are commensal on the skin and may be found in the nasopharynx, axillae and perineum of some individuals. They cause infections that include: boils, impetigo, wound infection, endocarditis, pneumonia, osteomyelitis, toxic shock syndrome and septicaemia. Staphylococci cause many nosocomial infections. The genus includes the major pathogen *Staphylococcus aureus*, which produces the enzyme coagulase; some strains produce a powerful exotoxin, and others are methicillin-resistant. ⇒ methicillin-resistant *Staphylococcus aureus*. *Staphylococcus epidermidis* is a skin commensal (non-coagulase producer). It infects wounds and increasingly causes infection involving intravascular devices, peritoneal dialysis catheters, valves, etc. Treatment is problematic as the microorganism has a natural resistance to many antibiotics.

staphyloma *n* a protrusion of the cornea or sclera of the eye—**staphylomata** *pl*.

starch *n* a polysaccharide formed from glucose molecules, the carbohydrate present in potatoes, rice and maize.

Starling's law of the heart states that the force of myocardial contraction is proportional to the length (stretching) of the ventricular muscle fibres. Increased stretching results in the next contraction being more powerful.

start-up costs the costs, such as the purchase of equipment that occur at the start of a project.

stasis *n* stagnation; cessation of motion.

static stretching a technique of muscle stretching used to increase range of motion; the muscle/muscle group is held at the end of its range of movement, in a static position for a period of time.

statins *npl* colloquial expression for HMG-CoA reductase inhibitors.

Statistical Package for the Social Sciences (SPSS) software package often used in the analysis of quantitative data.

statistical significance in research, an expression of how likely it is that a set of results happened by chance, e.g. 0.05, 0.01 and 0.001 levels. ⇒ *P* value.

statistics *n* scientific study of numerical data collection and its analysis and evaluation.

status *n* state; condition. *status asthmaticus* ⇒ severe acute asthma. *status epilepticus* describes epileptic attacks following each other almost continuously.

STD *abbr* sexually transmitted disease.

steatorrhoea *n* passage of pale, oily stool due to fat malabsorption.

Stein–Leventhal syndrome ⇒ polycystic ovary syndrome.

Steinmann's pin an alternative to the use of a Kirschner wire for applying skeletal traction to a limb. It has its own introducer and stirrup.

stellate *adj* star-shaped. *stellate ganglion* a large collection of nerve cells (ganglion) on the sympathetic chain in the root of the neck. *stellate ganglionectomy* surgical removal of the stellate ganglion.

Stellwag's sign occurs in Graves' disease: the person blinks infrequently and the eyelids are retracted. ⇒ exophthalmos.

stem cell a cell normally present in the bone marrow that is capable of developing into any of a full range of mature blood cells. They are the 'active ingredient' of bone marrow transplantations (also called stem cell transplants).

stenosis *n* a narrowing—**stenoses** *pl*, **stenotic** *adj*. *pyloric stenosis* **1** narrowing of the pylorus due to scar tissue formed during the healing of a peptic ulcer. **2** congenital hypertrophic pyloric stenosis due to a thickened pyloric sphincter muscle. ⇒ pyloromyotomy.

stent *n* device used to provide a shunt or keep a tube or vessel open. For example stent insertion into the bile duct to relieve obstructive jaundice, stenting the ureters to overcome urinary obstruction, and stenting the oesophagus for palliation of dysphagia caused by oesophageal cancer. *transjugular intrahepatic portasystemic stent shunting (TIPSS)* a stent placed between the hepatic portal vein and the hepatic vein in the liver to reduce hepatic portal pressure by providing a shunt between the hepatic portal and systemic circulations. Performed to prevent further bleeding from oesophageal varices.

stercobilin *n* the brown pigment of faeces; it is formed from stercobilinogen which is derived from the bile pigments.

stercobilinogen *n* faecal urobilinogen. It is formed by bacterial action on the bile pigment bilirubin. ⇒ urobilinogen.

stereopsis *n* ability to use both eyes together for depth perception.

stereotactic radiotherapy ⇒ radiosurgery.

stereotactic surgery electrodes and cannulae are passed to a predetermined point in the brain for physiological observation or destruction of tissue—**stereotaxy** *n*.

stereotype *n* a generalization about a behaviour, individual or a group; can be the basis for prejudice.

sterile *adj* free from micro-organisms—**sterility** *n*.

sterilization *n* **1** activity that kills or removes all types of micro-organisms including spores. It is accomplished by the use of heat, radiation, chemicals or filtration. **2** rendering incapable of reproduction.

sternal puncture insertion of a special guarded hollow needle with a stylet into the body of the sternum for aspiration of a bone marrow sample.

sternoclavicular *adj* pertaining to the sternum and the clavicle.

sternocleidomastoid muscle a strap-like neck muscle arising from the sternum and clavicle, and inserting into the mastoid process of temporal bone. (⇒ Figures 4, 5). ⇒ torticollis.

sternocostal *adj* pertaining to the sternum and ribs.

sternotomy *n* surgical division of the sternum.

sternum *n* the breast bone—**sternal** *adj*. ⇒ Figure 2.

steroids *npl* a large group of organic compounds (lipids) that have a common basic chemical structure: three 6-carbon rings and a 5-carbon ring. They include: cholesterol, bile salts, vitamin D precursors, sex hormones and the corticosteroid hormones.

sterol *n* chemicals with the basic steroid structure combined with an alcohol group such as cholesterol.

stertor *n* loud snoring; sonorous breathing—**stertorous** *adj*.

stethoscope *n* an instrument used for listening to the various body sounds, especially those of the heart and chest—**stethoscopic** *adj*, **stethoscopically** *adv*.

Stevens–Johnson syndrome severe variant of the allergic response—erythema multiforme. It is an acute hypersensitivity state and can follow a viral or bacterial infection, or drugs such as long-acting sulphonamides, some anticonvulsants and some antibiotics. In some cases no cause can be found. Lung complications during the acute phase can be fatal. Mostly it is a benign condition, and there is complete recovery.

STI *abbr* sexually transmitted infection.

stigma *n* a defining feature or characteristic of a person, or an action usually viewed in a negative way by others.

stigmata *n* marks of disease, or congenital abnormalities, e.g. facies of congenital syphilis—**stigma** *sing*.

stilette *n* a wire or metal rod for maintaining patency of hollow instruments.

stillbirth *n* birth of a baby, after 24 weeks' gestation, that shows no sign of life.

stillborn *n* born dead.

Still's disease term seldom used, having been superseded by systemic onset juvenile idiopathic arthritis. ⇒ juvenile idiopathic arthritis.

stimulant *adj*, *n* stimulating. An agent which excites or increases function.

stimulant laxative ⇒ laxatives. ⇒ Appendix 5.

stimulus *n* anything which excites functional activity in an organ or part.

stitch *n* **1** a sudden, sharp darting pain or spasm in the chest wall or abdomen, usually on the lower right hand side during exertion. **2** a suture.

Stokes–Adams syndrome a fainting (syncopal) attack, commonly transient, which occurs in patients with heart block. If severe, may take the form of a convulsion, or patient may become unconscious.

stoma *n* the mouth; any opening. ⇒ colostomy, ileostomy, urostomy—**stomata** *pl*, **stomal** *adj*.

stomach *n* the most dilated part of the digestive tube, situated between the oesophagus and the duodenum (⇒ Figure 18b); it lies in the epigastric, umbilical and left hypochondriac regions of the abdomen (⇒ Figure 18a). The wall is composed of four coats: serous, muscular, submucous and mucous. It produces gastric juice containing digestive enzymes, hydrochloric acid and mucus.

stomatitis *n* inflammation of the mouth. *angular stomatitis* fissuring in the corners of the mouth consequent upon riboflavin deficiency. Sometimes misapplied to: (a) the superficial maceration and fissuring at the labial commissures in perlèche and (b) the chronic fissuring at the site in older people with loose lower lip or poorly fitting dentures. *aphthous stomatitis* recurring crops of small ulcers in the mouth. ⇒ aphthae. *gangrenous stomatitis* ⇒ cancrum oris—**stomal** *adj*.

stone *n* calculus; a hardened mass of mineral matter.

stone bruise ⇒ heel bruise.

stool *n* faeces.

stove-in chest there may be multiple anterior or posterior fractures of the ribs (causing paradoxical respiration) and fractures of sternum, or a mixture of such fractures.

strabismus *n* (*syn* squint) abnormal position of the eyes relative to each other, such that the visual axes of the two eyes fail to meet at the object of regard. *comitant (or concomitant) strabismus* consistent deviation between the eyes in all positions of gaze. *convergent strabismus* when the eyes turn inwards. *divergent strabismus* when the eyes turn outwards. *latent strabismus* deviation only present when eyes are dissociated, e.g. by converging one eye. *manifest strabismus* deviation present without dissociation.

strain *n* **1** group of micro-organisms within the same species but with different characteristics. **2** the injury to the musculotendinous (muscle and tendon) unit resulting from excessive stretch or tension during physical activity.

strangulated hernia ⇒ hernia.

strangulation *n* constriction which impedes the circulation—**strangulated** *adj*.

strangury *n* a constant painful urge to micturate.

Strassman operation a plastic operation to make a bicornuate uterus a near normal shape.

Strategic Health Authority a body responsible for strategic health planning for a geographical area with a population of many millions (e.g. the English counties of Cambridgeshire, Norfolk and Suffolk). They are also responsible for the performance management of the PCTs within that area.

strategic management the management function concerned with longer-term future strategy. Financial and resource planning. ⇒ operational management.

stratified *adj* arranged in layers.

stratum *n* a layer or lamina, e.g. the various layers of the epithelium of the skin, i.e. stratum granulosum, stratum corneum.

strawberry tongue the tongue is thickly furred with projecting red papillae. As the fur disappears the tongue is vividly red like an overripe strawberry. A characteristic of scarlet fever.

strength *n* the maximum force or torque that can be developed during maximal voluntary contraction of muscle(s).

Streptobacillus *n* a genus of Gram-negative bacteria. *Streptobacillus moniliformis* causes a type of rat-bite fever in humans.

Streptococcus *n* a genus of bacteria. Gram-positive cocci, often occurring in chains. They have varying haemolytic ability, α, β and non-haemolytic, and some types produce powerful toxins. Some streptococci are commensal in the intestinal tract (*Streptococcus faecalis*) and respiratory tract (*Streptococcus viridans*). The commensal streptococci, together with the pathogens *Streptococcus pyogenes* and *Streptococcus pneumoniae*, cause serious infections that include: tonsillitis, scarlet fever, otitis media, erysipelas, endocarditis, wound infections, pneumonia, meningitis, urinary infection. Glomerulonephritis and rheumatic fever may follow some streptococcal infections. Group B streptococcus, an intestinal and vaginal commensal, may cause meningitis, pneumonia and septicaemia in neonates infected by bacteria present in the maternal genital tract. ⇒ Griffith's typing, Lancefield's groups, necrotizing fasciitis.

streptodornase *n* a proteolytic enzyme used with streptokinase to liquefy blood clot and pus.

streptokinase *n* a streptococcal enzyme. Used with streptodornase in wound management. Plasminogen activator. Used as a fibrinolytic drug in the management of several thromboembolic conditions including acute myocardial infarction and pulmonary embolism.

streptolysins *npl* exotoxins produced by streptococci. Streptolysin antibody may be measured as an indicator of recent streptococcal infection.

Streptothrix *n* a filamentous bacterium which shows true branching. ⇒ *Streptobacillus*.

stress *n* the response of an organism to any demand made upon it by agents threatening physical or emotional well-being. Selye described such agents as stressors, which could be physical, physiological, psychological or sociocultural. Stress may be either *distress*, a negative event which has long-term effects on health when it becomes chronic, or *eustress*, a more positive event that accompanies pleasurable excitement and euphoria. *stress management* a range of measures that reduce the negative effects of stress, such as relaxation techniques, biofeedback, etc., or reducing stress, e.g. delegation. ⇒ general adaptation syndrome.

stress fracture (*syn* fatigue fracture) a bone fracture resulting from repeated loading with relatively low magnitude forces. Can be caused by a number of factors including overtraining, incorrect biomechanics, fatigue, hormonal imbalance, poor nutrition and osteoporosis.

stressors *npl* factors that cause stress responses. They may be physical, physiological, psychological and sociocultural, and include: pain, cold, trauma and blood loss, heavy workload, a life crisis such as the death of a close relative, job loss, or serious illness. ⇒ burnout.

stretch reflex a short latency reflex often used to examine spinal cord function. The stimulus is a rapid stretch of muscle and the response is a contraction of muscle that is checked by reciprocal stretch of antagonistic muscle, e.g. in the knee jerk, contraction of the quadriceps muscles (agonists) is checked by contraction of the hamstring muscles (antagonists).

striae *npl* streaks; stripes; narrow bands. Occur when the abdomen enlarges such as with obesity, tumours and pregnancy, when the marks are called *striae*

gravidarum they are red at first and then become silvery-white. Striae may also occur as a side-effect of corticosteroid therapy—**stria** *sing*, **striated** *adj*.

stricture *n* a narrowing, especially of a tube or canal, due to scar tissue or tumour.

stricturoplasty *n* surgical reconstruction of a stricture by means of a longitudinal muscle-splitting incision and transverse suture repair, e.g. for the strictures of Crohn's disease.

stridor *n* a harsh breathing sound caused by turbulent airflow through constricted air passages—**stridulous** *adj*.

stroke *n* a popular term for cerebrovascular accident. Loss of blood supply to a part of the nervous system leading to permanent damage.

stroke volume (SV) the volume of blood pumped out of the heart by each ventricular contraction.

stroma *n* the interstitial or foundation substance of a structure.

Strongyloides *n* a genus of small intestinal nematode worms, e.g. *Strongyloides stercoralis*. They infect humans (natural host), but can infect dogs. ⇒ strongyloidiasis.

strongyloidiasis *n* infestation with the nematode *Strongyloides stercoralis*. It commonly occurs in the tropics and subtropics, but may also affect immunocompromised people, such as those with AIDS. Infection usually occurs through the skin from contaminated soil, but can be through the mucosae. There may be an itchy rash at the site of larval entry. The larvae migrate through the lungs and may cause respiratory symptoms as the larvae are coughed up in sputum. Some larvae are swallowed and lead to varying abdominal symptoms, e.g. pain, diarrhoea and malabsorption, as the female worm burrows into the intestinal mucosa and submucosa. Some individuals have allergic reactions such as wheezing.

strontium (Sr) *n* a metallic element present in bone. Isotopes of strontium are used in radionuclide scanning of bone. *strontium*^{90} a radioisotope with a half-life of 28 years produced during atomic explosions. It is dangerous when it becomes integrated within bone tissue where turnover is slow.

Stryker bed a proprietary bed. Designed to allow rotation of patients to the prone or supine position. Main uses include spinal injuries and burns.

student's elbow olecranon bursitis.

Student's paired test a parametric test for statistical significance. Used to test differences in mean values for two related measurements such as those obtained from the same subject. ⇒ Wilcoxon test.

Student's t test for independent groups a parametric test for statistical significance. Used to test differences in mean values of two groups. ⇒ Mann–Whitney test.

stupor *n* a state of marked impairment of, but not complete loss of, consciousness. The victim shows a gross lack of responsiveness, usually reacting only to noxious stimuli—**stuporous** *adj*.

Sturge–Weber syndrome (*syn* naevoid amentia) a genetically determined congenital ectodermosis, i.e. a capillary haemangioma above the eye may be accompanied by similar changes in vessels inside the skull giving rise to epilepsy and other cerebral manifestations.

St Vitus' dance ⇒ chorea.

stye *n* (*syn* external hordeolum) an abscess in the follicle of an eyelash.

styloid *adj* long and pointed; resembling a pen or stylus.

styptic *n* an astringent applied to arrest bleeding.

subacute *adj* neither acute nor chronic. Often the stage between the acute and chronic phases of disease. *subacute bacterial endocarditis* ⇒ endocarditis. *subacute combined degeneration of the spinal cord* a complication of untreated pernicious anaemia (PA) and affects the posterior and lateral columns.

subacute sclerosing panencephalitis (SSPE) a rare late complication of measles with progressive and fatal loss of neurological and cognitive function due to inflammation and destruction of brain tissue.

subarachnoid haemorrhage (SAH) the loss of blood from a vessel in the brain which leaks into the subarachnoid space. This is typically due to an intracerebral aneurysm or arteriovenous malformation and can be fatal. Blood is present in the cerebrospinal fluid (CSF).

subarachnoid space the space beneath the arachnoid membrane, between it and the pia mater. It contains cerebrospinal fluid.

subcarinal *adj* below a carina, usually referring to the carina tracheae.

subclavian *adj* beneath the clavicle. *subclavian artery* ⇒ Figure 9. *subclavian vein* ⇒ Figure 10.

subclinical *adj* insufficient to cause the classical identifiable disease.

subconjunctival *adj* deep to the conjunctiva—**subconjunctivally** *adv*.

subconscious *adj, n* that part of the mind outside the range of consciousness and full awareness, but still able to affect conscious mental or physical reactions.

subcostal *adj* beneath the rib.

subcutaneous *adj* beneath the skin—**subcutaneously** *adv*. *subcutaneous oedema* is demonstrable by the 'pitting' produced by pressure of the finger. *subcutaneous tissue* ⇒ Figure 12.

subdural *adj* beneath the dura mater; between the dura and arachnoid membranes.

subdural haematoma (SDH) the accumulation of blood beneath the dura lining the skull that can occur after head trauma. It develops slowly and may present as a space-occupying lesion with vomiting, papilloedema, fluctuating level of consciousness, weakness, usually hemiplegia on the opposite side to the clot. Finally there is a rise in blood pressure and a fall in pulse rate.

subendocardial *adj* immediately beneath the endocardium.

subhepatic *adj* beneath the liver.

subinvolution *n* failure of the gravid uterus to return to its normal size within a normal time after childbirth. ⇒ involution.

subjective *adj* internal; personal; arising from the senses and not perceptible to others. ⇒ objective *opp*.

sublimate *n* a solid deposit resulting from the condensation of a vapour.

sublimation *n* a mental defence mechanism whereby undesirable basic instinctive drives are unconsciously redirected to, and expressed through, personally approved and socially accepted behaviour, such as aggression redirected to sporting activity.

subliminal *adj* inadequate for perceptible response. Below the threshold of consciousness. ⇒ liminal.

sublingual *adj* beneath the tongue.

subluxation *n* incomplete dislocation of a joint.

submandibular *adj* below the mandible.

submaxillary *adj* below the maxilla.

submucosa *n* the layer of connective tissue beneath a mucous membrane—**submucous, submucosal** *adj*.

submucous *adj* beneath a mucous membrane. *submucous resection (SMR)* surgical correction of a deviated nasal septum.

suboccipital *adj* beneath the occiput; in the nape of the neck.

subperiosteal *adj* beneath the periosteum of bone.

subphrenic *adj* beneath the diaphragm.

subpoena *n* a court order requiring a person to appear as a witness (subpoena ad testificandum) or to bring documents/records (subpoena duces tecum).

substrate *n* chemical upon which a specific enzyme is active.

subsultus *n* muscular tremor. *subsultus tendinum* twitching of tendons and muscles particularly around the wrist in severe fever, such as typhoid.

subungual *adj* under a nail. *subungual exostosis* a small outgrowth of bone under the nail plate near to, or immediately distal to the free edge. It often affects the hallux of young people, and causes considerable pain. The nail becomes elevated and displaced from the nail bed. Radiographic examination is required for an accurate diagnosis. *subungual heloma (corn)* the development of a corn or keratinized lesion under the nail plate. It is a small yellowish-grey area and may occur on any part of the nail bed. It detaches the nail from the nail bed.

succussion *n* **1** splashing sound produced by fluid in a hollow cavity when the patient moves, e.g. liquid content of dilated stomach in pyloric stenosis. **2** a term in homeopathy. It describes the vigorous shaking of natural diluted substances.

sucrase *n* intestinal enzyme that converts sucrose to glucose and fructose.

sucrose *n* a disaccharide that is hydrolysed into glucose and fructose during digestion. It occurs naturally in sugar and is added to many manufactured foods. Frequent consumption of sucrose causes dental disease.

sudamina *n* sweat rash.

Sudan blindness ⇒ onchocerciasis.

sudden infant death syndrome (SIDS) (*syn* cot death) the unexpected sudden death of an infant, usually occurring overnight while sleeping in a cot, but may occur under other situations. The commonest mode of death in infants between the ages of 1 month and 1 year, neither clinical nor postmortem findings being adequate to account for death. Overheating, sleeping in the prone position, respiratory illness and infection, and being in an environment where people smoke have all been implicated as risk factors. Parents/carers are now recommended to put babies to sleep on their backs, at the foot of the cot to prevent them wriggling under bedclothes, not to overheat the room, not to smoke in the same room and seek advice from a health professional if the baby seems unwell.

sudor *n* sweat—**sudoriferous** *adj*.

sudorific *adj*, *n* (*syn* diaphoretic) describes an agent which induces sweating.

suggestibility *n* abnormal vulnerability to suggestion. May be increased in individuals who have dependence on others such as those in hospital and people with learning disability.

suggestion *n* the implanting in a person's mind of an idea which he or she accepts fully. In psychology suggestion may be used as a therapeutic measure during hypnosis.

suicide *n* intentional taking of one's own life. Usually related to depression and hopelessness. Attitudes to suicide are culturally determined, and stigma may be present in some communities. ⇒ deliberate self-harm, parasuicide.

sulcus *n* a furrow or groove, particularly those separating the gyri (convolutions) of the cerebral cortex—**sulci** *pl*.

sulphaemoglobin *n* (*syn* sulphmethaemoglobin) a sulphide oxidation product of haemoglobin, produced in vivo by certain drugs. It cannot transport oxygen or carbon dioxide, and not being reversible in the body, is an indirect poison.

sulphaemoglobinaemia *n* a condition of circulating sulphaemoglobin in the blood.

sulphate salt of sulphuric acid, e.g. magnesium sulphate.

sulphonamides *npl* a group of bacteriostatic antibacterial agents. They inhibit the formation of folic acid, which is needed for bacterial metabolism. ⇒ Appendix 5.

sulphones *npl* a group of synthetic antileprotic drugs, related to sulphonamides. ⇒ Appendix 5.

sulphonylureas *npl* a group of oral hypoglycaemic drugs derived from sulphonamides. ⇒ Appendix 5.

sulphur *n* an insoluble yellow powder. Used in topical preparations and baths for acne and other skin disorders.

sulphuric acid inorganic acid. Highly corrosive.

sunstroke *n* ⇒ heatstroke.

supercilium *n* the eyebrow—**superciliary** *adj*.

superego *n* one of the three main aspects of the personality (the others being the ego and id); part of the mind concerned with moral sanctions, inhibitions and self criticism; it functions at a partly conscious, but mostly unconscious level. Roughly equates to the 'conscience'.

superficial *adj* near the surface such as the superficial veins of the leg. *superficial bursitis* (*syn* Haglund's bumps, pump bumps, heel bumps, winter heel, and calcaneal (retro calcaneal) exostosis) an adventitious bursa found superficial to the insertion of the Achilles tendon. It is a common condition and mainly affects adolescent females. It is not seen in later life.

superinfection *n* infection that follows the elimination of the normal flora by antibiotic usage. This permits other micro-organisms, such as *Clostridium difficile*, to thrive in the intestine without competition from micro-organisms of the normal flora. ⇒ pseudomembranous colitis, *Pseudomonas*.

superior *adj* in anatomy, the upper of two parts—**superiorly** *adj*.

supernumerary *adj* in excess of the normal number; additional. *supernumerary bones* these include os trigonum, os tibial externum and os vesalii. Such abnormalities of sesamoid bones and supernumerary bones rarely directly cause problems in the paediatric foot but may result in soft tissue lesions. Their presence is confirmed radiographically. *supernumerary digits* ⇒ polydactyly.

superoxide ⇒ free radical.

supinate *vt* turn or lay face or palm upward ⇒ pronate *opp*—**supination** *n*.

supinator *n* that which supinates, usually applied to a muscle. ⇒ pronator *opp*.

supine *adj* **1** lying on the back with face upwards. **2** of the hand with palm upwards. ⇒ prone *opp*.

suppository *n* medicament in a base that melts at body temperature. Administered rectally.

suppression *n* **1** in psychology, a mental defence mechanism, whereby people voluntarily force difficult or painful thoughts out of the mind; it can precipitate mental health problems. **2** cessation of a secretion (e.g. urine) or a normal process (e.g. menstruation).

suppuration *n* the formation of pus—**suppurative** *adj*, **suppurate** *vi*.

supraclavicular *adj* above the clavicle.

supracondylar *adj* above a condyle. *supracondylar fracture* one affecting the lower end of the femur or humerus. The latter may interfere with the blood supply to the forearm. ⇒ Volkmann's ischaemic contracture.

supraorbital *adj* above the orbits. *supraorbital ridge* the ridge covered by the eyebrows.

suprapubic *adj* above the pubis.

suprarenal *adj* above the kidney. ⇒ adrenal.

suprasternal *adj* above the sternum.

supraventricular *adj* above the ventricles. Usually used to define an arrhythmia such as tachycardia originating in the atrial tissue. ⇒ Wolff–Parkinson–White syndrome.

surfactant *n* a mixture of phospholipids secreted by type II pneumocytes. It reduces surface tension in the alveoli, allows lung inflation and prevents alveolar collapse between breaths. ⇒ neonatal respiratory distress syndrome, pneumocytes.

surgery *n* that branch of medicine which treats diseases, deformities and injuries, wholly or in part, by manual or operative procedures.

surgical *adj* pertaining to surgery. *surgical emphysema* air in the subcutaneous tissue planes following the trauma of surgery or injury.

surgical dressings ⇒ wound dressings.

surrogate *n* a substitute for an object or person. *surrogate motherhood* where a woman agrees to have a child for an infertile couple. Surrogacy is allowed in the UK, but women may only receive reasonable financial expenses. There are, however, many informal arrangements for surrogacy.

survey *n* a data collection method. Includes: interview, postal, telephone, or via the internet.

susceptibility *n* the opposite of resistance. Includes a state of reduced capacity to deal with infection.

suspensory ligaments supporting or suspending such as that supporting the lens. ⇒ Figure 15.

suture *n, v* 1 the junction of cranial bones. 2 in surgery, a stitch or series of stitches used to appose the edges of a surgical or traumatic wound. Also describes the placement of such stitches. ⇒ ligature.

S v̄O₂ *abbr* mixed venous oxygen saturation.

swab *n* 1 a small piece of cotton wool or gauze. 2 a small piece of sterile cotton wool, or similar material, on the end of a shaft of plastic, wire or wood, inside protecting tube. It is used to collect material for microbiological examination.

swallowing *n* deglutition. Part voluntary and part involuntary activity with three stages: oral (buccal), pharyngeal and oesophageal. ⇒ dysphagia.

sweat *n* the secretion from the sweat (sudoriferous) glands. Contains water, electrolytes (mainly sodium and chloride) and waste. Sweat production is primarily concerned with temperature regulation but has a small excretory role. *sweat gland* ⇒ Figure 12, apocrine glands, eccrine.

sweat test used to measure the amount of sodium and chloride in sweat, to confirm a diagnosis of cystic fibrosis. The drug pilocarpine is introduced into the skin by iontophoresis to stimulate the sweat glands and induce sweating. The sweat is collected and tested.

sycosis barbae (*syn* barber's itch) a pustular folliculitis of the beard area in men.

sycosis nuchae a folliculitis at the nape of the neck which leads to keloid thickening (acne keloid).

symbiosis *n* a relationship between two or more organisms in which the participants are of mutual aid and benefit to one another. ⇒ antibiosis *opp*—**symbiotic** *adj*.

symblepharon *n* adhesion of the lid to the eyeball.

sympathetic nervous system part of the peripheral nervous system (PNS), it describes a division of the autonomic nervous system (ANS). It is composed of a chain of ganglia on either side of the vertebral column and nerve fibres having thoracolumbar outflow. It opposes the parasympathetic nervous system and is usually involved with body stimulation. Its action is augmented by adrenaline (epinephrine) and noradrenaline (norepinephrine).

sympathectomy *n* surgical excision of part of the sympathetic nervous system.

sympatholytic *n* an antagonist. A drug which impedes or opposes the effects of the sympathetic nervous system. ⇒ alpha (α)-adrenoceptor antagonists, beta (β)-adrenoceptor antagonists.

sympathomimetic *adj* an agonist. Producing effects similar to those produced by stimulation of the sympathetic nerves. ⇒ alpha (α)-adrenoceptor agonists, beta (β)-adrenoceptor agonists.

symphysis *n* a fibrocartilaginous union of bones such as the symphysis pubis—**symphyseal** *adj*.

symptom *n* a subjective phenomenon or manifestation of disease—**symptomatic** *adj*. *symptom complex* a group of symptoms which, occurring together, typify a particular disease or syndrome.

symptomatology *n* 1 the branch of medicine concerned with symptoms. 2 the combined symptoms typical of a particular disease.

Synacthen test ⇒ tetracosactide (Synacthen) test.

synapse *n* the gap between the axon of one neuron and the dendrites of another, or the gap between the axon and a gland or muscle. Most operate chemically but a few are electrical. The synapse permits the passage of an impulse across the gap. This is achieved chemically by the release of calcium ions and a neurotransmitter such as acetylcholine.

synapsis *n* during meiosis the pairing of homologous chromosomes.

synchronized intermittent mandatory ventilation (SIMV) mode of positive pressure ventilation in which the timing of the breaths is varied according to the patient's own respiratory effort.

synchysis scintillans cholesterol crystals in the vitreous of the eye, often following vitreous haemorrhage.

syncope *n* (*syn* faint) literally, sudden loss of strength. Caused by reduced cerebral circulation often following a fright, when vasodilation is responsible. May be symptomatic of cardiac arrhythmia, e.g. heart block.

syncytium *n* a mass of tissue with several nuclei. Boundaries between individual cells are absent or poorly defined.

syndactyly, syndactylism, syndactylia *n* (*syn* webbed toes, zygodactyly) a term applied to a total or partial fusion of adjacent digits. It is very common, usually bilateral and often familial. Multiple syndactyly occurs in hands and feet associated with other anomalies, as in Apert's syndrome, an autosomal dominant disorder–acrocephalosyndactyly. Treatment is not required for webbing of the toes—**syndactylous** *adj*.

syndrome *n* a group of symptoms and/or signs which, occurring together, produce a pattern or symptom complex, typical of a particular disease.

syndrome of inappropriate ADH secretion (SIADH) syndrome in which excessive antidiuretic hormone leads to water retention and low serum sodium.

synechia *n* abnormal union of structures, especially adhesion of the iris to the cornea in front, or the lens capsule behind—**synechiae** *pl*.

synergism, synergy *n* the harmonious working together of two agents, such as drugs, micro-organisms, muscles, etc.—**synergistic** *adj*.

synergist *n* an agent cooperating with another.

synergistic action that brought about by the cooperation of two or more muscles, neither of which could bring about the action alone.

synkinesis *n* the ability to carry out precision movements.

synovectomy *n* excision of synovial membrane.

synovial fluid the fluid secreted by the membrane lining a freely movable joint cavity.

synovial membrane ⇒ membrane.

synovioma *n* a tumour of synovial membrane—benign or malignant.

synovitis *n* inflammation of a synovial membrane.

synthesis *n* the process of compiling complex substances from less complex ones by chemical reactions—**synthetic** *adj*.

syphilide *n* a syphilitic skin lesion.

syphilis *n* a sexually transmitted infection caused by the spirochaete *Treponema pallidum* (ssp. *pallidum*). It may be congenital or acquired. *acquired syphilis* is contracted during sexual intercourse with an infected person. There are two main stages: (a) early, characterized by a primary lesion (chancre) at the site of entry into the body that heals within about one month, and may be followed by a generalized illness (secondary syphilis) characterized by a skin rash, fever, generalized lymph node enlargement, mucosal ulcers (snail track); (b) late (that may occur many years after the infection) with skin or visceral lesions (gumma), neurosyphilis (tabes dorsalis and general paralysis of the insane), or cardiovascular syphilis (including aneurysm formation in the ascending aorta). In many individuals there may be no clinical signs of syphilis (latent syphilis), the diagnosis being made on the basis of positive serological tests for *T. pallidum*. *congenital syphilis* the spirochaete is transmitted from mother to fetus via the placenta. The affected infant may exhibit characteristic features that include a generalized rash, generalized lymphadenopathy and hepatitis.

syringe *n* a device for injecting, instilling or withdrawing fluids. Consists of a cylindrical barrel to one end of which a hollow needle is attached, and a close-fitting plunger. *syringe driver* medical device for the continuous delivery of drugs intravenously or subcutaneously. Commonly used in palliative care to control symptoms including pain.

syringomyelia *n* an uncommon, progressive disease of the spinal cord of unknown cause, beginning mainly in early adult life. Cavitation and surrounding fibrous tissue reaction, in the upper spinal cord, interferes with sensation of pain and temperature, and sometimes with the motor pathways. The characteristic symptom is painless injury, particularly of the hands. Touch sensation is typically intact in the early stages. ⇒ Charcot's joint.

syringomyelocele *n* the most severe form of meningeal hernia (spina bifida). The central canal is dilated and the thinned-out posterior part of the spinal cord is in the hernia.

syrinx *n* a cyst-like cavity in the spinal cord.

systematic desensitization a technique that utilizes classical conditioning to treat anxiety disorders and phobias. ⇒ conditioning, desensitization.

systematic review a systematic approach to literature reviews of both published and unpublished material that lessens bias and random errors.

Système International d'Unités (SI) (International System of Units) system of measurement used for scientific, technical and medical purposes. There are seven base units: ampere, candela, kelvin, kilogram, metre, mole and second, and various derived units, e.g. pascal, becquerel, etc. ⇒ Appendix 2.

systemic circulation oxygenated blood leaves the left ventricle and, after flowing throughout the body, returns deoxygenated to the right atrium.

system for identifying motivated abilities (SIMA) a self-explanatory term. The tests are especially useful in diagnosing the level of mental deterioration.

systemic inflammatory response syndrome (SIRS) generalized inflammatory response, which may be triggered by a range of processes (e.g. poor perfusion). Features include; abnormal temperature, altered white cell count, increased respiratory rate and increased heart rate. SIRS and multiple organ dysfunction syndrome frequently occur together in critically ill patients.

systemic lupus erythematosus (SLE) a connective tissue disease where autoantibodies cause effects in many parts of the body, e.g. sun-exposed skin, lungs, heart and blood vessels, kidneys and joints. The aetiology is multifactorial. There may be skin changes with a typically butterfly-shaped facial rash, alopecia, pyrexia, pleurisy, pericarditis, alveolitis, arthritis and renal damage.

systemic sclerosis a multisystem connective tissue disease. The most characteristic features are scleroderma (thickening of the skin) and Raynaud's phenomenon. Most internal organs are affected.

systole *n* the contraction phase of the cardiac cycle, as opposed to diastole—**systolic** *adj*.

systolic murmur a cardiac murmur occurring between the first and second heart sounds due to valvular disease, e.g. mitral systolic murmur.

T

T₃ *abbr* **triiodothyronine.**

T₄ *abbr* **thyroxine.**

tabes *n* wasting away—**tabetic** *adj*. *tabes dorsalis* a variety of neurosyphilis characterized by a staggering gait and 'lightning' limb pains. ⇒ Charcot's joint, locomotor ataxia.

tabetic gait ⇒ gait.

taboo *n* a behaviour forbidden by individual societies, such as incest.

taboparesis *n* a form of neurosyphilis in which there are clinical features of both brain and spinal cord involvement.

tachycardia *n* excessively rapid action of the heart at rest (in excess of 100 beats per minute in adults). *paroxysmal tachycardia* a temporary but sudden marked increase in frequency of heart beats, because the conducting stimulus is originating in an abnormal focus.

tachyphasia *n* extreme rapidity of speech.

tachypnoea *n* abnormal frequency of respiration—**tachypnoeic** *adj*.

tactile *adj* relating to the sense of touch.

Taenia *n* a genus of flat, parasitic worms; cestodes or tapeworms. *Taenia saginata* larvae present in infested, undercooked beef. In the human (the definitive host) intestinal lumen they develop into the adult tapeworm, which by its four suckers attaches itself to the gut wall. *Taenia solium* has hooklets as well as suckers. The larvae are ingested in infested, undercooked pork; humans can also be the intermediate host for this worm by ingesting eggs, which develop into larvae in the stomach and pass via the intestinal wall to reach organs where they develop into cysts. In the brain these may cause seizures. ⇒ cysticercosis, cysticercus, *Echinococcus*.

taenia *n* a flat band. *taenia coli* three flat bands running the length of the large intestine and consisting of the longitudinal muscle fibres.

taeniacide *n* an agent that destroys tapeworms—**taeniacidal** *adj*.

talipes *n* any of a number of deformities of the foot and ankle. *talipes calcaneovalgus* a condition usually caused by intrauterine posture. The foot has been fixed in an upturned position with the sole against the uterine wall. Improvement and usually complete recovery occurs with active movement after birth. *talipes equinovarus* the heel is drawn up, the foot inverted and the hindfoot adducted—in the equinovarus position.

talus *n* the astragalus; situated between the tibia proximally and the calcaneus distally, thus directly bearing the weight of the body. It is the second largest bone of the ankle.

tampon *n* a plug used in the nose, vagina or other orifice to absorb blood or secretions. *tampon shock syndrome* ⇒ toxic shock syndrome.

tamponade *n* insertion of a tampon. ⇒ cardiac tamponade.

tapeworm *n* cestodes. They include *Taenia saginata* (beef tapeworm), *Taenia solium* (pork tapeworm) and *Diphyllobothrium latum* (fish tapeworm). Dogs and cats are the definitive host for the tapeworm *Dipylidium caninum*, which may cause human disease. ⇒ *Taenia*.

tapotement *n* (*syn* tapping) massage manipulations in which the hands strike, or percuss, the body alternately and rhythmically; used to eliminate secretions, as in postural drainage, and in an invigorating massage. It may involve: beating with loosely clenched fists, clapping using clapped hands and producing a deep-toned sound, hacking using the ulnar (little finger side) borders of the hands and fingers, and pounding with the ulnar sides of loosely clenched fists.

tapping *n* **1** ⇒ aspiration. **2** ⇒ tapotement.

tardive dyskinesia abnormal movements. Repeated involuntary movements of the face, trunk and limbs. Associated with the long-term use of typical neuroleptic drugs, particularly the phenothiazines.

target zone (*syn* training zone) the use of heart rate ranges to indicate the intensity of effort required during exercise programmes.

tarsal coalition (peroneal spastic flat foot) an anomaly in which adjacent tarsal bones are fused together. Fusion may be bony or cartilaginous. The most common occurs between the calcaneus and the navicular with union across the mid-tarsal joint. Talocalcaneal coalition also occurs.

tarsalgia *n* pain in the foot.

tarsometatarsal *adj* relating to the tarsal and metatarsal region.

tarsorrhaphy *n* suturing of the lids together.

tarsus *n* **1** the seven small bones of the foot (⇒ Figure 2). **2** the dense connective tissue found in each eyelid, contributing to its form and support—**tarsal** *adj*.

tartar *n* ⇒ calculus.

task *n* an autonomous, purposeful, component part of an activity.

taste *n* gustation. A chemical sense closely linked with smell. *taste buds* sensory receptors found on the tongue, epiglottis and pharynx.

Tay–Sachs disease (*syn* gangliosidosis) inherited lipid storage disease in which GM_2 ganglioside (carbohydrate-rich sphingolipid) accumulates within the nervous system. It is due to a deficiency of the enzyme β-N-acetylhexosaminidase and results in mental deterioration, blindness and death. The gene responsible is most commonly carried by individuals of Ashkenazic Jewish origins.

TB *abbr* tuberculosis.

TBI *abbr* ⇒ total body irradiation.

TCA *abbr* tricyclic antidepressants.

T cell ⇒ lymphocyte.

TCRE *abbr* transcervical resection of endometrium.

tears *npl* the secretion produced by the lacrimal gland. Tears contain the bactericidal enzyme lysozyme.

technetium (Tc) *n* a radioactive element. The isotope ^{99m}Tc derived from molybdenum is used in radionuclide imaging (scans).

teething *n* lay term for the discomfort during the eruption of the primary dentition in babies.

tegument *n* the skin or covering of the body.

telangiectasis *n* dilatation of small blood vessels.

telemetry *n* the electronic transmission of data including clinical measurement between distant sites. May be used for cardiac monitoring.

teletherapy *n* treatment with a radiation source that is distant from the patient such as cobalt–60 or X-rays—**teletherapeutic** *adj*, **teletherapeutically** *adv*.

telomeres *npl* protective regions of DNA at the ends of chromosomes that become shorter with age. Normally they stop chromosomal damage during cell division, but with increasing age the telomeres no longer function properly. Results eventually in genetic damage and cell death. ⇒ apoptosis.

temperament *n* the usual mental attitude of the person.

temple *n* that part of the head situated between the outer angle of the eye and the top of the pinna.

temporal *adj* relating to the temple. *temporal bones* one on each side of the skull below the parietal bone, containing the middle ear.

temporal arteritis also known as giant cell arteritis. Occurs in older people and mainly affects the external carotid artery and its branches, e.g. the temporal artery supplying the scalp. Blindness can ensue if there is thrombosis of the ophthalmic vessels. Early treatment with corticosteroids is effective.

temporomandibular *adj* relating to the temporal region or bone, and the lower jaw, such as the joint between the temporal bone and mandible.

temporomandibular joint (TMJ) syndrome pain in the region of the temporomandibular joint frequently caused by malocclusion of the teeth, resulting in malposition of the condylar heads in the joint and abnormal muscle activity, and by bruxism.

TEN *acron* toxic epidermal necrolysis.

Tenckhoff catheter commonest form of peritoneal dialysis catheter.

tendinitis *n* inflammation of a tendon.

tendon *n* a band of white, fibrous connective tissue that joins muscle to bone—**tendinous** *adj*.

tenesmus *n* painful, ineffectual straining to empty the bowel or bladder.

tenoplasty *n* a reconstructive operation on a tendon—**tenoplastic** *adj*.

tenorrhaphy *n* the suturing of a tendon.

tenosynovitis *n* inflammation of the thin synovial lining of a tendon sheath, as distinct from its outer fibrous sheath. It may be caused by mechanical irritation or by bacterial infection.

tenotomy *n* division of a tendon.

TENS *acron* transcutaneous electrical nerve stimulation.

tensile force force applied along the fibres of a tissue. Excessive tensile forces cause a tearing of the tissues as they are stretched beyond their normal length.

tentorium cerebelli a fold of dura mater between the cerebellum and cerebrum. Damage during birth may result in intracranial bleeding.

TEPP *abbr* tetraethyl pyrophosphate.

teratogen *n* anything capable of disrupting embryonic/fetal growth and producing malformation. Classified as drugs, poisons, radiations, physical agents such as ECT, infections, e.g. rubella and Rhesus and thyroid antibodies—**teratogenic, teratogenetic** *adj*, **teratogenicity, teratogenesis** *n*.

teratology *n* the scientific study of teratogens and their mode of action—**teratological** *adj*, **teratologist** *n*, **teratologically** *adv*.

teratoma *n* commonly a tumour of the testis or ovary. It is of embryonic origin and usually malignant. Some testicular tumours have both seminoma and teratoma components. The cure rate for germ cell tumours has increased 10-fold with use of platinum-based chemotherapy—**teratomata** *pl*, **teratomatous** *adj*.

termination of pregnancy (TOP) ⇒ abortion.

tertian *adj* recurring every 48 hours such as the fever in some types of malaria.

tertiary *adj* third in order. *tertiary care* highly specialized healthcare services accessed through indirect referral via secondary care. Deals usually with uncommon or rare conditions. The specialized hospital care is provided by a regional or national centre, e.g. spinal injuries, certain cancers. *tertiary prevention* ⇒ disease prevention.

testicle *n* ⇒ testis—**testicular** *adj*.

testis *n* a male gonad. One of the two glandular structures contained in the scrotum of the male (⇒ Figure 16); they produce spermatozoa and the male sex hormones. *undescended testis* the testis remains within the bony pelvis or inguinal canal. ⇒ cryptorchism—**testes** *pl*.

testosterone *n* the major androgen, a steroid hormone produced by the testes. It is responsible for the development of the male secondary sexual characteristics and reproductive functioning.

test-tube baby one produced by in vitro fertilization.

tetanus *n* **1** (*syn* lockjaw) disease caused by the bacterium *Clostridium tetani*, an anaerobic spore-forming micro-organism present in the intestine of domestic animals and humans, commonly found in soil, dust and manure. It produces a powerful exotoxin that affects the motor nerves causing muscle spasms, rigidity and convulsions. Active immunization with tetanus toxoid (TT) is available as part of routine programmes, as regular booster doses and when risk is increased. Tetanus immunoglobulin is available for passive immunization. ⇒ opisthotonos, risus sardonicus, trismus—**tetanic** *adj*. **2** in the contraction of muscle, the summation that increases the force of contraction by increasing the frequency of stimulation to the maximum to produce a sustained contraction.

tetany *n* condition of muscular hyperexcitability in which mild stimuli produce cramps and muscle spasms in the hands and feet (carpopedal spasm). It is due to a reduction in ionized calcium levels, for example as a result of alkalosis from hyperventilation or alkali ingestion, or hypoparathyroidism. ⇒ Chvostek's sign, Trousseau's sign.

tetracosactide (Synacthen) test a test of adrenocortical function. Adrenocortical insufficiency is indicated if the plasma cortisol concentration fails to rise following an intramuscular injection of tetracosactide (an ATCH analogue).

tetracyclines *npl* a group of broad spectrum antibiotics. Problems associated with the tetracyclines include superinfection with gastrointestinal disturbances, bacterial resistance and vitamin B deficiency. They are also deposited in teeth and bone and should not be prescribed for pregnant or lactating women, or for children because they can lead to discoloration of the second dentition and bone abnormalities. ⇒ Appendix 5.

tetradactylous *adj* having four digits on each limb.

tetraethyl pyrophosphate (TEPP) organophosphorous compound used as a commercial insecticide. Toxicity results from its powerful and irreversible anticholinesterase action.

tetralogy of Fallot ⇒ Fallot's tetralogy.

tetraplegia *n* (*syn* quadriplegia) paralysis of all four limbs—**tetraplegic** *adj*.

thalamotomy *n* usually operative (stereotaxic) destruction of a portion of thalamus. Can be done for intractable pain.

thalamus *n* a collection of grey matter at the base of the cerebrum. Sensory impulses from the whole body pass through the thalamus en route to the cerebral cortex—**thalami** *pl*, **thalamic** *adj*.

thalassaemia *n* a group of inherited haemoglobinopathies in which mutation or deletion of one or more globin genes results in an imbalance in the production of α and β globin molecules. Because it affects the deformability of the red cell, this imbalance leads to increased red cell breakdown and a failure of bone marrow red cell precursors to produce fully mature erythrocytes. This in turn leads to anaemia, the severity of which depends on the nature of the genetic defect. *beta thalassaemia* results most often from genetic mutations in the β globin genes. If both copies of the gene are affected (patient is homozygous for a mutation), a severe, transfusion-dependent anaemia, with jaundice and hepatosplenomegaly may result (beta thalassaemia major). By contrast, in the carrier (heterozygous) state where only one copy of the gene is mutated, there is often only a mild asymptomatic anaemia. The situation with *alpha thalassaemia* is more complex as there are four α globin genes, and the severity of alpha thalassaemia varies from asymptomatic, if only one gene is affected, to usually fatal in utero if four genes are affected (hydrops fetalis). Persons with three affected genes have so-called haemoglobin H disease and are often transfusion dependent.

thanatology *n* the scientific study of death, including its cause and diagnosis.

theca *n* an enveloping sheath, especially of a tendon, or the dura mater—**thecal** *adj*.

thenar *adj* relating to the palm (hand) and the sole (foot). *thenar eminence* the palmar eminence below the thumb.

therapeutic abortion ⇒ abortion.

therapeutic index an indicator of the difference between the therapeutic dose of a drug and a dose that causes toxicity. It can vary between individuals.

therapeutics *n* the branch of medicine concerned with the treatment of disease states—**therapeutic** *adj*, **therapeutically** *adv*.

therapy *n* treatment of a range of psychological or physical conditions. ⇒ occupational therapy, physiotherapy, speech and language therapy.

thermal *adj* pertaining to heat.

thermistor *n* a device used to detect very small changes in temperature.

thermogenesis *n* the production of heat—**thermogenetic** *adj*.

thermography *n* an investigation that detects minute temperature differences over different body areas by use of an infrared thermograph that is sensitive to radiant heat. The uses include the study of blood flow and detection of cancers, such as breast cancer.

thermolabile *adj* capable of being easily changed or destroyed by heat.

thermolysis *n* heat-induced chemical dissociation. Dissipation of body heat—**thermolytic** *adj*.

thermometer *n* an instrument for measuring temperature—**thermometric** *adj*. ⇒ clinical thermometer.

thermostable *adj* unaffected by heat. Remaining unaltered at a high temperature, which is usually specified—**thermostability** *n*.

thermotherapy *n* heat treatment. ⇒ hyperthermia.

thiamin(e) *n* a member of the vitamin B complex. It is concerned in carbohydrate, fat and alcohol metabolism. Deficiency causes beri-beri, mental confusion or cardiomyopathy. ⇒ Korsakoff's psychosis/syndrome, Wernicke's encephalopathy.

thiazide diuretics a group of diuretics that act on the first part of the distal tubule of the nephron. They reduce sodium and chloride reabsorption, which increases the amount of water, sodium and chloride excreted. ⇒ Appendix 5.

Thiersch skin graft ⇒ skin graft.

thoracentesis *n* aspiration of the pleural cavity.

thoracic *adj* pertaining to the thorax. *thoracic aorta* ⇒ Figure 9. *thoracic nerve* ⇒ Figure 11. *thoracic cage* framework of bones that protects the thoracic structures and provides muscle attachments. *thoracic duct* a channel conveying lymph (chyle) from the cisterna chyli in the abdomen to the left subclavian vein. *thoracic inlet syndrome* (*syn* cervical rib) a supernumerary rib in the cervical region, which may present no symptoms or it may press on nerves of the brachial plexus.

thoracoplasty *n* an operation on the thorax in which the ribs are resected to allow the chest wall to collapse and the lung to rest; previously used in the treatment of tuberculosis. Since the advent of antituberculous drugs it is extremely rare.

thoracoscope *n* an instrument which can be inserted into the pleural cavity through a small incision in the chest wall, to permit inspection of the pleural surfaces and division of adhesions by electric diathermy—**thoracoscopic** *adj*, **thoracoscopy** *n*.

thoracotomy *n* surgical exposure of the thoracic cavity.

thorax *n* the chest cavity—**thoracic** *adj*.

threadworm *n* Enterobius vermicularis. Tiny thread-like nematode worm that infests the intestine. ⇒ enterobiasis.

threatened abortion ⇒ miscarriage.

threonine *n* an essential (indispensable) amino acid.

thrill *n* vibration as perceived by the sense of touch.

thrombectomy *n* surgical removal of a thrombus from within a blood vessel.

thrombin *n* the active enzyme formed from prothrombin. Thrombin is formed during both the extrinsic and intrinsic coagulation pathways; it converts fibrinogen to fibrin. ⇒ coagulation, prothrombin, thromboplastin.

thromboangiitis *n* clot formation within an inflamed vessel. *thromboangiitis obliterans* ⇒ Buerger's disease.

thromboarteritis *n* inflammation of an artery with clot formation.

thrombocyte *n* (*syn* platelet) plays a part in the clotting of blood. ⇒ blood.

thrombocythaemia *n* a condition in which there is an increase in circulating blood platelets, which can encourage clotting within blood vessels. ⇒ myeloproliferative disorders, thrombocytosis.

thrombocytopenia *n* a reduction in the number of platelets in the blood, which can result in spontaneous bruising and prolonged bleeding after injury—**thrombocytopenic** *adj*.

thrombocytosis *n* an increase in the number of platelets in the blood. It may arise in reaction to infection, bleeding, inflammation or malignancy or may indicate the presence of a bone marrow disorder.

thromboembolic *adj* describes the phenomenon whereby a thrombus or clot detaches itself and is carried to another part of the body in the bloodstream to block a blood vessel there. ⇒ deep vein thrombosis, pulmonary embolus.

thromboendarterectomy *n* removal of a thrombus and atheromatous plaques from an artery.

thromboendarteritis *n* inflammation of the inner lining of an artery with clot formation.

thrombogenic *adj* capable of clotting blood—**thrombogenesis, thrombogenicity** *n*, **thrombogenically** *adv*.

thrombokinase *n* ⇒ thromboplastin.

thrombolytic *adj* pertaining to disintegration of a blood clot—**thrombolysis** *n*. *thrombolytic therapy* the attempted removal of preformed intravascular fibrin occlusions using fibrinolytic drugs, such as alteplase and streptokinase.

thrombophilia *n* an inherited or acquired tendency to develop venous thrombosis. ⇒ factor V Leiden.

thrombophlebitis *n* inflammation of the wall of a vein with secondary thrombosis within the involved segment—**thrombophlebitic** *adj*. *thrombophlebitis migrans* recurrent episodes of thrombophlebitis affecting short lengths of superficial veins: deep vein thrombosis is uncommon and pulmonary embolism rare.

thromboplastin *n* (*syn* thrombokinase) a substance released from damaged tissue to start the extrinsic coagulation pathway. *activated partial thromboplastin time (APTT)* a test of coagulation ability. *intrinsic thromboplastin* produced by the interaction of several factors during coagulation. More active than *tissue thromboplastin*, factor III of blood coagulation, which interacts with other factors in the formation of a fibrin clot.

thrombosis *n* the unwanted, intravascular formation of a blood clot—**thromboses** *pl*, **thrombotic** *adj*. ⇒ coronary thrombosis, deep vein thrombosis.

thromboxanes *npl* regulatory lipids derived from arachidonic acid (fatty acid). They are released from platelets and cause vasospasm and platelet aggregation during platelet plug formation. ⇒ haemostasis.

thrombus *n* an intravascular blood clot—**thrombi** *pl*.

thrush *n* ⇒ candidiasis.

thymectomy *n* surgical excision of the thymus gland.

thymocytes *npl* cells found in the dense lymphoid tissue of the thymus gland—**thymocytic** *adj*.

thymoma *n* a tumour arising in the thymus—**thymomata** *pl*.

thymopoietin *n* peptide hormone secreted by the thymus gland.

thymosin *n* peptide hormone secreted by the thymus gland.

thymus *n* a lymphoid gland lying behind the sternum and extending upward as far as the thyroid gland. It is well developed in infancy and attains maximum size during puberty; and then the lymphatic tissue is replaced by fatty tissue. It produces thymic hormones (thymosins and thymopoietin) that ensure the proper development of T lymphocytes. The autoimmune condition myasthenia gravis results from pathology of the thymus gland—**thymic** *adj*.

thyrocalcitonin *n* ⇒ calcitonin.

thyroglobulin *n* a colloid stored in the thyroid follicles used for the production of thyroxine.

thyroglossal *adj* pertaining to the thyroid gland and the tongue. *thyroglossal cyst* a retention cyst caused by blockage of the thyroglossal duct: it appears on one or other side of the neck. *thyroglossal duct* the embryonic passage from the thyroid gland to the back of the tongue. In this area thyroglossal cyst or fistula can occur.

thyroid *adj* pertaining to the thyroid gland. *thyroid antibody test* the presence and severity of autoimmune thyroid disease is diagnosed by the levels of thyroid-stimulating immunoglobulins in the blood. *thyroid cartilage* ⇒ Figure 6. *thyroid gland* a two-lobed endocrine gland, either side of the trachea. It secretes three hormones: triiodothyronine (T_3) and thyroxine (T_4) under pituitary control, which stimulate metabolism, and calcitonin from the follicular cells, which helps to regulate calcium and phosphate homeostasis. ⇒ hyperthyroidism, hypothyroidism. *thyroid-stimulating hormone (TSH)* pituitary hormone that stimulates the secretion of the thyroid hormones thyroxine and triiodothyronine. *thyroid-stimulating hormone assay* radioimmunoassay of the level of thyroid-stimulating hormone in the serum. Used in the diagnosis of hypothyroidism.

thyroidectomy *n* surgical removal of part or the whole of the thyroid gland.

thyroiditis *n* inflammation of the thyroid gland; can occur postpartum, following viral infection (De Quervain's), or due to autoimmune diseases. ⇒ Hashimoto's disease, Riedel's thyroiditis.

thyrotoxic crisis dramatic, sudden worsening of symptoms in a patient with hyperthyroidism; may occur immediately after thyroidectomy if the patient is insufficiently prepared prior to surgery.

thyrotoxicosis ⇒ hyperthyroidism.

thyrotrophic *adj* (describes) any substance that stimulates the thyroid gland, e.g. thyrotrophin (thyroid-stimulating hormone, TSH) secreted by the anterior pituitary gland.

thyroxine (T_4) *n* the principal hormone of the thyroid gland, it contains four atoms of iodine. It is essential for metabolism and development. Used in the treatment of hypothyroidism. ⇒ triiodothyronine.

TIA *abbr* transient ischaemic attack.

tibia *n* the shin bone; the larger of the two bones in the lower part of the leg; it articulates with the femur, fibula and talus. ⇒ Figures 2, 3.

tibial *adj* relating to the tibia, as in the artery and vein. ⇒ Figures 9, 10.

tibiofibular *adj* pertaining to the tibia and the fibula.

tic *n* purposeless involuntary, spasmodic muscular movements and twitchings, due partly to habit, but may be associated with a psychological factor.

tic douloureux (trigeminal neuralgia) spasms of excruciating pain in the distribution of the trigeminal nerve.

tick *n* a blood-sucking parasite, larger than a mite. Some of them are involved in the transmission of relapsing fever, typhus, etc.

tidal air/volume (TV) the volume of air that passes in and out of the lungs in normal breathing.

Tietze syndrome costochondritis. A self-limiting condition of unknown aetiology. There is no specific treatment. Differential diagnosis is myocardial infarction.

tinea *n* (*syn* ringworm) a fungal infection of the skin, hair or nails caused by a variety of dermatophytes: *Trichophyton, Epidermophyton* and *Microsporum*. Usually named for the area of the body affected, i.e. *tinea barbae*, the beard area; *tinea capitis*, the head; *tinea corporis* (circinata), the body; *tinea cruris* (dhobie itch), the groin; *tinea pedis*, the foot (athlete's foot); *tinea unguium*, the nails.

tine test a multiple puncture test using disposable equipment. The plastic holder has four small tines coated with undiluted tuberculin. The reaction is read in 48–72 h using a grading system.

tinnitus *n* an abnormal perception of buzzing, thumping or ringing sounds in the ears.

tissue *n* a collection of cells or fibres of similar function, forming a structure, often in a background stroma. *tissue plasminogen activator (t-PA)* a substance that activates plasminogens. *tissue respiration* ⇒ respiration.

titration *n* volumetric analysis using standard solutions to determine the concentration of a substance in solution.

titre *n* a standard of concentration per volume, as determined by titration. Unit of measure used to assess antibody concentration in serum.

TIVA *abbr* total intravenous anaesthesia.

TLS *abbr* tumour lysis syndrome.

TMJ *abbr* temporomandibular joint syndrome.

TNF *abbr* tumour necrosis factor.

TNM classification *abbr* tumour, node (lymph) and metastasis. ⇒ staging.

tobacco amblyopia toxic amblyopia.

tocography *n* process of recording uterine contractions using a tocograph or a parturiometer.

tocolytics *npl* a group of drugs that relax uterine muscle. They have a restricted role in the inhibition of preterm labour. ⇒ beta (β)-adrenoceptor agonists. ⇒ Appendix 5.

tocopherols *npl* group of chemicals with vitamin E activity which includes the important α-tocopherols. They are widely distributed in many foods and function as important antioxidants in biological membranes.

tocotrienols *npl* a group of chemicals that have vitamin E activity. They have similar biological action to tocopherols but are less potent.

tolerance *n* ability to endure the application or administration of a substance, usually a drug. ⇒ drug tolerance. *exercise tolerance* exercise undertaken without marked dyspnoea or pain. American Heart Association's classification of functional capacity: Class I—no symptoms with ordinary effort; Class II—slight disability with ordinary effort (usually subdivided into Class IIa—able to carry on with normal housework under difficulty—and Class IIb—cannot manage shopping or bed-making except very slowly); Class III—marked disability with ordinary effort which precludes any attempt at housework; Class IV—symptoms at rest or heart failure.

tomography *n* a technique of using X-rays to create an image of a specific, thin layer through the body (rather than the whole body)—**tomographic** *adj*, **tomogram** *n*, **tomograph** *n*, **tomographically** *adv*.

tone *n* a quality of sound, or the normal, healthy state of tension.

tongue *n* the mobile muscular organ situated in the mouth; it is concerned with mastication, swallowing, taste and speech. ⇒ strawberry tongue.

tonic *adj* used to describe a state of continuous muscular contraction, as opposed to intermittent contraction.

tonography *n* continuous measurement of blood, or intraocular, pressure. *carotid compression tonography* normally occlusion of one common carotid artery causes an ipsilateral fall of intraocular pressure. Used as a screening test for carotid insufficiency.

tonometer *n* an instrument for measuring intraocular pressure.

tonsillectomy *n* surgical removal of the palatine tonsils. *tonsillectomy position* the three-quarters prone position to prevent inhalation (aspiration) pneumonia and asphyxiation.

tonsillitis *n* inflammation of the tonsils.

tonsilloliths *npl* concretions arising in the body of the tonsil.

tonsillopharyngeal *adj* relating to the tonsils and pharynx.

tonsils *npl* small aggregations of lymphoid tissue located around the pharynx. Forming part of body defences they contain macrophages and are a site for lymphocyte proliferation. There are *lingual tonsils* under the tongue, *nasopharyngeal tonsils* located on the posterior wall of the nasopharynx (called adenoids when enlarged) and the *palatine tonsils* found in the oropharynx, one on each side in the fauces between the palatine arch—**tonsillar** *adj*. ⇒ Waldeyer's ring.

tooth *n* hard calcified structures in the mouth used for masticating food. Composed largely of dentine with enamel covering the crown and cementum covering the root surface. The pulp occupies the cavity at the core of the crown (pulp chamber) and the channel running along the length of the root (root canal). The primary (deciduous, milk) and secondary (permanent, adult) dentitions consist of 20 and 32 teeth, respectively—**teeth** *pl*. ⇒ canine tooth, Hutchinson's teeth, incisor tooth, molar tooth, premolar tooth, wisdom tooth.

TOP *abbr* termination of pregnancy.

tophus *n* a small, hard concretion forming on the ear lobe, on the joints of the phalanges, etc. in gout—**tophi** *pl*.

topical *adj* describes the local application of drugs to skin and mucous membrane—**topically** *adv*.

topography *n* a description of the regions of the body—**topographical** *adj*, **topographically** *adv*.

torsion *n* twisting. *torsion of the testis* twisting of the structures supporting the testis. The blood supply is disrupted and can result in testicular infarction.

torticollis *n* (*syn* wryneck) a painless contraction of one sternocleidomastoid muscle. The head is slightly flexed and drawn towards the contracted side, with the face rotated over the other shoulder.

total body irradiation (TBI) a treatment used in the treatment of some cancers, e.g. haemopoietic tissue. Usually carried out before a bone marrow transplant.

total intravenous anaesthesia (TIVA) general anaesthetic produced with intravenous drugs only and no gases.

total parenteral nutrition (TPN) ⇒ parenteral feeding.

total quality management (TQM) a whole organization approach to quality where all employees are expected to take responsibility for quality. It aims to ensure quality at every interface and improve effectiveness and flexibility throughout the organization.

Tourette's syndrome a disorder where affected individuals use obscene language and make rude gestures.

tourniquet *n* an apparatus for the compression of the blood vessels of a limb. Designed for compression of a main artery to control bleeding. It is also often used to obstruct the venous return from a limb and so facilitate the withdrawal of blood from a vein. Tourniquets vary from a simple rubber band to a pneumatic cuff.

Townsend index composite index of deprivation in the population. Sum of the standardized values of the percentages of households without cars, households not owner-occupied, overcrowded and unemployed in an electoral ward. The components (socio-economic variables) are drawn from census information.

toxaemia *n* a generalized poisoning of the body by the products of bacteria or damaged tissue—**toxaemic** *adj*.

toxic *adj* poisonous, caused by a poison. *toxic epidermal necrolysis (TEN)* a syndrome in which the appearance is of scalded skin with scaling, rash and hyperpigmentation. It can occur in response to adverse drug reactions, staphylococcal infection, systemic illness, and may be idiopathic. *toxic shock syndrome (TSS)* (*syn* tampon shock syndrome), a potential but rare complication of tampon use, but it does occur in non-menstruating women and men. It is caused by the toxins of the bacterium *Staphylococcus aureus* found at various sites including the perineal area in healthy people. Bacterial contamination of the tampon occurs and the bacteria multiply within the vagina. The bacterial toxins enter the bloodstream and cause pyrexia, vomiting and diarrhoea, rash, and sometimes life-threatening hypovolaemic shock.

toxicity *n* the quality or degree of being poisonous.

toxicology *n* the science dealing with poisons, their mechanisms of action and antidotes to them—**toxicological** *adj*, **toxicologically** *adv*.

toxin *n* a poison, usually bacterial that damages or kills cells. ⇒ endotoxin, exotoxin.

Toxocara *n* genus of nematode roundworm of the dog and cat, e.g. *Toxocara canis*. Humans can be infested. ⇒ toxocariasis.

toxocariasis *n* infestation with *Toxocara*. Infestation occurs by eating with hands contaminated from affected animals, especially puppies. The ova can exist for several months in soil contaminated by infected faeces from dogs or cats. Because the worms cannot develop properly in humans (incorrect host) the larvae move through the body before dying. This can lead to problems in the liver and the eye: fever, hepatomegaly and possible blindness.

toxoid *n* a toxin altered in such a way that it has lost its poisonous properties but retained its antigenic properties. *toxoid antitoxin* a mixture of toxoid and homologous antitoxin in floccule form, used as a vaccine, e.g. in immunization against diphtheria.

Toxoplasma a genus of protozoon, e.g. *Toxoplasma gondii*. The definitive host is the domestic cat and other felines and rodents are the intermediate host. It can cause serious infections in humans and other mammals, e.g. sheep. ⇒ toxoplasmosis.

toxoplasmosis *n* infection with *Toxoplasma gondii*. Infected animals contaminate the environment with faeces containing cysts. Human infection occurs through environmental contact, such as gardening, playing and cleaning cat litter trays, or by contacting infected animals, or by eating undercooked meat. Most infections are symptomless or may cause a mild illness with tiredness and myalgia. There is serious disease in immunocompromised individuals, e.g. AIDS patients, who develop encephalitis and eye involvement. It is possible to be infected from a donated organ during transplant surgery. Primary toxoplasmosis during pregnancy can lead to the disease being passed to the fetus via the placenta. This is extremely serious and can lead to stillbirth or an infant with problems such as microcephaly or hydrocephaly, convulsions, or liver damage, thrombocytopenia and purpura or eye involvement. Infants who survive may have learning disability and develop encephalitis, liver cirrhosis and blindness.

TPN *abbr* total parenteral nutrition.

trabeculae *npl* the septa or fibrous bands projecting into the interior of an organ, e.g. the spleen—**trabecula** *sing*, **trabecular** *adj*.

trabeculectomy *n* operation used to reduce intraocular pressure by creating a drainage channel from the anterior chamber of the eye to the subconjunctival space.

trabeculotomy *n* operation for congenital glaucoma. Creation of a channel from the canal of Schlemm into the anterior chamber.

trace elements elements that are present in very small amounts in the tissues and known to be essential for normal metabolism (e.g. copper, cobalt, manganese, fluorine).

tracer *n* a substance or instrument used to gain information. Radioactive tracers are used in the diagnosis of some cancers, e.g. brain, and thyroid disease.

trachea *n* (*syn* windpipe) the fibrocartilaginous tube lined with ciliated mucosa passing from the larynx to the bronchi (⇒ Figure 6). It is about 115 mm long and about 25 mm wide—**tracheal** *adj*.

tracheitis *n* inflammation of the trachea; most commonly the result of a viral infection such as the common cold.

trachelorrhaphy *n* operative repair of a uterine cervical laceration.

tracheobronchial *adj* pertaining to the trachea and the bronchi.

tracheobronchitis *n* inflammation of the trachea and bronchi. ⇒ bronchitis.

tracheo-oesophageal *adj* pertaining to the trachea and the oesophagus. *tracheo-oesophageal fistula* usually occurs in conjunction with oesophageal atresia. The fistula usually connects the distal oesophagus to the trachea.

tracheostomy *n* surgical opening between the front of the neck and the trachea to create an artificial airway. It is kept open with a tracheostomy tube—**tracheostome** *n*.

tracheotomy *n* vertical slit in the anterior wall of the trachea at the level of the third and fourth cartilaginous rings.

trachoma *n* an eye disease caused by infection with *Chlamydia trachomatis*, which is transmitted by flies. It is common in communities with sparse water and therefore poor facial hygiene. It is characterized by a chronic, scarring, follicular conjunctivitis which may lead to corneal scarring and blindness. Infection occurs through contact, during birth when a baby may become infected from vaginal secretions, or from unhygienic use of personal articles. Also called trachoma inclusion conjunctivitis (TRIC)—**trachomatous** *adj*.

traction *n* a drawing or pulling on the patient's body to overcome muscle spasm and to reduce or prevent deformity. A steady pulling exerted on some part (limb or head) by means of weights, pulleys and cords in conjunction with a variety of splints or frames. *skeletal traction* applied on a bone by means of a wire or pin passed through the lower fragment. *skin traction or extension* involves the application of weights to foam or extension plaster attached to the skin. ⇒ beam, Braun's frame, hoop traction, halopelvic traction.

tractotomy *n* incision of a nerve tract. Surgical relief of intractable pain, using stereotactic measures.

tragus *n* the projection in front of the external auditory meatus—**tragi** *pl*.

trait *n* an individual physical or mental characteristic which is inherited or develops.

training *n* in sports medicine describes a deliberate scheme or programme to assist learning and/or improve fitness. The four principles of training are: specificity, individual differences, overload and reversibility. Training programmes will vary depending on the nature of the sport being trained for and the goals to be achieved.

trance *n* a term used for hypnotic sleep and for certain self-induced hysterical stuporous states.

tranquillizers *npl* drugs that relieve anxiety or deal with psychotic symptoms without excessive sedation. ⇒ anxiolytics, neuroleptics (antipsychotics). ⇒ Appendix 5.

transabdominal *adj* through the abdomen—**transabdominally** *adv.*

transactional analysis a form of psychotherapy based on the theory that interrelationships between people can be analysed in terms of transactions with each other as representing 'child', 'adult' and 'parent'. The aim is to give the adult ego decision-making power over the child and parent egos.

transaminases ⇒ aminotransferases.

transamniotic *adj* through the amniotic membrane and fluid, as a transamniotic transfusion of the fetus for haemolytic disease.

transcervical resection of endometrium (TCRE) a hysteroscopic procedure of removing the endometrium in cases of menorrhagia.

transcription *n* first stage in protein synthesis where genetic information is transferred from DNA to mRNA. ⇒ translation.

transcutaneous *adj* through the skin, for example monitoring, e.g. oxygen saturation by pulse oximetry, or drug absorption.

transcutaneous electrical nerve stimulation (TENS) a method of non-invasive pain control using pads placed either side of the spine to apply a mild electric current from a battery-operated device, which can be controlled by the patient for pain relief. Used for the control of chronic pain symptoms.

transdermal *adj* through the skin. A drug administration system using patches, creams and gels. Thus drugs delivered in this way, e.g. hormone replacement, avoid first pass metabolism in the liver.

transducer *n* device that converts one form of energy into another to facilitate its electrical transmission.

transection *n* the cutting across or mechanical severance of a structure.

transfer RNA (tRNA) ⇒ ribonucleic acid.

transferrin *n* a protein that binds iron for safe transport in the blood.

transfrontal *adj* through the frontal bone; an approach used for hypophysectomy.

transfusion *n* the introduction of fluid into the tissue or into a blood vessel. *blood transfusion* the intravenous replacement of lost or destroyed blood by compatible citrated human blood. Also used for severe anaemia with deficient blood production. Fresh blood from a donor or stored blood from a blood bank may be used. It can be given 'whole', or as plasma-depleted blood (packed-cell transfusion). If incompatible blood is given, severe reaction follows. ⇒ blood groups. *intrauterine transfusion* of the fetus endangered by Rhesus incompatibility. Red cells are transfused directly into the abdominal cavity of the fetus, on one or more occasions. This enables the induction of labour to be postponed until a time more favourable to fetal welfare.

transient ischaemic attack (TIA) a brief loss of neurological function as a result of a disturbance of blood supply that lasts for minutes to hours.

transillumination *n* the transmission of light through the sinuses for diagnostic purposes.

translation *n* the second stage of protein synthesis in which tRNA and rRNA translate the base sequence required to make a new protein. ⇒ transcription.

translocation *n* transfer of a chromosomal segment to a different site on the same chromosome (shift) or to a different chromosome. Can be a cause of congenital abnormality.

translucent *adj* in between transparent and opaque.

translumbar *adj* through the lumbar region. Route used for injecting aorta prior to aortography.

transmethylation *n* a process in which methyl groups are donated by amino acids and transferred to other compounds.

transmigration *n* ⇒ diapedesis.

transmural *adj* through the wall, e.g. of an organ etc.—**transmurally** *adv.*

transnasal *adj* through the nose—**transnasally** *adv.*

transonic *adj* allowing the passage of ultrasound.

transperitoneal *adj* across or through the peritoneal cavity. ⇒ dialysis, laparoscopy.

transplacental *adj* through the placenta—**transplacentally** *adv.*

transplant *n* customarily refers to the surgical operation of grafting an organ, which has been removed from a cadaver that has been declared brain dead, or from a living relative. If the recipient's malfunctioning organ is removed and the transplant is placed in its bed, it is referred to as an *orthotopic transplant* (e.g. liver and heart). If the transplanted organ is not placed in its normal anatomical site the term *heterotopic transplant* is used—**transplantation** *n*, **transplant** *vt.*

transplantation *n* ⇒ graft.

transrectal *adj* through the rectum. *transrectal ultrasonography (TRUS)* method used to perform an ultrasound examination of the prostate—**transrectally** *adv.*

trans-sphenoidal *adj* through the sphenoid bone; an approach used for hypophysectomy.

transthoracic *adj* across or through the chest, as in transthoracic needle biopsy of a lung mass.

transudate *n* a fluid that has passed out of the cells either into a body cavity (e.g. ascitic fluid in the peritoneal cavity) or to the exterior (e.g. serum from the surface of a burn).

transurethral *adj* through the urethra. ⇒ prostatectomy.

transvaginal *adj* through the vagina—**transvaginally** *adv.*

transventricular *adj* through a ventricle. Term used mainly in cardiac surgery—**transventricularly** *adv.*

transverse colon ⇒ Figure 18b.

transverse plane a horizontal plane that divides the body into superior and inferior parts. Also called the horizontal plane.

transvesical *adj* through the urinary bladder—**transvesically** *adv.*

trapezius large muscle of the neck and thorax (⇒ Figures 4, 5).

trauma *n* bodily injury—**traumatic** *adj.* ⇒ post-traumatic stress disorder.

traumatologist *n* a doctor or nurse who specializes in traumatology.

traumatology *n* the branch of medicine dealing with injury—**traumatological** *adj*, **traumatologically** *adv.*

Trematoda *n* a class of parasitic flukes which include many human pathogens such as the *Schistosoma* of schistosomiasis.

tremor *n* rhythmic movement disorder that can affect any part of the body but typically the hands and which can be seen in Parkinson's disease. *intention tremor* a type of tremor that becomes manifest as the hand approaches the target, typically seen in disease of the cerebellum.

trench foot (*syn* immersion foot) occurs in frostbite or other conditions of exposure when local blood supply is impaired and secondary bacterial infection is present.

Trendelenburg's position lying on an operating or examination table, with the head lowermost and the legs raised.

Trendelenburg's sign a test of the stability of the hip, and particularly of the ability of the hip abductors (gluteus medius and minimus) to steady the pelvis upon the femur. Normally, when one leg is raised from the ground the pelvis tilts upwards on that side, through the hip abductors of the standing limb. If the abductors are inefficient (e.g. in poliomyelitis, severe coxa vara and developmental dysplasia of the hip), they are unable to sustain the pelvis against the body weight and it tilts downwards instead of rising.

trephine *n* an instrument with sawlike edges for removing a circular piece of tissue, such as the cornea or skull.

Treponema *n* a genus of slender spiral-shaped bacteria that are actively motile. Best visualized with dark-ground illumination. Cultivated in the laboratory with great difficulty. *Treponema carateum* causes pinta; *Treponema pallidum* causes syphilis; *Treponema pertenue* causes yaws.

Treponema pallidum haemagglutination assay (TPHA) *n* a specific serological test for syphilis and other treponemal diseases.

treponematosis *n* any treponemal diseases.

treponemicide *n* lethal to *Treponema*—**treponemicidal** *adj.*

Trexler isolator a flexible film, negative pressure, bed isolator for dangerous infections such as viral haemorrhagic disease.

triacylglycerol *n* triglyceride.

triage *n* a system of priority classification of patients in any emergency situation.

TRIC *abbr* trachoma inclusion conjunctivitis. ⇒ trachoma.

triceps *n* the three-headed muscle on the back of the upper arm (⇒ Figures 4, 5).

trichiasis *n* abnormal ingrowing eyelashes.

Trichinella a genus of parasitic nematode worms, e.g. *Trichinella spiralis* a parasite of pigs and rats that causes human disease. ⇒ trichinosis.

trichinosis *n* also called trichiniasis. Caused by eating undercooked pork infected with *Trichinella spiralis* (the trichina worm). The female worms in the small intestine produce larvae which invade the body and, in particular, form cysts in skeletal muscles; usually causes diarrhoea, nausea, colicky pain, fever, facial oedema, muscle pains and stiffness.

trichomonacide *n* an agent that is lethal to the protozoa belonging to the genus *Trichomonas*.

Trichomonas *n* a genus of motile protozoan parasites; e.g. *Trichomonas vaginalis* causes vaginitis in females and urethral infection in males. The organism is easily recognized by wet microscope preparations of the discharge. ⇒ trichomoniasis.

trichomoniasis *n* inflammation of the vagina (urethra in males) caused by the protozoan *Trichomonas vaginalis*.

Trichophyton *n* a genus of fungi affecting the skin and nails.

trichophytosis *n* infection with a species of the fungus *Trichophyton*, e.g. ringworm of the hair or skin.

trichuriasis *n* infestation with *Trichuris trichiura*. Infestation occurs from ingesting contaminated soil or food. Usually produces few symptoms but heavy infestation may cause blood-stained diarrhoea.

Trichuris *n* a genus of nematode worms. *Trichuris trichiura* (whipworm). ⇒ trichuriasis.

tricuspid *adj* having three cusps. *tricuspid valve* the right atrioventricular valve of the heart.

tricyclic antidepressants a group of antidepressant drugs. They act by inhibiting the uptake of the neurotransmitters serotonin (5-hydroxytryptamine) and noradrenaline (norepinephrine). ⇒ Appendix 5.

trigeminal *adj* triple; separating into three sections, e.g. the trigeminal nerve, the fifth cranial nerve, which has three branches, ophthalmic, maxillary and mandibular. *trigeminal neuralgia* ⇒ tic douloureux.

trigger finger a condition in which the finger can be actively bent but cannot be straightened without help; usually due to tenosynovitis of the flexor tendon sheath resulting in thickening or nodules which prevent free gliding.

trigger point a hypersensitive fibrous band of tissue.

triglyceride *n* triacylglycerol. A lipid with three fatty acids and a glycerol molecule. The major source of stored energy in the body.

trigone *n* a triangular area, especially applied to the bladder base, bounded by the ureteral openings at the back and the urethral opening at the front—**trigonal** *adj*.

triiodothyronine (T$_3$) *n* a thyroid hormone that plays a part in maintaining the body's metabolic processes. It contains three iodine atoms and is formed from thyroxine.

trimester *n* a period of 3 months. Applied especially to pregnancy.

triple antigen ⇒ triple vaccine.

triple test blood test offered to pregnant women. It measures alphafetoprotein, unconjugated oestriol and total hCG in maternal serum and is used early in pregnancy to predict the estimated risk of conditions such as Down's syndrome. ⇒ amniocentesis, chorionic villus sampling.

triple vaccine contains diphtheria, tetanus and pertussis antigens. Offered as part of a routine immunization programme.

triploid *adj* possessing three chromosomal sets (3n). ⇒ genome, haploid, polyploidy.

trismus *n* spasm in the muscles of mastication such as that occurring in tetanus.

trisomy *n* the presence of three chromosomes where normally they would be paired. Results in an increase in the chromosome number by one (single trisomy), e.g. to 47 in humans. *trisomy 18* ⇒ Edward syndrome. *trisomy 21* ⇒ Down's syndrome.

trocar *n* a pointed rod which fits inside a cannula.

trochanters *npl* two processes, the larger one (greater *trochanter*) on the outer, the other (lesser *trochanter*) on the inner side of the femur between the neck and shaft; they provide attachment for muscles—**trochanteric** *adj.*

trochlea *n* any part which is like a pulley in structure or function—**trochlear** *adj.*

trochlear nerves the fourth pair of cranial nerves. They innervate the muscle that moves the eyeball in an outwards and downward direction.

trophic *adj* pertaining to nutrition.

trophoblast *n* cells covering the embedding ovum and concerned with the nutrition of the ovum, invasion of the endometrium and secretion of hCG—**trophoblastic** *adj.*

tropia *n* manifest strabismus. May be used as a suffix.

tropical sprue chronic malabsorption of unknown aetiology occurring in residents or visitors to tropical regions.

tropomyosin *n* one of the proteins located in the thin filaments of a muscle myofibril.

troponin *n* one of the proteins present in a muscle myofibril. ⇒ cardiac enzymes.

Trousseau's sign a test for latent tetany. Spasm of the forearm muscle is observed, within 3–4 minutes of inflating a cuff on the upper arm to a pressure above the systolic blood pressure. ⇒ carpopedal spasm, Chvostek's sign.

Trypanosoma *n* a genus of parasitic protozoa. Their life cycle alternates between blood-sucking arthropods and vertebrate hosts. A limited number of species are pathogenic to humans. ⇒ trypanosomiasis.

trypanosomiasis *n* disease caused by infection with *Trypanosoma*. In Africa these include: *Trypanosoma rhodesiense* or *Trypanosoma brucei gambiense*. Both are transmitted by the bite of infected tsetse flies. The disease caused by *T. brucei gambiense* is usually chronic. Central nervous system involvement causes headache, confusion, insomnia, daytime sleepiness and eventual coma and death. ⇒ sleeping sickness. Infection with *T. rhodesiense* is more acute, with myocarditis, hepatitis, pleural effusion and central nervous system involvement that leads to coma, tremors and death. In South America, trypanosomiasis is also known as Chagas' disease. It is

caused by *Trypanosoma cruzi* transmitted by bugs.

trypsin *n* active proteolytic enzyme. ⇒ trypsinogen.

trypsinogen *n* inactive form of trypsin secreted by the pancreas. Activated by enterokinase (enteropeptidase).

tryptophan *n* one of the essential (indispensable) amino acids necessary for growth. It is a precursor of serotonin. Nicotinamide is synthesized from tryptophan.

tsetse fly a fly of the genus *Glossina*, the vector of *Trypanosoma* in Africa. The *Trypanosoma* are transferred to new hosts, including humans, in the salivary juices when the fly bites for a blood meal.

TSS *abbr* toxic shock syndrome.

tubal *adj* pertaining to a tube. *tubal abortion* ⇒ miscarriage. *tubal ligation* tying of both uterine (fallopian) tubes as a means of sterilization. *tubal pregnancy* ⇒ ectopic pregnancy.

tubercle *n* **1** a small rounded prominence, usually on bone. **2** the specific lesion produced by *Mycobacterium tuberculosis*.

tuberculide, tuberculid *n* a small lump. Metastatic manifestation of tuberculosis, producing a skin lesion, e.g. papulonecrotic tuberculide, rosacea-like tuberculide.

tuberculin *n* a sterile extract of either old tuberculin or refined purified protein derivative (PPD) formed from *Mycobacterium tuberculosis*. Utilized in skin testing for tuberculosis or before administration of BCG. ⇒ Heaf test, Mantoux reaction.

tuberculoid *adj* resembling tuberculosis. One of the two types of leprosy.

tuberculoma *n* a caseous tubercle, usually large, its size suggesting a tumour.

tuberculosis (TB) *n* chronic granulomatous infection caused by *Mycobacterium tuberculosis* (human type). Incidence, especially of multidrug resistant tuberculosis (MDR-TB) is increasing, in Asia and Africa, in association with poverty and homelessness, and in those who are immunocompromised. Bovine tuberculosis is endemic in cattle and transmitted to humans by drinking infected milk. Pasteurization of milk and monitoring of dairy herds are the mainstays of disease control. *M. avium intracellulare (MAI)* is an atypical mycobacterium, which may infect severely immunocompromised individuals (such as those with advanced AIDS). Tuberculosis causes systemic effects such as pyrexia, night sweats and weight loss, plus those dependent upon the site, e.g. cough in lung disease, haematuria in renal TB.

tuberosity *n* a bony prominence.

tuberous sclerosis (*syn* epiloia) an inherited disorder characterized by cognitive defects, skin lesions and epilepsy.

tubo-ovarian *adj* pertaining to or involving both tube and ovary, e.g. tubo-ovarian abscess.

tubule *n* a small tube. *collecting tubule* straight tube in the kidney medulla conveying urine to the renal pelvis. *convoluted tubule* coiled tube in the kidney cortex. *renal tubule* part of a nephron. *seminiferous tubule* coiled tube in the testis.

tularaemia *n* (*syn* deer-fly fever, rabbit fever, tick fever) an infection of mammals and birds caused by the bacterium *Francisella tularensis*; transmitted by bites from ticks and flies. Humans acquire the infection either from ticks or from handling infected animal carcasses, such as rabbits. Skin ulceration at the inoculation site is followed by painful lymphadenopathy and fever with constitutional upset. Rarely it causes septicaemia and complications that include pneumonia—**tularaemic** *adj.*

tumescence *n* a state of swelling; turgidity.

tumor *n* swelling; usually used in the context of being one of the five classical signs and symptoms of inflammation, the others being calor, dolor, loss of function and rubor.

tumour *n* a swelling. A mass of abnormal tissue which resembles the normal tissues in structure, but which fulfils no useful function and which grows at the expense of the body. Benign, simple or innocent tumours are encapsulated, do not infiltrate adjacent tissue or cause metastases and are unlikely to recur if removed—**tumorous** *adj. malignant tumour* not encapsulated, infiltrates adjacent tissue and causes metastases. ⇒ cancer.

tumour lysis syndrome (TLS) may occur following intensive chemotherapy treatment for some haematological malignancies. As cancer cells are destroyed there is release of cellular breakdown products. This results in metabolic problems (e.g.

hyperkalaemia, hypocalcaemia, hyperuricaemia, hyperphosphataemia) that may cause renal failure and possibly circulatory and respiratory failure.

tumour marker chemical detected in the serum that may be associated with a specific cancer or sometimes nonmalignant diseases. They include: alphafetoprotein, Ca-125, carcinoembryonic antigen and prostate specific antigen. They may be used for monitoring disease progress and efficacy of treatment, but are of limited use for population screening.

tumour necrosis factor (TNF) a cytokine that is toxic to cancer cells and activates other leucocytes. It causes profound metabolic effects that include inflammatory responses, pyrexia and weight loss.

tunica *n* a lining membrane; a coat. *tunica adventitia* the outer coat of an artery or vein. *tunica intima* the lining of an artery or vein. *tunica media* the middle muscular coat of an artery or vein.

TUR/TURP *abbr* transurethral resection of prostate.

turbinate *adj* shaped like an inverted cone. *turbinate bone* three on either side forming the lateral nasal walls. Also called nasal conchae.

turbinectomy *n* removal of a nasal turbinate bone.

turf toe a colloquial expression used in sports medicine to describe the sprain and subsequent inflammation of the first metatarsophalangeal joint.

turgid *adj* swollen; firmly distended, as with blood by congestion—**turgescence** *n*, **turgidity** *n*.

Turner syndrome a condition of multiple congenital abnormalities in females, with infantile genital development, webbed neck, cubitus valgus and, often, aortic coarctation. The ovaries are almost completely devoid of germ cells and there is failure of pubertal development. Subjects with Turner syndrome have a single sex chromosome, the X, and thus only 45 chromosomes in their body cells.

tussis *n* a cough.

tylosis *n* ⇒ keratosis.

tympanic *adj* pertaining to the tympanum. *tympanic membrane* (eardrum) separates the outer from the middle ear. *tympanic thermometer* accurate body temperature recorded by means of an electronic probe introduced into the external auditory canal.

tympanites, tympanism *n* (*syn* meteorism) abdominal distension due to accumulation of gas in the intestine.

tympanoplasty *n* reconstructive operation on the middle ear designed to improve hearing or prevent otorrhoea in ears damaged by chronic suppurative otitis media—**tympanoplastic** *adj*.

tympanum *n* the cavity of the middle ear.

type I error (α error) in research, rejecting a null hypothesis that is true.

type II error (β error) in research, not rejecting a null hypothesis that is false.

typhoid fever an infectious enteric fever usually spread by contamination of food, milk or water supplies with *Salmonella typhi*, either directly by sewage, indirectly by flies or by faulty personal hygiene. Symptomless carriers harbouring the micro-organism in the gallbladder and excreting it in faeces are the main source of outbreaks of disease in the UK. The average incubation period is 10–14 days. A progressive febrile illness marks the onset of the disease, which develops as the micro-organism invades lymphoid tissue, including that of the small intestine (Peyer's patches), to profuse diarrhoeal (pea soup) stools which may become frankly haemorrhagic; ultimate recovery usually begins at the end of the third week. A rose-coloured rash may appear on the upper abdomen and back at the end of the first week. Immunization is available for travellers to regions where the infection is endemic. ⇒ paratyphoid.

typhus *n* an acute infectious disease characterized by high fever, a skin eruption and severe headache. It is a disease of war, famine or catastrophe, being spread by lice, ticks or fleas. It is only sporadic in Britain. Epidemic typhus is caused by the rickettsia *Rickettsia prowazekii*. ⇒ rickettsial fevers.

tyramine *n* an amine present in several foodstuffs, especially cheese, meat and vegetable extracts. It has a similar effect in the body to adrenaline (epinephrine); consequently patients taking drugs in the monoamine oxidase inhibitor (MAOI) group should not eat foods containing tyramine such as cheese, otherwise a dangerously high blood pressure may result.

tyrosine *n* a conditionally essential (indispensable) amino acid required for growth. Combines with iodine to form the hormone thyroxine. If phenylalanine intake is restricted, as in phenylketonuria (PKU), the diet needs supplementing with tyrosine.

tyrosinosis *n* due to abnormal metabolism of tyrosine: excess parahydroxyphenylpyruvic acid is excreted in the urine.

U

ulcer *n* destruction of either mucous membrane or skin from whatever cause, producing a crater or indentation. An inflammatory reaction occurs and if it penetrates a blood vessel bleeding ensues. If the ulcer is in the lining of a hollow organ it can perforate through the wall.

ulcerative *adj* pertaining to or of the nature of an ulcer. *ulcerative colitis* superficial inflammatory condition affecting the colon. It always involves the rectum and spreads continuously for a variable distance. Long-standing disease predisposes to colorectal cancer. ⇒ colitis, inflammatory bowel disease.

ulcerogenic *adj* capable of producing an ulcer.

Ullrich syndrome ⇒ Noonan syndrome.

ulna *n* the inner bone of the forearm. ⇒ Figure 2.

ulnar *adj* pertaining to the ulna as in artery, vein and nerve ⇒ Figures 9, 10, 11.

ultrafiltration *n* filtration under pressure; e.g. in haemofiltration where the blood is filtered under pressure.

ultrasonic *adj* relating to mechanical vibrations of very high frequency.

ultrasonography *n* formation of a visible image from the use of ultrasound. A controlled beam of sound is directed into the relevant part of the body. The reflected ultrasound is used to build up an electronic image of the various structures of the body. Routinely offered during pregnancy to monitor progress and detect fetal and placental abnormalities. ⇒ ultrasound. *diagnostic ultrasonography* information is derived from echoes which occur when a controlled beam of sound energy crosses the boundary between adjacent tissues of differing physical properties. *real-time ultrasonography* an ultrasound imaging technique involving rapid pulsing to enable continuous viewing of movement to be obtained, rather than stationary images—**ultrasonograph** *n*, **ultrasonographically** *adv*.

ultrasound *n* sound waves with a frequency of over 20 000 Hz, not audible to the human ear.

ultraviolet rays (UV) short wavelength electromagnetic rays outside the visible spectrum.

umbilical cord the cord connecting the fetus to the placenta. It contains a vein and two arteries.

umbilical hernia ⇒ hernia.

umbilicated *adj* having a central depression.

umbilicus *n* (*syn* navel) the abdominal scar left by the separation of the umbilical cord after birth—**umbilical** *adj*.

unconsciousness *n* state of being unconscious; insensible. ⇒ Glasgow Coma Scale.

underclass *n* a group who are deprived, disenfranchised and marginalized in society, such as rough sleepers.

undulant fever brucellosis.

unguentum *n* ointment.

unicellular *adj* consisting of only one cell.

unilateral *adj* relating to or on one side only—**unilaterally** *adv*.

uniocular *adj* pertaining to, or affecting, one eye.

uniovular *adj* (*syn* monovular) pertaining to one ovum, as uniovular twins (identical, same sex). ⇒ binovular *opp*.

unipara *n* a woman who has borne only one child. ⇒ primipara—**uniparous** *adj*.

unit cost an average cost for a specific activity, e.g. a surgical procedure, or a home visit. It is calculated by dividing the total cost of the service by the number of outputs.

univariate statistics descriptive statistics that analyse one variable, such as frequency distributions.

universal precautions the routine infection control precautions taken during contact, or the possibility of contact, with blood and body fluids, such as wearing gloves. ⇒ infection.

upper respiratory tract infection (URTI) the upper respiratory tract is the commonest site of infection in all age groups. The infections include rhinitis—usually viral—sinusitis, tonsillitis, adenoiditis, pharyngitis, otitis media and croup (laryngitis), often involving the tonsils and cervical lymph nodes. Such infections seldom require hospital treatment, but epiglottitis can be rapidly fatal.

urachus *n* the stemlike structure connecting the bladder with the umbilicus in the fetus; after birth it becomes a fibrous cord situated between the apex of the bladder and the umbilicus, known as the median umbilical ligament—**urachal** *adj*.

uraemia *n* a syndrome in which accumulation of endogenous waste products due to renal failure causes symptoms, particularly nausea, lethargy and anorexia—**uraemic** *adj*.

urate *n* any salt of uric acid.

urea *n* the main nitrogenous end product of protein metabolism; produced in the liver it is excreted in the urine.

urea breath test a non-invasive test for the diagnosis of *Helicobacter pylori* in the stomach.

urease *n* bacterial enzyme that splits urea.

ureter *n* the tube passing from each kidney to the bladder for the conveyance of urine (⇒ Figures 19, 20); its average length is 25–30 cm—**ureteric, ureteral** *adj*.

ureterectomy *n* excision of a ureter.

ureteritis *n* inflammation of a ureter.

ureterocolic *adj* pertaining to the ureter and colon, usually indicating anastomosis of the two structures.

ureteroileal *adj* pertaining to the ureters and ileum as in the anastomosis necessary in ileal conduit.

ureterolith *n* a calculus in the ureter.

ureterolithotomy *n* surgical removal of a stone from a ureter.

ureterolysis *n* surgical technique of freeing encased ureters.

ureterostomy *n* the formation of a permanent fistula through which the ureter discharges urine. ⇒ cutaneous, ileal conduit.

ureterosigmoidostomy *n* operation to implant a ureter into the sigmoid colon.

ureterovaginal *adj* pertaining to the ureter and vagina.

ureterovesical *adj* pertaining to the ureter and urinary bladder.

urethra *n* the passage from the bladder through which urine is excreted (⇒ Figure 19)—**urethral** *adj*.

urethral syndrome symptoms of urinary infection although the urine is sterile when withdrawn by catheter.

urethritis *n* inflammation of the urethra. *non-specific urethritis* ⇒ non-gonococcal urethritis.

urethrocele *n* prolapse of the urethra, usually into the anterior vaginal wall.

urethrography *n* radiological examination of the urethra. Can be an inclusion with cystography either retrograde (ascending) or during micturition—**urethrographic** *adj*, **urethrogram** *n*, **urethrograph** *n*, **urethrographically** *adv*.

urethrometry *n* measurement of the urethral lumen using a urethrometer—**urethrometric** *adj*, **urethrometrically** *adv*.

urethroplasty *n* any reconstructive operation on the urethra.

urethroscope *n* an instrument designed to allow visualization of the interior of the urethra—**urethroscopic** *adj*, **urethroscopy** *n*, **urethroscopically** *adv*.

urethrotomy *n* incision into the urethra; usually part of an operation for stricture.

urethrotrigonitis *n* inflammation of the urethra and the trigone of the urinary bladder. ⇒ trigone.

uric acid substance formed during purine metabolism, which is present in nucleic acids and some foods and beverages. Uric acid is excreted in the urine and may give rise to kidney stones. High levels of uric acid in the blood may be due to faulty excretion of uric acid, excessive cell breakdown, or associated with high purine intake. ⇒ gout.

uricosuric agents drugs that enhance renal excretion of uric acid. ⇒ Appendix 5.

uridrosis *n* excess of urea in the sweat; it may be deposited on the skin as fine white crystals.

urinalysis *n* examination of the urine.

urinary *adj* pertaining to urine. *urinary bladder* a muscular distensible bag situated in the pelvis (⇒ Figures 16, 19). It receives urine from the kidneys via two ureters and stores it until micturition occurs. *urinary system* comprises two kidneys, two ureters, one urinary bladder and one urethra. The kidneys produce urine of variable content; the ureters convey the urine to the bladder, which stores it until there is sufficient volume to elicit reflex emptying or the desire to pass urine and it is then conveyed to the exterior by the urethra. ⇒ Figures 19, 20. *urinary tract infection (UTI)* the second most prevalent infection in hospital, but the most common hospital-acquired infection. It occurs most frequently in the presence of an indwelling catheter. It is most commonly caused by the bacterium *Escherichia coli*, suggesting that self-infection via the periurethral route is a common pathway.

urination *n* ⇒ micturition.

urine *n* the clear straw-coloured fluid excreted by the kidneys. Urine contains water, nitrogenous waste and electrolytes. Normally adults produce about 1500 mL every 24 h, but this depends on fluid intake, activity and age. Usually slightly acidic (pH 6.0), but varies between 4.5 and 8.0. The specific gravity is usually within the range 1005–1030.

urinogenital *n* ⇒ urogenital.

urinometer *n* an instrument for estimating the specific gravity of urine.

urobilin *n* a brownish pigment excreted in the faeces. Formed by the oxidation of urobilinogen.

urobilinogen *n* (*syn* stercobilinogen) a pigment formed from bilirubin in the intestine by bacterial action. It may be reabsorbed into the circulation and converted back to bilirubin in the liver and re-excreted in the bile or urine.

urobilinuria *n* the presence of increased amounts of urobilin in the urine. Evidence of increased production of bilirubin in the liver, e.g. after haemolysis.

urodynamics *n* the method used to study bladder function. ⇒ cystometry.

urogenital *adj* (*syn* urinogenital) pertaining to the urinary and the genital organs.

urography *n* radiographic visualization of the renal pelvis and ureter by injection of a contrast medium. The medium may be injected into the bloodstream whence it is excreted by the kidney (intravenous urography) or it may be injected directly into the renal pelvis or ureter by way of a fine catheter introduced through a cystoscope (retrograde or ascending urography)—**urographic** *adj*, **urogram** *n*, **urographically** *adv*. *intravenous urography (IVU)* demonstration of the urinary tract following an intravenous injection of an opaque medium.

urokinase *n* an enzyme which dissolves fibrin clot. It is used therapeutically in vitreous haemorrhage (eye), thrombosed arteriovenous shunts and other thromboembolic conditions.

urologist *n* a person who specializes in disorders of the female urinary tract and the male genitourinary tract.

urology *n* that branch of biomedical science which deals with disorders of the female urinary tract and the male genitourinary tract—**urological** *adj*, **urologically** *adv*.

uropathy *n* disease in any part of the urinary system.

urostomy *n* the collective term for cutaneous ureterostomy, ileal conduit, ureterosigmoidostomy.

URTI *abbr* upper respiratory tract infection.

urticaria *n* (*syn* nettlerash, hives) skin eruption characterized by multiple, circumscribed, smooth, raised, pinkish, itchy weals, developing very suddenly, usually lasting a few days and leaving no visible trace. The cause is unknown in most cases. ⇒ angio-oedema. *factitial urticaria* ⇒ dermographia.

uterine *adj* pertaining to the uterus. *uterine supports* muscles of the pelvic floor, the peritoneum and various ligaments; pubocervical, round, transverse cervical (Mackenrodt's or cardinal) and the uterosacral ligaments that hold the uterus in the correct anteverted and anteflexed position. *uterine tubes* (*syn* fallopian tubes, oviducts) two tubes opening out of the upper part of the uterus. Each measures 10 cm and the distal end is fimbriated (⇒ Figure 17) and lies near the ovary. They are the site of fertilization and they convey the ovum to the uterus.

uteroplacental *adj* pertaining to the uterus and placenta.

uterorectal *adj* pertaining to the uterus and the rectum.

uterosacral *adj* pertaining to the uterus and sacrum.

uterosalpingography *n* (*syn* hysterosalpingography) radiological examination of the uterus and uterine tubes involving retrograde introduction of an opaque medium during fluoroscopy. Used to investigate patency of uterine (fallopian) tubes. Is being superseded by ultrasound examination.

uterovaginal *adj* pertaining to the uterus and the vagina.

uterovesical *adj* pertaining to the uterus and the urinary bladder.

uterus *n* the womb (⇒ Figure 17); a hollow muscular organ into which the ovum is received through the uterine (fallopian) tubes and where it is retained during development, and from which the fetus is expelled through the vagina. ⇒ bicornuate—**uteri** *pl*, **uterine** *adj*.

UTI *abbr* urinary tract infection.

utilitarianism *n* ethical theory that holds that an action should always produce more benefits than harm. It aims to provide the greatest good for the majority of individuals. ⇒ deontological.

utricle *n* a little sac or pocket. A fluid-filled sac in the internal ear. Part of the vestibular apparatus. ⇒ saccule.

uvea *n* the pigmented middle coat of the eye, includes the iris, ciliary body and choroid—**uveal** *adj*.

uveitis *n* inflammation of the uvea.

uvula *n* the central tag hanging down from the free edge of the soft palate.

uvulectomy *n* excision of the uvula.

uvulitis *n* inflammation of the uvula.

uvulopalatopharyngoplasty *n* operation on the soft palate for relief of snoring.

V

vaccination *n* originally described the process of inoculating persons with discharge from cowpox to protect them from smallpox. Now applied to the inoculation of any antigenic material for the purpose of producing active artificial immunity.

vaccines *npl* suspensions or products of infectious agents, used chiefly for producing active immunity. ⇒ BCG, Hib, MMR, Sabin, Salk, triple vaccine.

vaccinia *n* a pox virus causing disease in cattle. Used when it is necessary to provide immunity against smallpox such as in laboratory staff.

vacuum extractor 1 an instrument used to assist delivery of the fetus. **2** an instrument used as a method of terminating pregnancy.

VADAS *abbr* voice activated domestic appliance system.

vagal *adj* pertaining to the vagus nerve.

vagina *n* literally, a sheath; the musculo-membranous passage extending from the cervix uteri to the vulva (⇒ Figure 17)—**vaginal** *adj*.

vaginismus *n* painful muscular spasm of the vaginal walls resulting in dyspareunia or painful coitus.

vaginitis *n* inflammation of the vagina.

vaginosis *n* vaginal infection caused by a proliferation of commensal micro-organisms such as *Gardnerella vaginalis*.

vagolytic *adj, n* that which neutralizes the effect of a stimulated vagus nerve.

vagotomy *n* surgical division of the vagus nerves; done in conjunction with gastroenterostomy in the treatment of peptic ulcer, or with pyloroplasty.

vagus nerve the tenth cranial nerve, composed of both motor and sensory fibres, with a wide distribution in the neck, thorax and abdomen, sending important parasympathetic branches to the heart, lungs, stomach, etc.—**vagi** *pl*, **vagal** *adj*.

valgus, valga, valgum *adj* exhibiting angulation away from the midline of the body, e.g. hallux valgus.

validity (external) a term that indicates the degree to which research findings can be generalized to other populations and in other settings.

validity (internal) in research, a term that indicates the extent to which a method or test measures what it intends to measure.

valine *n* an essential (indispensable) amino acid.

Valsalva manoeuvre the maximum intra-thoracic pressure achieved by forced expiration against a closed glottis; occurs in such activities as lifting heavy objects, changing position and during defaecation: the glottis narrows simultaneously with contraction of the abdominal muscles.

value for money (VFM) a means of obtaining the best quality of service within the resource allocation. It involves economy, efficiency and effectiveness.

values *npl* the individual and personal view of the worth of an idea or specific behaviour. Principles of living which are refined from life experiences that guide behaviour. *value systems* an accepted set of values, conduct and way of behaving in a particular social group. ⇒ beliefs, secular beliefs.

valve *n* a fold of membrane in a passage or tube permitting the flow of contents in one direction only—**valvular** *adj*.

valvoplasty *n* a plastic operation on a valve, usually reserved for the heart; to be distinguished from valve replacement or valvotomy—**valvoplastic** *adj*.

valvotomy, valvulotomy *n* incision of a stenotic valve, by custom referring to the heart, to restore normal function.

valvulitis *n* inflammation of a valve, particularly in the heart.

valvulotomy *n* ⇒ valvotomy.

vancomycin-resistant enterococci (VRE) enterococci such as *Enterococcus faecium* that have developed resistance to vancomycin (a glycopeptide antibiotic). ⇒ *Enterococcus*.

Van den Bergh's test estimation of serum bilirubin. Direct positive reaction (conjugated) occurs in obstructive and hepatic jaundice. Indirect positive reaction (unconjugated) occurs in haemolytic jaundice.

vanillylmandelic acid (VMA) a metabolite of adrenaline (epinephrine) which is excreted in the urine.

variable *n* a research term that describes any factor or circumstance that is part of the study. *confounding variable* one that affects the conditions of the independent variables unequally. *dependent variable* one that depends on the experimental conditions. *independent variable* the variable conditions of an experimental situation, e.g. control or experimental. *random variable* background factors such as environmental conditions that may affect any conditions of the independent variables equally.

variance *n* a mathematical term used in statistics. The distribution range of a set of results around the mean. ⇒ standard deviation.

varicella *n* ⇒ chickenpox—**varicelliform** *adj*.

varicella-zoster immunoglobulin (VZIG) polyclonal immunoglobulin (largely IgG) from donors exposed to varicella-zoster.

Contains high concentrations of specific antibody, and used to convey passive immunity to varicella.

varicella-zoster virus (VZV) herpesvirus causing chickenpox (varicella) and shingles (herpes zoster).

varices *npl* dilated, tortuous (or varicose) veins. ⇒ oesophageal varices, varicose veins—**varix** *sing*.

varicocele *n* varicosity of the veins of the pampiniform plexus in the spermatic cord.

varicose ulcer (*syn* gravitational ulcer) ⇒ venous ulcer.

varicose veins dilated veins, the valves of which become incompetent so that blood flow may be reversed. Most commonly found in the lower limbs where they can result in a gravitational ulcer; in the rectum, when the term 'rectal varices' (haemorrhoids) is used; and in the lower oesophagus, when they are called oesophageal varices.

variola *n* ⇒ smallpox.

varioloid *n* attack of smallpox modified by previous vaccination.

varix *n* ⇒ varices.

varus, vara, varum *adj* displaying displacement or angulation towards the midline of the body, e.g. coxa vara.

vas *n* a vessel—**vasa** *pl*. *vas deferens (deferent duct)* the excretory duct of the testis. *vasa vasorum* the minute nutrient vessels of the artery and vein walls.

vascular *adj* supplied with vessels, especially referring to blood vessels.

vascularization *n* the acquisition of a blood supply; the process of becoming vascular.

vasculitis *n* (*syn* angiitis) inflammation of a blood vessel.

vasculotoxic *adj* any substance or agent that causes harmful changes in blood vessels.

vasectomy *n* surgical excision of all or part of the vas deferens, usually for sterilization.

vasoconstriction *n* narrowing of the lumen of a blood vessel.

vasoconstrictor *n* any agent causing vasoconstriction.

vasodilation *n* widening of the lumen of a blood vessel.

vasodilator *n* any agent causing vasodilation.

vasoepididymostomy *n* anastomosis of the vas deferens to the epididymis.

vasomotor *adj* relating to nerves and muscles that control vessel lumen size. *vasomotor centre (VMC)* a centre, located in the medulla oblongata. Concerned with controlling lumen size of peripheral arterioles. It operates through sympathetic activity in response to baroreceptor signals.

vasopressin *n* formed in the hypothalamus and stored in the posterior lobe of the pituitary gland. It is the antidiuretic hormone (ADH).

vasopressor *n* a drug which increases blood pressure. Usually by constricting arterioles but not always.

vasospasm *n* constricting spasm of vessel walls—**vasospastic** *adj*.

vasovagal reflex stimulation of the vagus nerve that results in a rapid fall in blood pressure and heart rate. Frequently associated with the transient loss of consciousness (vasovagal syncope) caused by insufficient blood reaching the brain, pallor, nausea and sweating. May be caused by stimulation of the soft palate (gag reflex), Valsalva manoeuvre, pain or emotional episodes.

VBI *abbr* vertebrobasilar insufficiency.

vector *n* a carrier of disease, e.g. tick.

vegan *n* a person who excludes all animal flesh and products from their diet, so does not eat meat, fish, eggs or dairy produce. Protein is provided by nuts and pulses. The diet can be nutritionally adequate but may be deficient in iron and vitamin B_{12}.

vegetarian ⇒ lacto-ovovegetarian, lacto-vegetarian.

vegetations *npl* growths or accretions composed of fibrin and platelets occurring on the edge of the cardiac valves in endocarditis.

vegetative *adj* relating to the non-sporing stage of a bacterium.

vein *n* a vessel conveying blood from the capillaries back to the heart. It has the same three coats as an artery, the inner one modified to form valves—**venous** *adj*.

vellus hair short downy hair found on most hair bearing parts of the body except scalp, axillae and external genitalia.

vena cava one of two large veins emptying into the right atrium of the heart. ⇒ Figures 8, 10.

veneer *n* in dentistry, a thin restoration that covers the surface of a tooth, usually made from composite resin or porcelain.

venepuncture *n* insertion of a needle into a vein.

venereal *adj* pertaining to or caused by sexual intercourse.

venereal disease research laboratory (VDRL) test a non-specific serological test for syphilis.

venereology *n* the study and treatment of sexually transmitted infections.

venesection *n* (*syn* phlebotomy) a clinical procedure whereby blood is removed via venepuncture. It is used in the treatment of iron overload, e.g. haemochromatosis and occasionally acutely for congestive heart failure.

venography *n* (*syn* phlebography) radiological examination of the venous system involving injection of an opaque medium. Mostly replaced by ultrasound—**venographic** *adj*, **venogram** *n*, **venograph** *n*, **venographically** *adv*.

venom *n* a poisonous fluid produced by some snakes, spiders and scorpions.

venotomy *n* incision of a vein. ⇒ venesection.

venous *adj* pertaining to the veins.

venous ulcer (*syn* gravitational ulcer) ulcer with a venous cause. They usually occur close to the ankle or between ankle and knee. There is often brown staining to the skin and dermatitis. Ulcers are large and shallow with large amounts of exudate. They frequently occur in people who have a history of deep vein thrombosis or varicose veins. They are difficult to treat effectively.

ventilation *n* the supply of fresh air. Also used to describe the mechanical process of breathing. ⇒ pulmonary ventilation. *ventilation perfusion ratio (V/Q)* the ratio between gases in the alveoli (alveolar ventilation) and blood flow in the pulmonary capillaries (pulmonary perfusion).

ventilator *n* specialized equipment for mechanically inflating a patient's lungs. Used to support or replace the patient's own breathing. Known colloquially as a 'life support machine'.

Ventouse extraction use of the vacuum extractor in obstetrics.

ventral *adj* pertaining to the abdomen or the anterior surface of the body—**ventrally** *adv*.

ventricle *n* a small belly-like cavity—**ventricular** *adj*. *ventricle of the brain* four cavities filled with cerebrospinal fluid within the brain. *ventricle of the heart* the two lower muscular chambers of the heart. (⇒ Figure 8).

ventricular fibrillation (VF) a serious cardiac arrhythmia where uncoordinated ventricular activity fails to produce any output of blood into the circulation. A common cause of sudden death following myocardial infarction. ⇒ cardiac arrest.

ventricular tachycardia (VT) a very serious ventricular arrhythmia characterized by a rapid ventricular rate of 140–200 per minute. It may lead to cardiac arrest, ventricular fibrillation or pulseless ventricular tachycardia.

ventriculocysternostomy *n* artificial communication between cerebral ventricles and subarachnoid space. One of the drainage operations for hydrocephalus.

ventriculostomy *n* an artificial opening into a ventricle. Usually refers to a drainage operation for hydrocephalus.

ventrosuspension *n* fixation of a displaced uterus to the anterior abdominal wall.

Venturi effect a principle of gas behaviour used for the mixing and delivery of gases, such as oxygen masks. ⇒ Venturi mask.

Venturi mask an oxygen therapy mask designed to direct atmospheric air to mix it with a given flow of prescribed oxygen. A variety of masks are available that allow the administration of oxygen at different concentrations.

venule *n* a small vein.

Veress needle a sharp needle with a blunt ended trochar which has a lateral hole; it is used for a pneumoperitoneum. When the trochar projects from the needle, the gut is pushed safely away from the needle point.

vermicide *n* an agent which kills intestinal worms—**vermicidal** *adj*.

vermiform *adj* wormlike. *vermiform appendix* the vestigial, hollow, wormlike structure attached to the caecum.

vermifuge *n* an agent that expels intestinal worms.

vernix caseosa the fatty substance which covers and protects the skin of the fetus.

verocytotoxin *n* powerful enterotoxin produced by enterohaemorrhagic *Escherichia coli* such as *E. coli* 0157.

verruca *n* ⇒ wart, condyloma—**verrucae** *pl*, **verrucous, verrucose** *adj*.

version *n* turning—applied to the manoeuvre to alter the position of the fetus in utero. *cephalic version* turning the child so that the head presents. *external cephalic version (ECV)* the conversion of a transverse into a head presentation to facilitate labour. The technique is safer with the use of ultrasound and tachographic monitoring. *internal version* is turning the child by one hand in the uterus, and the other on the patient's abdomen. *podalic version* turning the child to a breech presentation. This version may be external or internal.

vertebra *n* one of the irregular bones making up the spinal column—**vertebrae** *pl*, **vertebral** *adj*.

vertebral column (*syn* spinal column) made up of 33/34 vertebrae, articulating with the skull above and the pelvic girdle below. The vertebrae are so shaped that they enclose a cavity (spinal canal, neural canal) which houses the spinal cord.

vertebrobasilar insufficiency (VBI) a poorly understood condition in which there is thought to be transient disturbances in the blood flow to the brainstem.

vertex *n* the top of the head.

vertical transmission transmission of disease from mother to fetus, via the placenta, during delivery or via breast milk, e.g. HIV.

vertigo *n* giddiness, dizziness—**vertiginous** *adj*.

very-low-density lipoprotein (VLDL) ⇒ lipoprotein.

vesical *adj* pertaining to the urinary bladder.

vesicle *n* **1** a small bladder, cell or hollow structure. **2** a skin blister—**vesicular** *adj*, **vesiculation** *n*.

vesicostomy ⇒ cystostomy.

vesicoureteric *adj* pertaining to the urinary bladder and ureter. *vesicoureteric reflux (VUR)* retrograde passage of urine up the ureters following a rise of pressure within the bladder. It can cause pyelonephritis.

vesicovaginal *adj* pertaining to the urinary bladder and vagina.

vesiculitis *n* inflammation of a vesicle, particularly the seminal vesicles.

vesiculopapular *adj* pertaining to or exhibiting both vesicles and papules.

vesiculopustular *adj* pertaining to or exhibiting both vesicles and pustules.

vessel *n* a tube, duct or canal, holding or conveying fluid, especially blood and lymph.

vestibule *n* **1** the middle part of the internal ear, lying between the semicircular canals and the cochlea. **2** the triangular area between the labia minora. **3** the area of the mouth between the lips and the gums/teeth—**vestibular** *adj*.

vestibulocochlear *adj* relating to the vestibule and the cochlear. *vestibulocochlear nerve* auditory nerve. The eighth pair of cranial nerves. There are two branches: the vestibular, which transmits impulses from the vestibular apparatus of the ear to the cerebellum, and the cochlear, which transmits impulses from the cochlea in the ear to the auditory cortex situated in the temporal lobe of the cerebrum.

vestibulo-ocular reflex compensatory eye movement stimulated by head movement to stabilize gaze in space.

vestigial *adj* pertaining to a rudimentary structure, a remnant of something formerly present.

viable *adj* capable of living a separate existence—**viability** *n*.

vibration *n* a form of massage manipulation. A fine tremor transmitted through the hands and finger tips to body cavities in order to move fluids and gases.

vibration syndrome (*syn* Raynaud's phenomenon) ⇒ hand-arm vibration syndrome.

vibration—whole body arises from use of equipment in which the worker is supported by the vibrating machinery, e.g. a vehicle seat or ship's deck. The cardiovascular system is affected, with an increase in heart rate and interference with circulation; musculoskeletal problems are common particularly involving the spine. Fatigue and poor concentration are also thought to be significant.

Vibrio *n* a genus of curved, motile microorganisms. *Vibrio cholerae* causes cholera.

vicarious *adj* substituting the function of one organ for another. *vicarious liability* describes the liability of the employer for the wrongful acts of an employee committed during the course of employment.

villus *n* a microscopic fingerlike projection; found in the mucosa of the small intestine or on the outside of the chorion of the embryonic sac—**villi** *pl*, **villous** *adj*.

vinca alkaloids a group of cytotoxic drugs extracted from the periwinkle plant. They prevent mitosis and cell division by inhibiting microtubule formation. ⇒ cytotoxic. ⇒ Appendix 5.

Vincent's angina (*syn* ulcerative gingivitis) infection of the mouth or throat by mixed bacteria. To be differentiated from Ludwig's angina.

viraemia *n* the presence of virus in the blood—**viraemic** *adj*.

viral haemorrhagic fevers fevers occurring mainly in tropical areas; they are often transmitted by mosquitoes or ticks; they may have a petechial skin rash. They include: chikungunya, ebola, dengue, Lassa fever, Marburg disease, Rift Valley fever and yellow fever.

viral hepatitis ⇒ hepatitis.

virement *n* financial term meaning to move money from one expenditure category to another.

viricidal *adj* lethal to a virus—**viricide** *n*.

virilism *n* the appearance of secondary male characteristics in the female.

virologist *n* an expert in viruses and viral diseases.

virology *n* the study of viruses and the diseases caused by them—**virological** *adj*.

virulence *n* infectiousness; the disease-producing power of a micro-organism and its power to overcome host resistance—**virulent** *adj*.

viruses *npl* a diverse group of micro-organisms which are only visible using electron microscopy. They contain either DNA or RNA, and can only replicate within the host cell. Viruses infect humans, animals, plants and other micro-organisms (bacteriophages). Diseases caused by viruses in humans include: colds, influenza, measles, rabies, hepatitis, chickenpox, poliomyelitis, dengue and AIDS. Some viruses are associated with cancer of the cervix, Burkitt's lymphoma and some types of leukaemia. ⇒ Epstein–Barr virus, human T-cell lymphotropic virus, human papilloma virus.

viscera *n* the internal organs—**viscus** *sing*, **visceral** *adj*.

viscid *adj* sticky, glutinous, may be used to describe sputum, mucus, etc.

visual *adj* pertaining to vision. *visual acuity* measure of the ability of the eye to resolve detail. ⇒ Snellen chart. *visual field* also called field of vision. The area in which objects can be seen without moving the eye. In binocular vision, the overlap of the fields of both eyes across the nose allows perception of depth (stereoscopic vision).

vital capacity (VC) the amount of air expelled from the lungs after a deep inspiration. ⇒ forced vital capacity.

vitallium *n* an alloy used in the manufacture of nails, plates, etc., used in orthopaedic and other surgical procedures.

vitalograph *n* apparatus for measuring the forced vital capacity.

vital signs monitor apparatus that automatically records and displays physiological measurements such as blood pressure and ECG.

vitamin A (*syn* retinol) a fat-soluble anti-infective substance present in all animal fats. In its provitamin form, β-carotene, it is present in carrots, cabbage, lettuce, tomatoes and other fruits and vegetables: in the body it is converted into retinol. It is essential for healthy skin and mucous membranes: it aids night vision. Deficiency can result in stunted growth, night blindness and xerophthalmia and is an important cause of blindness in certain parts of the world, e.g. India.

vitamin B any one of a group of water-soluble vitamins—the vitamin B complex, all chemically related and often occurring in the same foods. ⇒ biotin, cobalamins, folate, nicotinic acid, pantothenic acid, pyridoxine, riboflavin, thiamin.

vitamin B_1 thiamin diphosphate or thiamin pyrophosphate. It occurs in wheatgerm, wheat products, yeast extracts, meat and fortified breakfast cereals. Functions as a coenzyme in carbohydrate metabolism. Deficiency results in beri-beri and Wernicke–Korsakoff syndrome. ⇒ Korsakoff's syndrome, Wernicke's encephalopathy.

vitamin B_2 riboflavin. Occurs in most foods, the best sources are milk, milk products, offal and fortified breakfast cereals. It functions as part of the coenzymes flavin mononucleotide (FMN) and flavin adenine dinucleotide (FAD) involved in the oxidation chain occurring in mitochondria. ⇒ oxidative phosphorylation. Deficiency symptoms are angular stomatitis, cheilosis and anaemia.

vitamin B₆ pyridoxine. Occurs in unprocessed cereal foods, vegetables, meat and eggs. It functions as a coenzyme in protein metabolism. Deficiency symptoms include general weakness, peripheral neuropathy, dermatitis, glossitis and impaired immunity.

vitamin B₁₂ cobalamins. Occurs in meat, eggs, milk and cheese. It functions as a coenzyme in protein metabolism. Deficiency may develop in vegans and symptoms include megaloblastic anaemia and neurological dysfunction. ⇒ pernicious anaemia.

vitamin C ⇒ ascorbic acid.

vitamin D a fat-soluble vitamin needed for the absorption of calcium and the calcification of the skeleton. It occurs in two forms—cholecalciferol (vitamin D₃) formed by the action of ultraviolet radiation on 7-dehydrocholesterol, which occurs naturally in the skin, and ergocalciferol (vitamin D₂, calciferol) formed by the action of ultraviolet radiation on ergosterol, which occurs naturally in plants. Occurs in oily fish, eggs, fortified margarine. Deficiency leads to rickets and osteomalacia.

vitamin E a group of chemically related compounds known as tocopherols and tocotrienols. It is an intracellular fat-soluble antioxidant and maintains the stability of polyunsaturated fatty acids and other fat-like substances. It is thought that deficiency results in muscle degeneration, a haemolytic blood disease, and is associated with the ageing process. *vitamin E deficiency syndrome* occurs in small infants, less than 2 kg and under 35 weeks gestation. Diagnosis at between 6 and 11 weeks reveals low haemoglobin and reticulocytosis; there is good response to vitamin E including a rise in haemoglobin and loss of oedema. The condition is aggravated by giving iron. Deficiency in older children results in cerebellar ataxia and is associated with abetalipoproteinaemia.

vitamin K occurs in three forms—phylloquinone, menaquinones and menadione.

Phylloquinone occurs in green vegetables and menaquinones are produced by bacteria in the gastrointestinal tract. It is required for the synthesis of several clotting factors. Deficiency leads to reduced blood clotting.

vitamins *npl* organic substance or group of substances that have specific biochemical functions in the body. They are either fat-soluble—vitamins A, D, E and K, or water-soluble—vitamin B complex and vitamin C. They are essential for normal metabolism and are provided by the diet. Some vitamins can also be synthesized in the body, e.g. vitamin D. Their absence causes deficiency diseases.

vitiligo *n* a skin disease of probable autoimmune origin characterized by areas of complete loss of pigment, often on the face and hands.

vitrectomy *n* surgical removal of the vitreous humour from the vitreous chamber.

vitreous *adj* resembling glass. *vitreous chamber* the cavity inside the eyeball and behind the lens. *vitreous humour (body)* the jelly-like substance contained in the vitreous chamber (⇒ Figure 15).

vocal cords membranous folds stretched anteroposteriorly across the larynx. Sound is produced by their vibration as air from the lungs passes between them.

vocational assessment the objective evaluation of a person's ability to perform a specific job consistently and competently. This may include the identification of the need for training or the provision of compensatory techniques.

voice activated domestic appliance system (VADAS) a microprocessor and voice input system that allows people with severe physical impairments to control their environment and live as independently as possible.

volatile *adj* evaporating rapidly. *volatile anaesthetic agent* drug in the form of a liquid which when vaporized induces general anaesthesia.

volition *n* the will to act—**volitional** *adj*.

Volkmann's ischaemic contracture a flexion deformity of the wrist and fingers from fixed contracture of the flexor muscles in the forearm. The cause is ischaemia of the muscles by injury or obstruction to the brachial artery, near the elbow.

volt (V) *n* the derived SI unit (International System of Units) for electromotive force (also known as potential difference or electrical potential).

voluntary *adj* under the control of the will; free and unrestricted, as opposed to reflex or involuntary.

voluntary sector the organizations controlled and run by volunteers, e.g. Samaritans, MIND. Many have charitable status, some receive grants from government, and some employ professionals and other paid staff to facilitate their work.

volvulus *n* torsion of a loop of intestine, so as to occlude the lumen causing intestinal obstruction.

vomit *n* ejection of the stomach contents through the mouth and sometimes the nose; sickness.

vomiting centre a centre in the medulla oblongata that has overall control of vomiting. It responds to various stimuli such as those from the gastrointestinal organs.

vomiting of pregnancy ⇒ hyperemesis.

vomitus *n* vomited matter.

von Recklinghausen's disease (*syn* Recklinghausen's disease) describes two conditions: (a) osteitis fibrosa cystica—the result of hyperparathyroidism leading to decalcification of bones and formation of cysts; (b) multiple neurofibromatosis—the tumours can be felt beneath the skin along the course of nerves. There may be pigmented spots (café au lait) on the skin and neurofibroma in the endocrine glands and the gastrointestinal tract.

von Willebrand's disease an inherited bleeding disease due to deficiencies relating to the von Willebrand factor in plasma. The inheritance is autosomal dominant, affecting both sexes. Essentially a disorder of the primary haemostatic mechanism with abnormal platelet–endothelial cell interaction. In rare, severe cases von Willebrand's disease results in a clotting defect resembling haemophilia.

vulva *n* the external genitalia of the female—**vulval** *adj*.

vulvectomy *n* excision of the vulva.

vulvitis *n* inflammation of the vulva.

vulvodynia *n* chronic painful vulval discomfort such as burning, rawness and stinging. Previously regarded by many as a psychogenic condition, vulvodynia is an organic disease that presents with surface changes or as an aberration of sensory function in which surface changes may be absent.

vulvovaginal *adj* pertaining to the vulva and the vagina.

vulvovaginitis *n* inflammation of the vulva and vagina.

vulvovaginoplasty *n* operation for congenital absence of the vagina, or acquired disabling stenosis—**vulvovaginoplastic** *adj*.

VUR *abbr* vesicoureteric reflux.

VZIG *abbr* varicella-zoster (hyperimmune) immunoglobulin.

W

Waldeyer's ring a lymphoid tissue circle surrounding the pharynx. ⇒ tonsils.

walking aids walking sticks, crutches, tripods and various types of metal frame that allow people to regain or retain independence for walking.

Wallace's rule of nine a method of calculating the percentage of burn area using standard body maps.

warm-up *n* techniques used to increase local muscle and core body temperature prior to vigorous exercise. Can be either active or passive and may be specific to the sport or exercise about to be performed.

wart *n* verruca. *common warts* are due to human papilloma virus (HPV) and usually occur on the hands or feet. *seborrhoeic warts* (*syn* basal cell papilloma) the brown, greasy warts seen in older people, commonly on the chest or back. *plane warts* flat small papules commonly seen on the face or hands in children.

waterbrash ⇒ pyrosis.

Waterhouse–Friderichsen syndrome shock with widespread skin haemorrhages occurring in meningitis, especially meningococcal. There is bleeding in the adrenal glands.

watt (W) *n* derived SI unit (International System of Units) for electrical power.

WBC *abbr* white blood cell (leucocyte). ⇒ blood.

weal *n* a superficial swelling, characteristic of urticaria, nettle-stings, etc.

Weber's test a tuning fork test for the interpretation of asymmetric deafness.

Weil–Felix test a non-specific agglutination reaction used in the diagnosis of rickettsial disease, e.g. typhus.

Weil's disease serious bacterial disease caused by infection with spirochaetes of the genus *Leptospira* such as *Leptospira icterohaemorrhagica*. Transmission is via the infected urine of rats and other animals. ⇒ leptospirosis.

wen *n* ⇒ sebaceous.

Wernicke's encephalopathy a level of impaired consciousness and thinking due to thiamin(e) deficiency and which is therefore most commonly seen in long-term alcohol misuse.

Wertheim's hysterectomy a radical and extensive operation performed for cancer of the cervix, where the uterus, cervix, upper vagina, uterine (fallopian) tubes, ovaries and regional lymph nodes are removed.

Western blot also known as immunoblotting, a process of identifying antigens in a mixture using specific antibodies. The antigens are separated using an electrophoretic technique, transferred to a sheet of nitrocellulose, and then identified by radio- or enzyme-labelled antibodies.

Wharton's jelly embryonic connective tissue contained in the umbilical cord.

wheezing *n* a whistling or rasping breathing sound. Associated with the bronchospasm of asthma and other conditions.

Whipple's operation radical operation sometimes performed for cancer of the head of pancreas. It involves: partial pancreatectomy, and excision of the pylorus, duodenum and bile duct with a gastrojejunostomy, choledochojejunostomy and pancreaticojejunostomy.

whipworm *n Trichuris trichiura*. ⇒ trichuriasis.

white leg thrombophlebitis occurring in women after childbirth.

white matter white nerve tissue of the CNS, the myelinated fibres. ⇒ grey matter.

white muscle a term used to describe muscle consisting mainly of fast-twitch fibres. It is white because there is very little myoglobin and a less abundant blood supply than in red muscle.

whitlow *n* acute paronychia or purulent infection of the finger pulp. ⇒ paronychia.

WHO *abbr* World Health Organization.

whooping cough ⇒ pertussis.

Widal test an agglutination reaction for typhoid fever.

Wilcoxon test a statistical test used as a non-parametric alternative to Student's paired test.

Wilms tumour the commonest abdominal tumour of childhood, and one which usually affects the kidneys. Usually diagnosed during the preschool period. Prognosis is uncertain and depends on the stage of the tumour and child's age at onset of diagnosis and treatment. ⇒ nephroblastoma.

Wilson's disease rare inherited hepaticolenticular degeneration. Due to disturbance of copper metabolism with copper deposition in various organs, such as the liver and basal nuclei (ganglia). Associated with dementia, tremor, chorea, cirrhosis, portal hypertension and liver failure. Treatment is with penicillamine, which binds the copper. Relatives with the disease should have prophylactic penicillamine, even if they have no symptoms. ⇒ Kayser–Fleischer ring.

windpipe *n* ⇒ trachea.

wisdom tooth lay term for the molar tooth placed eighth from the midline in the secondary dentition. The last teeth to erupt.

Wolfe graft ⇒ skin graft.

wolffian ducts primitive embryonic ducts that, under the influence of testosterone, become the genitourinary structures in the genetically male embryo. ⇒ mullerian ducts.

Wolff–Parkinson–White (WPW) syndrome an arrhythmia resulting from an abnormal conduction pathway between the atria and ventricles. Usually results in a supraventricular tachycardia.

womb *n* the uterus.

Wood's light special ultraviolet light used for the detection of fungal diseases such as ringworm.

woolsorter's disease ⇒ anthrax.

work *n* productive, purposeful engagement in physical and cognitive activities by individuals in order to support themselves and their dependants, and make a useful contribution to society.

work-related upper limb disorder (WRULD) occurs as a result of prolonged persistent repetitive overuse of the upper limb with maintenance of static postures. It is common in keyboard workers, production workers and telephonists. The soft tissues in the shoulders, arms, wrists and hands are affected, leading to various diagnoses, e.g. tendinitis, tenosynovitis, carpal tunnel syndrome and tennis elbow. It can be prevented by adequate ergonomic-based risk assessment of the workplace.

World Health Organization (WHO) health organization that coordinates health activity and promotes public health worldwide. Established through a 'declaration' during the United Nations Conference on International Organization held in San Francisco in 1945. A number of disparate health organizations were joined together under the aegis of the United Nations with a headquarters in Geneva, Switzerland.

worms *npl* ⇒ cestode, nematodes, trematoda.

wound *n* most commonly used when referring to injury to the skin or underlying tissues or organs by a blow, cut, missile or stab. It also includes injury to the skin caused by chemicals, cold, friction, heat, pressure and radiation. Wounds may be acute, e.g. surgical, or chronic such as pressure ulcers. Wounds are usually classified as being clean, clean contaminated, contaminated or dirty. ⇒ incised wound, laceration, penetrating wound.

wound drains most commonly used in surgical wounds. They may be inserted as treatment, e.g. to drain pus, or prophylactically, e.g. to prevent haematoma formation. Drains may be attached to a vacuum system or suction apparatus, producing a closed system of wound suction.

wound dressings a variety of proprietary materials applied to surgical or medical wounds, e.g. leg ulcers. Modern dressings should be permeable to water vapour and gases but not to bacteria or liquids, thus retaining serous exudate. They do not adhere to the wound surface and can be removed without damage to new tissue.

wound healing there are four stages/phases in normal wound healing: haemostasis, inflammation, proliferation and maturation, which may take many months. Wound healing may be delayed by local factors, e.g. mechanical stress, inadequate blood supply, or by general factors that include: malnutrition, ageing, drugs such as corticosteroids, etc. ⇒ angiogenesis, epithelialization, granulation, moist wound healing. Wound healing may be by *first/primary intention* in a clean wound with the edges in apposition. There is minimal scarring and deformity; *second intention* when the wound edges are not in apposition, the gap must be filled by granulation tissue before epithelialization can take place; or by *third intention* when a wound is left open until local factors such as infection have been treated before the wound edges are brought together.

WPW *abbr* Wolff–Parkinson–White syndrome.

wrinkle *n* furrow or skin crease, increase in number with ageing.

wrist *n* the carpus (⇒ Figure 2). *wrist drop* paralysis of the muscles which raise the wrist, caused by damage to the radial nerve.

wryneck *n* ⇒ torticollis.

X

xanthelasma *n* a variety of xanthomas. *xanthelasma palpebrarum* small yellowish plaques on the eyelids.

xanthine *n* an intermediate product formed during the breakdown of nucleic acids to uric acid. It is excreted in the urine.

xanthinuria *n* rare inherited disorder in which xanthine oxidase enzyme is lacking, resulting in excessive urinary xanthine and hypoxanthine in place of uric acid.

xanthogranulomatous pyelonephritis a granulomatous reaction within the kidney usually secondary to chronic infection and stone disease.

xanthoma *n* nodules showing a yellow discoloration—**xanthomata** *pl*.

X chromosome sex chromosome that is paired in genetic females. Present in every oocyte and in half of spermatozoa. ⇒ sex-linked, Y chromosome.

xenograft (*syn* heterograft) a graft between individuals of two different species.

xenon (Xe) *n* a rare inert gas.

Xenopsylla *n* a genus of fleas. *Xenopsylla cheopis* is the rat flea that transmits diseases, including bubonic plague.

xeroderma, xerodermia *n* dryness of the skin ⇒ ichthyosis. *xeroderma pigmentosum* (*syn* Kaposi's disease) a rare inherited skin condition where there is severe photosensitivity to ultraviolet radiation. It is characterized by the formation of freckles, keratoses, telangiectases and malignant skin tumours. Those affected must avoid exposure to ultraviolet radiation.

xerophthalmia *n* dryness and ulceration of the cornea which may lead to blindness. Can be associated with lack of vitamin A.

xerosis *n* dryness. *xerosis conjunctivae* ⇒ Bitot's spots.

xerostomia *n* dry mouth.

X-linked agammaglobulinaemia (XLA) a primary (inherited) immunodeficiency affecting boys. A gene mutation results in absent B cells and hence absent immunoglobulin production.

X-linked hyper-IgM syndrome (XHIM) a primary (inherited) immunodeficiency affecting boys. There is defective antibody production, particularly very high IgM levels, and impaired cellular immunity.

X-rays *npl* short wavelength, penetrating rays of electromagnetic spectrum, produced by electrical equipment. The word is popularly used to mean radiographs.

XXY syndrome Klinefelter syndrome.

xylose absorption test a test for malabsorption. Xylose is given orally and its urinary excretion is measured. Less than 16% excretion indicates malabsorption.

Y

yaws *n* a contact disease of children, particularly in Africa, characterized by crops of infectious skin lesions, and later, periostitis. Caused by *Treponema pallidum* (ssp. pertenue). ⇒ bejel, pinta.

Y chromosome sex chromosome found only in the genetic male. It is shorter than the X chromosome and has fewer major genes.

yeast *n* a unicellular fungus some of which are human pathogens, e.g. *Candida albicans*, *Cryptococcus neoformans*.

yellow card reporting in the UK a system for reporting suspected adverse drug reactions to the Committee on Safety of Medicines (CSM) and Medicines Control Agency. Cards are supplied at the back of the current BNF.

yellow fever an acute febrile illness of tropical areas, caused by a group B arbovirus and spread by a mosquito (*Aedes aegypti*). There is fever, headache, nausea and vomiting, gastrointestinal bleeding, jaundice, petechial haemorrhages, backache and anuria.

Yersinia *n* a genus of Gram-negative bacilli, e.g. *Yersinia pestis*, the cause of plague.

yin and yang the philosophy of complementary therapies, such as acupuncture and shiatsu. They describe a dynamic, symbiotic relationship between active and passive energy forces believed to be present in the universe (true Qi) and the human body (Qi). Keeping equilibrium between the two aspects is important in maintaining health.

yoga *n* complementary therapy that utilizes breathing techniques, postures and exercises to relax, reduce stress and generally enhance well-being.

yolk *n* nutrient of the ovum. *yolk sac* early embryonic structure, provides a site for very early blood cell formation.

yttrium 90 (^{90}Y) a substance emitting beta particles with a half-life of 64 h. Implantations of this in bone wax are left in the pituitary fossa after hypophysectomy for breast cancer. Also used in a number of interstitial cancer treatments.

Z

Ziehl–Neelsen stain (ZN) a microbiological staining technique used in the identification of acid-fast bacilli, e.g. *Mycobacterium tuberculosis*.

ZIFT *abbr* zygote intrafallopian tube transfer.

zinc (Zn) *n* a metallic element needed by the body in small amounts for certain enzyme reactions, insulin storage, cell multiplication and wound healing. Phytates in the diet can reduce absorption. *zinc oxide* a widely used mild astringent, present in calamine lotion and cream and several other dermatological applications.

Zollinger–Ellison syndrome gastrin-secreting tumour of the pancreatic islets resulting in hypersecretion of gastric acid, fulminating ulceration of the oesophagus, stomach and duodenum and jejunum. Diagnosed by high basal gastric acid secretion and elevated fasting serum gastrin levels.

zona *n* a zone; a girdle; herpes zoster. *zona pellucida* membrane around the oocyte.

zones *npl* a term used in reflexology. The suggestion is that inborn Qi energy flows through different zones (reflexes) that end in the feet or hands.

zonule *n* **1** small zone, belt or girdle. Zonula. **2** suspensory ligament attaching the periphery of the lens of the eye to ciliary body.

zoonosis *n* disease in humans transmitted from animals, e.g. anthrax, rabies—**zoonoses** *pl*.

zoster *n* herpes zoster.

zygoma *n* the cheekbone—**zygomatic** *adj*.

zygote *n* the fertilized ovum. The diploid cell derived from the fusion after fertilization of the female and male nuclei, each of which has the haploid, chromosome complement.

zygote intrafallopian tube transfer (ZIFT) a technique used in assisted conception where the fertilized conceptus is transferred laparoscopically into the uterine (fallopian) tube.

zymogen *n* a proenzyme. An inactive precursor of a proteolytic enzyme, e.g. a clotting factor. May be activated by another enzyme.

Appendices

Appendix 1

Illustrations of major body systems

Acknowledgements

Figures 1, 2, 3, 6, 7, 8, 9, 10, 12, 13, 14, 15, 16, 17, 18(b) and 20 are reproduced with permission from Waugh A, Grant A (2001) *Ross and Wilson Anatomy and Physiology in Health and Illness*, 9th edn, Churchill Livingstone, Edinburgh.

Figure 18(a) is reproduced from Brooker C (2002) *Mosby Nurse's Pocket Dictionary*, 32nd edn, Mosby, Edinburgh.

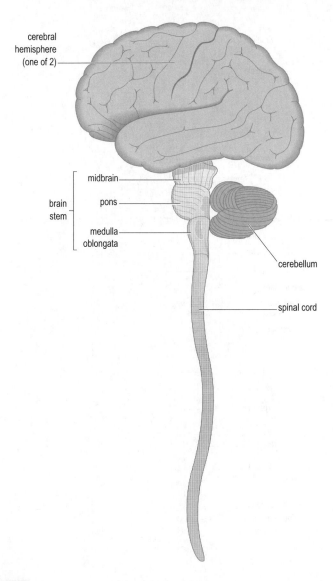

cerebral
hemisphere
(one of 2)

brain
stem

midbrain

pons

medulla
oblongata

cerebellum

spinal cord

Figure 1 Brain and spinal cord (central nervous system)

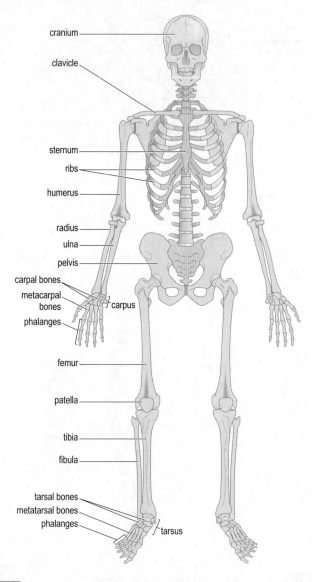

cranium
clavicle
sternum
ribs
humerus
radius
ulna
pelvis
carpal bones
metacarpal bones
carpus
phalanges
femur
patella
tibia
fibula
tarsal bones
metatarsal bones
phalanges
tarsus

Figure 2 Skeleton—front view

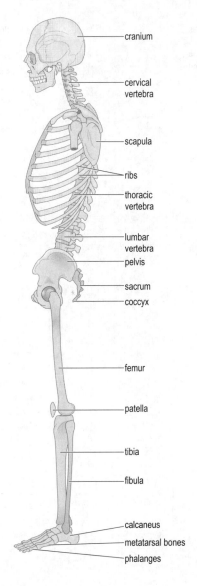

cranium

cervical
vertebra

scapula

ribs

thoracic
vertebra

lumbar
vertebra

pelvis

sacrum

coccyx

femur

patella

tibia

fibula

calcaneus

metatarsal bones

phalanges

Figure 3 Skeleton—side view

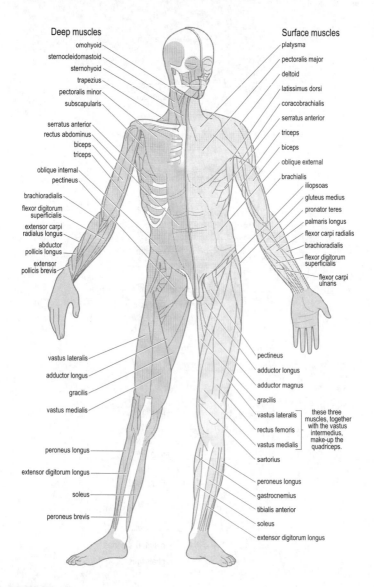

Deep muscles

- omohyoid
- sternocleidomastoid
- sternohyoid
- trapezius
- pectoralis minor
- subscapularis
- serratus anterior
- rectus abdominus
- biceps
- triceps
- oblique internal
- pectineus
- brachioradialis
- flexor digitorum superficialis
- extensor carpi radialus longus
- abductor pollicis longus
- extensor pollicis brevis
- vastus lateralis
- adductor longus
- gracilis
- vastus medialis
- peroneus longus
- extensor digitorum longus
- soleus
- peroneus brevis

Surface muscles

- platysma
- pectoralis major
- deltoid
- latissimus dorsi
- coracobrachialis
- serratus anterior
- triceps
- biceps
- oblique external
- brachialis
- iliopsoas
- gluteus medius
- pronator teres
- palmaris longus
- flexor carpi radialis
- brachioradialis
- flexor digitorum superficialis
- flexor carpi ulnaris
- pectineus
- adductor longus
- adductor magnus
- gracilis
- vastus lateralis
- rectus femoris
- vastus medialis
- sartorius
- peroneus longus
- gastrocnemius
- tibialis anterior
- soleus
- extensor digitorum longus

these three muscles, together with the vastus intermedius, make-up the quadriceps.

Figure 4 Muscles—front view

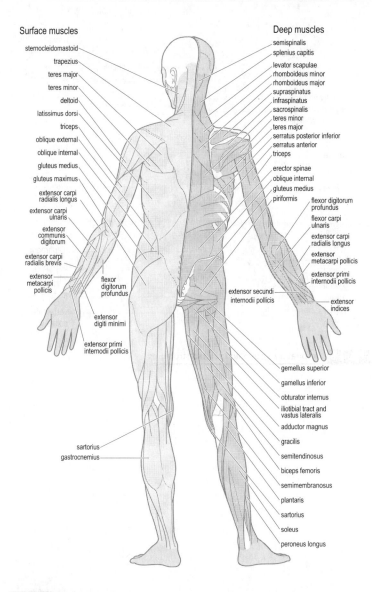

Surface muscles

- sternocleidomastoid
- trapezius
- teres major
- teres minor
- deltoid
- latissimus dorsi
- triceps
- oblique external
- oblique internal
- gluteus medius
- gluteus maximus
- extensor carpi radialis longus
- extensor carpi ulnaris
- extensor communis digitorum
- extensor carpi radialis brevis
- extensor metacarpi pollicis
- flexor digitorum profundus
- extensor digiti minimi
- extensor primi internodii pollicis
- sartorius
- gastrocnemius

Deep muscles

- semispinalis
- splenius capitis
- levator scapulae
- rhomboideus minor
- rhomboideus major
- supraspinatus
- infraspinatus
- sacrospinalis
- teres minor
- teres major
- serratus posterior inferior
- serratus anterior
- triceps
- erector spinae
- oblique internal
- gluteus medius
- piriformis
- flexor digitorum profundus
- flexor carpi ulnaris
- extensor carpi radialis longus
- extensor metacarpi pollicis
- extensor primi internodii pollicis
- extensor secundi internodii pollicis
- extensor indices
- gemellus superior
- gamellus inferior
- obturator internus
- iliotibial tract and vastus lateralis
- adductor magnus
- gracilis
- semitendinosus
- biceps femoris
- semimembranosus
- plantaris
- sartorius
- soleus
- peroneus longus

Figure 5 Muscles—back view

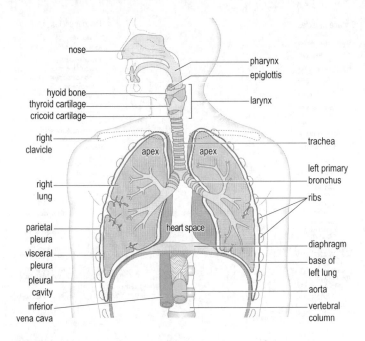

Figure 6 Respiratory system and related structures

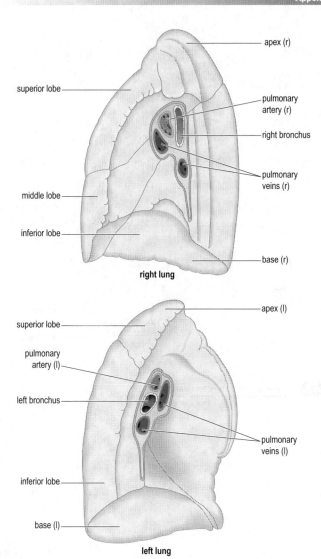

apex (r)

superior lobe

pulmonary artery (r)

right bronchus

pulmonary veins (r)

middle lobe

inferior lobe

base (r)

right lung

apex (l)

superior lobe

pulmonary artery (l)

left bronchus

pulmonary veins (l)

inferior lobe

base (l)

left lung

Figure 7   Respiratory system—lungs showing lobes, airways and vessels (medial views)

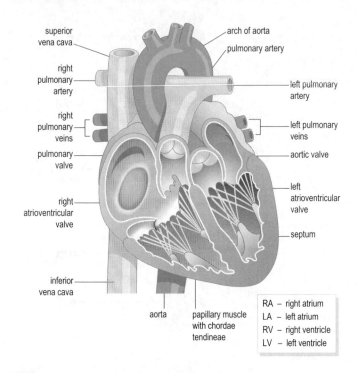

superior vena cava

right pulmonary artery

right pulmonary veins

pulmonary valve

right atrioventricular valve

inferior vena cava

arch of aorta

pulmonary artery

left pulmonary artery

left pulmonary veins

aortic valve

left atrioventricular valve

septum

aorta

papillary muscle with chordae tendineae

RA – right atrium
LA – left atrium
RV – right ventricle
LV – left ventricle

Figure 8 Circulatory system—the heart

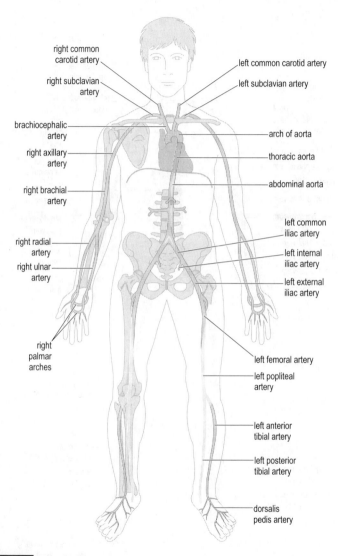

right common carotid artery

right subclavian artery

brachiocephalic artery

right axillary artery

right brachial artery

right radial artery

right ulnar artery

right palmar arches

left common carotid artery

left subclavian artery

arch of aorta

thoracic aorta

abdominal aorta

left common iliac artery

left internal iliac artery

left external iliac artery

left femoral artery

left popliteal artery

left anterior tibial artery

left posterior tibial artery

dorsalis pedis artery

Figure 9 Circulatory system—arteries

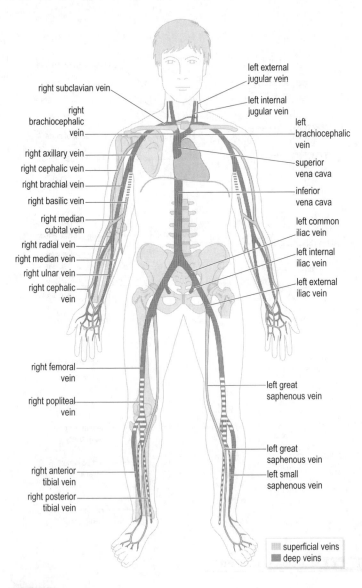

Figure 10 Circulatory system—veins

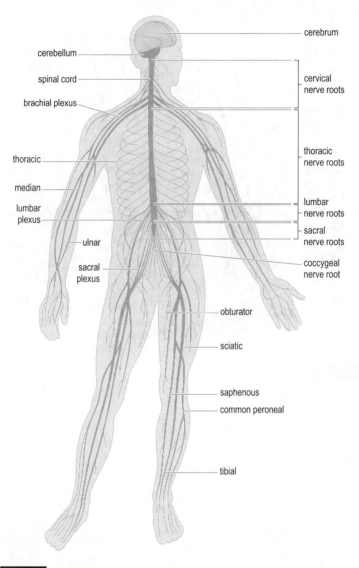

cerebrum

cerebellum

spinal cord

brachial plexus

cervical
nerve roots

thoracic

median

lumbar
plexus

thoracic
nerve roots

lumbar
nerve roots

sacral
nerve roots

ulnar

sacral
plexus

coccygeal
nerve root

obturator

sciatic

saphenous

common peroneal

tibial

Figure 11 Nervous system

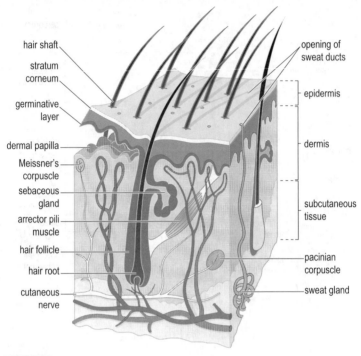

hair shaft
stratum corneum
germinative layer
dermal papilla
Meissner's corpuscle
sebaceous gland
arrector pili muscle
hair follicle
hair root
cutaneous nerve

opening of sweat ducts
epidermis
dermis
subcutaneous tissue
pacinian corpuscle
sweat gland

Figure 12 Skin

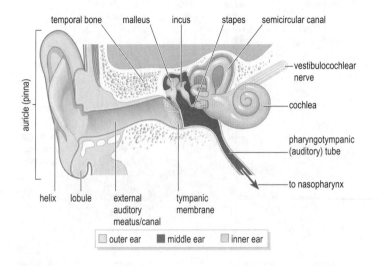

Figure 13 Ear

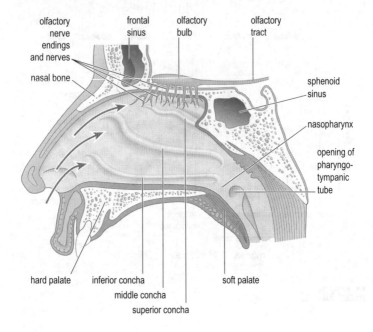

olfactory nerve endings and nerves

frontal sinus

olfactory bulb

olfactory tract

nasal bone

sphenoid sinus

nasopharynx

opening of pharyngo-tympanic tube

hard palate

inferior concha

middle concha

superior concha

soft palate

Figure 14 Nose

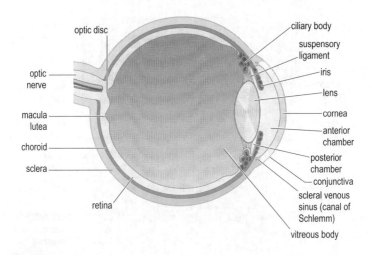

Figure 15 Eye

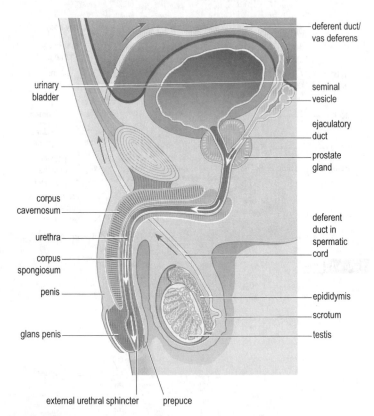

deferent duct/
vas deferens

urinary
bladder

seminal
vesicle

ejaculatory
duct

prostate
gland

corpus
cavernosum

deferent
duct in
spermatic
cord

urethra

corpus
spongiosum

penis

epididymis

scrotum

glans penis

testis

external urethral sphincter   prepuce

Figure 16 Male reproductive system
(showing route taken by spermatozoa during ejaculation)

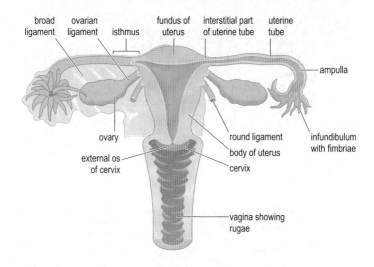

Figure 17 Female reproductive system

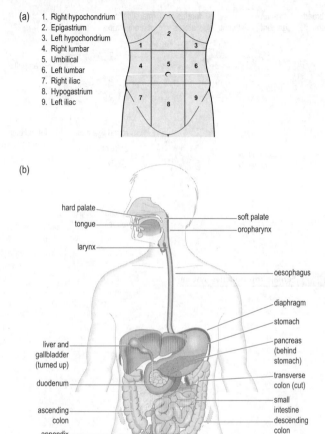

(a)
1. Right hypochondrium
2. Epigastrium
3. Left hypochondrium
4. Right lumbar
5. Umbilical
6. Left lumbar
7. Right iliac
8. Hypogastrium
9. Left iliac

(b)

hard palate
tongue
larynx
soft palate
oropharynx
oesophagus
diaphragm
stomach
pancreas (behind stomach)
liver and gallbladder (turned up)
duodenum
transverse colon (cut)
small intestine
descending colon
ascending colon
appendix
sigmoid colon
rectum

Figure 18 (a) Abdominal regions. (b) Digestive system

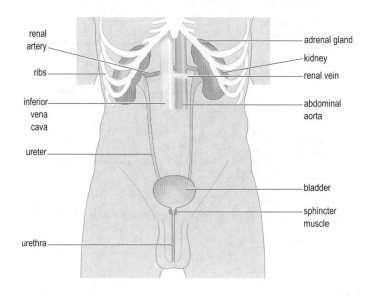

renal artery
ribs
inferior vena cava
ureter
urethra

adrenal gland
kidney
renal vein
abdominal aorta
bladder
sphincter muscle

Figure 19 Urinary system

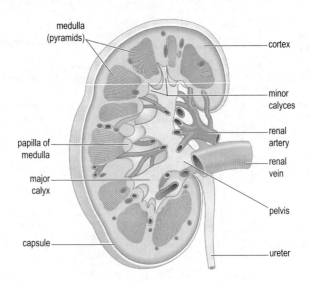

Figure 20 Urinary system—the kidney

SI units and the metric system

Acknowledgement
Conversion scales are taken from Goodsell D (1975) Coming to terms with SI metric. *Nursing Mirror* 141: 55–59 and are reproduced by kind permission of the author and *Nursing Mirror*.

Système International (SI) Units

At an international convention in 1960, the General Conference of Weights and Measures agreed to promulgate an International System of Units, frequently described as SI or Système International. This is merely the name for the current version of the metric system, first introduced in France at the end of the 18th century.

In any system of measurement, the magnitude of some physical quantities must be arbitrarily selected and declared to have unit value. These magnitudes form a set of standards and are called *base units*. All other units are *derived units*.

The SI measurement system is used for medical, scientific and technical purposes in most countries and comprises seven base units with several derived units. Each unit has its own symbol and is expressed as a decimal multiple or submultiple of the base unit by use of the appropriate prefix; for example, millimetre is one thousandth of a metre.

Base units

Name of SI Unit	Symbol for SI Unit	Quantity
metre	m	length
kilogram	kg	mass
second	s	time
mole	mol	amount of substance
ampere	A	electric current
kelvin	$^{\circ}$K	thermodynamic temperature
candela	cd	luminous intensity

Derived units

Derived units are obtained by dividing or multiplying any two or more of the seven base units.

Name of SI unit	Symbol for SI unit	Quantity
joule	J	work, energy, quantity of heat
pascal	Pa	pressure
newton	N	force
watt	W	power
volt	V	electrical potential, potential difference, electromotive force
hertz	Hz	frequency
becquerel	Bq	radioactivity
gray	Gy	adsorbed dose of radiation
sievert	Sv	dose equivalent

Decimal multiples and submultiples

The metric system uses multiples of 10 to express number.

Multiples and submultiples of the base unit are expressed as decimals and the following prefixes are used:

The most widely used prefixes are kilo, milli and micro:

$0.000\,001\ g = 10^{-6}\ g = 1$ microgram (microgram is used in full for drug prescriptions to avoid dose errors)

Multiples and submultiples of units

Multiplication factor		Prefix	Symbol
1 000 000 000 000	10^{12}	tera	T
1 000 000 000	10^{9}	giga	G
1 000 000	10^{6}	mega	M
1 000	10^{3}	kilo	k
100	10^{2}	hecto	h
10	10^{1}	deca	da
0.1	10^{-1}	deci	d
0.01	10^{-2}	centi	c
0.001	10^{-3}	milli	m
0.000 001	10^{-6}	micro	μ
0.000 000 001	10^{-9}	nano	n
0.000 000 000 001	10^{-12}	pico	p
0.000 000 000 000 001	10^{-15}	femto	f
0.000 000 000 000 000 001	10^{-18}	atto	a

Rules for using units

a. The symbol for a unit is unaltered in the plural and should not be followed by a full stop except at the end of the sentence:

5 cm *not* 5 cm. or 5 cms.

b. The decimal sign between digits is indicated by a full stop positioned near the line. No commas are used to divide large numbers into groups of three, but a half-space (whole space in typing) is left after every third digit. If the numerical value of the number is less than 1 unit, a zero should precede the decimal sign:

> 0.123 456 *not* .123,456

c. The SI symbol for 'day' (i.e. 24 hours) is 'd', but urine and faecal excretion of substances should preferably be expressed as 'per 24 hours':

> g/24 h

d. 'Squared' and 'cubed' are expressed as numerical powers and not by abbreviation:

> square centimetre is cm^2 *not* sq cm.

Commonly used measurements

a. The SI base unit for temperature is the kelvin; however, temperature is expressed as degrees Celsius (°C).

> 1° Celsius = 1° Centigrade

b. The calorie is replaced by the joule:

> 1 calorie = 4.2 J
> 1 kilocalorie (dietetic 'large' Calorie) = 4.2 kilojoules

The energy of food or individual requirements for energy are measured in kilojoules (kJ), but in practice the kilocalorie (kcal) is still in common use.

c. The SI base unit for amount of substance is the mole (mol). The concentration of many substances is expressed in moles per litre (mol/L) or millimoles per litre (mmol/L), which replaces milliequivalents per litre (mEq/L). Some exceptions exist and include: haemoglobin and plasma proteins expressed in grams per litre (g/L). Enzyme activity is expressed in International Units (IU, U or iu).

d. The SI unit of pressure is the pascal (Pa), and the kilopascal (kPa) replaces millimetres of mercury pressure (mmHg) for blood pressure and blood gases.

> 1 mmHg = 133.32 Pa
> 1 kPa = 7.5006 mmHg

However, blood pressure is still widely measured in mmHg pressure, cerebrospinal fluid (in mmH_2O) and central venous pressure (in cmH_2O).

e. Volume is calculated by multiplying length, width and depth. The SI unit for length, the metre (m), is not appropriate, as a cubic metre is not practical for most purposes. The volume of a 10 cm cube; the litre (L), is used instead. The millilitre (mL) is commonly used in clinical practice.

Weights and measures

Linear measure

1 kilometre (km)	= 1000 metres (m)
1 metre (m)	= 100 centimetres (cm) or 1000 millimetres (mm)
1 centimetre (cm)	= 10 millimetres (mm)
1 millimetre (mm)	= 1000 micrometres (µm)
1 micrometre (µm)	= 1000 nanometres (nm)

Conversions

Metric	Imperial
1 metre (m)	= 39.370 inches (in)
1 centimetre (cm)	= 0.3937 inches (in)
30.48 centimetres (cm)	= 1 foot (ft)
2.54 centimetres (cm)	= I inch (in)

Volume

1 litre (L)	= 1000 millilitres (mL)
1 millilitre (mL)	= 1000 microlitres (μL)

Conversions

Metric	Imperial
1 litre (L)	= 1.76 pints (pt)
568.25 millilitres (mL)	= 1 pint (pt)
28.4 millilitres (mL)	= 1 fluid ounce (fl oz)

Weight (mass)

1 kilogram (kg)	= 1000 grams (g)
1 gram (g)	= 1000 milligrams (mg)
1 milligram (mg)	= 1000 micrograms (μg)
1 microgram (μg)	= 1000 nanograms (ng)

NB. to avoid any confusion with milligram (mg) the word microgram should be written in full on prescriptions.

Conversions

Metric	Imperial
1 kilogram (kg)	= 2.204 pounds (lb)
1 gram (g)	= 0.0353 ounce (oz)
453.59 grams (g)	= 1 pound (lb)
28.34 grams (g)	= 1 ounce (oz)

Temperature

$$°\text{Fahrenheit} = \left(\frac{9}{5} \times x°\text{C}\right) + 32$$

$$°\text{Centigrade} = \frac{5}{9} \times (x°\text{F} - 32)$$

where x is the temperature to be converted

Conversion scales for certain chemical pathology tests and units of measurement

Chemical pathology Blood plasma

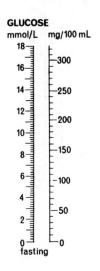

GLUCOSE

mmol/L mg/100 mL

fasting

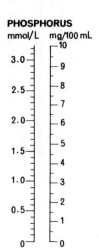

PHOSPHORUS

mmol/L mg/100 mL

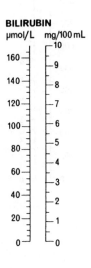

BILIRUBIN

µmol/L mg/100 mL

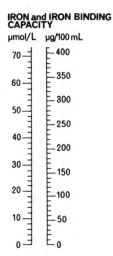

IRON and IRON BINDING CAPACITY

µmol/L µg/100 mL

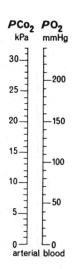

PCO_2 **PO_2**

kPa mmHg

arterial blood

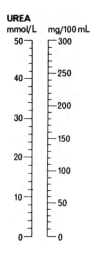

UREA

mmol/L mg/100 mL

CREATININE
μmol/L   mg/100 mL

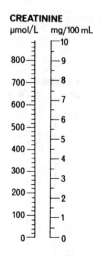

URATE (Uric acid)
mmol/L   mg/100 mL

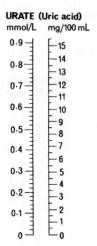

CALCIUM
mmol/L   mg/100 mL

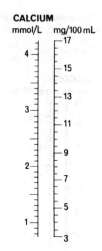

CHOLESTEROL
mmol/L   mg/100 mL

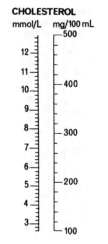

TRIGLYCERIDES
mmol/L   mg/100 mL

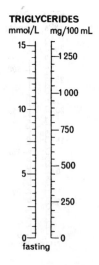

fasting

PROTEINS
(Total and albumin)
g/L   g/100 mL

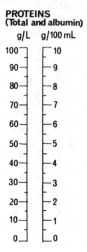

PBI

nmol/L   µg/100 mL

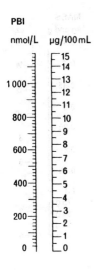

CORTISOL

nmol/L   µg/100 mL

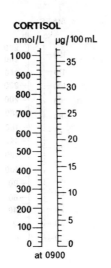

at 0900

Urine
OESTRIOL
('Oestrogens')

µmol/24 h   mg/24 h

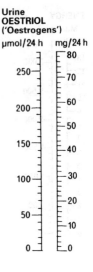

General measurements

HEIGHT

cm   inches

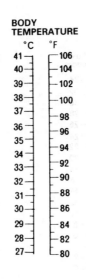

BODY
TEMPERATURE

°C   °F

ROOM
TEMPERATURE

°C   °F

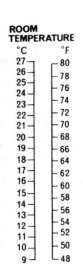

347

ENERGY

| MJ | kcal |

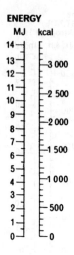

MASS

| kg | lb |

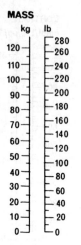

MASS

| kg and g | oz |

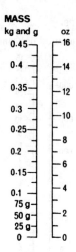

VOLUME

| mL | fluid ounces |

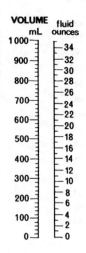

VOLUME

| L | pints |

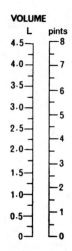

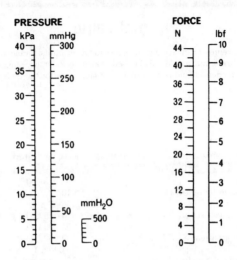

349

Normal values

The values below represent an 'average' reference range, in adults, for blood, cerebrospinal fluid, faeces and urine, and should only be used as a guide. Reference ranges vary between laboratories and readers should consult their own laboratory for those used locally.

Blood   350
CSF   352
Faeces   352
Urine   352

Blood—biochemistry (venous serum unless otherwise stated)

Test	Reference range
Acid phosphatase	0.1–0.6 U/L
Alanine aminotransferase (ALT)	10–40 U/L
Albumin	36–47 g/L
Alkali phosphatase	40–125 U/L
Amylase	90–300 U/L
Aspartate aminotransferase (AST)	10–35 U/L
Base excess	−2 to +2
Bicarbonate (arterial blood analysis)	22–28 mmol/L
Bilirubin—total	2–17 μmol/L
Caeruloplasmin	150–600 mg/L
Calcium	2.1–2.6 mmol/L
Chloride	97–106 mmol/L
Cholesterol (total)	Less than 5.2 mmol/L ideal 5.2–6.5 mmol/L mild 6.5–7.8 mmol/L moderate greater than 7.8 mmol/L severe
HDL cholesterol	
Female	0.6–1.9 mmol/L
Male	0.5–1.6 mmol/L
$PaCO_2$ (arterial blood analysis)	4.6–6.0 kPa
Copper	13–24 μmol/L
Cortisol (at 08.00 h)	160–560 nmol/L
Creatine kinase (total)	
Female	30–150 U/L
Male	30–200 U/L
Creatinine	60–120 μmol/L
Ferritin	
Female	14–150 μg/L
Male	17–300 μg/L
Gamma-glutamyl transferase (GGT)	
Female	30–150 U/L
Male	30–200 U/L
Globulins	24–37 g/L
Glucose (venous blood, fasting)	3.6–5.8 mmol/L
Glycosylated haemoglobin (HbA_1)	4–6%
Hydrogen ion concentration (arterial blood analysis)	35–44 nmol/L

(continued)

Blood—biochemistry (venous serum unless otherwise stated) (Continued)

Test	Reference range
Iron	
Female	10–28 μmol/L
Male	14–32 μmol/L
Iron-binding capacity total (TIBC)	45–70 μmol/L
Lactate (arterial blood)	0.3–1.4 mmol/L
Lactate dehydrogenase (total)	230–460 U/L
Lead (whole blood)	
Adults	Less than 1.7 μmol/L
Children	Less than 1.2 μmol/L
Magnesium	0.75–1.0 mmol/L
Osmolality	275–295 mosmol/kg
Oxygen saturation	More than 97%
PaO_2 (arterial blood analysis)	10.0–13.3 kPa
pH (arterial blood analysis)	7.35–7.45
Phosphate (fasting)	0.8–1.4 mmol/L
Potassium (plasma)	3.3–4.7 mmol/L
Potassium (serum)	3.6–5.0 mmol/L
Protein (total)	60–80 g/L
Sodium	135–143 mmol/L
Thyroxine (free)	10–27 pmol/L
Triiodothyronine	1.0–2.6 nmol/L
Transferrin	2.0–4.0 g/L
Triglycerides	0.45–2.0 mmol/L
Urea	2.5–6.4 mmol/L
Uric acid	
Female	0.09–0.36 mmol/L
Male	0.1–0.45 mmol/L
Vitamin A	0.7–3.5 μmol/L
Vitamin C	23–57 μmol/L
Zinc	11–22 μmol/L

Blood—haematology

Activated partial thromboplastin time (APTT)	30–40s
Bleeding time (Ivy)	2–8 min
Erythrocyte sedimentation rate (ESR) (adult)	
Female	0–7 mm/h
Male	0–5 mm/h
	NB. Older people may have higher values
Fibrinogen	1.5–4.0 g/L
Folate (serum)	2.0–9 μg/L
Haematocrit see PCV	
Haemoglobin	
Female	115–165 g/L (11.5–16.5 g/dL)
Male	130–180 g/L (13–18 g/dL)
Haptoglobins	0.3–2.0 g/L

(continued)

Blood—haematology (Continued)

Mean cell haemoglobin (MCH)	27–32 pg
Mean cell haemoglobin concentration (MCHC)	30–35 g/dL
Mean cell volume (MCV)	78–94 fL
Packed cell volume (PCV)	
Female	0.35–0.47 (35–47%)
Male	0.40–0.54 (40–54%)
Platelets	150–400×10⁹/L
Prothrombin time	11–14s
Red cell count	
Female	3.8–5.3×10¹²/L
Male	4.5–6.5×10¹²/L
Reticulocytes (adults)	25–85×10⁹/L
White cells	
Total	4.0–11.0×10⁹/L
Differential	
Neutrophils	2.0–7.5×10⁹/L
Eosinophils	0.04–0.4×10⁹/L
Basophils	0.02–0.10×10⁹/L
Lymphocytes	1.5–4.0×10⁹/L
Monocytes	0.2–0.8×10⁹/L

Cerebrospinal fluid

Pressure (adult)	50–200 mm water
Cells	0–5 mm³
Glucose	2.5–4.0 mmol/L
Protein	100–400 mg/L
Chloride	120–170 mmol/L

Faeces

Fat content (daily output on normal diet)	less than 7 g/24 h
Fat (as stearic acid)	11–18 mmol/24 h

Urine

Albumin/creatinine ratio (ACR)	less than 3.5 mg
(used to detect microalbuminuria)	albumin/mmol creatinine
Albumin excretion rate (AER)	less than 20 µg
(used to detect microalbuminuria)	albumin/min
Calcium (depends on diet)	up to 12 mmol/24 h
	(normal diet)
Copper	0.2–0.6 µmol/24 h
Cortisol	9–50 µmol/24 h
Creatinine	10–20 mmol/24 h
5-Hydroxyindole-3-acetic	15–60 µmol/24 h
acid (5HIAA)	
Metadrenaline	0.3–1.7 µmol/24 h
Magnesium	3.3–5.0 mmol/24 h
Normetadrenaline	0.4–3.4 µmol/24 h

(continued)

Urine (Continued)

Oxalate	
Female	40–320 mmol/24 h
Male	80–490 mmol/24 h
Phosphate	15–50 mmol/24 h
pH	4–8
Potassium (depends on intake)	25–100 mmol/24 h
Protein (total)	no more than 0.3 g/L
Sodium (depends on intake)	100–200 mmol/24 h
Urate	1.2–3.0 mmol/24 h
Urea	170–500 mmol/24 h

Nutrients

The maintenance of health requires the correct intake of nutrients for the production of energy and the molecules needed for cell growth and repair. These nutrients are the energy-yielding macronutrients—carbohydrate (including non-starch polysaccharide), protein and fat; and the micronutrients—vitamins (water-soluble and fat-soluble) and minerals (including trace elements).

Macronutrients

Nutrient and energy value	RNI (DoH 1991)	Sources	Action/ functions	Deficiency	Excess	Special points
Carbohydrate 1 g yields 16 kJ (3.75 kcal)	A minimum of 47% of total daily energy intake should be provided by carbohydrate this should include no more than 10% as non-milk extrinsic sugars. The RNI for non-starch polysaccharide is 18 g/d	Rice, pasta, noodles, chapatti, bread, breakfast cereals, sugar, yam, plantain and potato	Provides energy for metabolic processes	Weight loss, ketosis	Obesity, hypertrigly-ceridaemia	Diets high in carbohydrate tend to be low in fat
Protein 1 g yields 17 kJ (4 kcal)	Female 45 g/d Male 55 g/d	Meat, fish, eggs, nuts, pulses, dairy products, tofu, and Quorn	A component of all body tissues; energy source in some situations	Retarded growth; weight loss and muscle wasting, poor wound healing; impaired immune system; fat deposition in the liver	Possible link with loss of minerals from bone and age-related deterioration in renal function	Protein content of Western diets usually higher than the RNI
Fat 1 g yields 37 kJ (9 kcal)	Should not exceed 33% of total daily energy intake and of this no more than 10% should be saturated fatty acids	Pastry, cakes, biscuits, chocolate and crisps, cooking oils, ghee, margarine, fried foods, full fat dairy products, meat, oily fish, seeds, nuts	Source of energy, energy storage, absorption of fat-soluble vitamins, synthesis of steroid hormones, integrity of nerve and cell membranes, insulation	Weight loss; deficiency of EFAs can lead to neurological damage	Obesity; increased risk of many conditions including cardiovascular disease and some cancers	The normal development of the nervous system depends on two essential fatty acids— linoleic acid and alpha-linolenic acid

Micronutrients: Vitamins—water-soluble

Vitamin	RNI (DoH 1991)	Sources	Action/functions
Vitamin B group:			
(i) B₁ Thiamin(e)	0.4 mg/1000 kcal	Fortified breakfast cereals, yeast extract, vegetables, fruit, wholegrain cereals, milk, liver, eggs, pork	Coenzyme for carbohydrate metabolism
(ii) B₂ Riboflavin	Female 1.1 mg/d Male 1.3 mg/d	Milk, milk products, offal, yeast extract, fortified breakfast cereals	Coenzyme for the metabolism of carbohydrate, fat and protein
(iii) B₃ Niacin (nicotinic acid and nicotin-amide)	6.6 mg/1000 kcal as nicotinic acid equivalents	Meat, fish, yeast extract, pulses, wholegrains, forti-fied breakfast cereals	Energy metabolism, as part of coenzymes NAD and NADP involved in oxidation and reduction reactions
(iv) B₅ Pantothenic acid	None set	Widespread in food, e.g. liver, eggs, yeast, vegetables, pulses, cereals	Protein, fat, carbohydrate and alcohol metabolism
(v) B₆ Pyridoxine	Female 1.2 mg/d Male 1.4 mg/d	Meat, fish, eggs, some vegetables, wholegrains	Amino acid metabolism. Needed for haemoglobin production
(vi) Biotin	None set	Widely distributed in many foods, e.g. offal, egg yolk, legumes, etc. Can be synthesized by intestinal bacteria	Essential in fat metabolism
(vii) B₁₂ Cobalamins	15 μg/g of protein	Animal products, meat, eggs, fish dairy products, yeast extract	Essential for red blood cell formation and nerve myelination. Needed for folate use
(viii) Folates (folic acid)	200 μg/d	Green leaf vegetables, bread, fortified breakfast cereals, yeast extract, liver	Red blood cell production, DNA synthesis
Vitamin C— ascorbic acid	40 mg/d	Citrus fruits, kiwi fruit, blackcurrants; green peppers, green leaf vegetables; potato; strawberries; tomatoes. Content decreases with storage	Collagen synthesis, formation of bones, connective tissue, teeth. Iron absorp-tion for red blood cell production. Acts as an antioxidant

Deficiency	Excess	Special points
Beri-beri; neuritis; mental confusion; fatigue; poor growth in children. Wernicke–Korsakoff syndrome occurring with alcohol misuse	Headache, insomnia, irritability, contact dermatitis	Requirement related to the amount of carbohydrate intake
Fissures at corner of mouth; tongue inflammation; corneal vascularization	Large quantities are not absorbed thus preventing toxicity	Destroyed by sunlight
Pellagra—dermatitis, diarrhoea and dementia	Liver damage, skin irritation	Also synthesized from the amino acid tryptophan
Vomiting, insomnia	Not reported	
Rare; metabolic abnormalities and convulsions	Peripheral nerve damage	Requirement is related to protein intake
Rare; dermatitis, hair loss, nausea, fatigue and anorexia. May be seen in patients having long-term total parenteral nutrition and where large quantities of raw egg are eaten	None known	
Megaloblastic anaemia. Irreversible spinal cord damage	Not reported	Requires the intrinsic factor produced by the stomach for absorption; only found in foods of animal origin; therefore, strict vegetarians and vegans require a dietary supplement
Megaloblastic anaemia; growth retardation	Can mask the megaloblastic anaemia of B_{12} deficiency	Supplement recommended prior to conception and during first 3 months of pregnancy to reduce the incidence of neural tube defects
Sore mouth and gums; capillary bleeding; scurvy; delayed wound healing, scar breakdown	Diarrhoea; oxalate stones in kidneys	Destroyed by cooking in the presence of air and by plant enzymes released when cutting and grating raw food

Micronutrients: Vitamins—fat-soluble

Vitamin	RNI (DoH 1991)	Sources	Action/functions	Deficiency	Excess	Special points
Vitamin A— retinol	Female 600 µg/d Male 700 µg/d	As retinol in liver, kidney, oily fish, egg yolk, full fat dairy produce. As the provitamin carotenes in green, yellow, orange and red fruit and vegetables, e.g. broccoli, carrots, apricots, mangoes, sweet potatoes and tomatoes	Visual pigments in retina, aids night vision. Normal growth and development of tissues; essential for healthy skin and mucosae. Acts as an antioxidant	Poor growth; rough, dry skin and mucosae; xerophthalmia and eventual blindness; increased risk of infection; poor night vision	High doses are teratogenic	Synthesized in the body from carotenes present in the diet
Vitamin D— cholecalciferol and ergosterol	10 µg/d for the house-bound	Oily fish, egg yolk, butter, fortified margarine; action of ultraviolet rays (sunlight) on the provitamin (7-dehydro-cholesterol) in the skin	Calcium and phosphorus homeostasis	Rickets (children); osteomalacia (adults)	Rare; weight loss and diarrhoea	Produced in the body by action of sunlight on a provitamin in the skin, deficiency develops in those who are not exposed to sun, for example the housebound

Vitamin E—tocopherols and toco-trienes	None set	Wheat germ, vegetable oils, nuts, seeds, egg yolk, cereals, dark green vegetables	An antioxidant. Protects against cell membrane damage	Haemolytic anaemia, can develop in premature infants and malabsorption syndrome	Breast pain, muscle weakness, gastrointestinal disorders	Requirement is increased with increased intake of PUFAs
Vitamin K—phyllo-quinones and mena-quinones	None set	Green leafy vegetables, fruit and dairy products	Needed for the production of prothrombin and other coagulation factors	Impaired clotting; liver damage	Not yet observed from naturally occurring vitamin	Synthesized by intestinal bacteria so deficiency unusual; can occur in new-borns (haemorrhagic disease of the newborn) and those on anticoagulant therapy

Micronutrients—minerals

Mineral and chemical symbol	RNI (DoH 1991)	Sources	Action/functions	Deficiency	Excess	Special points
Calcium—Ca	700 mg/d	Milk and milk products, green leafy vegetables, soya beans, white bread and hard water	Strengthening the skeleton and teeth; blood coagulation; normal neuro-muscular function	Osteomalacia; rickets; tetany. Reduced bone density; osteoporosis	Calcium deposits in soft tissue, hypercalcaemia	Absorption helped by vitamin D and parathyroid hormone
Iodine—I	140 µg/d	Seafood: iodized salt; milk and milk products, meat and eggs	Production of the thyroid hormones: thyroxine and triiodothyronine	Goitre; retarded growth; impaired brain development; congenital abnormalities	Goitre and hyperthyroidism	Some vegetables contain goitrogens that inhibit iodine absorption
Iron—Fe	Female 14.8 mg/d Male 8.7 mg/d	Liver, kidney, red meat, egg yolk, wholegrains, pulses, dark green vegetables, dried fruit, treacle, cocoa, molasses	Component of haemo-globin, myoglobin and many enzymes	Iron deficiency anaemia. Poor growth; impaired intellectual development	Liver damage	Absorption is aided by vitamin C and inhibited by phytates and tannins
Magnesium—Mg	Female 270 mg/d Male 300 mg/d	Cereals, milk, nuts, seeds, and green vegetables	Cofactor for many enzymes essential for carbohydrate and protein metabolism; important role in calcium homeo-stasis and skeletal development. Neuromuscular function	Unlikely, mainly in cases of chronic malabsorption and chronic renal failure when it will accompany hypocalcaemia	Unlikely from dietary sources	Absorption inhibited by phytate

Potassium—K	3500 mg/d	Fruit, vegetables, meat, wholegrains	Major intracellular electrolyte; influences muscle contraction and nerve excitability. Regulation of acid–base balance	Muscular weakness; depression; confusion; arrhythmias; cardiac arrest	Hyperkalaemia, cardiac arrest	Kidney controls secretion and absorption; deficiency is rare due to poor dietary intake but can occur following prolonged use of diuretics and purgatives
Sodium—Na	1600 mg/d	Table salt, milk, meat, vegetables, sauces, pickles, processed foods and snacks, cheese	Major extracellular electrolyte; important for regulating water balance. Regulation of acid–base balance	Weakness; cramp; faintness	Oedema, hypertension	Lost through fever, sweat and diarrhoea
Zinc—Zn	Female 7.0 mg/d Male 9.5 mg/d	Red meats, eggs, wholegrains	Cofactor needed for many enzymes. Structural role in some proteins; wound healing; functioning of immune system; sexual and physical development	Fatigue; retarded growth and sexual maturity	Nausea, vomiting, fever, or anaemia with chronic excess	Present in all tissues

Plus other minerals and trace elements (needed in minute quantities) that include: chloride; copper; chromium; fluoride; phosphorus as phosphates; manganese; molybdenum and selenium

Further reading

Barker H (2002) *Nutrition/dietetics for Healthcare*. 10th edn. Edinburgh: Churchill Livingstone.
COMA Annual Report 1999–2000 at www.doh.gov.uk/pub/docs/doh/coma99.pdf

Reference

Department of Health (DoH) (1991) *Report on Health and Social Subjects 41. Dietary Reference Values for Food energy and Nutrients for the United Kingdom*. London: HMSO.

Drugs—the law, measurement and drug groups in common use

Helen Richmond

Drugs and the law

The main Acts governing the use of medicines in the UK are the Medicines Act 1968, the Misuse of Drugs Act 1971 and the Medicinal Products: Prescription by Nurses Act 1992.

There are considerable changes concerning the extension of independent prescribing by nurses, and plans to increase supplementary prescribing by nurses and pharmacists. Readers are advised to check new legislation that may affect practice.

The Medicines Act 1968

This Act identifies doctors, dentists and veterinary surgeons as the only appropriate practitioners to prescribe medicines and states:

No person shall administer (otherwise than to himself) any such medicinal product unless he is an appropriate practitioner or a person acting in accordance with an appropriate practitioner.

The Medicines Act 1968 deals with drugs in three groups:

- Prescription only medicines (POM) include most of the potent drugs in common use, from antidepressants to hypoglycaemics. They are only supplied or administered to a patient on the instructions of the appropriate practitioner (a doctor or dentist) and from an approved list for a nurse prescriber. NB. Excludes controlled drugs (see below).

- Pharmacy only medicines (P) are licensed drugs supplied under the control and supervision of a registered pharmacist. Examples include ibuprofen, antihistamines and glyceryl trinitrate.

- General sales list medicines (GSL) are those commonly used drugs such as aspirin and paracetamol, available through any retail outlet such as supermarkets.

All drugs in hospital are supplied on prescription so the distinctions of POM, P and GSL medicines do not apply.

The Medicines Act 1968 also makes provision for various other substances such as potent herbal medicines (not available for unrestricted sale to the public) used in complementary therapies. However, many homeopathic preparations, food supplements, herbal and traditional medicines from non-European countries are not presently covered by the licensing process.

The Misuse of Drugs Act 1971

This Act imposes controls on those drugs liable to produce dependence or cause harm if misused. It prohibits certain activities in relation to controlled drugs (CD). Only doctors and dentists can prescribe CDs.

However, the Misuse of Drugs (Notification of and Supply to Addicts) Regulations 1973 state that medical practitioners may not prescribe, administer or supply CDs to addicted persons as a means of treating their addiction, unless specifically licensed to do so.

The Misuse of Drugs (Supply to Addicts) Regulations 1997 revoked the requirement for prescribers to provide the Home Office with information about drugs addicts, but there is an expectation that practitioners will report cases of drug misuse to the local Drug Misuse Database.

CDs are divided into three classes that reflect the level of harm caused by each drug if misused. The three classes are as follows:

Legal class	Examples
Class A (most harm)	Alfentanil, cocaine, diamorphine (heroin), dipanone, lysergide (LSD), methadone, methylenedioxy-methamfetamine (MDMA or ecstasy), morphine, opium, pethidine NB: and Class B drugs when they are in injectable form
Class B (intermediate)	Oral amphetamines, barbiturates, *cannabis, *cannabis resin, codeine, ethylmorphine, pentazocine
Class C (least harm)	Certain drugs related to amphetamines (e.g. benzfetamine). Most benzodiazepines. Androgenic and anabolic steroids, and growth hormone

*In the UK the reclassification of cannabis to a class C drug is currently underway. The necessary legislation is likely to be in place by July 2003.

Further to the 1971 Act, the Misuse of Drugs Regulations 1985 identifies those who may supply and possess controlled drugs while acting in their professional capacity and ordains the conditions under which these activities may be carried out.

Midwives unlike nurses are licensed to 'administer' controlled drugs and obtain controlled drugs (pentazocine lactate, pethidine hydrochloride) under legislation. They are exempt from prescribing. The legislation covering them is: The Statutory Instrument 1997 Number 1830 and the prescription only medium (Human Use Order 1997). Midwives are referred to in Section 5 Part 3 of this legislation. In addition, this states that the other drugs (prescription only medicines) a midwife may administer are: ergometrine maleate, lidocaine (lignocaine) hydrochloride, naloxone hydrochloride, oxytocin (natural and synthetic), phytonenadione (vitamin K) and promazine hydrochloride.

The administration shall be only in the course of their professional practice. In the case of promazine hydrochloride and lidocaine (lignocaine) hydrochloride; these shall only be administered to a woman during childbirth. Further guidance for midwives is recorded in the Midwives Rules.

The Misuse of Drugs Regulations 1985 further subdivides drugs into five schedules (see p. 365). Each schedule details the requirements for import, export, production, supply, possession, prescribing and record keeping. Health professionals should be familiar with those relating to drugs in Schedules 2 and 3.

Controlled drug prescription rules
Prescriptions for controlled drugs are required to fulfil the following conditions:

- They must be hand-written.
- The name and the address of the patient must be clearly written in ink.
- The dosage form must be hand written, e.g. tablets, and the strength must be specific.
- The total quantity of the preparation, or the number of dose units, in both words and figures, must be stated.
- The dose must be stated.
- If for dental treatment, this must be stated clearly.

Schedule	Examples
Schedule 1	Drugs that are often used illegally, e.g. cannabis and hallucinogens such as lysergide. Possession and supply are only permitted with Home Office authority.
Schedule 2	Addictive drugs including: amfetamine, cocaine, diamorphine (heroin), morphine, pethidine, secobarbital, glutethimide. The prescription, safe custody and storage of Schedule 2 CDs must fulfil the full controlled drug requirements, which includes maintaining registers.
Schedule 3	Barbiturates (except secobarbital), buprenorphine, diethylpropion, flunitrazepam, mazidol, meprobamate, pentazocine, phentermine and temazepam. Schedule 3 CDs are subject to special prescription requirements (except phenobarbital, temazepam) but not safe custody (with exceptions, e.g. temazepam). Registers do not need to be kept, only invoices for 2 years.
Schedule 4	Schedule 4 CDs are subject neither to controlled drug prescription rules nor to safe custody. Part II includes: benzodiazepines except flunitrazepam and temazepam, and pemoline. Part I includes: anabolic steroids, clenbuterol, chorionic gonadotrophin (HCG), somatropin.
Schedule 5	Schedule 5 includes medicines, such as some cough mixtures, that by virtue of their strength are exempt from most CD regulations except the keeping of invoices for 2 years.

Pharmacists are not allowed to dispense the drug unless all of the above is correct. Accurate records must be kept by general practitioners, dentists, and hospital staff of all purchases, amounts of the drugs issued and dosages given.

Storage of controlled drugs

- There should be a special locked cupboard for CDs. This should be a locked cupboard within a locked cupboard, which is attached to the wall.

- In hospital the keys to the cupboard are kept on the person in charge of the ward, or deputy.

- Supplies can be obtained by prescription signed by a medical officer, and the drugs can only be given under written instructions.

- Ward stocks of CDs in frequent use can be ordered in special CD order books. A qualified practitioner must sign each order.

- A careful written record of each dose given to a patient must be kept. This record must state: the patient's name, the time the drug was administered and the dosage. The practitioner (usually a nurse) giving the drug, and another nurse who has checked the source of the drug as well as the dosage against the prescription signs the record.

All containers used for CDs must bear special labels to distinguish them clearly. A hospital pharmacist must check the contents of the CD cupboard at regular intervals against the record books. Any discrepancies must be fully investigated.

Medicinal Products: Prescription by Nurses Act 1992

This Act, together with subsequent amendments to the Pharmaceutical Services regulations, allows registered health visitors and district nurses, who have their qualification recorded on the NMC register, to become nurse prescribers, after completing appropriate educational programmes. Practitioners whose prescribing status is denoted on the register, and who are approved within their employment setting, may prescribe from the *Nurse Prescribers' Formulary* (NPF). Nurse prescribers must comply with the current legislation and be accountable for their practice.

Prescriptions written by nurse prescribers should:

- Be written legibly in ink.
- Be dated.
- State patient's full name and address.
- Be signed in ink by the prescriber.
- Include age and date of birth.

Also recommended:

- Dose and dose frequency should be stated.
- Unnecessary use of decimal point should be avoided.
- Strength of the preparation should be stated.
- Quantity should be carefully specified.
- Names of medicines should be written clearly using generic titles or non-proprietary names.
- Directions should be in English.

In the case of children: Children's age should always be stated on the product.

NB. Changes from April 2002 have sanctioned the extension of independent nurse prescribing, whereby certain nurses (after specific preparation and training) may prescribe from the *Nurse Prescribers' Extended Formulary*, which includes some POMs. Details are available from the Department of Health web site (www.doh.gov.uk/nurseprescribing) and further information is contained in the Department of Health publication *Extended Independent Nurse Prescribing within the NHS in England: A guide to implementation* (DoH 2002).

Further reading and information sources

British Medical Association and the Royal Pharmaceutical Society of Great Britain. *British National Formulary*. London (revised twice yearly—March and September). Also available online at: www.bnf.org.uk.

British Medical Association and the Royal Pharmaceutical Society of Great Britain in association with Community Practitioners' and Health Visitors' Association and the Royal College of Nursing (2002–2003) *Nurse Prescribers' Formulary*. Edited by Dinesh K Mehta.

Department of Health (2002) *Extended Independent Nurse Prescribing within the NHS in England: A guide to implementation*. London: Department of Health.

McCormick C (2002) Midwives and Patient Group Direction. *British Journal of Midwives* 10(5): 286–287. www.legislation.HMSO.gov.uk/si/si1997/1971830

Drug measurement

SI units are used for drug doses and concentrations and patient data (including weight, height and body surface area), drug levels in the body and other measurements (see Appendix 2). It is important to collect relevant and accurate patient data before calculating the amount of drug required. This is particularly so in infants and children.

Weight

Grams (g) and milligrams (mg) are the units most often used for drug doses. Where the dose is less than 1 gram it should be expressed in milligrams, e.g. 500 mg, rather than 0.5 g. Doses less than 1 mg should be expressed in micrograms, e.g. 250 micrograms, rather than 0.25 mg. Whenever drugs are prescribed in micrograms, the units should be written in full, i.e. trandolapril 500 micrograms, as the use of the abbreviations μg or mcg may in practice be mistaken for mg, which is one thousand times greater.

Where drug doses are tailored to the size of the person they are usually described in unit dose per kilogram of body weight, e.g. mg/kg or μg/kg. This method of dosage is frequently used for infants and children.

Volume

Almost all measurements of volume used in prescription and drug administration are in litres (L or l) and millilitres (mL or ml).

Concentration

There are several methods used for expressing concentration of dosages of a medicine in liquid form.

- Unit weight per unit volume—describes the unit weight of a drug contained in unit volume, e.g. 1 mg in 1 mL, 20 mg in 5 mL. Examples include prochlorperazine injection 12.5 mg/mL, phenoxymethylpenicillin oral solution 125 mg/5 mL.

- Percentage (weight in volume)—describes the weight of a drug expressed in grams which is contained in 100 mL of solution. For example, lidocaine (lignocaine) hydrochloride injection 2%, which contains 2 g in each 100 mL of solution or 200 mg (0.2 g) in each 10 mL or 20 mg (0.02 g) in each mL, etc.

- Percentage (weight in weight)—describes the weight of a drug expressed in grams which is contained in 100 g of a semisolid or solid medicament such as creams or ointments. For example, fusidic acid ointment 2%, which contains 2 g of fusidic acid in 100 g of ointment.

- Volume containing one part—a few liquids and some gases containing drugs in very low concentrations are often described as containing 1 part per x units of volume. For liquids: 'parts' are equal to grams and volume to millimetres, e.g. adrenaline (epinephrine) intramuscular or subcutaneous injection 1 in 1000, which contains 1 g in 1000 mL (1 mg in 1 mL) or expressed as a percentage (w/v)—0.1%.

- Molar concentration—drugs in liquid form are very occasionally expressed in molar concentration. A mole is the molecular weight of a drug expressed in grams, and one molar (1 M) solution contains this weight dissolved in each litre. The millimole (mmol) is often used to describe a medicinal product; e.g. sodium chloride 10 mmol in 10 mL indicates a solution containing the molecular weight of sodium chloride in milligrams × 10 dissolved in 10 mL of solution.

Body height and surface area

Where precise dosages need to be tailored to individual needs, dosages may be expressed in terms of microgram, milligram or gram per unit of body surface area. For example, cytotoxic drugs and drugs given to infants and children. Body surface area is expressed as square metres (m^2) and drug dosages as units/m^2, e.g. methotrexate 15 mg/m^2.

Acknowledgement

The measurement section was adapted from Henney CR et al (1995) *Drugs in Nursing Practice*, 5th edn. Churchill Livingstone, Edinburgh, with permission.

Drug groups in common use

Drug groups and subgroups	Examples	Indications
Alpha-adrenoceptor agonists (alpha stimulants)		
1. Alpha$_1$ receptor agonist	1. Phenylephrine (selective agonist)	1. Acute hypotension
2. Alpha$_2$ receptor agonist	2. Clonidine (selective agonist)	2. Hypertension, migraine
Alpha-adrenoceptor antagonists (alpha blockers)		
1. Alpha$_1$ receptor antagonist	1. Doxazosin (selective antagonist)	1. Benign prostatic hyperplasia, hypertension
2. Alpha$_{1,2}$ receptor antagonist	2. Phenoxybenzamine (non-selective).	2. Phaeochromocytoma (with other drugs)
Anabolic steroids	Nandrolone, stanozolol	Aplastic anaemia, pruritus in palliative care
Analgesics		
1. Non-opioids (see also NSAIDs)	1. Aspirin, paracetamol	1. Mild to moderate pain, e.g. simple headache, pyrexia
2. Opioids	2. Diamorphine, dihydrocodeine, fentanyl, morphine, etc.	2. Moderate to severe pain, e.g. palliative care
Angiotensin-converting enzyme inhibitor (ACE inhibitor)	Captopril, ramipril, etc.	Diabetic nephropathy, heart failure, hypertension, myocardial infarction
Antacids	Aluminium hydroxide, magnesium trisilicate	Dyspepsia
Anthelmintics	1. Levamisole	1. Roundworm
	2. Mebendazole	2. Hookworm, roundworm, threadworm, whipworm
	3. Piperazine	3. Roundworm, threadworm
	4. Praziquantel	4. Tapeworm
	5. Tiabendazole	5. Strongyloidiasis
Antiandrogens	1. Cyproterone acetate	1. Male hypersexuality, prostate cancer, acne and hirsutism in women
	2. Finasteride.	2. Benign prostatic hyperplasia.

(continued)

Drug groups in common use (Continued)

Drug groups and subgroups	Examples	Indications
Antiarrhythmics		
1. Supraventricular arrhythmias	1(a). Digoxin	1(a). Atrial fibrillation and flutter, etc.
	1(b). Verapamil	1(b). Supraventricular tachycardia etc.
2. Ventricular arrhythmias	2. Lidocaine (lignocaine)	2. Ventricular tachycardia
3. Used for both supraventricular and ventricular arrhythmias	3. Amiodarone.	3. Atrial fibrillation and flutter, ventricular tachycardia, etc.
Antibiotics (antibacterials)		
1. Aminoglycosides	1. Gentamicin	1. Septicaemia, acute pyelonephritis, meningitis, etc.
2. Antituberculosis	2. Ethambutol, isoniazid, pyrazinamide, rifampicin (in combination)	2. Tuberculosis
3. Carbapenems	3. Meropenem	3. Aerobic and anaerobic Gram-positive and Gram-negative bacteria
4. Cephalosporins	4. Cefaclor	4. Otitis media, respiratory infections, sinusitis, urinary infection, etc.
5. Fluoroquinolones	5. Ciprofloxacin	5. Gastrointestinal infection, e.g. typhoid, gonorrhoea, respiratory infection, urinary infection, etc.
6. Glycopeptides	6. Vancomycin	6. Endocarditis, pseudomembranous colitis, Gram-positive cocci infections including MRSA
7. Macrolides	7. Erythromycin	7. In place of penicillin in hypersensitive patients, campylobacter enteritis, pneumonia, syphilis, etc.

(continued)

Drug groups in common use (Continued)

Drug groups and subgroups	Examples	Indications
8. Penicillins	8(a). Ampicillin (broad spectrum)	8(a). Bronchitis, gonorrhoea, otitis media, urinary infections
	8(b). Flucloxacillin (beta-lactamase resistant)	8(b). Cellulitis, endocarditis (staphylococcal), otitis externa, pneumonia, etc.
9. Sulphonamides and trimethoprim	9. Co-trimoxazole	9. Pneumonia caused by *Pneumocystis carinii*, toxoplasmosis, etc.
10. Tetracyclines	10. Doxycycline	10. Chlamydial infections, brucellosis, rickettsia, mycoplasma. Also for periodontal disease, chronic bronchitis, etc.
Anticoagulants		
1. Coumarins	1. Warfarin	1. Deep vein thrombosis, pulmonary embolus, and patients with mechanical prosthetic heart valves
2. Heparin	2. Standard and low molecular weight heparin	2. Treatment and prophylaxis of deep vein thrombosis and pulmonary embolus, etc.
Antidepressants		
1. Monoamine oxidase inhibitors (MAOI)	1. Phenelzine	1. Depressive illness
2. Selective serotonin reuptake inhibitors (SSRI)	2. Fluoxetine	2. Depressive illness, obsessive-compulsive disorder, etc.
3. Tricyclic antidepressants (TCA)	3. Amitriptyline	3. Depressive illness, bedwetting in children
Antidiarrhoeals	Codeine phosphate, loperamide (antimotility drugs)	Adjuncts to rehydration in acute diarrhoea
Antiemetics		Nausea and vomiting:
1. Cannabinoids	1. Nabilone	1. Caused by cytotoxic chemotherapy
2. D_2-receptor antagonists	2. Metoclopramide	2. Caused by gastrointestinal disorders, radiation and chemotherapy

(continued)

Drug groups in common use (Continued)

Drug groups and subgroups	Examples	Indications
3. H$_1$-receptor antagonists	3. Cinnarizine	3. Motion sickness, vestibular disorders
4. 5-HT$_3$-receptor antagonists	4. Ondansetron	4. Caused by chemotherapy, radiation and postoperatively
5. Muscarinic antagonists	5. Hyoscine	5. Motion sickness
Antiepileptic (anticonvulsant)	Phenytoin	Epilepsy control
Antifungal	Fluconazole	Candidiasis, cryptococcal meningitis in AIDS patients
Antihistamine	Chlorphenamine (chlorpheniramine)	Hay fever, emergency treatment of anaphylactic reactions
Antihypertensives		
1. Vasodilator See: alpha-adrenoceptor antagonists, ACE inhibitors, beta-adrenoceptor antagonists, calcium channel blockers, diuretics	1. Hydralazine	1. Hypertension, heart failure
Anti-inflammatory drugs See: analgesics, NSAIDs		
Antileprotic	Dapsone (a sulphone), rifampicin	Leprosy
Antimalarial	Chloroquine, mefloquine, proguanil, quinine, etc.	Malaria—chemoprophylaxis and treatment (drug choice depends on the degree of risk and the extent of drug resistance in the area, side-effects and drug efficacy and user features such as age)
Antioestrogens	1. Clomifene	1. Female infertility
	2. Exemestane, goserelin, tamoxifen	2. Breast cancer
Antiparkinson	1. Co-beneldopa (levodopa plus benserazide)	1. Parkinsonism
	2. Orphenadrine	2. Parkinsonism, drug-induced extrapyramidal effects

(continued)

Drug groups in common use (Continued)

Drug groups and subgroups	Examples	Indications
Antiplatelet drugs	Aspirin, clopidogrel, dipyridamole, tirofiban	Prophylaxis of cerebrovascular disorders and myocardial infarction and thromboembolism in patients with a prosthetic heart valve. Peripheral arterial disease. Prevention of infarction in unstable angina, etc.
Antiprotozoal	Metronidazole	Infection with *Trichomonas vaginalis*
Antipsychotics See: neuroleptics		
Antipyretics See: NSAIDs	Aspirin	Pyrexia
Antispasmodics	Dicycloverine hydro-chloride, mebeverine hydrochloride	Gastrointestinal smooth muscle spasm
Antithyroid	Carbimazole	Hyperthyroidism
Antivirals	Aciclovir	Herpes simplex, varicella-zoster
1. Nucleoside reverse transcriptase inhibitors	1. Zidovudine	1. HIV infection (with other antiviral drugs)
2. Protease inhibitors	2. Ritonavir	2. Progressive or advanced HIV infection (used in combination with nucleoside reverse transcriptase inhibitors)
3. Non-nucleoside reverse transcriptase inhibitors	3. Efavirenz	3. HIV infection (with other antiviral drugs)
Anxiolytics Benzodiazepines	Diazepam	Short term for anxiety and insomnia, status epilepticus, alcohol withdrawal (acute), etc.
Beta-adrenoceptor agonists (beta stimulants, sympathomimetics)		
1. Beta$_1$ receptor agonists	1. Dobutamine (selective agonist, positive inotrope)	1. Cardiogenic shock, etc.
2. Beta$_2$ receptor agonists	2. Salbutamol (selective agonist)	2. Bronchodilator in asthma, etc.

(continued)

Drug groups in common use (Continued)

Drug groups and subgroups	Examples	Indications
Beta-adrenoceptor antagonists (beta blockers)		Hypertension, angina, arrhythmias, anxiety and glaucoma
1. Beta$_1$ receptor antagonists	1. Atenolol (selective antagonist)	
2. Beta$_{1,2}$ receptor antagonists	2. Propranolol (non-selective)	
Bisphosphonates	Disodium etidronate	Paget's disease, osteoporosis, hypercalcaemia of cancer
Bronchodilators See: beta-adrenoceptor agonists, muscarinic antagonists		
Calcium channel blockers (antagonists)	Verapamil (a negative inotrope)	Angina, arrhythmias, hypertension
Chelating agents	Desferrioxamine	Poisoning with iron salts, treatment for iron overload, e.g. repeated blood transfusion in thalassaemia
Corticosteroids	Prednisolone	Asthma, inflammatory bowel disease, malignant disease, rheumatoid arthritis, etc.
Cytotoxic agents		
1. Alkylating agent	1. Chlorambucil	1. Chronic lymphocytic leukaemia, Hodgkin's disease, ovarian cancer etc.
2. Antimetabolite	2. Methotrexate	2. Acute lymphoblastic leukaemia, non-Hodgkin's lymphoma, solid tumours, etc.
3. Antitumour antibiotic	3. Doxorubicin	3. Acute leukaemia, lymphomas, solid tumour
4. Vinca alkaloids	4. Vincristine	4. Acute leukaemias, lymphomas, lung and breast cancer, etc.
5. Etoposide	5. Etoposide	5. Small cell cancer of the bronchus, testicular cancer and lymphomas

(continued)

Drug groups in common use (Continued)

Drug groups and subgroups	Examples	Indications
6–9. Other anticancer drugs	6. Cisplatin	6. Ovarian and testicular cancers
	7. Paclitaxel	7. Ovarian and some lung cancers
	8. Irinotecan hydrochloride	8. Colorectal cancer (metastatic)
	9. Tretinoin.	9. Acute promyelocytic leukaemia
Decongestant	Pseudoephedrine (oral), ephedrine hydrochloride (nasal drops), etc.	Nasal congestion
Diuretics		
1. Carbonic anhydrase inhibitors (weak diuresis with systemic use)	1. Acetazolamide	1. Glaucoma
2. Loop diuretic	2. Furosemide (frusemide)	2. Oedema, heart failure, oliguria due to renal failure
3. Osmotic diuretic	3. Mannitol	3. Cerebral oedema, glaucoma
4. Potassium sparing	4. Amiloride	4. Oedema, conservation of potassium with other diuretics
5. Thiazide	5. Bendroflumethiazide (bendrofluazide)	5. Heart failure, hypertension.
Fibrinolytic drugs	Streptokinase reteplase, alteplase	Deep vein thrombosis, pulmonary embolus, arterial thromboembolism, acute myocardial infarction, etc.
H_2-receptor antagonists	Ranitidine	Peptic ulceration, gastro-oesophageal reflux, etc.
HMG-CoA reductase inhibitors (statins)	Pravastatin	Hypercholesterolaemia, hyperlipidaemia, prevention of coronary events in patients with CHD, etc.
$5\text{-}HT_1$ agonists	Sumatriptan	Migraine (treatment)
Hypnotics	Zaleplon	Insomnia (short-term only)
Hypoglycaemics (oral)		Diabetes
1. Alpha-glucosidases inhibitor	1. Acarbose	
2. Biguanides	2. Metformin	
3. Sulphonylureas	3. Glipizide	
Immunosuppressants	Azathioprine, ciclosporin	Organ transplantation

(continued)

Drug groups in common use (Continued)

Drug groups and subgroups	Examples	Indications
Inotropes—positive	1. Digoxin (a cardiac glycoside; see also antiarrhythmics)	1. Heart failure
	2. Dopamine	2. Cardiogenic shock after cardiac surgery or infarction
Inotropes—negative (see calcium channel blockers)		
Insulin	Short-acting—soluble Intermediate/long-acting—insulin zinc suspension and biphasic isophane insulin	Diabetes
Laxatives (aperients)		Constipation
1. Bulk-forming laxatives	1. Ispaghula, methylcellulose	
2. Faecal softeners	2. Arachis oil (enema)	
3. Osmotic laxative	3. Lactulose	
4. Stimulant	4. Senna	
Mucolytics	Dornase alpha (inhaled)	Cystic fibrosis
Muscarinic agonists (parasympathomimetic)	Pilocarpine	Raised intraocular pressure. Dry mouth, e.g. following radiotherapy. Dry eyes and mouth in Sjögren's syndrome
Muscarinic antagonists (antimuscarinic, parasympatholytic)	Ipratropium bromide	Bronchodilation in reversible chronic obstructive pulmonary disease
Mydriatics	Tropicamide	Pupil dilatation for ophthalmic examination
Neuroleptics (antipsychotics)		Disturbed individuals, e.g. agitated depression. Short-term treatment of severe anxiety. Long-term management of schizophrenia
1. Typical, e.g. phenothiazines	1. Fluphenazine	
2. Atypical, e.g. dibenzodiazepines	2. Clozapine	
Nitrates	Glyceryl trinitrate (sublingual, transdermal)	Angina

(continued)

Drug groups in common use (Continued)

Drug groups and subgroups	Examples	Indications
NSAIDs		Pain relief, antipyretic, reduction of inflammation and stiffness in arthritis, etc.
1. Fenamates	1. Mefenamic acid	
2. Oxicams	2. Piroxicam	
3. Propionic acids	3. Ibuprofen	
4. Pyrazolones	4. Azapropazone	
5. Salicylates (See analgesics)	5. Aspirin (also antiplatelet)	
Opioids See: analgesics		
Oxytocics	Oxytocin	Induction of labour, prevention and treatment of postpartum haemorrhage, etc.
Prostaglandins	Dinoprostone (PGE_2)	Induction of labour, termination of pregnancy
Proton pump inhibitors	Omeprazole	Peptic ulceration, part of regimen for eradicating *Helicobacter pylori*, etc.
Retinoids (See: cytotoxic agents—tretinoin)	1. Acitretin 2. Isotretinoin	1. Severe psoriasis 2. Acne
Selective (o)estrogen receptor modulators (SERMS)	Raloxifene	Prevention and treatment of postmenopausal osteoporosis.
Tocolytics See: beta adrenoceptor agonists	Terbutaline sulphate	Uncomplicated premature labour (24–33 weeks gestation)
Tranquillizers See: anxiolytics, neuroleptics		
Uricosuric	Probenecid	Prevention of gout

(Readers should be aware that some drugs used as examples for a particular drug group may also have other uses; for example, acetazolamide, a carbonic anhydrase inhibitor, is occasionally used as a second-line antiepileptic drug.)

Abbreviations—medical terms, degrees, diplomas, organizations

AA	Alcoholics Anonymous
AAA	abdominal aortic aneurysm
AAMI	age-associated memory impairment
ABGs	arterial blood gases
ACE	angiotensin-converting enzyme
ACh	acetylcholine
ACTH	adrenocorticotrophic hormone
ADH	antidiuretic hormone
ADHD	attention deficit hyperactivity disorder
ADLs	activities of daily living
ADP	adenosine diphosphate
ADPKD	adult dominant polycystic kidney disease
ADRs	adverse drug reactions
AFB	acid-fast bacilli
AFP	alphafetoprotein
AHF	antihaemophilic factor
AID	artificial insemination using donor semen
AIDS	acquired immune deficiency syndrome
AIH	artificial insemination using husband's (partner's) semen
AIMLS	Associate of the Institute of Medical Laboratory Sciences
AIMSW	Associate of the Institute of Medical Social Workers
ALD	adrenoleucodystrophy
ALG	antilymphocyte globulin
ALS	(1) advanced life support (2) amyotrophic lateral sclerosis
ALT	alanine aminotransferase
AMA	antimitochondrial antibody
AMI	acute myocardial infarction
AMP	adenosine monophosphate
ANA	antinuclear antibody
ANCA	anti-neutrophil cytoplasmic antibody
ANOVA	analysis of variance
ANS	autonomic nervous system
APD	automated peritoneal dialysis
APEL	Accreditation (Assessment) of Prior Experiential Learning
APKD	adult polycystic kidney disease
APL	Accreditation (Assessment) of Prior Learning
APTT	activated partial thromboplastin time
ARC	AIDS related complex
ARDS	acute respiratory distress syndrome
ARF	(1) acute renal failure (2) acute respiratory failure
ARM	artificial rupture of membranes
ARSH	Associate of the Royal Society of Health
ASO	antistreptolysin O
AST	aspartate aminotransferase

(continued)

ASW	approved social worker
ATN	acute tubular necrosis
ATP	adenosine triphosphate
BA	Bachelor of Arts
BACUP	British Association of Cancer United Patients
BAL	bronchial alveolar lavage
BASc	Bachelor of Applied Science
BASW	British Association of Social Workers
BBA	born before arrival
BBB	blood–brain barrier
BBV	blood-borne virus
BC, BCh, BChir	Bachelor of Surgery
BCG	bacille Calmette–Guérin
BChD	Bachelor of Dental Surgery
BDA	(1) British Dental Association
	(2) British Dietetic Association
BDS	Bachelor of Dental Surgery
BDSc	Bachelor of Dental Science
BID	brought in dead
BIH	benign intracranial hypertension
BIPAP	biphasic positive airways pressure
BLS	basic life support
BM	Bachelor of Medicine
BMA	British Medical Association
BME	benign myalgic encephalomyelitis
BMedSc	Bachelor of Medical Science
BMI	body mass index
BMR	basal metabolic rate
BMT	bone marrow transplant
BN	Bachelor of Nursing
BNF	British National Formulary
BP	(1) blood pressure (2) British Pharmacopoeia
BPH	benign prostatic hyperplasia
BPharm	Bachelor of Pharmacy
Bq	becquerel
BRM	biological response modifier
BRSC	British Red Cross Society
BSc	Bachelor of Science
BSc (Soc Sc-Nurs)	Bachelor of Science (Nursing)
BSChB	Bachelor of Surgery
BSE	(1) bovine spongiform encephalopathy
	(2) breast self-examination
BSL	British sign language
BVMS	Bachelor of Veterinary Medicine and Surgery
CAL	computer assisted learning
cAMP	cyclic adenosine monophosphate
CAPD	continuous ambulatory peritoneal dialysis
CAPE	Clifton Assessment Procedures for the Elderly
CAT	computed axial tomography
CATS	Credit Accumulation Transfer Scheme
CBA	cost-benefit analysis

(continued)

CBF	cerebral blood flow
CCF	congestive cardiac failure
CCK	cholecystokinin
CCPNS	cell cycle phase non-specific
CCPS	cell cycle phase specific
CCU	coronary care unit
CD	controlled drug
cd	candela
CDC	Centers for Disease Control and Prevention
CDH	congenital dislocation of the hip
CEA	carcinoembryonic antigen
CF	cystic fibrosis
CFM	cerebral function monitor
CFT	complement fixation test
CGM	continuous glucose monitoring
CHART	continuous hyperfractionated accelerated radiotherapy
ChB	Bachelor of Surgery
ChD	Doctor of Surgery
CHD	coronary heart disease
CHF	congestive heart failure
CHI	(1) Commission for Health Improvement
	(2) creatinine height index
CIN	cervical intraepithelial neoplasia
CINAHL	Cumulative Index to Nursing and Allied Health Literature
CJD	Creutzfeldt–Jakob disease
CMChM	Master of Surgery
CMO	Chief Medical Officer
CMV	cytomegalovirus
CNO	Chief Nursing Officer
CNS	(1) central nervous system (2) clinical nurse specialist
CO	cardiac output
COC	combined oral contraceptive
COMA	Committee on Medical Aspects of Food Policy
COPD	chronic obstructive pulmonary disease
COSHH	Control of Substances Hazardous to Health
COT	College of Occupational Therapists
CPAP	continuous positive airways pressure
CPD	continuing professional development
CPH	Certificate in Public Health
CPK	creatine kinase/phosphokinase
CPM	continuous passive motion
CPN	Community Psychiatric Nurse
CPP	cerebral perfusion pressure
CPR	cardiopulmonary resuscitation
CRCP	Certificant of the Royal College of Physicians
CRCS	Certificant of the Royal College of Surgeons
CREST	calcinosis, Raynaud's phenomenon,
	(o)esophageal dysfunction, sclerodactyly and telangiectasis
CRF	(1) chronic renal failure (2) corticotrophin-releasing factor
CRP	C-reactive protein (test)
CSF	(1) cerebrospinal fluid (2) colony stimulating factor
CSII	continuous subcutaneous insulin infusion

(continued)

CSM	Committee on Safety of Medicines
CSP	Chartered Society of Physiotherapists
CSSD	central sterile supplies department
CSSU	central sterile supply unit
CT	(1) computed tomography (2) cerebral tumour (3) coronary thrombosis
CTG	cardiotocography
CV	curriculum vitae
CVA	cerebrovascular accident
CVID	common variable immunodeficiency
CVP	central venous pressure
CVS	(1) cardiovascular system (2) chorionic villus sampling
CVVH	continuous veno-venous haemofiltration
CVVHD	continuous veno-venous haemodiafiltration
CXR	chest X-ray
DA	Diploma in Anaesthetics
DADL	domestic activities of daily living
D and C	dilatation and curettage
D and E	dilatation and evacuation
DAv Med	Diploma in Aviation Medicine
Db	decibel
DBO	Diploma of the British Orthoptic Council
DCh	Doctor of Surgery
DCH	Diploma in Child Health
DChD	Doctor of Dental Surgery
DCM	Diploma in Community Medicine
DCMT	Diploma in Clinical Medicine of Tropics
DCP	Diploma in Clinical Pathology
DCPath	Diploma of the College of Pathologists
DCR	Diploma, College of Radiographers
DDH	developmental dysplasia of the hip
DDM	Diploma in Dermatological Medicine
DDO	Diploma in Dental Orthopaedics
DDR	Diploma in Diagnostic Radiology
DDS	Doctor of Dental Surgery
DFHom	Diploma of the Faculty of Homoeopathy
DGO	Diploma in Gynaecology and Obstetrics
DHyg	Doctor of Hygiene
DIC	disseminated intravascular coagulation
DIH	Diploma in Industrial Health
DipCD	Diploma in Child Development
DipCOT	Diploma of the College of Occupational Therapists
DipEd	Diploma in Education
DipHE	Diploma in Higher Education
DipPharmMed	Diploma in Pharmaceutical Medicine
DipRG	Diploma in Remedial Gymnastics
DipTP	Diploma for Teachers of Physiotherapy
DLO	Diploma in Laryngology and Otology
DM	Doctor of Medicine
DMD	Doctor of Dental Medicine
DMedRehab	Diploma in Medical Rehabilitation
DMJ	Diploma in Medical Jurisprudence

(continued)

DMR	Diploma in Medical Radiology
DMRD	Diploma in Medical Radiodiagnosis
DMRE	Diploma of Medical Radiology and Electrology
DMRT	Diploma in Medical Radiotherapy
DMS	(1) Director of Medical Services,
	(2) Doctor of Medicine and Surgery
DMSA	Diploma in Medical Services Administration
DMV	Doctor of Veterinary Medicine
DNA	deoxyribonucleic acid
DO	Diploma in Ophthalmology
DO_2	oxygen delivery
DObstRCOG	Diploma of the Royal College of Obstetricians and Gynaecologists
DOMS	(1) delayed onset muscle soreness
	(2) Diploma in Ophthalmic Medicine and Surgery
DOrth	Diploma in Orthodontics
DPA	Diploma in Public Administration
DPD	Diploma in Public Dentistry
2,3-DPG	2,3-diphosphoglycerate
DPH	Diploma in Public Health
DPM	Diploma in Psychological Medicine
DPhil	Doctor of Philosophy
DPhysMed	Diploma in Physical Medicine
DR	Diploma in Radiology
DRCOG	Diploma of the Royal College of Obstetricians and Gynaecologists
DRCPath	Diploma of the Royal College of Pathologists
DRM	Diploma in Radiation Medicine
DRVs	dietary reference values
DS	Doctor of Surgery
DSc	Doctor of Science
DSH	deliberate self-harm
DSM	Diploma in Social Medicine
DSSc	Diploma in Sanitary Science
DTCD	Diploma in Tuberculosis and Chest Diseases
DTCH	Diploma in Tropical Child Health
DTD	Diploma in Tuberculous Diseases
DTH	Diploma in Tropical Hygiene
DTM	Diploma in Tropical Medicine
DTMH	Diploma in Tropical Medicine and Hygiene
DTPH	Diploma in Tropical Public Health
DV&D	Diploma in Venereology and Dermatology
DVT	deep vein thrombosis
EAR	estimated average requirement
EBM	(1) evidence-based medicine (2) expressed breast milk
EBP	evidence-based practice
EBV	Epstein–Barr virus
ECF	extracellular fluid
ECG	electrocardiogram
ECMO	extracorporeal membrane oxygenation
ECoG	electrocochleography
ECT	electroconvulsive therapy

(continued)

ECV	external cephalic version
EDD	expected date of delivery
EEG	electroencephalogram
EFAs	essential fatty acids
EHEC	enterohaemorrhagic *Escherichia coli*
EIA	exercise induced asthma
EIEC	enteroinvasive *Escherichia coli*
ELISA	enzyme-linked immunosorbent assay
EMD	electromechanical dissociation
EMF	electromotive force
EMG	electromyography
EMRSA	epidemic methicillin-resistant *Staphylococcus aureus*
ENT	ear, nose and throat
EOG	electro-oculogram
EPEC	enteropathic *Escherichia coli*
EPOC	excess post-exercise oxygen consumption
ERCP	endoscopic retrograde cholangiopancreatography
ERG	electroretinogram
ERPC	evacuation of retained products of conception
ESP	extrasensory perception
ESPs	extended scope physiotherapy practitioners
ESR	erythrocyte sedimentation rate
ESRD	end-stage renal disease
ESWL	extracorporeal shock wave lithotripsy
ETCO$_2$	end-tidal carbon dioxide
ETEC	enterotoxigenic *Escherichia coli*
EUA	examination under anaesthetic
FACA	Fellow of the American College of Anesthetists
FACC	Fellow of the American College of Cardiology
FACD	Fellow of the American College of Dentists
FACDS	Fellow of the Australian College of Dental Surgeons
FACG	Fellow of the American College of Gastroenterology
FACO	Fellow of the American College of Otolaryngology
FACOG	Fellow of the American College of Obstetricians and Gynecologists
FACP	Fellow of the American College of Physicians
FACR	Fellow of the American College of Radiologists
FACS	Fellow of the American College of Surgeons
FAGO	Fellow in Australia in Obstetrics and Gynaecology
FANZCP	Fellow of the Australian and New Zealand College of Psychiatrists
FAS	fetal alcohol syndrome
FBPsS	Fellow of the British Psychological Society
FCAP	Fellow of the College of American Pathologists
FCCP	Fellow of the American College of Chest Physicians
FCMS	Fellow of the College of Medicine and Surgery
FCOT	Fellow of the College of Occupational Therapists
FCP	Fellow of the College of Clinical Pharmacology
FCPath	Fellow of the College of Pathologists
FCPS	Fellow of the College of Physicians and Surgeons
FCPSA	Fellow of the College of Physicians and Surgeons of South Africa

(*continued*)

FCRA	Fellow of the College of Radiologists of Australasia
FCS	Fellow of the Chemical Society
FCSP	Fellow of the Chartered Society of Physiotherapists
FDS	Fellow in Dental Surgery
FESS	functional endoscopic sinus surgery
FETC	Further Education Teaching Certificate
FEV	forced expiratory volume
FFARCS	Fellow of the Faculty of Anaesthetists of the Royal College of Surgeons
FFCM	Fellow of the Faculty of Community Medicine
FFD	Fellow of the Faculty of Dental Surgeons
FFDRCS	Fellow of the Faculty of Dental Surgery of the Royal College of Surgeons
FFHom	Fellow of the Faculty of Homeopathy
FFR	Fellow of the Faculty of Radiologists
FIBiol	Fellow of the Institute of Biology
FICS	Fellow of the International College of Surgeons
FIMLS	Fellow of the Institute of Medical Laboratory Sciences
FiO$_2$	fractional inspired oxygen concentration
FLCO	Fellow of the London College of Osteopathy
FLCOM	Fellow of the London College of Osteopathic Medicine
FPA	Family Planning Association
FPCert	Family Planning Certificate
FPS	Fellow of the Pharmaceutical Society
FRACDS	Fellow of the Royal Australasian College of Dental Surgery
FRACGP	Fellow of the Royal Australian College GP
FRACO	Fellow of the Royal Australasian College of Ophthalmologists
FRACP	Fellow of the Australasian College of Physicians
FRACR	Fellow of the Royal Australasian College of Radiologists
FRACS	Fellow of the Australasian College of Surgeons
FRANZCP	Fellow of the Royal Australian and New Zealand College of Psychiatrists
FRCD	Fellow of the Royal College of Dentists
FRCGP	Fellow of the Royal College of General Practitioners
FRcn	Fellow of the Royal College of Nursing
FRCOG	Fellow of the Royal College of Obstetricians and Gynaecologists
FRCP	Fellow of the Royal College of Physicians
FRCPA	Fellow of the Royal College of Pathologists Australasia
FRCPath	Fellow of the Royal College of Pathologists
FRCPE	Fellow of the Royal College of Physicians, Edinburgh
FRCPsych	Fellow of the Royal College of Psychiatrists
FRCR	Fellow of the Royal College of Radiologists
FRCRA	Fellow of the Royal College of Radiologists Australasia
FRCS	Fellow of the Royal College of Surgeons
FRCSE	Fellow of the Royal College of Surgeons, Edinburgh
FRFPS	Fellow of the Royal Faculty of Physicians and Surgeons
FRIPHH	Fellow of the Royal Institute of Public Health and Hygiene
FRMS	Fellow of the Royal Microscopical Society
FRS	Fellow of the Royal Society
FRSH	Fellow of the Royal Society of Health
FRSM	Fellow of the Royal Society of Medicine

(continued)

FSH	follicle stimulating hormone
FSR(R)	Fellow of the Society of Radiographers (Radiography)
FSR(T)	Fellow of the Society of Radiographers (Radiotherapy)
FTA-Abs	fluorescent treponemal antibody absorbed test
FVC	forced vital capacity
GAS	general adaptation syndrome
GBM	glomerular basement membrane
GCS	Glasgow Coma Scale
GDS	geriatric depression scale
GFR	glomerular filtration rate
GGT	gamma-glutamyl transferase
GH	growth hormone
GI	gastrointestinal
GIFT	gamete intrafallopian transfer
GMC	General Medical Council
GMS	general medical services
GP	general practitioner
G6PD	glucose-6-phosphate dehydrogenase
GPI	general paralysis of the insane
GSL	general sales list
GUM	genitourinary medicine
GVHD	graft versus host disease
Gy	gray
HAI	hospital acquired infection
HAV	hepatitis A virus
HAVS	hand-arm vibration syndrome
Hb	haemoglobin
HBIG	hepatitis B immunoglobulin
HBV	hepatitis B virus
HCA	healthcare assistant
HCG (hCG)	human chorionic gonadotrophin
HCV	hepatitis C virus
HDL	high-density lipoprotein
HDU	high dependency unit
HHNK	hyperglycaemic hyperosmolar non-ketotic (coma)
Hib vaccine	*Haemophilus influenzae* type B vaccine
HIV	human immunodeficiency virus
HLA	human leucocyte antigen
HONK	hyperosmolar non-ketotic (coma)
HPV	human papilloma virus
HRmax	maximum heart rate
HRT	hormone replacement therapy
HSDU	hospital sterilization and disinfection unit
HSSU	hospital sterile supply unit
HSV	herpes simplex virus
5-HT	5-hydroxytryptamine
HTLV	human T-cell lymphotropic virus
HUS	haemolytic uraemic syndrome
HV	health visitor
HVCert	Health Visitor's Certificate
HVT	Health Visitor Teacher

(continued)

IABP	intra-aortic balloon pump
IADL	instrumental activities of daily living
IBD	inflammatory bowel disease
IBS	irritable bowel syndrome
ICD	International Classification of Diseases
ICE	ice, compress and elevation
ICF	intracellular fluid
ICP	intracranial pressure
ICSH	interstitial cell stimulating hormone
ICSI	intracytoplasmic sperm injection
ICU	intensive care unit
IDDM	insulin dependent diabetes mellitus
IFN	interferon
Ig	immunoglobulin
IHD	ischaemic heart disease
IL	interleukin
IMLS	Institute of Medical Laboratory Sciences
IMRT	intensity modulated radiotherapy
IOP	intraocular pressure
IPE	interprofessional education
IPPV	intermittent positive pressure ventilation
IQ	intelligence quotient
ITP	idiopathic thrombocytopenic purpura
ITU	intensive therapy unit
IUCD	intrauterine contraceptive device
IUD	intrauterine device
IUGR	intrauterine growth restriction/retardation
IV	intravenous
IVC	inferior vena cava
IVF	in vitro fertilization
IVI	intravenous infusion
IVIG	intravenous immunoglobulin
IVU/IVP	intravenous urogram/pyelogram
J	joule
JCA	juvenile chronic arthritis
JGA	juxtaglomerular apparatus
JVP	jugular venous pressure
kJ	kilojoule
KP	keratic precipitates
LASER	light amplification by stimulated emission of radiation
LCPS	Licentiate of the College of Physicians and Surgeons
LDH	lactate dehydrogenase
LDL	low-density lipoprotein
LDS	Licentiate in Dental Surgery
LDSc	Licentiate in Dental Science
LE	lupus erythematosus
LEA	Local Education Authority
LFT	liver function test
LGVCFT	lymphogranuloma venereum complement fixation test

(continued)

LH	luteinizing hormone
LLCO	Licentiate London College Osteopathy
LM	Licentiate in Midwifery
LMP	last menstrual period
LMS	Licentiate in Medicine and Surgery
LMSSA	Licentiate in Medicine and Surgery of the Society of Apothecaries of London
LOA	left occipitoanterior
LOC	level of consciousness
LOP	left occipitoposterior
LP	lumbar puncture
LRCP	Licentiate of the Royal College of Physicians
LRCPE	Licentiate of the Royal College of Physicians of Edinburgh
LRCS	Licentiate of the Royal College of Surgeons
LRCSE	Licentiate of the Royal College of Surgeons of Edinburgh
LRNI	lower reference nutrient intake
LRTI	lower respiratory tract infection
LSA	Licentiate of the Society of Apothecaries of London
LSD	lysergic acid diethylamide
LSM	Licentiate of the School of Medicine
LTM	long-term memory
LTOT	long-term oxygen therapy
LVAD	left ventricular assist device
LVF	left ventricular failure

MA	Master of Arts
MAC	(1) *Mycobacterium avium* complex (2) mid-arm circumference
MAI	*Mycobacterium avium intracellulare*
MAOI	monoamine oxidase inhibitor
MB	Bachelor of Medicine
MBA	Master of Business Administration
MBBS	Bachelor of Medicine, Bachelor of Surgery
MBC	maximal breathing capacity
MBChB	Bachelor of Medicine, Bachelor of Surgery
MBIM	Member of the British Institute of Management
MC	Master of Surgery
MCA	Medicines Control Agency
MCB	Master of Clinical Biochemistry
MCh	Master of Surgery
MCH	mean cell haemoglobin
MCHC	mean cell haemoglobin concentration
MChD	Master of Dental Surgery
MChir	Master of Surgery
MChOrth	Master of Orthopaedic Surgery
MChOtol	Master of Otology
MChS	Member of the Society of Chiropodists
MClSc	Master of Clinical Science
MCommH	Master of Community Health
MCP	multiple cosmetic phlebectomy
MCPath	Member of the College of Pathologists
MCPS	Member of the College of Physicians and Surgeons

(*continued*)

MCSP	Member of the Chartered Society of Physiotherapists
MCV	mean cell volume
MD	Doctor of Medicine
MDA	Medical Devices Agency
MDD	Doctor of Dental Medicine
MDS	Master of Dental Surgery
MDSc	Master of Dental Science
MDM	mental defence mechanism
MDR-TB	multidrug resistant tuberculosis
ME	myalgic encephalopathy
MEd	Master of Education
MFCM	Member of the Faculty of Community Medicine
MFHom	Member of the Faculty of Homoeopathy
MFOM	Member of the Faculty of Occupational Medicine
mg	milligram
MHC	major histocompatibility complex
MHyg	Master of Hygiene
MIBiol	Member of the Institute of Biology
MIH	Master of Industrial Health
mL	millilitre
MLC	multi-leaf collimation
MLCO	Member of the London College of Osteopathy
MLCOM	Member of the London College of Osteopathic Medicine
MLNS	mucocutaneous lymph node syndrome
MLSO	Medical Laboratory Scientific Officer
mm	millimetre
MMed	Master of Medicine
MMedSci	Master of Medical Science
mmHg	millimetres of mercury
mmol	millimole
MMR	measles, mumps and rubella (vaccine)
MMSE	Mini Mental State Examination
MO	(1) Master of Obstetrics (2) Medical Officer
MO&G	Master of Obstetrics and Gynaeology
MODS	multiple organ dysfunction syndrome
MODY	maturity onset diabetes of the young
MOH	Medical Officer of Health
mol	mole
MPH	Master of Public Health
MPhil	Master of Philosophy
MPS	Member of the Pharmaceutical Society
MPsyMed	Master of Psychological Medicine
MRad	Master of Radiology
MRC	Medical Research Council
MRCGP	Member of the Royal College of General Practitioners
MRCOG	Member of the Royal College of Obstetricians and Gynaecologists
MRCP	Member of the Royal College of Physicians
MRCPath	Member of the Royal College of Pathologists
MRCPsych	Member of the Royal College of Psychiatrists
MRCS	Member of the Royal College of Surgeons
MRCVS	Member of the Royal College of Veterinary Surgeons

(continued)

MRI	magnetic resonance imaging
mRNA	messenger ribonucleic acid
MRO	Member of the Register of Osteopaths
MRSA	methicillin-resistant *Staphylococcus aureus*
MRSH	Member of the Royal Society of Health
MS	(1) Master of Surgery (2) multiple sclerosis (3) musculoskeletal system
MSA	Member of the Society of Apothecaries
MSH	melanocyte stimulating hormone
MSP	Munchausen syndrome by proxy
MSRG	Member of the Society of Remedial Gymnasts
MSR(R)	Member of the Society of Radiographers (Radiography)
MSR(T)	Member of the Society of Radiographers (Radiotherapy)
MSU	midstream specimen of urine
MSW	Medical Social Worker
MT	Midwifery Teacher
N	newton
NACNE	National Advisory Committee on Nutrition Education
NAD	nicotinamide adenine dinucleotide
NADP	nicotinamide adenine dinucleotide phosphate
NAI	non-accidental injury
NAMCW	National Association for Maternal and Child Welfare
NAWCH	National Association for the Welfare of Children in Hospital
NBM	nil (nothing) by mouth
NCSC	National Care Standards Commission
NCVQ	National Council for Vocational Qualifications
NDN	National District Nurse Certificate
NEC	necrotizing enterocolitis
ng	nanogram
NG	nasogastric
NGF	nerve growth factor
NGU	non-gonococcal urethritis
NHL	non-Hodgkin's lymphoma
NHS	National Health Service
NICE	National Institute for Clinical Excellence
NICU	Neonatal Intensive Care Unit
NIDDM	non-insulin dependent diabetes mellitus
NIPPV	non-invasive positive pressure ventilation
nm	nanometre
NMC	Nursing and Midwifery Council
NMR	nuclear magnetic resonance
NNU	neonatal unit
NPF	Nurse Prescribers' Formulary
NPN	non-protein nitrogen
NRDS	neonatal respiratory distress syndrome
NREM	non-rapid eye movement (sleep)
NSAIDs	non-steroidal anti-inflammatory drugs
NSCLC	non-small cell lung carcinoma
NSFs	National Service Frameworks

(*continued*)

NSP	non-starch polysaccharide
NSU	non-specific urethritis
NVQ	National Vocational Qualification

OAE	otoacoustic emission
OBLA	onset of blood lactate accumulation
OBS	organic brain syndrome
ODA	operating department assistant
ODP	operating department practitioner
OHNC	Occupational Health Nursing Certificate
OND	Ophthalmic Nursing Diploma
ORS	oral rehydration solution
ORT	oral rehydration therapy
OT	occupational therapy/therapist
OTC	over-the-counter (medicines)

Pa	pascal
$PaCO_2$	partial pressure of carbon dioxide in arterial blood
$PACO_2$	partial pressure of carbon dioxide in alveolar air
PACS	picture archiving communication system
PADL	personal activities of daily living
PAFC	pulmonary artery flotation catheter
PAL	physical activity level
PALS	paediatric advanced life support
PAO	peak acid output
PaO_2	partial pressure of oxygen in arterial blood
PAO_2	partial pressure of oxygen in alveolar air
PAOP	pulmonary artery occlusion pressure
Pap	Papanicolaou smear test
PAR	physical activity ratio
PAWP	pulmonary artery wedge pressure
PBD	peak bone density
PBM	peak bone mass
PCA(S)	patient controlled analgesia (system)
PCEA	patient controlled epidural analgesia
PCM	protein-calorie malnutrition
PCO_2	partial pressure of carbon dioxide
PCOS	polycystic ovary syndrome
PCP	*Pneumocystis carinii* pneumonia
PCR	polymerase chain reaction
PCT	Primary Care Trust
PCV	packed cell volume
PCWP	pulmonary capillary wedge pressure
PDP	personal development plan
PE	pulmonary embolus
PEEP	positive end expiratory pressure
PEFR	peak expiratory flow rate
PEG	percutaneous endoscopic gastrostomy
PEM	protein-energy malnutrition
PET	positron emission tomography
PGD	preimplantation genetic diagnosis
PGDRS	psychogeriatric dependency rating scale

(continued)

PGL	persistent generalized lymphadenopathy
pH	hydrogen ion concentration
Ph	Philadelphia chromosome
PHC	primary health care
PhD	Doctor of Philosophy
PHLS	Public Health Laboratory Services
PI	performance indicator
PICC	peripherally inserted central catheter
PICU	Paediatric Intensive Care Unit
PID	(1) pelvic inflammatory disease (2) prolapsed intervertebral disc
PKU	phenylketonuria
PMB	postmenopausal bleeding
PMS	premenstrual syndrome
PNF	proprioceptive neuromuscular facilitation
PNI	psychoneuroimmunology
PNS	peripheral nervous system
POAG	primary open angle glaucoma
POM	prescription only medicine
POMR	problem-orientated medical record
PONV	postoperative nausea and vomiting
POP	(1) progestogen only pill (2) plaster of Paris
PPLO	pleuropneumonia-like organism
PPS	pelvic pain syndrome
PPV	positive pressure ventilation
PR	(1) per rectum (2) peripheral resistance
PRL	prolactin
PRP	panretinal photocoagulation
PSA	prostate specific antigen
PT	(1) physiotherapist (2) prothrombin
PTC	percutaneous transhepatic cholangiography
PTCA	percutaneous transluminal coronary angioplasty
PTH	parathyroid hormone
PTSD	post-traumatic stress disorder
PUFA	polyunsaturated fatty acid
PUO	pyrexia of unknown origin
PUVA	psoralen plus ultraviolet light A
PV	per vagina
PVD	peripheral vascular disease
QALYs	quality-adjusted life years
RADAR	Royal Association for Disability and Rehabilitation
RADC	Royal Army Dental Corps
RAMC	Royal Army Medical Corps
RAS	reticular activating system
RAST	radioallergosorbent test
RBC	red blood cell
RCT	randomized controlled trial
RDA	recommended daily allowance
RDS	respiratory distress syndrome
REF	renal erythropoietic factor
REM	rapid eye movement (sleep)

(continued)

RES	reticuloendothelial system
RG	remedial gymnast
RGN	Registered General Nurse
Rh	Rhesus
RHD	rheumatic heart disease
RHV	Registered Health Visitor
RICE	rest, ice, compress, elevation
RIHSA	radioiodinated human serum albumin
rINN	Recommended International Non-proprietary Name
RIP	raised intracranial pressure
RM	Registered Midwife
RMN	Registered Mental Nurse
RMO	(1) registered medical officer (2) resident medical officer
RN	Registered Nurse
RNA	ribonucleic acid
RNI	reference nutrient intake
RNIB	Royal National Institute for the Blind
RNID	Royal National Institute for the Deaf
RNMH	Registered Nurse for the Mentally Handicapped
RNT	Registered Nurse Tutor
RO	reality orientation
ROA	right occipitoanterior
ROM	(1) range of motion (2) resisted range of movement
ROP	right occipitoposterior
RPR	rapid plasma reagin test
rRNA	ribosomal ribonucleic acid
RSCN	Registered Sick Children's Nurse
RSI	repetitive strain injury
RSV	respiratory syncytial virus
RTA	(1) renal tubular acidosis (2) road traffic accident
RVF	right ventricular failure
SAD	seasonal affective disorder
SAH	subarachnoid haemorrhage
SAID	specific adaptation to imposed demands
SANDS	Stillbirth and Neonatal Death Society
StAAA	St Andrew's Ambulance Association
StJAA	St John Ambulance Association
StJAB	St John Ambulance Brigade
SaO_2	arterial oxygen saturation
SARA	sexually acquired reactive arthritis
SCAT	sheep cell agglutination test
SCBU	special care baby unit
SCC	(1) spinal cord compression (2) squamous cell carcinoma
SCID	severe combined immunodeficiency
SCM	State Certified Midwife
SD	standard deviation
SDA	specific dynamic action
SDH	subdural haematoma
SE	standard error
SERMs	selective (o)estrogen receptor modulators

(continued)

SGA	small for gestational age
SGOT	serum glutamic oxaloacetic transaminase (aspartate aminotransferase)
SGPT	serum glutamic pyruvic transaminase (alanine aminotransferase)
SHO	Senior House Officer
SI Units	Système International d'Unités
SIADH	syndrome of inappropriate antidiuretic hormone
SIB	self-injurious behaviour
SIDS	sudden infant death syndrome
SIMA	system for identifying motivated abilities
SIMV	synchronized intermittent mandatory ventilation
SIRS	systemic inflammatory response syndrome
SLE	systemic lupus erythematosus
SLT	speech and language therapist
SMBG	self-monitoring blood glucose
SMBR	standardized morbidity ratio
SMR	(1) standardized mortality ratio (2) submucous resection
SNB	sentinel node biopsy
SPMSQ	Short Portable Mental State Questionnaire
SPSS	Statistical Package for Social Sciences
SRCh	State Registered Chiropodist
SRN	State Registered Nurse
SSPE	subacute sclerosing panencephalitis
SSRIs	selective serotonin reuptake inhibitors
STD	sexually transmitted disease
STI	sexually transmitted infection
STM	short-term memory
Sv	sievert
SV	stroke volume
SVQs	Scottish Vocational Qualifications
T_3	triiodothyronine
T_4	thyroxine
$t_{1/2}$	half-life
TB	tuberculosis (tubercle bacillus)
TBI	total body irradiation
TCA	tricyclic antidepressant
TCRE	transcervical resection of endometrium
TEN	toxic epidermal necrolysis
TENS	transcutaneous electrical nerve stimulation
TEPP	tetraethyl pyrophosphate
TIA	transient ischaemic attack
TIBC	total iron binding capacity
TIPSS	transjugular intrahepatic portasystemic stent shunting
TIVA	total intravenous anaesthesia
TLS	tumour lysis syndrome
TMJ	temporomandibular joint syndrome
TNF	tumour necrosis factor
TNM	tumour, node (lymph), metastasis
TOP	termination of pregnancy
tPA	tissue plasminogen activator
TPHA	*Treponema pallidum* haemagglutination assay

(*continued*)

TPN	total parenteral nutrition
TPR	temperature, pulse, respiration
TQM	total quality management
TRIC	trachoma inclusion conjunctivitis
tRNA	transfer ribonucleic acid
TRUS	transrectal ultrasonography
TSF	triceps skinfold thickness
TSH	thyroid-stimulating hormone
TSS	toxic shock syndrome
TT	tetanus toxoid
TUR	transurethral resection of the prostate
TV	tidal volume

URTI	upper respiratory tract infection
USS	ultrasound scan
UTI	urinary tract infection

v	volt
VADAS	voice activated domestic appliance system
VBI	vertebrobasilar insufficiency
VC	vital capacity
VDRL	venereal disease research laboratory (test)
VF	ventricular fibrillation
VFM	value for money
VLDL	very-low-density lipoprotein
VMA	vanillylmandelic acid
VMC	vasomotor centre
VO_2	oxygen consumption
V/Q	ventilation perfusion ratio
VRE	vancomycin resistant enterococci
VSO	Voluntary Service Overseas
VT	ventricular tachycardia
VUR	vesicoureteric reflux
VZIG	varicella-zoster hyperimmune immunoglobulin
VZV	varicella-zoster virus

W	watt
WBC	white blood cell
WHO	World Health Organization
WPW	Wolff–Parkinson–White (syndrome)
WRULD	work-related upper limb disorder

| XLA | X-linked agammaglobulinaemia |
| XHIM | X-linked hyper-IgM syndrome |

| ZIFT | zygote intrafallopian tube transfer |
| ZN | Ziehl–Neelsen (stain) |

Useful addresses including web sites

Acne Support Group
First Floor, Howard House, The Runway
South Ruislip
Middlesex HA4 6SE
www.m2w3.com/acne/

Action for Sick Children
300 Kingston Road
London SW20 8LX
www.actionforsickchildren.org

Action on Smoking and Health (ASH)
109 Gloucester Place
London W1H 4EJ
www.ash.org.uk

Age Concern (England)
1268 London Road
London SW16 4ER
www.ageconcern.org.uk

Alcoholics Anonymous
PO Box 1
Stonebow House, Stonebow
York YO1 2NJ
www.alcoholics-anonymous.org.uk

Alzheimer's Society
Gordon House, 10 Greencoat Place
London SW1P 1PH
www.alzheimers.org.uk

Arthritis Care
18 Stephenson Way
London NW1 2HD
www.arthritiscare.org.uk

Breast Cancer Care
Kiln House, 210 New King's Road
London SW6 4NZ
www.breastcancercare.org.uk

British Allergy Foundation
Deepdene House, 30 Bellegrove Road
Welling
Kent DA16 3BY
www.allergyfoundation.com/

**British Association for Cancer
United Patients BACUP**
3 Bath Place, Rivington Street
London EC2 3JR
www.cancerbacup.org.uk

British Colostomy Association
15 Station Road
Reading RG1 1LG
www.bcass.org.uk

British Deaf Association
1–3 Worship Street
London EC2A 2AB
www.bda.org.uk

British Heart Foundation
14 Fitzharding Street
London W1H 4DH
www.bhf.org.uk

British Liver Trust
Ransomes Europark
Ipswich
Suffolk IP3 9QG
www.britishlivertrust.org.uk

British National Formulary
www.bnf.org.uk

British Organ Donor Society
Balsham
Cambridge CB1 6DL
www.argonet.co.uk/body/

British Pregnancy Advisory Service
Austy Manor, Wootton Wawen
Solihull
West Midlands B95 6BX
www.bpas.org

British Red Cross
9 Grosvenor Crescent
London SW1X 7EJ
www.redcross.org.uk

British Society of Hearing Therapists
Hearing Centre, Yardley Green Unit
East Birmingham Hospital
Birmingham B9 5PX
www.hearingtherapy.org

Cancer Research UK
PO Box 123
Lincoln's Inn Fields
London WC2A 3PX
www.cancerresearchuk.org

Capability (formerly Spastics Society)
12 Park Crescent
London W1N 4EQ

Cardiomyopathy Association
40 The Metro Centre, Tolpits Lane
Watford
Herts WD1 8SB
www.cardiomyopathy.org

Carers UK
20–25 Glasshouse Yard
London EC1A 4JS
www.carersonline.org.uk

Centre for Evidence Based Medicine
http://cebm.jr2.ox.ac.uk

Chartered Society of Physiotherapists
14 Bedford Row
London WC1R 4ED
www.csp.org.uk

Cochrane Library
www.cochrane.co.uk

Coeliac Society
PO Box 220
High Wycombe
Bucks HP11 2HY
www.coeliac.co.uk

College of Occupational Therapists
106–114 Borough High Street
London SE1 1LB
www.cot.co.uk

**Commission for Health
Improvement (CHI)**
www.chi.gov.uk

Commission for Racial Equality
Elliot House, 10–12 Allington Street
London SW1E 5EH
www.cre.gov.uk

**Committee on Safety of Medicines and
Medicines Control Agency**
www.mca.gov.uk

Coronary Prevention Group (CPG)
2 Taviton Street
London WC1H 0BT
www.healthnet.org.uk

Cruse
Cruse House, 126 Sheen Road
Richmond
Surrey TW9 1UR
www.crusebereavementcare.org.uk

Department of Health
Richmond House, 79 Whitehall
London SW1A 2NS
www.doh.gov.uk

Department of Health
(Northern Ireland)
Dundonald House
Upper Newtownards Road
Belfast BT4 3SB

Diabetes UK
10 Queen Anne Street
London W1M 0BD
www.diabetes.org.uk

Digestive Disorders Foundation
2 Andrew's Place
London NW1 4LB
www.digestivedisorders.org.uk

Disabled Living Foundation
380–384 Harrow Road
London W9 2HU
www.dlf.org.uk

Eating Disorders Association
103 Prince of Wales Road
Norwich NR1 1DW
www.edauk.com/

**Epilepsy Action (British Epilepsy
Association)**
New Anstey House, Gate Way Drive
Leeds LS3 1BE
www.epilepsy.org.uk

Equal Opportunities Commission
Arndale House, Arndale Centre
Manchester M4 5EQ
www.eoc.org.uk

General Medical Council
178 Great Portland Place
London W1W 5JE
www.gmc-uk.org

Guide Dogs for the Blind Association
Hillfields
Burghfield Common
Reading
Berkshire RG7 3YG
www.gdba.org.uk

Guillain–Barré Syndrome Society
GBS Support Group, LCC Offices
Eastgate
Sleaford NG34 7EB
www.gbs.org.uk

Headway—brain injury association
2 Tavistock Place
London WC1H 9RA
www.headway.org.uk

Health Development Agency
Trevelyan House, 30 Great Peter Street
London SW1P 2HW
www.hda-online.org.uk

Health & Safety Executive
Rose Court, 2 Southwark Bridge
London SE1 9HS
www.hse.gov.uk

Health Service Commissioner
13th Floor Millbank
Millbank Tower
London SW1P 4QP
www.health.ombudsman.org.uk

Haemophilia Society
Chesterfield House, 385 Euston Road
London NW1 3AU
www.haemophilia.org.uk

Ileostomy & Internal Pouch Support Group
Amblehurst House
PO Box 23
Mansfield NG18 4TT
www.ileostomypouch.demon.co.uk

Institute of Complementary Medicine
PO Box 194
London SE16 7QZ
www.icmedicine.co.uk

International Glaucoma Association (IGA)
108c Warner Road
London SE5 9HQ
www.iga.org.uk

King's Fund
11–13 Cavendish Square
London W1M 0AN
www.kingsfund.org.uk

Leukaemia Care Society
2 Shrubbery Ave
Worcester WR1 1QH
www.leukaemiacare.org.uk

Leukaemia Society
14 Kingfisher Court
Venny Bridge, Pinhoe
Exeter EX4 8JN
www.leukaemiasociety.org.uk

Macmillan Cancer Relief
89 Albert Embankment
London SE1 7UQ
www.macmillan.org.uk

Malcolm Sargent Cancer Fund for Children
14 Abingdon Road
London W8 6AF

Marie Curie Cancer Care
28 Belgrave Square
London SW1X 8QG
www.mariecurie.org.uk

Medical Devices Agency
www.medical-devices.gov.uk

Mencap
123 Golden Lane
London EC1Y 0RT
www.mencap.org.uk

Ménière's Society (UK)
98 Maybury Rd
Woking
Surrey GU21 5HX
www.menieres.co.uk

Meningitis Research Foundation
Midland Way
Thornbury
Bristol BS35 2BS
www.meningitis.org.uk

Migraine Action Association
Unit 6, Oakley Hay Lodge Business Park
Great Folds Way
Great Oakley
Northants NN18 9AS
www.migraine.org.uk

MIND—National Association for Mental Health
Granta House, 15–19 Broadway
London E15 4BQ
www.mind.org.uk

Multiple Sclerosis Society
National Centre, 372 Edgware Road
London NW2 6ND
www.mssociety.org.uk

Muscular Dystrophy Campaign (MDC)
7–11 Prescott Place
London SW4 6BS
www.muscular-dystrophy.org

National Aids Trust
196 Old Street
London EC1V 9FR
www.nat.org.uk

National Asthma Campaign
Providence House, Providence Place
London N1 0NT
www.asthma.org.uk

National Care Standards Commission (NCSC)
www.carestandards.gov.uk

National Childbirth Trust (NCT)
Alexandra House, Oldham Terrace
London W3 6NH
www.nctpregnancyandbabycare.com

National Eczema Society
Hill House, Highgate Hill
London N19 5NA
www.eczema.org.uk

National Institute for Clinical Excellence (NICE)
www.nice.org.uk

National Osteoporosis Society
PO Box 10
Radstock
Bath BA3 3YB
www.nos.org.uk

National Society for the Prevention of Cruelty to Children (NSPCC)
42 Curtain Road
London EC2A 3NH
www.nspcc.org.uk

NHS Centre for Reviews and Dissemination (York)
www.york.ac.uk/inst/crd/

Nursing and Midwifery Council
23 Portland Place
London W1N 3AF
www.nmc-uk.org

Parkinson's Disease Society
215 Vauxhall Bridge Road
London SW1V 1EJ
www.parkinsons.org.uk

Royal Association for Disability and Rehabilitation (RADAR)
Unit 12, City Forum
250 City Road
London EC1V 8AF
www.radar.org.uk

Royal National Institute for the Blind (RNIB)
224 Great Portland Place
London W1N 6AA
www.rnib.org.uk

Royal National Institute for the Deaf (RNID)
19–23 Featherstone Street
London EC1Y 8SL
www.rnid.org.uk

Royal Society for the Prevention of Accidents (RoSPA)
Cannon House
Priory Queensway
Birmingham B4 6BS
www.rospa.co.uk

Royal Society for the Promotion of Health
38a St Georges Drive
London SW1Y 4BH
www.rsph.org

St John Ambulance Association & Brigade
1 Grosvenor Crescent
London SW1X 7EF
www.sja.org.uk

Samaritans
UK National number:
Tel 0345 90 90 90 (Lo-call)
www.samaritans.org.uk

Scoliosis Association (UK)
2 Ivebury Court, 325 Latimer Road
London W10 6RA
www.sauk.org.uk

Scottish Health Department
St Andrew's House, Regent Road
Edinburgh EH1 3DE
www.scotland.gov.uk

**Scottish Intercollegiate Guidelines
Network (SIGN)**
www.sign.ac.uk

Sickle Cell Society
54 Station Road
Harlesden
London NW10 4UA
www.sicklecellsociety.org

Society & College of Radiographers
2 Carriage Row, 183 Eversholt Street
London NW1 1BU
www.sor.org

Society of Chiropodists & Podiatrists
53 Welbeck Street
London W1M 7HE
www.scpod.org

**Stillbirth & Neonatal Death Society
(SANDS)**
28 Portland Place
London W1N 4DE
www.uk-sands.org/

Stroke Association
123–127 Whitecross Street
London EC1Y 8JJ
www.stroke.org.uk

Terrence Higgins Trust
52–54 Grays Inn Road
London WC1X 8JU
www.tht.org.uk

**UK National Poisons Information
Services**
www.doh.gov.uk/npis.htm

UK Thalassaemia Society
19 The Broadway, Southgate Circus
London N14 6PH
www.ukts.org

VSO
317 Putney Bridge Road
London SW15 2PN
www.vso.org.uk

World Health Organization
Avenue Appia
1211 Geneva 27
Switzerland
www.who.org

Chemical symbols and formulae

Aluminium	Al
Ammonia	NH_3
Ammonium	NH_4
Barium	Ba
Cadmium	Cd
Calcium	Ca
Carbon	C
Carbonic acid	H_2CO_3
Caesium	Cs
Carbon dioxide	CO_2
Chloride	Cl
Chromium	Cr
Cobalt	Co
Copper	Cu
Fluorine	F
Gold	Au
Helium	He
Hydrochloric acid	HCl
Hydrogen	H_2
Hydrogen carbonate (bicarbonate)	HCO_3
Hydrogen phosphate	HPO_4
Hydroxide	OH
Iodine	I
Iridium	Ir
Iron	Fe
Lead	Pb
Lithium	Li
Magnesium	Mg
Magnesium sulphate	$MgSO_4$
Manganese	Mn
Mercury	Hg
Molybdenum	Mo
Nickel	Ni
Nitrogen	N
Nitrate	NO_3
Nitric acid	HNO_3
Oxygen	O_2
Phosphate	PO_4
Phosphorus	P
Potassium	K
Potassium chloride	KCl
Radium	Ra
Selenium	Se
Silicon	Si
Silver	Ag
Sodium	Na

(continued)

Sodium chloride	NaCl
Sodium hydroxide	NaOH
Sodium hydrogen carbonate (bicarbonate)	$NaHCO_3$
Strontium	Sr
Sulphate	SO_4
Sulphur	S
Sulphuric acid	H_2SO_4
Technetium	Tc
Thallium	Tl
Vanadium	V
Water	H_2O
Xenon	Xe
Yttrium	Y
Zinc	Zn

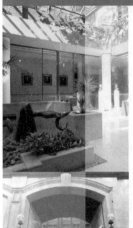

Books from The Royal Society of Medicine Press

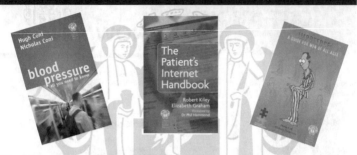

Blood Pressure: All You Need to Know by *Hugh Coni* and *Nick Coni*
This is a clear, easy-to-understand account of blood pressure and how to keep it under control. Comprehensive and well-illustrated, this book is an ideal information resource for individuals and their families suffering from high or low blood pressure. Nurses and GPs will also find this a useful guide.

£14.95, 1-85315-536-5, 148pp, paperback, October 2002, www.rsm.ac.uk/pub/bkconi.htm

The Patient's Internet Handbook by *Robert Kiley* and *Elizabeth Graham*
This book introduces the reader to the wealth of health information on the Internet. An A-Z section lists key Web addresses, patient support groups and email discussion lists for over 100 common conditions.

Jam-packed with search tips, medical databases and advice, this painstakingly researched book is invaluable. Health and Fitness Magazine

To swim successfully in the huge ocean of medical information that is out there on the Internet you definitely need webbed fingers! This superb book will be those webbed fingers that will get you through the tangle of information quickly, successfully and rewardingly.
Claire Rayner, President of the Patients Association

£9.95, 1-85315-498-9, 302pp, paperback, October 2001, www.patient-handbook.co.uk

Impotence: A Guide for Men of All Ages by *Philip Kell* and *Wallace Dinsmore*
Written by two leading experts, and endorsed by the Impotence Association, the UK's leading patient support group for this problem, this book answers all of the questions that men may have about their condition but are too embarrassed to ask.

This book will answer all your questions and provide reassurance that the problem can be treated. Top Sante Magazine

£9.95, 1-85315-402-4, 64pp, paperback, September 2001, www.rsm.ac.uk/pub/bkkell.htm

How to order books

Contact our distributors
Marston Book Services
PO Box 269, Abingdon
Oxfordshire, OX14 4YN
Tel +44 (0)1235 465 500
Fax +44 (0)1235 465 555

online at

www.rsmpress.co.uk

From our catalogue
To receive a catalogue featuring all our books and journals please e-mail
rsmpublishing@rsm.ac.uk
or call +44 (0)20 7290 3926